MCQs in Surgery

An Ultimate Solution for the Super Speciality Exam in Surgery

MCQs in Surgery
An Ultimate Solution for the Super Speciality Exam in Surgery

Vinod Kumar Nigam
MBBS MS FICS FIAGES
Associate Director
Department of General and Minimal Access Surgery
Max Hospital
Gurugram, Haryana, India

Siddharth Nigam
MBBS MS FIAGES FALS (Robotic)
Senior Consultant
Department of General and Minimal Access Surgery
Max Hospital
Gurugram, Haryana, India

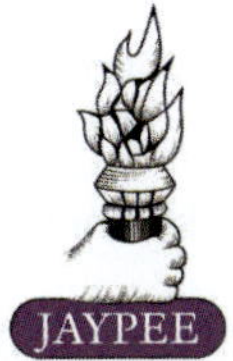

JAYPEE BROTHERS MEDICAL PUBLISHERS
The Health Sciences Publisher
New Delhi | London

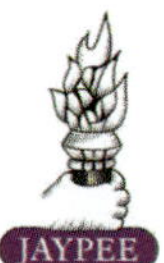

Jaypee Brothers Medical Publishers (P) Ltd

Headquarters
EMCA House, 23/23-B
Ansari Road, Daryaganj
New Delhi 110 002, India
Landline: +91-11-23272143, +91-11-23272703
+91-11-23282021, +91-11-23245672
e-mail: jaypee@jaypeebrothers.com

Corporate Office
4838/24, Ansari Road, Daryaganj
New Delhi 110 002, India
Phone: +91-11-43574357
Fax: +91-11-43574314
e-mail: jaypee@jaypeebrothers.com

Overseas Office
JP Medical Ltd.
83, Victoria Street, London
SW1H 0HW (UK)
Phone: +44-20 3170 8910
e-mail: info@jpmedpub.com

EU GPSR Authorised Representative
Logos Europe, 9 rue Nicolas Poussin
17000, La Rochelle, France
Phone: +33 (0) 6 67 93 73 78
e-mail: contact@logoseurope.eu

Website: www.jaypeebrothers.com
Website: www.jaypeedigital.com

Inquiries for bulk sales may be solicited at: jaypee@jaypeebrothers.com

MCQs in Surgery: An Ultimate Solution for the Super Speciality Exam in Surgery

First Edition: **2026**

ISBN: 978-93-6616-115-0

Printed in India

Dedicated to

Students

Preface

"Real knowledge is to know the extent of one's ignorance"

– Confucius

In today's world, he who has knowledge rules. Students must acquire knowledge both for appearing in competitive examination and for their own development. Medical understanding of diseases is fast improving. The surgical procedures are also developing at a high pace with the trend toward minimally invasive surgery. It is becoming difficult to accommodate all in one small and handy book which can be taken to wards, to bedsides of patients, and to clinics for ready reference. That is why we thought of taking out one topic in one volume and include everything about that subject, from anatomy to recent advancements.

The sole purpose of this book is to provide everything about MCQs for preparing for competitive examinations in one book. We hope that this will be helpful to undergraduate and postgraduate students, as well as to practicing surgeons and to those who are interested in acquiring knowledge about surgery. Surgery is one of the most important and common topics in the field of medicine. The book is primarily written for clinical students, surgeons, and higher surgical trainees. This book will be helpful to those who require an understanding of the basic sciences and essential principles of surgery while dealing with the diseases requiring surgery.

This book is also designed to be a reference book for family practice doctors and for the doctors in other specialties who are interested to know about surgery. We are sure that this book will have the greatest appeal among its readers who want to enhance their knowledge. There is a vast difference between this book and any other textbook of surgery and MCQ books. This is a book about surgery having an extensive description with a view to have the pathophysiology, anatomy, clinical problems, differential diagnosis, management, and operative details in simple language and an easy-to-understand manner. The book has simple, informative, and easy-to-practice line diagrams which will be very helpful to the students. Photographs of the patients, investigative procedures, and operations are chosen carefully to explain the salient points rather than just filling the space. Unnecessary text, diagrams, and photographs are avoided to reduce confusion.

The clinical material in this book is from our day-to-day clinical practice. To avoid a monotonous design and text, the book has many quotations. These quotations are to keep interest and enthusiasm of readers alive in reading the book. Care is taken to explain the operative procedures step-by-step to make it short, simple, easy to understand, and quick to refer. Recent advancements and modern trends make the reader aware of what is recent and what is obsolete. Mnemonics, questions and answers, and MCQs are important for students and will also enhance the knowledge of surgeons. At the end of each chapter, there is an exhaustive list of references which is important for readers who wishes to know more.

Vinod Kumar Nigam
Siddharth Nigam

Acknowledgments

"Knowledge is of no value unless you put it into practice."

– Anton Chekhov

It is not easy to prepare the book of MCQs for any subject solely by one individual, it is a team effort. We are thankful to all our colleagues who helped us by providing valuable information, suggestions, and photographs used in this book. We thank Dr Kunal Nigam for helping us write anatomy and other basic sciences. Dr Madhur Arora helped us by drawing beautiful line diagrams and searching the medical literature and bibliography. Dr Charvi Chawla deserves thanks for proofreading and suggestions. Mrs Kumud acted as the backbone for allowing me to take as much time as required from personal life to devote in writing this book without any complaints. She also did an excellent job of proofreading the book. Mr Vipin Sharma earns my thanks and gratitude for transcription of the manuscript.

We are extremely thankful to Shri Jitendar P Vij (Group Chairman), Mr Ankit Vij (Managing Director), Mr MS Mani (Group President), Ms Pooja Bhandari [Director—Production (Books and Journals)], and Ms Kajal Keshri (Development Editor) of M/s Jaypee Brothers Medical Publishers (P) Ltd, New Delhi, India, for constant encouragement.

Contents

SECTION 1: Preparation for Entrance Examinations

SECTION 2: Basic Principles of Surgery

SECTION 3: Surgical Diseases of Skin and Subcutaneous Tissue

SECTION 4: Head and Neck

SECTION 5: Breast

SECTION 6: Endocrine

SECTION 7: Gastrointestinal Diseases

SECTION 8: Genitourinary

SECTION 9: Vascular System

SECTION 10: Oncology

SECTION 11: Transplantation

SECTION 12: Pediatric Surgery

SECTION 13: Miscellaneous

SECTION 1

Preparation for Entrance Examinations

1. How to Increase your Retention while Preparing for Examinations?
2. How to Prepare for these Entrance Examinations?
3. How to Attempt the Entrance Examination Paper?
4. How to Keep Healthy and Avoid Anxiety and Stress during Exam Preparations?
5. How to be Motivated and have a Positive Attitude?
6. What should be the Daily Routine during Preparations for these Entrance Exams?

CHAPTER 1 How to Increase your Retention while Preparing for Examinations?

MNEMONICS

"Memory is the mother of all wisdom."

– Aeschylus

A mnemonic is a memory device or tool. A mnemonic is a word, sentence, or poem used to help remember a rule, name, etc. Mnemonic is a model for learning. These are good ways to remember difficult points for students who are trying to remember new or even old, difficult items, especially when preparing for an examination or entrance test. A mnemonic can be a word or sentence created by using the first letter of each word.

The mnemonics collectively known as the Ancient Art of Memory, were discovered in 447 BC by the Greek poet Simonides and were adequately described by Cicero, Quintilian, and Pliny.

In the word, Mnemonic, the "M" letter is silent. If "Mn" appears at the beginning of a word, it means "memory" for the Greek Goddess of Memory: Mnemosyne. Mnemonics are also called "Memoria technical" or "Memory technique." For making a mnemonic in your study to remember certain items, first write all the items and then write the first letter of each word separately, and then try to make the word easy to remember, and if it is funny, it will further help in remembering. The words chosen to form a mnemonic are usually not related to the topic, you wish to remember, so the relation between mnemonic and the topic is not important. It is also observed that when a student starts using mnemonics in his/her studies, they get significant improvement in memorizing the subjects. Mnemonics help students retain information and recall it easily. *Mnemonic must be simple and uncomplicated.*

Mnemonics are used in medicine as instruments to remember medical knowledge for the long term. Various medical terms and facts that are difficult to remember can be remembered for a long time with the help of mnemonics. A mnemonic couplet to help students learn the names of cranial nerves has been in use in the United States since the mid-19th century.

Mn: TIC-TAC (differential diagnosis of appendicular mass)
- T = Ileocecal TB
- I = Iliac lymphadenitis
- C = Crohn's disease
- T = Tumor, carcinoma of cecum
- A = Amebic typhlitis and actinomycosis
- C = Twisted ovarian cyst

Example of mnemonic: A commonly used mnemonic to remember during taking history for a sickness.

- *SAMPLE:*
  - S = Signs and symptoms
  - A = Allergies
  - M = Medications
  - P = Pertinent medical history
  - L = Last ins and outs
  - E = Events
- *Murphy's triad: Mnemonic (Mn):* PVP
  - P = Pain in abdomen
  - V = Vomiting
  - P = Pyrexia
- *Etiology of appendicitis (common causes):*
  - *Mn:* DR SODA
    - D = Diet
    - R = Racial, familial, and geographical factors
    - S = Socioeconomical level
    - O = Obstruction of the appendix by fecalith and worms
    - D = Diseases of the cecum; cancer, Crohn's disease, and tuberculosis
    - A = Abuse of purgative

- *Alvarado scoring:*
  - M = Migrating right iliac fossa (RIF) pain
  - A = Anorexia
  - N = Nausea and vomiting
  - T = Tenderness RIF
  - R = Rebound tenderness
  - E = Elevated temperature (>37.3°C)
  - L = Leukocytosis
  - S = Shift to left (segmental neutrophils) (>75%)

- *Ochsner-Sherren regimen:*
  - A = Aspiration—Ryle's tube
  - B = Bowel care—no purgatives
  - C = Charts for pulse/temperature/blood pressure (BP)/size of mass
  - D = Drugs, antibiotics
  - E = Exploration is avoided in the appendicular mass
  - F = Fluids, IV
- *Common differential diagnosis of acute appendicitis:*
  - *Mn:* PUNAM TRIPS MRCP
    - P = Perforated peptic ulcer
    - U = Ureteric colic
    - N = Nonspecific mesenteric lymphadenitis
    - A = Acute gastroenteritis
    - M = Mittelschmerz
    - T = Torsion of ovarian cyst
    - R = Regional ileitis
    - I = Intestinal obstruction
    - P = Pancreatitis
    - S = Salpingitis
    - M = Meckel's diverticulitis
    - R = Ruptured ectopic gestation
    - C = Cholecystitis
    - P = Pyelonephritis
- *Clinical features of carcinoid syndrome:*
  - *Mn:* DABAR
    - D = Diarrhea
    - A = Attack of bronchial asthma due to histamine
    - B = Increased borborygmi
    - A = Attack of flushing of the face, induced by alcohol
    - R = Reddish blue hue (cyanosis) due to histamine

- *Important signs of acute appendicitis:*
  - *Mn:* Remember Best Teachers Certify [2(R) 2(B) 2(T) 2(C) MCH]
  - R = Rebound tenderness
  - R = Rovsing sign
  - B = Bed shaking test of Bapat
  - B = Baldwin's test
  - T = Tenderness in RIF
  - T = Tenderness in digital rectal examination (DRE)
  - C = Cope's psoas test
  - C = Cope's obturator test
  - M = Muscle guarding
  - C = Cough sign
  - H = Hyperesthesia in Sherren's triangle

- *Complications of acute appendicitis:*
  - *Mn:* GAPSAP
    - G = Generalized peritonitis
    - A = Appendicular abscess
    - P = Perforated appendix
    - S = Septicemia
    - A = Appendicular lump
    - P = Portal pyemia
- *Important tumors of the appendix:*
  - *Mn:* CAP
    - C = Carcinoid tumor
    - A = Adenocarcinoma
    - P = Pseudomyxoma peritonei (PMP)
- *Complications of appendicectomy:*
  - *Mn:* 2 (PACIF)
    - P = Portal pyemia
    - P = Paralytic ileus
    - A = Abscess, pelvic and intraperitoneal
    - A = Adhesions, postoperative
    - C = Complication of any operation, wound infection
    - C = Complication of any operation, hemorrhage
    - I = Intestinal obstruction, acute
    - I = Inguinal hernia, right
    - F = Fecal fistula
    - F = Future stump appendicitis
- *Two layers of subcutaneous tissue in RIF:*
  - *Mn:* CS (C comes before S as the alphabet)
    - C = Camper's superficial fatty layer
    - S = Scarpa's deep membranous layer
- *Names of three Taenia coli:*
  - *Mn:* MOL
    - M = Taenia mesocolica
    - O = Taenia omentalis
    - L = Taenia libera

Key points

Mnemonic is one of the best ways to remember and retain items while studying.

SUGGESTED READING

1. Alvarado A. A practical score for the early diagnosis of acute appendicitis. Ann Emerg Med.1986;15(5):557-64.
2. Lanska DJ. On old Olympus? Oliver Wendell Holmes and the origin and evolution of a mnemonic couplet for the cranial nerves. J Hist Neurosci. 2022;31(1):20-9.
3. Patten BM. The history of memory arts. Neurology. 1990;40(2):346-52.

POMODORO METHOD OF STUDYING

"One day we will be more creative, more productive, and yet more relaxed."

– Francesco Cirillo

I have been using my own technique for studies since I was admitted to medical college. I felt that the medical studies were very hard and tiring. This technique helped me a lot in my studies. So, I used my technique for my son, also, who was getting tired and bored due to the pressure to study continuously. I thought for a while and decided that he should be given breaks during his study time and must use time breaks to do the things he enjoys best, such as reading comics and watching TV. I believe in the old proverb, "All work and no play makes Jack a dull boy." My technique, which is based on the basics of the Pomodoro technique, did wonders for him.

> My younger son, who is now a Consultant ENT Surgeon, was in class X and was to appear after 2 months for the board examination. His exam preparations were not up to the mark. I sat with him and charted out a plan. It was a proper study plan with two breaks of 15 minutes each for meditation and visualization, and two breaks for watching TV, so that he could refresh. The preparations went as planned. Exams started. In the examination hall, he used to do meditation for 2 minutes after the distribution of the question paper and then started writing the answers. He did well and scored very good marks. We gave due credit to his hard work, but I felt that the meditation, visualization, and relaxing breaks were also a help.

POMODORO TECHNIQUE

The Pomodoro technique was developed by Francesco Cirillo in the late 1980s. Pomodoro is an Italian word meaning a tomato. Francesco Cirillo was a university student when he developed it. Francesco Cirillo used a kitchen timer for this technique, which looked like a tomato **(Fig. 1)**. This technique advises working for some time and then getting a short break.

The original Pomodoro technique has the following six steps:

1. Decide on the task to be done.
2. Set the Pomodoro timer (for 25 minutes)
3. Work on the task.
4. End work when the timer rings and take a short break (5–10 minutes)

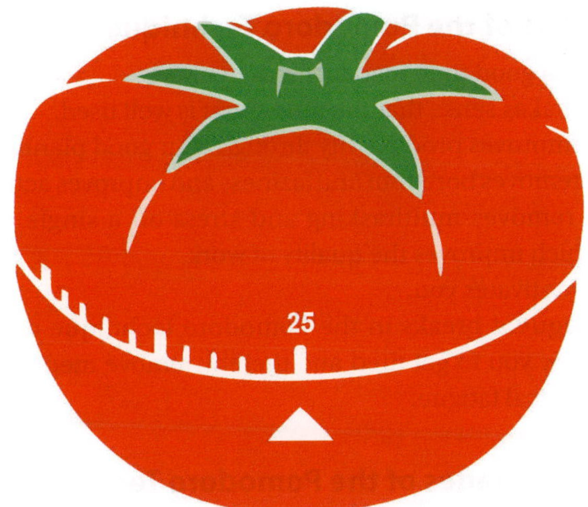

Fig. 1: Tomato (Pomodoro) timer.

5. If you have finished fewer than three pomodoros, go back to step 2 and repeat until you go through all three pomodoros.
6. After three pomodoros are done, take the fourth pomodoro and then take a long break (typically 20–30 minutes). Once the long break is finished, return to step 2.

   Four pomodoros make a set, and there is a long break between two sets, usually 20–30 minutes. It is a time management method.

> Three main principles of Pomodoro technique:
> 1. Plan your pomodoro schedule properly.
> 2. Select what to do during breaks of your liking.
> 3. Stick to the clock.

Three main benefits of the Pomodoro technique:

1. It improves positivity, self-confidence, and willpower that *you can do*.
2. It improves concentration and focus, avoiding distractions.
3. Long hours of study feel easy and interesting.

Three important fields in which a student can use the Pomodoro technique:

1. In daily study.
2. In preparation for examinations and competition.
3. In reducing weight by exercises that you feel are now not boring.

Benefits of the Pomodoro Technique

- It is a good time management method.
- It makes sense that the time spent is well used.
- It improves productivity through your good planning.
- It removes boredom and laziness and improves activity.
- It removes multitasking and stress on a single task, which improves the quality of work.
- It motivates you.
- Frequent breaks in the Pomodoro technique do not allow you to get tired and thereby remove mental and physical fatigue.

Disadvantages of the Pomodoro Technique

Fixed work and break times sometimes make you feel rigid and stressed.

The Pomodoro technique can be helpful in work that are of long duration and boring if done continuously, such as:

- Study
- Preparation for competitive examinations, such as the National Eligibility cum Entrance Test (NEET)
- Weight reduction exercises
- Any work where you can get easily distracted and usually love to postpone due to boring subjects.
- It is good for homework for students.
- Any goal to accomplish, such as preparing for sports tournaments, such as school or state-level sports competitions, and even for the Olympics, Asian games, World Cup, etc.

> One can even make certain changes in Pomodoro technique practice, such as changing breaks to 10 minutes from 5 minutes. I do practice the Pomodoro technique for writing my research papers with a 10-minute break when I go jogging, and 25–30 minutes I write sitting at the table. The break intervals are called Pomodoro. This technique, with the help of a break, reduces the work time, so it helps in focusing on the work more easily and without getting bored.

Cirillo suggests, "Specific cases should be handled with common sense: If you finish a task while the Pomodoro is still ticking, the following rule applies: If a Pomodoro begins, it has to ring. It is a good idea to take advantage of the opportunity for overlearning, using the remaining portion of the Pomodoro to review or repeat what you have done, make small improvements, and note what you have learned until the Pomodoro rings."

A lucid chart makes it the best tool for study for students **(Fig. 2)**.

There are three very important factors that make you to fulfill your goals, which the Pomodoro technique provides. These are:

1. It motivates you to do the job with interest and focus. You feel that in this way you can do any work efficiently and completely.
2. It improves your willpower and thus accountability and determination.
3. It makes you happy and hopeful, preventing mental exhaustion, which improves the quality and quantity of your work. It makes or at least makes you feel, that this job is not that hard and is easy.

> I have developed the habit of doing spot jogging during breaks while doing my work with Pomodoro technique but one can select a work of his liking to do during breaks or can change the job in different breaks. You can choose any of the following:
> - Spot jogging
> - Yoga
> - Meditation
> - Deep abdominal breathing
> - Exercise
> - Reading
> - Relaxing
> - Listening to music
> - Maintaining silence

Three achievements by a student using the Pomodoro technique for study:

1. Time used well.
2. Anxiety and stress of study and examinations have reduced a lot.
3. Gaining confidence that nothing is impossible for me.

> Nicolas Vega published through *culture and media* that with an Oscar-winning career spanning >80 films over four decades, Tom Honks knows a thing or two about making movies. But when it came time for 66-year-old to sit down and write his first novel, Hanks needed help. In a recent profile in the Atlantic, the "Saving Private Ryan" star revealed that he used the famous Pomodoro technique to crank out his 448-page book. "The Making of Another Major Motion Picture Masterpiece" under the guidelines set out by the time management strategy.

A 2014 report in the *Harvard Business Review* found that experimenters who tried out the technique saw that their initial expectations were regularly exceeded when it came to improving productivity, reducing distractions

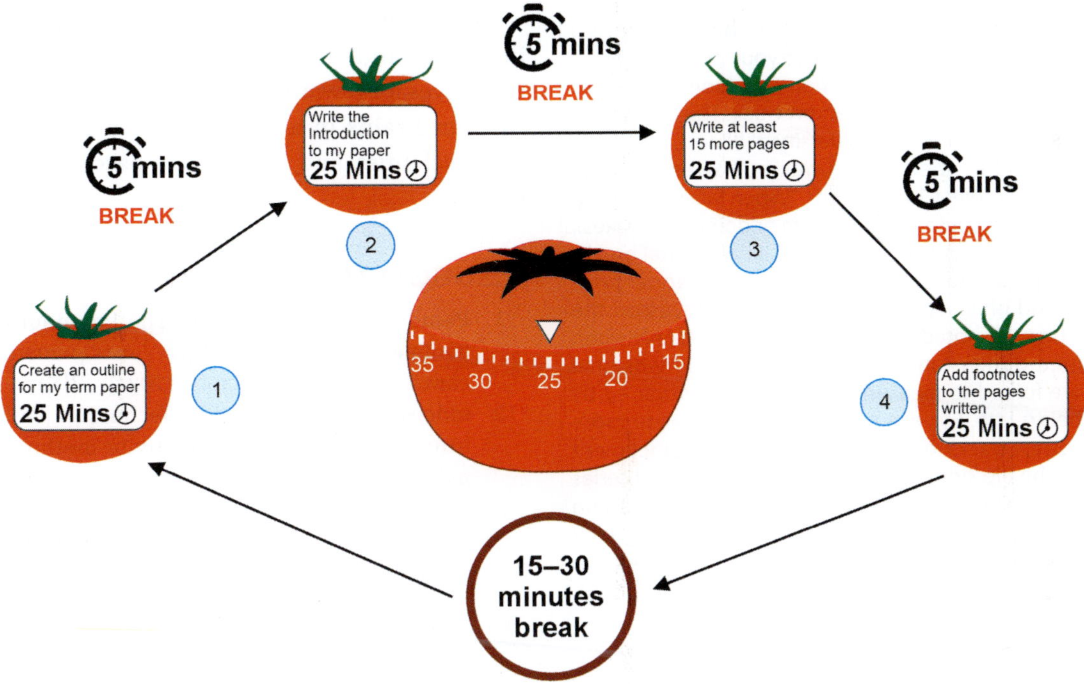

Fig. 2: Pomodoro technique.

from technology, and building a more reliable work process. Tanya Dalton writes in Entrepreneur, why the Pomodoro technique is failing you that a few CEOs who have referenced it as a helpful technique include Shama Hyder, Founder, and CEO of Zen Media; Kat Cohen, Founder, and CEO of Tribe Builder Media while the theory behind the Pomodoro technique is solid, giving yourself focused, blocks of time to dive into important work is extremely powerful. The problem is that the times are way too short.

Meditation can be a good selection for breaks. Meditation gives even very young children power over their thinking and their emotions, not by repressive self-control, but by enhanced self-understanding and self-acceptance. Fontana and Slack advocate meditation as a gentle and effective means of overcoming a wide variety of psychological and behavioral problems, such as anxiety, hyperactivity, and aggression, and they have backed this up with case histories. They also see meditation as a much more general tool, applicable to all children and bringing the following benefits:

Among other even more tangible benefits that can also accrue to a young child by way of meditation is an overall improvement in performance, a method by which to avoid negative developments such as hyperactivity, disobedience, and violent and abusive behavior, and a reduction of the risk of developing coronary artery disease in later life. Meditation should also be started at an early age to prevent against various diseases that make their first appearance during childhood. Children should therefore be taught a simple form of meditation, such as concentration on breathing, from the age of 10 years. They should do it for 5–10 minutes/day, if possible, after school or at any mutually convenient hour. We must teach children to use the Pomodoro technique in study and use meditation during time breaks. This will help children by:

Physical relaxation, improved concentration, increased tranquility and ability to deal with stress, improved awareness, improved creativity, and improved memory.

Masooma Memon writes in "The science behind Pomodoro technique and how it helps supercharge your productivity", a study published in the journal Cognition concludes that short breaks help keep your attention span on track. The study lead and psychology professor at the University of Illinois, Alejandro Lleras explained that the mind tunes out after working consistently on one project. In his words, "When faced with long tasks (such as studying before a final exam or doing your taxes), it is best to impose brief breaks on yourself. Brief mental breaks will actually help you stay focused on your task!" Nobel prize winner (1927) and philosopher, Henry Bergson, discussed the perception of time. He noted that time induced stress only when it wore its three-dimensional mask. In its three-dimensional aspect, you are forced to measure time, which is triggered by the idea of being late. For example, time would cause more stress when you are tracking it before a deadline for a document that is due. On the flip side, viewing time as a sequenced series of events such as having a shower, eating breakfast, heading to work, and so on does not cause stress. And, this is exactly how the Pomodoro technique beats time-related stress.

The Pomodoro technique's approach of dividing work into "do" and "break" sessions increases your brain's incentives for reward. In their book "The Distracted Mind: Ancient Brains in a High-Tech World," Dr Gazzaley, a neuroscientist, and Dr Rosen, a psychologist, talk about this.

SUGGESTED READING

1. Pomodoro technique.com. The Pomodoro® Technique. [Online] Available from https://www.pomodorotechnique.com/ [Last accessed October, 2024].
2. todoist.com. The Pomodoro Technique. [Online] Available https://todoist.com/productivity-methods/pomodoro-technique [Last accessed October, 2024].
3. www.developgoodhabits.com [Online] Available from /https://www.developgoodhabits.com/pomodoro-technique [Last accessed October, 2024].

How to Prepare for these Entrance Examinations?

"Research shows that we need to take a break and decompress so we can be at our best at work"

– Tina Halles

Preparation for a competitive entrance examination requires dreaming, devotion, dedication, and proper preparation. The following points are to be kept in mind while preparing for such examinations:

- *Plan the setting of study area and accessories:* Table, chair, light, may be a table lamp.
- Write a schedule for your study.
- Always set goals for the primary study of the course and revisions.
- Write hours of study and must stick to it. Hours of study are not important; regularity is more important.
- Make your synopsis notes with points only to revise easily.
- Revise the course at least three times before the examination.
- Make a list of dates to finish the primary study and revisions.
- Test yourself every week, whatever part of your course finished. For testing yourself, especially for multiple choice questions (MCQs), open the book on any page and give answers to the questions. For self-testing, every time open a different chapter. Self-testing ideally should be done three times a week for best results.
- Before going to bed, revise your diary synopsis. During sleep, your brain redesigns the information, which improves memory and attaining power.
- Teach others, and speak to your colleagues about whatever you have studied, which will improve your retaining power.
- Do not move ahead of something you are not able to understand in your studies.
- Ask somebody or check on the net, or book. The habit of skipping a difficult item or moving ahead without solving it is a bad and costly habit.
- Be away from distractions. Study in a quiet and isolated place, where there is no distraction. Distractions interfere not only with memory but also with retainment of memory.
- Learn time management skills. Do not waste time on unnecessary things.
- After studying for some time, give a treat to yourself according to the Pomodoro technique.

How to Attempt the Entrance Examination Paper?

"In this game, everyone needs a break to refuel, recharge, and jump back in full-throttle."

– Helen Edwards

When you are served with the examination paper or online questionnaire, go ahead according to the following plan:

- Do not jump and start answering. Devote 2 minutes for doing deep abdominal breathing, which will relax you and prepare you to answer better.

First attempt easy questions while going through the questionnaire. Do not go through the questionnaire initially, but as you go through, go on answering the questions which are easy and you know that you are 100% right. It will save the time and you will be able to complete the paper in time.

- By following the above point, you will be able to get time to revise your answers.

How to Keep Healthy and Avoid Anxiety and Stress during Exam Preparations?

"Learned persons, may we live in your company for a 100 years. Let not our bodies decay before that period, in which old age, our sons become fathers in turn. Break ye not in the midst of our course of fleeting life."

– Yajur Veda

I feel that success can be achieved by concentrating on five pillars of health. They are:

1. Diet
2. Exercise
3. Meditation, stress management and deep abdominal breathing
4. Sleep
5. Happiness

DIET

A low-fat vegetarian diet is the ideal diet. Dr Dean Ornish, Head of Preventive Medicine Research Institute at Sausalito, California, published his study in "Lancet Oncology" recommending lifestyle changes such as a diet rich in fiber, vegetables, whole grains, legumes, and soy products, moderate exercise, and stress management for a healthy and longer life. Sheldon G Sheps of the Mayo Clinic found that a diet of fruits, vegetables, grains, and leads to a lengthening of life span; whereas, unprocessed foods, such as whole wheat flour, vegetables, fresh fruit, and low-fat dairy products cause considerable reduction in blood pressure, which is a silent killer. Processed foods such as chocolates, cakes, and cookies mainly provide calories, and excessive consumption causes diabetes, obesity, and coronary artery disease. Free radicals are unstable and highly active compounds. Oxidation and other chemical reactions involving oxygen produce maximum free radicals. Free radicals damage cells and cause aging. Other than normal metabolism, some external substances also produce free radicals, such as tobacco, alcohol, environmental pollutants, radiation, and fatty diets. The human body produces antioxidant enzymes that oppose free radicals. Vitamins C and E, selenium, carotenes, and flavonoids are good antioxidants. A healthy, plant-based, nutritious, balanced, and light diet keeps the student alert, sharp, full of energy, and with good memory. It removes tiredness and negativity.

EXERCISE

Nothing better can be said for the importance of exercise in our lives than the statement of Edward Stanley, US Congressman, "Those who think have no time for bodily exercise will sooner or later have to make time for illness."

Regular physical exercise is important for maintaining good health. Daily 15–20 minutes of brisk walking will do the needful, any extra exercise is a bonus. Exercise consumes calories and avoids the conversion of any extra calories into fats, strengthens the heart for pumping blood, reduces resting heart rate and blood pressure, increases basal metabolic rate, and brings feelings of well-being due to the release of endorphins. Weight lifting pushes calcium into bones and prevents osteoporosis.

Professor Olstansky, University of Illinois, says a good pair of walking shoes is the single most important product to be purchased for antiaging. Most exercises do not require much of equipment, except a good pair of sneakers and willpower. Aerobic exercises such as walking, jogging, skipping, swimming, and cycling improve the body's flexibility, oxygen processing, production of antioxidants, relaxation of body and mind. Exercise has an antiaging effect, which also helps a healthy mind and body, required for a successful life.

Yoga is very beneficial and improves the physical, mental, and spiritual aspects of life. It improves the body's flexibility, well-being, and relaxation and boosts the immune system. It gives both external and internal massage to the body.

Light aerobic exercises such as brisk walking and jogging are best for a student during the preparation for a competitive exam, as they improve concentration and mental positivity.

MEDITATION AND STRESS MANAGEMENT

Dr Herbert Benson, the Co-Founder of the Mind/Body Clinic of Harvard Medical School, mentions in his book, "The Relaxation Response," that stress raises blood pressure, increases heart rate, and makes breathing rapid while lowering the body's immune response. The opposite can, however, be achieved by repeating a prayer, a word, sound, phrase, or movement, and disregarding other thoughts, meditation in short.

According to Dr Benson, "the relaxation response is a great longevity tool, since deep relaxation promotes greater oxygenation of blood and tissues and causes the adrenal glands to switch their production of age-accelerating hormones, adrenaline and cortisol to dehydroepiandrosterone (DHEA) a steroid hormone which reduces the risk of heart disease, increases well-being, fights serious infections and prolongs life." The relaxation response of the body reduces stress at a cellular level, thereby slowing down the aging process.

Regular meditation, even for 10 minutes daily, helps in relaxing the mind and improving mental concentration and retaining power with positivity and hope, which is required by a student appearing for the exam.

The world's longest-living people are from Sardinia (Italy), Okinawa (Japan), and Loma Linda (California, USA). Two striking features among them, they follow a plant-based diet and lead a stress-free life.

Technique of Deep Abdominal Breathing

When we are under stress, we breathe from the chest, and it is shallow breathing. When we breathe from the diaphragm (abdominal), it is deep breathing. Shallow or chest breathing utilizes 10–15% of lung capacity, so there is less oxygen in the blood, and also less vitality and freshness.

- Stand or sit, or lie down.
- Inhale deeply from the diaphragm, pushing out the abdomen without moving your chest, and count 1, 2, 3, and 4 slowly in your mind while inhaling.
- Hold your breath by counting from 1 to 16 in your mind.
- Exhale by pushing the abdomen in and not moving the chest, and counting from 1 to 8 in your mind.
- Repeat it five times.

SLEEP

About 6–8 hours of sleep are essential for the body's health, as during sleep, the body and mind relax and repair themselves. Sleep deprivation leads to illnesses. Sleep hormone, melatonin, is also an excellent antioxidant, improving mental health. Melatonin production deteriorates with age, and sleeping in a dark room improves its production. Hence, avoid sleeping disturbing factors, such as light, coffee, alcohol, tea, and large meals before sleep.

6 hours of sleep is required for the student who is preparing for a competition, as it helps in reducing anxiety and stress, and improves concentration.

HAPPINESS

Happiness is the ultimate goal of our lives. It gives comfort to the body and brings peace to the soul. But happiness is not found outside the body or soul, it resides within. Recognize the happiness lying deep inside you and feel it. Do not search for it in worldly possessions. Do good deeds. Wealth and fame cannot bring lifelong happiness. That is a state of mind.

Inner serenity, contentment, and happiness remove the fear of aging, illness, and death, leading to better health and success. There is clear evidence of the mind influencing the body. Happiness and positive thinking release helpful chemical substances that strengthen the immune system and ward off diseases, and help with antiaging.

Happiness improves the immunity of our body, thus avoiding falling sick during this important time of preparation for a competition.

CHAPTER 5

How to be Motivated and have a Positive Attitude?

"Believe you can and you are halfway there."

– Theodore Roosevelt

You must be hopeful and positive about the results of your examination, but it must be supported with hard work and regularity:

- You should be hopeful without any doubt.
- Remind yourself that you will be successful, daily, at least once.
- Fight those negative thoughts.
- Keep the company of positive people.
- Follow your goal with your heart.
- Read success stories of others.
- Practice visualization for success.

Believing in yourself is essential to achieving your goal.

CHAPTER 6

What should be the Daily Routine during Preparations for these Entrance Exams?

"My purpose is to lift your spirit and motivate you."

– Mavis Staples

No one can succeed without a goal and its follow-through. The following points are to be kept in mind while preparing for entrance exams:

- Make a chart of your daily routine.
- The program of daily routine should be realistic.

> - About 8–10 hours of study in a day for 2–3 months with concentration, devotion, and without distraction is sufficient to prepare for any examination.
> - Pomodoro method must be included in your daily routine, which gives you sufficient relaxation and satisfaction, improving your chances of success.

- Making a realistic program for study and following it with control of desires is a good way to prepare for exams.

Basic Principles of Surgery

CHAPTER 7

Wounds and Healing

"It is when we start working together that the real healing takes place."

– David Hume

NORMAL WOUND HEALING

A wound is a breach in the continuity of a surface, skin, or mucus membrane. Healing of a wound is an attempt to restore the continuity and replace the lost tissues. Healing of a wound may produce scarring, which may be in the form of adhesions or contractures. The following factors are affecting the healing of a wound:

- Site of the wound
- Size of the wound
- Loss of the tissue—amount and site
- Wound-causing mechanism—surgical, crush, and road traffic accident (RTA)
- Arterial or venous insufficiency
- History of radiation
- Pressure point
- Malnutrition or deficiencies, or smoking
- Diabetes mellitus (DM)
- Use of steroids
- Immune deficiency
- Acquired immunodeficiency syndrome (AIDS)

> *Stages of wound healing:*
> - Inflammatory phase
> - Proliferative phase
> - Remodeling phase/maturing phase

INFLAMMATORY PHASE

It starts immediately after the creation of the wound and it goes progresses for 2–3 days. Bleeding, thrombus formation, and sticking of platelets happen, which leads to the stoppage of bleeding. Then platelets release cytokines, histamine, serotonin, and prostaglandins, leading to the arrival of inflammatory cells. Macro phases act as scavengers, removing dead tissue and microorganisms. This phase has signs of redness, swelling, heat, and pain (Rubor, Tumor, Calor, and Dolor; Latin words).

PROLIFERATIVE PHASE

This phase is for the preparation of wound healing and continues from the third day to the third week. This phase is typically having two events:

1. Fibroblast activity with the production of collagen and ground substance.
2. New blood vessel growth.

These two processes of the proliferative phase form granulation tissue.

Remodeling Phase/Maturing Phase

This phase replaces collagen type III with collagen type I. Wound vascularity slows down, and wound contraction starts. This phase goes on for weeks.

As a routine, wound healing happens in above mentioned three phases. Wound closure and healing can be divided into three groups that are discussed here:

> 1. *Healing by primary intention:* Happens when wound edges are closed, leading to a minimum scar.
> 2. *Healing by secondary intention:* When the wound is not closed, it heals by granulation and epithelialization. The scar so formed is poor.
> 3. *Healing by tertiary intention:* When a wound is not closed, and closure is done after some time.

Important substances released during wound healing are ADP (adenosine diphosphate), PDGF (platelet-derived growth factor), TGFβ (transforming growth factor beta), and PMN (polymorphonuclear leukocytes).

Bone is healed by the formation of callus by periosteal and endosteal proliferation. A callus is an immature bone that gradually converts to mature bone. **Nerves** regenerate after injury after **Wallerian (Augustus Volney Waller, 1816–1870, French Physiologist)** degeneration. The nerve traumatic degeneration occurs distal to the wound as Wallerian degeneration and proximal to the wound up to the last node of Ranvier (Louis Antoine Ranvier, 1835–1922, French Physician and Histologist, described in 1878). Tendons heal by intrinsic and extrinsic mechanisms by which cells and nutrients reach to the site of injury.

TYPES OF WOUNDS

Wounds are classified as tidy and untidy wounds. Untidy wounds contain contaminated tissues, and we aim to convert an untidy wound into a tidy wound by making it decontaminated.

Tidy Wounds

These are clean wounds with healthy tissues and without the loss of tissue. Most of the tidy wounds are incised wounds.

Untidy Wounds

These are contaminated wounds with loss of tissue and may have crushed, devitalized, or broken tissues.

Debridement is the procedure of removing dead, damaged, or infected tissues to improve healing *(Dominique Jean Larrey, 1766-1842, French Surgeon of Napoleon's Army, introduced the term debridement).*

Wound: Breach in the continuity of the skin or epithelium surface.

Simple wound: Only skin and subcutaneous tissue are involved.

Complex wound: Involves underlying nerves, vessels, and tendons with devitalized tissue.

> *Classification of surgical wounds:*
> - *Class I:* Clean wound—lipoma removal incision.
> - *Class II:* Clean/contaminated wounds—planned and elective gastrointestinal surgery incisions.
> - *Class III:* Contaminated wounds—intestinal stoma formation.
> - *Class IV:* Dirty wounds—Fournier's gangrene debridement.

Degloving

Skin and subcutaneous fat are stripped by avulsion from the underlying fascia.

Leaving neurovascular structures, tendons, or bone exposed.

Compartment Syndrome

It occurs in closed limb injury characterized by excessive pain, severe pain on compartment muscle movement, low sensation distal to the injury, and lastly, absence of pulse. Fasciotomy is done to relieve the pressure by placing longitudinal incisions from the skin up to the fascia.

High Pressure Injuries

It is caused by the use of high-pressure devices used for watering and painting, etc. The tissue damage is due to pressure and the toxicity of the substance used. Treatment is debridement with proper exposure.

> *Wound closure:*
> - *Primary closure*—clean wounds and the least contaminated.
> - *Secondary closure*—high risk of infection, or infected wounds.
> - *Delayed primary closure*—highly contaminated wounds.

Chronic Wounds

A wound that takes more than normal healing time, such as venous ulcers on the leg, chronic infection (TB), neoplastic [Marjolin's (Jean-Nicholas Marjolin, 1780–1850, French Surgeon described in 1828) ulcer], bed sores (pressure sores). Pressure sores commonly occur at the sacrum, ischium, and greater trochanter. Pressure sores can be divided into four stages:

- *Stage 1:* Erythema without breach in the skin.
- *Stage 2:* Partial thickness skin loss.
- *Stage 3:* Full thickness skin loss.
- *Stage 4:* Full thickness skin loss involving deeper tissues.

External pressure higher than 30 mm Hg (capillary occlusive pressure) hampers skin blood flow and leads to necrosis and ulceration.

SCARRING AND CONTRACTURES

Scar

- The maturation phase of wound healing leads to the formation of scar.
- *Immature scar (pink, raised, hard, and itchy):* As the collagen matures and becomes denser, the scar becomes almost acellular, as fibroblast and blood vessels reduce—the scar becomes paler, flattens, softer and itching diminishes tensile strength of the scar increases; maximum at 12th week (after 3 months)

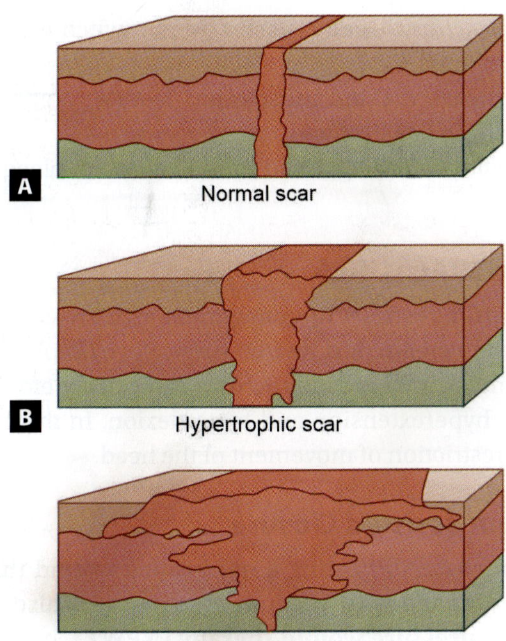

Figs. 1A and B: Types of scars.

postinjury; represent approximately 80% of uninjured skin strength.
- *Types of scars:* Atrophic scar, hypertrophic scar, and keloid **(Figs. 1A and B)**.

> Tensile strength of normal human tissue cannot be achieved by any type of wound healing. The tensile strength after the best wound healing will reach a maximum up to 70–80% of normal human tissue tensile strength.

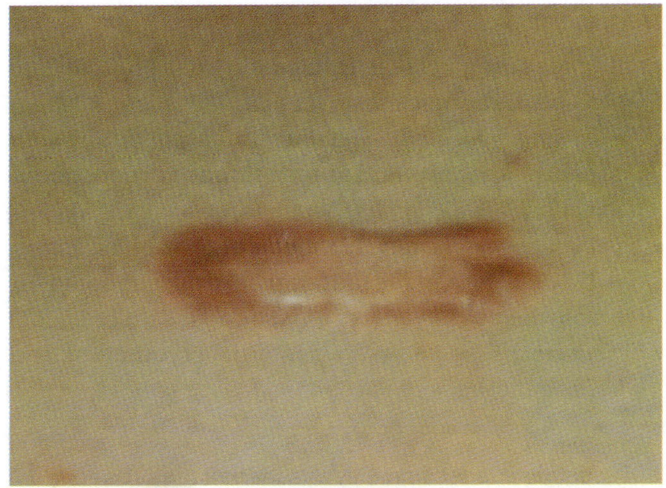
Fig. 2: Hypertrophic scar on chest.

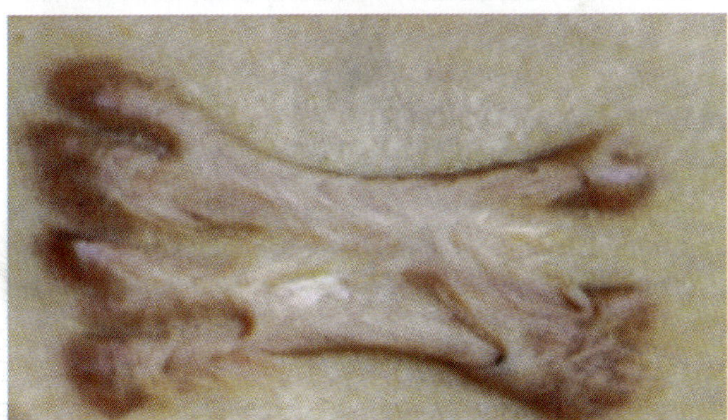
Fig. 3: Keloid on the chest wall.

Atrophic Scar

These are flat, shallow depressions that remain below the uppermost layer of skin. Loss of collagen from the skin due to injury is the cause. Ice pick scars, boxcar scars, and rolling scars are the types of atrophic scars.

Hypertrophic Scar

Common in children and does not go beyond the wound margin. Mainly develop on flexor surfaces **(Fig. 2)**, occur approximately within 3 months after injury, and subside with time.

Keloid

Excessive scar tissue that extends beyond the boundaries of the original incision or wound **(Fig. 3)**.

Etiology

Unknown; genetic predisposition, more common in blacks.
- *Associated with:* Elevated levels of growth factors; deeply pigmented skin.
- *Common in certain areas of the body:* Above clavicle, upper extremities, on the trunk, face (especially seen in a triangle whose boundaries are xiphisternum and each shoulder tip).

Histology

- Excess collagen and hypervascularity; contains disorganized type I and III collagen.
- Thicker collagen bundles from acellular node-like structures.

Treatment

- Keloids rarely regress with time, often refractory to medical and surgical intervention.
- *First-line treatment:* Silicones in combination with pressure therapy and intralesional corticosteroid injection
- *Refractory cases (after 12 months of therapy):* Excision + postoperative radiotherapy (external beam or brachytherapy).
- *New treatment modalities:* Internal cryotherapy and 5% imiquimod.

> *Tissue glues:*
> - Tissue glues are commonly cyanoacrylate polymers, i.e., SurgiSeal and Dermabond (n-butyl-2-cyanoacrylate).
> - The tensile strength after tissue glue application on a wound is low initially, but gradually increases and reaches a maximum at 1 week after repair.

WOUND STRENGTH

- At the end of the first week, wound strength is approximately 10% of that of unwounded skin.
- Strength increases rapidly over the next 4 weeks.
- This rate of increase then slows at approximately the third month after the original incision and reaches a plateau at about 70–80% of the tensile strength of unwounded skin, a condition that may persist for life.

> The recovery of tensile strength results from the excess of collagen synthesis over collagen degradation during the first two months of healing and later from structural modulation of *collagen fibers (cross-linking, increased fiber size)* after collagen synthesis ceases. Over the first three weeks, strength, and collagen content both increase but after 21 days collagen content remains static and only wound strength increases.

Suture marks may be minimized by using monofilament sutures that are removed early (3–5 days). Sutures inserted under tension will leave marks. The wound can be strengthened post suture removal by the use of steri strips. Fine sutures (6/0 or smaller) placed close to the wound margins tend to leave less scarring. Subcuticular suturing avoids suture marks on either side of the wound or incision.

MUSCLE VIABILITY IS DETECTED BY 4C

1. *Color:* Dead muscle has a dark, unhealthy color and has lost its sheen.
2. *Contractility:* Dead muscles do not twitch when held by forceps.
3. *Consistency:* Dead muscle has lost its turgor and is mushy in consistency.
4. *Capillary bleeding:* Dead muscle does not bleed at cut ends.

CONTRACTURES

Contracture restricts the movement as it crosses a joint or a flexion crease. It is treated surgically by Z-plasty, skin graft, and skin flaps. Contractures can cause deformities, such as hyperextension and hyperflexion. In the neck, it causes restriction of movement of the head.

Vacuum-assisted Closure

It is a method of healing a nonhealing wound through sealed dressing with vacuum creation. It is also called **negative pressure wound therapy (NPWT)**. It works by creating a vacuum that draws out fluid from the tissues of the wound and also increases the blood flow of the wound, which enhances the healing. Vacuum pressure is kept at about –1 to –5 mm Hg. It can be done continuously or intermittently.

Mechanism of Action

- Withdraws fluid, thus reducing edema
- **Micro deformation** causes cellular proliferation
- **Macro deformation** causes contraction of the wound, leading to closure of the wound
- Avoids infection as the wound is healed
- Gives a healing environment to the wound as it keeps the wound moist and comfortable

Contraindications

- Malignancy
- Osteomyelitis
- Infected fistula

FACTORS DELAYING WOUND HEALING

Local Factors Related to Wound, Mn = IF HIM

I = Infection
F = Foreign body
H = Hematoma
I = Ischemia
M = Movement

General factors, Mn = DR MADS

D = Diabetes
R = Radiation
M = Malnutrition
A = Age (old)
D = Deficiency (vitamin A, C, iron, and zinc)
S = Steroids

SOME IMPORTANT QUESTIONS

Q1. The vitamin that has an inhibitory effect on wound healing is:
a. Vitamin A
b. Vitamin E
c. Vitamin C
d. Vitamin B-complex

Ans. b

Q2. A clean incised wound heals by:
a. Primary intention
b. Secondary intention
c. Excessive scarring
d. None of the above

Ans. a

Q3. The tensile strength of the wound reaches that of normal tissue by:
a. 6 weeks
b. 2 months
c. 4 months
d. 6 months

Ans. None

Q4. A clean wound has the maximum strength of the wound on:
a. 3–4 days
b. 8–9 days
c. 11–12 days
d. 13–18 days

Ans. d

Q5. The tensile strength of the wound becomes normal after:
a. 6 weeks
b. Never
c. 4 months
d. 6 months

Ans. b

Q6. Which of the following is true about keloids?
a. Wide local excision is the treatment of choice
b. Collagen is the same, but arranged haphazardly
c. Will not spread beyond the wound site
d. More amount of growth factors

Ans. d

Q7. The following statement about keloids is true:
a. Elevated levels of growth factor are not seen
b. Extended excision is the treatment of choice
c. It does not extend beyond the wound
d. It will have more collagen and vascularity

Ans. d

Q8. First-line treatment for keloid is:
a. Intralesional injection of keloid
b. Local steroid
c. Radiotherapy
d. Wide excision

Ans. a

Q9. The following statement about keloids is true:
a. They do not extend into normal skin
b. Local recurrence is common after excision
c. They often undergo malignant changes
d. They are more common in whites than in blacks

Ans. b

Q10. Keloid formation is not seen over:
a. Ear
b. Face
c. Eyelids
d. Neck

Ans. c

Q11. If suture marks are to be avoided, skin sutures should be removed by:
a. 72 hours
b. 1 week
c. 2 weeks
d. 3 weeks

Ans. b

Q12. In an open injury during toileting and debridement, muscle viability is detected by:
a. Color of the muscle
b. Muscle size
c. Muscle function
d. Muscle contractility
e. Punctate bleed spots on the cut edge

Ans. a and e

Q13. The tensile strength of the wound starts and increases after:
a. Immediate suture of the wound
b. 3–4 days
c. 7–10 days
d. 6 months

Ans. b

Q14. Primary closure of incised wounds must be done within:
a. 2 hours
b. 4 hours
c. 6 hours
d. 12 hours
e. 16 hours

Ans. c

Q15. A patient had a lacerated, untidy wound on the leg and attended the casualty after 2 hours. His wound should be:
a. Sutured immediately
b. Debrided and sutured immediately

c. Debrided and sutured secondarily
d. Cleaned and dressed

Ans. b

Q16. Delayed wound healing is seen in all, *except*:

a. Malignancy b. Hypertension
c. Diabetes d. Infection

Ans. b

Q17. What causes a clean-contaminated wound?

a. Elective open cholecystectomy for cholelithiasis
b. Herniorrhaphy
c. Mastectomy with axillary node dissection
d. Abscess of the appendix

Ans. a

Q18. In a classification of contaminated wounds, which of the following are included?

a. Resection of unprepared bowel
b. Perforated appendix resection
c. Resection of intestinal fistula
d. Inguinal hernia repair
e. Hysterectomy

Ans. a and b

Q19. Which one of the following statements is true regarding keloids?

a. Commonly seen on eyelids, genitalia, palms, and soles
b. Tend to occur 3 months to one year after the initial insult
c. All these statements are true
d. Commonly extend into the underlying subcutaneous tissue

Ans. b

Q20. A drug used for intralesional injection for keloid is:

a. Prednisolone b. Triamcinolone
c. Androgen d. Hydrocortisone

Ans. b

MULTIPLE CHOICE QUESTIONS

Grade I	*Simple*

Q1. Wound healing is affected by: (PGI Dec 2007)

a. Age
b. Nutrition
c. Dryness or wetness of the wound
d. Drugs
e. Temperature

Q2. True about chronic wound: (PGI Nov 2009)

a. Found in diabetes mellitus (DM)
b. Always require surgical treatment
c. May be associated with vascular compromise
d. Monofilament sutures prevent infection
e. Any wound that does not heal within 3 months

Q3. The following are required for wound healing, *except*: (All India 1993)

a. Zinc b. Copper
c. Vitamin C d. Calcium

Q4. True about hypertrophied scar is: (PGI Dec 2008)

a. Grows beyond the original wound
b. Pigmented
c. Develops within 2–6 weeks
d. Pruritis present

Q5. Preferred time for prophylactic antibiotic administration for surgery: (PGI June 2009)

a. 1 day before surgery
b. IM 6 hours before surgery
c. At the time of induction of anesthesia
d. IV during surgery
e. Orally given the night before

Q6. The best skin graft for an open wound is: (All India 1993)

a. Isograft b. Homograft
c. Allograft d. Autograft

Q7. Regarding antibiotics, true facts are: (PGI June 2006)

a. No prophylaxis for clean contaminated surgery
b. No prophylaxis for gastric ulcer surgery
c. Prophylaxis for colorectal surgery
d. Local irrigation with an antibiotic is contraindicated when systemic antibiotics are given

Q8. Which of these scoring systems is helpful in assessing the severity of wound infection? (AIIMS Nov 1996)

a. Southampton grading scale
b. American Society of Anesthesiologists (ASA) classification
c. Glasgow score
d. Appearance, Pulse, Grimace, Activity, and Respiration (APGAR)

Grade II	Difficult

Q1. Prevention of wound infection is done by: (PGI June 2005)

a. Preop shaving
b. Preop antibiotic therapy
c. Monofilament suture
d. Wound apposition

Q2. Cell not involved in the healing of a clean wound: (PGI Nov 2011)

a. Macrophages
b. Platelet
c. Fibroblasts
d. Polymorphonuclear leukocytes
e. Myofibroblasts

Q3. All are true about keloid, *except*: (PGI Dec 2007)

a. Grows beyond would margin
b. Excess collagen deposition
c. Precancerous leading to cancer
d. More common in females
e. Whites are at high risk

Q4. The patient has a lacerated, untidy wound on the leg and attended the casualty after 2 hours. His wound should be: (AIIMS 1984)

a. Sutured immediately
b. Debrided and sutured immediately
c. Debrided and sutured secondarily
d. Cleaned and dressed

Q5. Best management of a contaminated wound with necrotic material is: (AIIMS Nov 2013)

a. Broad-spectrum antibiotics
b. Debridement
c. Control of blood sugar
d. Gas gangrene serum

Q6. Which of the following is a scoring system for the severity of wound infection, and is particularly useful for surveillance and research: (UPSC 2009)

a. APGAR score
b. Glasgow scoring system
c. Southampton grading system
d. ASA classification

Q7. Which one of the following organisms is not associated with synergic gangrene: (UPSC 2009)

a. *Escherichia*
b. *Staphylococcus*
c. *Clostridium*
d. *Peptostreptococcus*

Grade III	Most difficult

Q1. True about wound healing: (PGI June 2009)

a. Infected wound heals by primary intention
b. The deep dermal wound heals by scar formation.
c. Wound contraction is found in healing by secondary intention
d. The more intense inflammatory response is in primary intention

Q2. True statement(s) regarding hypertrophic scar: (PGI Dec 2008)

a. Grow beyond the wound margin
b. More common in females
c. Not familial
d. Rarely subsides
e. Not race-related

Q3. The most common site of hypertrophic keloid is: (AIIMS Nov 1993)

a. Face
b. Leg
c. Presternal area
d. Arm

Q4. Gastrojejunostomy is an example of: (JIPMER 1998)

a. Clean contaminated wound
b. Clean an uncontaminated wound
c. Unclean, uncontaminated wound
d. Unclean contaminated wound

Q5. A surgeon decides to operate on a patient with carcinoma cecum and perform a right hemicolectomy through a midline laparotomy approach. You have been instructed to prepare the parts of the patient for surgery. What will you do? (AIIMS May 2016)

a. Thigh Clean and drape from rib cage to inguinal regions
b. Clean and drape from the umbilicus to the midthigh
c. Clean and drape from chin to knee
d. Clean and drape from the level of the nipple to mid

ANSWERS

Grade I: 1. a, b, d, e; 2. a, c, d, e; 3. None; 4. c, d; 5. c; 6. d; 7. c; 8 a

Grade II: 1. b, c, d; 2. b, e; 3. c, e; 4. b; 5. b; 6. c; 7. c

Grade III: 1. b, c; 2. c, e; 3. c; 4. a; 5. d

MODEL QUESTIONS

Q1. Keloid is best treated:

a. Intralesional injection of triamcinolone
b. Wide excision and grafting
c. Wide excision and suturing
d. Deep X-ray therapy

Ans. a

Q2. Vacuum-assisted closure is contraindicated in:

a. Chronic osteomyelitis
b. A large amount of necrotic tissue with eschar.
c. Abdominal wound
d. Surgical wound dehiscence

Ans. b

Q3. Degloving injury is:

a. Surgeon made the wound
b. Lacerated wound
c. Blunt injury
d. Avulsion injury
e. Abrasive wound

Ans. d

Q4. The criteria for the viability of muscle are all, *except*:

a. Color
b. Intact fascia
c. Contractibility
d. Bleeding on cutting

Ans. c

Q5. Which management of an open wound was seen 12 hours after the injury?

a. Suturing
b. Debridement and suture
c. Secondary suturing
d. Heal by granulation

Ans. b

Q6. In a sutured surgical wound, the process of epithelialization is completed within:

a. 24 hours
b. 48 hours
c. 72 hours
d. 96 hours

Ans. b

Q7. Factors that may adversely affect the healing of wounds include all the following, *except*:

a. Exposure to UV light
b. Exposure to radiation
c. Obstructive jaundice
d. Advanced neoplasia

Ans. a

Q8. The maximum collagen content of the wound reaches on:

a. Between the third and sixth day
b. Between the 6th and 15th day
c. Between the 17th and 21st day
d. Between 21st and 24th day

Ans. c

Q9. A patient with a grossly contaminated wound presents 12 hours after an accident; his wound should be managed by:

a. Thorough cleaning and primary repair
b. Thorough cleaning with debridement of all dead and devitalized tissue without primary closure
c. Primary closure over a drain.
d. Covering the defect with a split skin graft after cleaning

Ans. b

Q10. Fibroblasts in healing wounds are derived from:

a. Local mesenchyme
b. Epithelium
c. Endothelium
d. Vascular fibrosis

Ans. a

Q11. True statement regarding hypertrophic scar:

a. Usually occurs across the flexural areas
b. Does not improve with time
c. Overgrows its boundaries
d. Develops months after surgery

Ans. a

Q12. A keloid scar is made up:

a. Dense collagen
b. Loose fibrous tissue
c. Granulomatous tissue
d. Loose areolar tissue

Ans. a

Q13. What is true about keloids?

a. It appears immediately after surgery
b. It appears a few days after surgery
c. It is limited in its distribution
d. It is common among old people

Ans. b

Q14. All of the following are principles of negative pressure wound therapy (NPWT), *except*:

a. Stabilization of wound environment
b. Clearance of infection
c. Macrodeformation of the wound
d. Decreased edema

Ans. b

Q15. NPWT is used in:

a. Bed sore in sacrum after debridement
b. After amputation, negative suction
c. Osteomyelitis
d. Unexplored fistulas

Ans. a

Q16. In the treatment of hand injuries, the greatest priority is:

a. Repair of tendons
b. Restoration of skin cover
c. Repair of nerves
d. Repair of blood vessels

Ans. d

Q17. "Limb salvage" primarily depends on:

a. Vascular injury
b. Skin cover
c. Bone injury
d. Nerve injury

Ans. a

Q18. Degloving injury:

a. Separation of skin only
b. Separation of skin + subcutaneous tissue
c. Separation of skin + subcutaneous tissue + fascia exposing
d. Separation of the tendon, exposing the bone

Ans. b

CHAPTER 8

Shock and Blood Transfusion

"The blood is the life"

– Bram Stoker

INTRODUCTION

The most common cause of death is shock. "Shock is a systemic stage of low tissue perfusion that is inadequate for normal cellular respiration."

When tissue perfusion is low then cells cannot receive the required amount of oxygen so they turn from aerobic to anaerobic metabolism. The products of anaerobic metabolism are carbon dioxide and lactic acid, the collection of these two leads to "metabolic acidosis." Ultimately cellular lysis or disintegration happens due to release of autodigestive lysosomes.

Tissue ischemia due to any reason leads to stimulation of immune and coagulation systems and activation of complement and prime neutrophils leading to endothelium damage which makes it leaky allowing fluid to leak and form edema.

EFFECTS ON BODY SYSTEMS

- *Heart and vascular system:* Sympathetic activity increases leading to tachycardia and vasoconstriction.
- *Respiratory system:* Increased sympathetic activity along with acidosis increases the rate of respiration leading to compensatory respiratory alkalosis.
- *Kidneys:* Low perfusion leads to low urine output. Renin-angiotensin-aldosterone axis activation leads to more sodium and water absorption.
- *Endocrine system:* The hypothalamus releases vasopressin and rennin-angiotensin leading to more reabsorption of water. Cortisol release is increased leading to sodium and water resorption.

CLASSIFICATION OF SHOCK

Mn = H-CODE:

- *H* = Hypovolemic shock
- *C* = Cardiogenic shock
- *O* = Obstructive shock
- *D* = Distributive shock
- *E* = Endocrine shock

Hypovolemic Shock

Hypovolemic shock is due to a reduced circulating volume. Hypovolemia may be due to *hemorrhagic* **or** *nonhemorrhagic* causes. Nonhemorrhagic causes include poor fluid intake (dehydration), excessive fluid loss due to vomiting, diarrhea, urinary loss (e.g., diabetes), evaporation, or "third spacing" where fluid is lost into the gastrointestinal tract and interstitial spaces, for example, in bowel obstruction or pancreatitis.

Types of Hemorrhagic Shocks

According to Advanced Trauma Life Support (ATLS), hemorrhagic shock is classified in four classes according to volume of blood loss and clinical features:

1. *Class I:* Loss of 0–15% of blood volume
2. *Class II:* Loss of 15–30% of blood volume
3. *Class III:* Loss of 30–40% of blood volume
4. *Class IV:* Loss of >40% of blood volume

Classes I and II are compensated, whereas Class III is decompensated, and Class IV is refractory.

Important Points

- Most common type of shock—hypovolemic
- *Mechanism:* Reduced intravascular volume → Reduced venous return and cardiac output → inadequate tissue perfusion → oliguria → anuria.
- Lactic acidosis → metabolic acidosis → tachypnea.

Activation of the compensatory mechanism, which includes increased production of epinephrine and norepinephrine, leads to cold and clammy skin, tachycardia, sweating, and low blood pressure (BP).

Cardiogenic Shock

Cardiogenic shock is due to the primary failure of the heart to pump blood to the tissues.

Obstructive Shock

There is a reduction in preload due to mechanical obstruction of cardiac filling. Common causes of obstructive shock include cardiac tamponade, tension pneumothorax, massive pulmonary embolus, or air embolus.

Distributive Shock

Distributive shock describes the pattern of cardiovascular responses characterizing a variety of conditions, including septic shock, anaphylaxis, and spinal cord injury.

Endocrine Shock

Endocrine shock may present as a combination of hypovolemic, cardiogenic, or distributive shock. Causes of endocrine shock include hypo- and hyperthyroidism and adrenal insufficiency.

Compensated Shock

When the body is able to continue maintaining normal or near normal blood flow to the vital organs, heart, lungs, liver, kidneys, and brain, it maintains cellular perfusion and respiration. A compensatory state of shock if insulted by delayed attention can lead to multiple organ failure and death. Ischemia-reperfusion syndrome, if it continues for >12 hours, will increase multiple organ failure and mortality.

Decompensated Shock

When the body fails to compensate, the tissue perfusion and cellular respiration in vital organs. This happens when blood volume loss becomes 30–40%.

TYPES OF SHOCK

- *Mild shock:* Mild anxiety, tachycardia, normal BP, conscious, normal urine output, respiratory rate, and lactic acidosis.
- *Moderate shock:* Drowsy, tachycardia, mild hypotension, increased respiratory rate, reduced urine output, and lactic acidosis.
- *Severe shock:* Comatose, tachycardia, severe hypotension, labored respiration, anuric, and lactic acidosis.

Multiple Organ Failure

When two or more organ systems fail. No specific treatment. Supportive treatment is required to various systems. Mortality is approximately 60%. Lung develops acute respiratory distress syndrome (ARDS), Kidneys develop acute renal insufficiency, Heart leads to failure, and clotting becomes abnormal (coagulopathy).

Monitoring of Patients in Shock

- Pulse
- Blood pressure
- Urine output
- Cardiac output
- Serum lactate
- Pulse oximetry
- Electrocardiogram (ECG)

Fluid Response to a Patient in Shock

In a shock patient, one of the most important therapies is rapid fluid administration. A patient can respond in any of the following ways:

- Responding
- Transient responding—responds early but fails within 20 minutes.
- Nonresponding

Intravenous Fluids

Crystalloid solutions: Normal saline, Hartmann's solution (Alexis Frank Hartmann, American pediatrician, describe the solution, 1898–1964), Ringer's lactate solution (Sidney Ringer, 1835–1910, Professor of Clinical Medicine, University College Hospital, London, UK).

Hemorrhage

Moderate to severe hemorrhage causes hypovolemic shock, leading to acute traumatic coagulopathy (ATC). In a higher percentage of trauma, ATC starts quickly within minutes and increases mortality tremendously, approximately four times.

- *Primary hemorrhage:* Immediately after injury or surgery.
- *Reactionary hemorrhage:* It is a delayed hemorrhage occurring within 24 hours due to the dislodgement of a clot.
- *Secondary hemorrhage:* Due to sloughing of a vessel wall, occurring 7–14 days after injury.

Classes of Hemorrhagic Shock

- *Class I:* <15% blood volume loss
- *Class II:* 15–30%
- *Class III:* 30–40%
- *Class IV:* >40%

> - *1901: Carl Landsteiner (1868–1943, Professor of Pathology and Anatomy, University of Vienna, Austria, awarded Nobel prize for Physiology or Medicine in 1930)* discovers the ABO system.
> - *1926:* The British Red Cross instituted the first blood transfusion service.
> - *1939:* The Rhesus system was identified and recognized.

SHOCK INDEX

Heart rate/systolic blood pressure—if higher than 0.9, then the mortality rate is significant.

Modified Shock Index

Heart rate/mean arterial pressure—a very sensitive index.

ANTISHOCK GARMENT

An antishock garment is required in hypovolemic shock, such as a lady with postpartum hemorrhage after delivery in a village clinic.

ANAPHYLACTIC SHOCK

- Anaphylactic shock happens with mismatched blood transfusions (BTs).
- Release of histamine → vasodilatation → blood pooling → warm extremities.

WARM SEPTIC SHOCK

Warm septic shock happens in sepsis → hyperdynamic circulation → extremities are warm.

COLD SEPTIC SHOCK

Cold septic shock happens late in sepsis → endotoxins depress heart muscles, extremities are cold.

SYSTEMIC INFLAMMATORY RESPONSE SYNDROME (CHRONIC INFLAMMATORY RESPONSE SYNDROME)

It is the body's response to inflammation. Happens in infection and non-infection inflammation. It is caused by interleukin-1 (IL-1), interleukin-6 (IL-6), and tumor necrosis factor alpha (TNF-α).

SEQUENTIAL ORGAN FAILURE ASSESSMENT SCORE

Sequential Organ Failure Assessment (SOFA) score is for organ failure assessment in sepsis.

QUICK SEQUENTIAL ORGAN FAILURE ASSESSMENT SCORE

Quick sequential organ failure assessment (QSOFA) score happens in sepsis and depends upon heart rate, systolic blood pressure, and altered mental state.

MULTIPLE ORGAN DYSFUNCTION SYNDROME

Multiple organ dysfunction syndrome (MODS) happens when more than two organ systems fail, in sepsis.

Sepsis

Mn: FAT-O-BLU

- *F* = Fluid
- *A* = Antibiotics
- *T* = Time within sixty minutes
- *O* = Oxygen
- *B* = Blood culture
- *L* = Lactate
- *U* = Urine output

FUNCTIONS OF CITRATE STORING SOLUTION FOR BLOOD

It acts as an anticoagulant by calcium chelation and also decreases glycolysis.

BLOOD AND ITS PRODUCTS

- Whole blood
- *Packed red cells:* 330 mL/unit, stored in saline, adenine, glucose, and mannitol (SAG-M) solution, with a shelf life of 5 weeks.
- *Fresh frozen plasma (FFP):* Rich in coagulation factors, shelf life 2 years, first-line therapy in coagulopathic hemorrhage.

- *Cryoprecipitate:* Supernatant precipitate of FFP, rich in factor VIII and fibrinogen.
- *Platelets:* Platelet concentrate, 250×10^9/L, shelf life 5 days.
- *Prothrombin complex concentrates (PCC):* Prepared from pooled plasma, contains factors II, IX, and X.
- *Autologous blood:* Blood drawn from the patient who is going for surgery before 3 weeks. Cell-saver washes and collects red blood cells (RBCs) from spilled blood during surgery and returns to the patient.

> *Transfusion trigger:* Blood transfusion above 6 g/dL is nowadays not advised as it may increase morbidity and mortality. 6 g/dL is now an acceptable limit for a patient who is not bleeding and not going for major surgery.

Massive Blood Transfusion

- Replacing the whole body's circulating blood within 24 hours.
- >10 units of blood in 24 hours.
- Five units in 5 hours.

Complications of Blood Transfusion

Mn = IF I EAT

- *I* = Incompatibility BT reaction
- *F* = Fever
- *I* = Infection
- *E* = Air embolism
- *A* = Allergy
- *T* = Thrombophlebitis

> Recent studies have elaborated on blood and its product transfusion policy in active hemorrhage. If one unit of red cell is given then it is better to also give one unit of FFP and one unit of platelets. Dilutional coagulopathy is reduced in this plan.

Complications of Massive Blood Transfusion

Mn = $CH_4\,OM$

- *C* = Coagulopathy
- *H* = Hypocalcemia
- *H* = Hyperkalemia
- *H* = Hypokalemia
- *H* = Hypothermia
- *O* = Fluid over load
- *M* = Metabolic

> **Transfusion Protocols**
>
> - *Blood transfusion should commence within 30 minutes of removing blood bags from refrigerators because of the increased risk of bacterial contamination.*
> - *Whole blood or packed RBC transfusion must be completed within 4 hours.*
> - Platelet and FFP transfusions should be completed within 20 minutes.
> - The transfusion set should have a standard filter of 170 µm.
> - Usual transfusion needle size should be of 18–19G.

Whole blood—1 unit contains 450 mL and is not used generally, but when massive bleeding occurs as in open heart surgery. It is also used when total exchange of blood is required in a neonate.

Red Blood Cells (Packed Red Blood Cells)

Red blood cells are stored at 1–6°C; the mean life of transfused RBCs is 35 days. *1 unit contains 180–200 mL.* It contains RBCs, some leukocytes, and a small quantity of plasma. One unit transfer increases hemoglobin (Hb) by 1 g/dL and 3% of hematocrit.

Platelet Concentrates

- One unit contains 50–70 mL
- Platelets are the only blood products that are stored at room temperature, 20–24°C (survival is 4–5 days).
- One unit of platelet increases the count by 5,000–10,000.
    - The threshold for prophylactic platelet transfusion is 10,000/mm^3 platelets/µL of blood
    - For invasive procedures, 50,000/mm^3 platelets is the usual target level.
    - Platelet count should be 1,00,000/mm^3 before accepting the patient for surgery.
- *Blood platelets in stored blood are nonfunctional after 24 hours.*

Fresh-frozen Plasma

1 unit contains 200–250 mL. It contains plasma proteins, coagulation factors, antithrombin, and protein C and S. It increases coagulation factors by 2%. Each unit contains 400 mg of fibrinogen and one unit of activity of each of the clotting factors.

- FFP should not be routinely used to expand blood volume.

- *FFP:* An acellular component that does not transmit intracellular infections, e.g., cytomegalovirus (CMV).
- *Factor V and VIII* are diminished.

Indications of Fresh-frozen Plasma Use

- Thrombocytic thrombocytopenic purpura
- Coagulopathies, such as in warfarin-induced

Cryoprecipitate

- *Cryoprecipitate is a source of fibrinogen, factor VIII, and non-Willebrand factor (non-vWF).*
- It is ideal for supplying fibrinogen to the volume-sensitive patient.
- Stored at ≤−18°C
    - 1 unit of cryoprecipitate, 10–15 mL, contains 80–145 units of Factor VIII and 250 mg of fibrinogen.
    - Cryoprecipitate is pooled from many donors, so there are maximum chances of disease transmission among all blood products.
- *Cryoprecipitate may also supply vWF to patients with dysfunctional (type II) or absent (type III) von Willebrand factor.*

Dextran

- It induces rouleaux of RBCs and this interferes with blood grouping and cross-matching procedures; hence, the need for a blood sample beforehand.
- It interferes with platelet function; hence it is recommended that the total volume of dextran should not exceed 1,000 mL.
    - Low-molecular-weight (LMW) dextran (short-acting) prevents sludging of RBCs in vessels and renal shutdown in severe hypotension and it is less likely to induce rouleaux formation than high-molecular weight (HMW) dextran (long-acting).

Arterial Injury

- Laceration → vasoconstriction → increase in laceration size → bleeds more.
- Transection of artery → coagulation → plug → bleeds less.

Excess heparin in the syringe can lead to:

- Reduction of pH
- Reduction of partial pressure of carbon dioxide in arterial blood ($PaCO_2$)
- Reduction of hydrogencarbonate (HCO_3)

TRALI: Transfusion-related acute lung injury—it is a condition of acute, noncardiogenic pulmonary edema associated with hypoxia that occurs during or after a transfusion.

TACO: Transfusion-associated circulatory overload—it is a common transfusion reaction in which pulmonary edema develops primarily due to volume excess or circulating overload.

TACO is caused by circulatory overload; TRALI is not.

RED BLOOD CELL TRANSFUSION GUIDELINE/CRITERIA

- <6 g/dL Hb—transfusion
- 6–8 g/dL Hb—transfusion if waiting for surgery
- >8 g/dL Hb—no transfusion

Some important points in blood transfusion are as follows:

- Blood used within 14 days of donation works well.
- WBCs and platelets are quickly destroyed within 24 hours.
- Microaggregation from white blood cells (WBCs), platelets, fibrin, and thrombin can be partially filtered by the microfilter of the blood transfusion set (filter size 20 µm and microaggregate size 20–70 µm).
- A feeling of heat and pain along the vein happens in transfusion reactions in conscious patients.
- Low urine output also happens in transfusion reactions in conscious patients.
- Blood to be transfused at the rate of five drops per minute for 10 minutes, then increased to 30–40 drops per minute, to be finished in 4 hours.
- After a massive blood transfusion, 2 mL of 10% calcium gluconate is required per 500 mL of blood.
- Approximately a clenched fist is equal to 500 mL of blood clot.

ANTICOAGULANTS

Anticoagulants used in whole blood are ACD (Acid Citrate Dextrose) (21 days maximum storage time)

Citrate phosphate dextrose adenine-1 (CPD-1)—35 days maximum storage time, saline adenine glucose mannitol (SAGM)—2 days

Actions of Anticoagulants

Ingredients

- *Adenine:* Synthesis of ATP
- *Glucose:* Glycolysis leading to the production of ATP
- *Sodium diphosphate*—maintaining normal pH
- *Citrate:* Chelates with calcium and prevents coagulation

SUGGESTED READING

1. In: Williams NS, O'Connell PR, McCaskie AW (Eds). Bailey & Love's Short Practice of Surgery, 27th edition. Florida: CRC Press; 2018. p. 13.

SOME IMPORTANT QUESTIONS

Q1. The most common blood transfusion reaction is:

a. Febrile nonhemolytic transfusion reaction (FNHTR)
b. Hemolysis
c. Transmission of infections
d. Electrolyte imbalance

Ans. a

Q2. After a blood transfusion, the Febrile nonhemolytic transfusion reaction FNHTR occurs due to:

a. WBCs
b. Antibodies against donor leukocytes and HLA Ag
c. Allergic reaction
d. Infection

Ans. b

Q3. Massive transfusion results in:

a. Disseminated intravascular coagulation (DIC)
b. Allergic reaction
c. Hemolysis
d. Thrombocytopenia

Ans. a, b, and d

Q4. Half-life of factor VIII is:

a. 6 hours
b. 8 hours
c. 12 hours
d. 36 hours

Ans. b

Q5. Cryoprecipitate is a rich source of:

a. Thromboplastin
b. Factor VIII
c. Factor X
d. Factor VII

Ans. b

Q6. Vasovagal shock is due to:

a. Pooling of blood in the lower limbs
b. Major operation
c. Head injury
d. Infected wound

Ans. a

Q7. Neurogenic shock is due to:

a. Spinal anesthesia
b. Trauma
c. Brain abscess
d. Hypertension

Ans. a

Q8. Which metabolism happens in hypovolemic shock?

a. Aerobic metabolism
b. Anaerobic metabolism
c. Catabolism metabolism
d. Endomorph metabolism

Ans. b

Q9. Death in burns within 2 days occurs due to:

a. Cardiogenic shock
b. Hypovolemic shock
c. Neurogenic shock
d. Renal damage

Ans. b

Q10. Causes of cardiogenic shock:

a. Injury
b. Cardiac failure
c. Infection
d. Pulmonary embolism

Ans. d

Q11. A man dies after burns in the second week due to:

a. Hypovolemic shock
b. Cardiogenic shock
c. Septic shock
d. Neurogenic shock

Ans. c

Q12. Which acid is produced during anaerobic metabolism?

a. Acetic acid
b. Salicylic acid
c. Lactic acid
d. Hydrochloric acid

Ans. c

Q13. What does cardiogenic shock produce?

a. Respiratory acidosis
b. Metabolic acidosis
c. Respiratory alkalosis
d. Hyaluronic acidosis

Ans. b

Q14. The normal central venous pressure (CVP) is:

a. 2–4 cm of saline
b. 5–8 cm of saline
c. 10–15 cm of saline
d. 15–20 cm of saline

Ans. b

Q15. Oliguria is called when:

a. <200 mL/day in adults
b. <500 mL/day in adults
c. <1500 mL/day in adults
d. <2,000 mL/day in adults

Ans. b

MULTIPLE CHOICE QUESTIONS

Grade I | **Simple**

Q1. How long can blood be stored with citrate phosphate dextrose adenine (CPDA)? (JIPMER 2003)
a. 12 days
b. 21 days
c. 28 days
d. 48 days

Q2. Mismatched blood transfusion in an anesthetic patient present is: (PGI June 2000)
a. Hyperthermia and hypertension
b. Hypotension and bleeding from the site of the wound
c. Bradycardia and hypertension
d. Tachycardia and hypertension

Q3. In a patient with thrombocytopenia, what is the target platelet count after transfusion to perform an invasive procedure? (AIIMS May 2015)
a. 30,000
b. 40,000
c. 50,000
d. 60,000

Q4. With reference to fresh frozen plasma (FFP), which one of the following statements is not correct? (UPSE 2008)
a. It is used as a volume expander
b. It is stored at –40°C to –50°C
c. It is a source of coagulation factors
d. It is given in a dose of 12–15 mL/kg body weight

Q5. Best blood product to be given to a patient with multiple clotting factor deficiency with active bleeding: (AIIMS May 2015)
a. Whole blood
b. Packed red blood cells (RBCs)
c. FFP
d. Cryoprecipitate

Q6. Which one of the following blood fractions is stored at –40°C? (UPSC 2006)
a. Cryoprecipitate
b. Human albumin
c. Platelet concentrate
d. Packed red cells

Q7. Platelets can be stored at: (AIIMS Nov 2005)
a. 20–24°C for 5 days
b. 20–24°C for 8 days
c. 4–8°C for 5 days
d. 4–8°C for 8 days

Grade II | **Difficult**

Q1. All of the following infections may be transmitted via blood transfusion, *except*: (AIIMS May 2009)
a. Parvo B-19
b. Hepatitis G
c. Dengue virus
d. Cytomegalovirus

Q2. Which of the following investigations should be done immediately to best confirm a nonmatched blood transfusion reaction? (All India 2010)
a. Indirect Coombs test
b. Direct Coombs test
c. Antibody in the patient's serum
d. Antibody in donor serum

Q3. Which of the following statements about acute hemolytic blood transfusion reaction is true? (PGI June 2004)
a. Complement-mediated hemolysis is seen
b. Type III hypersensitivity is responsible for most cases
c. Rarely life-threatening
d. Renal blood flow is always maintained
e. No need to stop the transfusion

Q4. Massive blood transfusion is defined as: (PGI 1995)
a. 350 mL in 5 minutes
b. 500 mL in 5 minutes
c. 1 L in 5 minutes
d. Whole blood volume

Q5. Storage period of 35 days for blood is seen with: (AIIMS 2017)
a. CPD
b. CPDA-1
c. ACD
d. CP2D

Q6. Massive blood transfusion is defined as: (PGI 1995)
a. Whole blood volume in 24 hours
b. Half blood volume in 24 hours
c. 40% blood volume in 24 hours
d. 60% blood volume in 24 hours

Q7. All of the following are major complications of massive transfusion, *except*: (All India 2006)
a. Hypokalemia
b. Hypothermia
c. Hypomagnesemia
d. Thrombocytopenia

Grade III	*Most difficult*

Q1. Which of the following is the least likely complication after a massive blood transfusion? (AIIMS 2009)

a. Hyperkalemia
b. Citrate toxicity
c. Hypothermia
d. Metabolic acidosis

Q2. Blood components products are: (PGI Dec 2005)

a. Whole blood
b. Platelets
c. FFP
d. Leukocyte reduced RBC
e. All of the above

Q3. A man is rushed to the casualty, nearly dying after a massive blood loss in an accident. There is not much time to match blood groups, so the physician decides to order one of the following blood groups. Which one of the following blood groups should the physician decide? (AIIMS June 2004)

a. O negative
b. O positive
c. AB positive
d. AB negative

Q4. True about blood transfusions: (PGI June 98)

a. Antigen "D" determines Rh positivity.
b. The febrile reaction is due to human leukocyte antigen (HLA) antigens.
c. Anti-D is a naturally occurring antibody.
d. Cryoprecipitate contains all coagulation factors.

Q5. Massive transfusion in previously healthy adult males can cause hemorrhage due to: (PGI 1998)

a. Increased t-PA
b. Dilutional thrombocytopenia
c. Vitamin K deficiency
d. Decreased fibrinogen

Q6. Indications of FFP is/are: (PGI Nov 2011)

a. Hypovolemia
b. Nutritional supplement
c. Coagulation factor deficiency
d. Warfarin toxicity
e. Hypoalbuminemia

Q7. Cryoprecipitate contains: (MCI March 2009)

a. Factor II
b. Factor V
c. Factor VIII
d. Factor IX

ANSWERS

Grade I: 1. c; 2. b; 3. c; 4. a; 5. c; 6. a; 7. a

Grade II: 1. c; 2. b; 3. a; 4. d; 5. b; 6. a; 7. a

Grade III: 1. d; 2. e; 3. a; 4. a and b; 5. b; 6. c and d; 7. c

MODEL QUESTIONS

Q1. Fresh hold blood transfusion is done within how much time of collection?

a. Immediately
b. 1 hour
c. 4 hours
d. 24 hours

Ans. d

Q2. One unit of fresh blood arises the hemoglobin% concentration by:

a. 0.1 g%
b. 1 g%
c. 2 g%
d. 2.2 g%

Ans. b

Q3. Which of the following is a better indicator of the need for transfusion?

a. Urine output
b. Hematocrit
c. Color of skin
d. Clinical examination

Ans. b

Q4. Heparin reduced the volume of which ingredient if it is in the bottle for blood gas analysis?

a. pCO_2
b. HCO_3
c. pH
d. All of the above

Ans. d

Q5. Blood grouping and cross-matching are a must before infusion of:

a. Gelatin
b. Dextran
c. Albumin
d. FFP

Ans. b

Q6. Blood grouping and cross-matching are a must prior to infusion of:

a. Gelatin
b. Albumin
c. Dextran
d. Haemaccel

Ans. c

Q7. In cholecystectomy, FFP should be given:
a. Just before the operation
b. At the time of operation
c. 6 hours before operation
d. 12 hours after the operation

Ans. a

Q8. Collection of blood for cross-matching and grouping is done before administration of which plasma expander?
a. Hydroxyl ethyl starch
b. Dextran
c. Mannitol
d. Haemaccel

Ans. b

Q9. True about FFP is the following, *except*:
a. Good source of all coagulation factors
b. Prepared from a single unit of blood
c. Coagulation factor levels are equal to plasma
d. None of the above

Ans. a

Q10. Rosenthal's syndrome is seen in a deficiency of factor:
a. II
b. V
c. IX
d. XI

Ans. d

Q11. Cryoprecipitate contains all, *except*:
a. Factor VIII
b. Factor IX
c. Fibrinogen
d. VWF

Ans. b

Q12. The maximum life of a transfused RBC is:
a. 12 hours
b. 24 hours
c. 20 days
d. 50 days

Ans. d

Q13. Blood platelets in stored blood do not remain functional after:
a. 24 hours
b. 36 hours
c. 48 hours
d. 60 hours

Ans. a

Q14. Stored plasma is deficient in:
a. Factors 7 and 8
b. Factors 2 and 5
c. Factors 5 and 8
d. Factors 7 and 9

Ans. c

CHAPTER 9

Metabolic Response to Injury

"There is a circumstance attending accidental injury that does not belong to the disease, namely that the injury done, has in all cases a tendency to produce both the deposition and means of cure."

– John Hunter

(The Father of Scientific Surgery, he inoculated himself with Syphilis contents in 1767)

INTRODUCTION

Homeostasis is a state of equilibrium and balance in human body. It is a phenomenon that keeps the functions of the organisms under control. Homeostasis mainly involves all vital organs to achieve this state: The brain and nerves, heart and vessels, lungs, kidneys, liver, and spleen.

Claude Bernard (Claude Bernard, 1813–1878, French physiologist), was of the view that various body systems act to maintain internal constancy.

Walter Cannon (Walter Bradford Cannon, 1871–1945, American Physiologist) defined homeostasis as the coordinated physiological process that maintains the most of steady states of the organism, meaning the complex homeostatic responses involving the brain, nerves, heart, lungs, kidneys, and spleen work to maintain body consistency.

John Hunter (John Hunter, 1728–1793, a British Surgeon) was regarded as "The father of scientific surgery, he was of the opinion that responses to injury are, in general, beneficial to the host and allow healing/survival.

RESPONSE TO INJURY

It is a graded response; the greater the injury, the greater is the response. It is a combination of physiological, metabolic, and immunological reactions.

Intermediate severity trauma of an elective surgery → rise in temperature, heart rate, respiratory rate, total lung capacity (TLC), and energy expenditure.

Major trauma/sepsis → systemic inflammatory response syndrome (SIRS), hypermetabolism, catabolism, and even multiple organ dysfunction syndrome (MODS).

Compensatory anti-inflammatory response syndrome (CARS) was proposed by Roger Bone (Roger Bone, 1941–1997) in 1997, which is a deactivation of the immune system during major traumas, which helps restore homeostasis.

Preoperative, operative, and postoperative care and services help to maintain homeostasis. *In seriously injured or seriously compromised patients, critical care with an expert critical care team helps in resuscitation and homeostasis maintenance.* The body's response from the neurological system and endocrine system towards serious illness and severe trauma helps in acute and chronic phases (pituitary hormones and cortisol, and adrenaline help for a small period in the acute phase, whereas hypothalamic activity helps in the chronic phase).

Systemic inflammatory response syndrome (SIRS): It is a response, especially in severe trauma such as a crush or mutilating injury. It is created by *cytokines:*
- Interleukin-1 (IL-1)
- IL-6
- Tumor necrosis factor (TNF)-alpha

Sir David Cuthbertson (Sir David Cuthbertson, 1900–1989, British biochemist) divided metabolic response to injury into two phases, the Ebb and Flow phases.
Injury → Ebb phase → metabolic stress response to surgery, flow phase → recovery
Injury → shock → catabolism → anabolism
These phases usually happen after an injury is created by the body's response system. Initially, the body goes into a shock phase lasting for a few hours, leading to the destruction of various cells and changes leading to catabolism, which goes on for a few days. This phase of catabolism is followed by a phase of reconstruction that is called the phase of anabolism. During this phase body tries to recover from the effects of severe trauma, which takes a few weeks to get back to the original state.

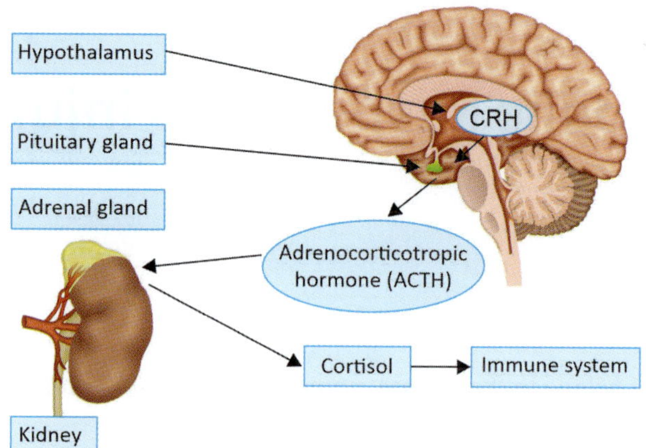

Fig. 1: Metabolic response to injury.

> The body itself has inbuilt protective systems to preserve homeostasis and help in survival during a massive or moderate injury by causing immobility, loss of appetite, and catabolism. Skeletal muscles also help to provide proteins for metabolic response to injury in the form of amino acids. It results in limitation of movement, especially walking and running, leading to pneumonia, and this may increase the incidence of death.

In the process of metabolic response **(Fig. 1)** to major injury, catabolism mainly affects fat and muscles. Surprisingly, in spite of catabolism, the body weight increases due to an increase in the extracellular spaces of the body.

HYPOTHERMIA

In major trauma, hypothermia develops, which increases the chances of cardiac arrhythmias and catabolism, leading to increased chances of severe morbidity and delay in recovery.

STARVATION

During starvation, glucose is needed to survive. Initially, the glycogen of the liver gets converted into glucose. This is done to maintain the cerebral energy metabolism. Intravenous dextrose and normal saline are essential in a fasting patient after major surgery. It is also important that one must not advise unnecessary starvation.

Physiological response to injury:

- Rest
- Immobility, as movement delays healing
- Anorexia
- Catabolism

Why do neuroendocrine changes happen after trauma?

Major trauma provokes a neuroendocrine response that is displayed by activation of sympathetic-adrenomedullary system through the hypothalamus, leading to changes in synthesis and secretion of various pituitary hormones and so changes in secretion of adrenal, thyroid, and pancreatic hormones.

- To provide essential factors for survival
- To postpone anabolism
- To optimize host defense

The Cori (Carl Ferdinand Cori, 1896–1984, and Gerty Theresa Cori, 1896-1957, they were American husband and wife, pharmacologist and biochemist) cycle is also known lactic acid cycle. During the Cori cycle, lactic acid is produced in muscles and is converted to glucose by the liver and moved back to the muscles to be metabolized again. Both were awarded the Nobel Prize for Physiology or Medicines in 1945 for their discovery of how glycogen is catalytically converted.

CHANGES IN SKELETAL MUSCULAR PROTEIN METABOLISM AFTER MAJOR TRAUMA

Under normal conditions, the muscle breakdown and synthesis (1–2%/day) remain constant to maintain muscle bulk in the body. After major trauma, wasting of skeletal muscle occurs due to:

- To provide amino acids for metabolic support to vital or central organs.
- Can cause immobility, which is good for healing in a severely traumatized patient.
- *Activation of ubiquitin proteasome pathway of muscle:* Protein → ubiquitin → proteasome → Amino acids.

Hepatic acute phase protein response: About >50% of the body protein turnover happens in the liver (10–20%) and muscles (1–2%) after major trauma, as:

- *Positive reactants (CRP):* Plasma concentration increases.
- *Negative reactants (albumin):* Plasma concentration decreases.

What happens to body composition after major trauma?

- The body's fat and skeletal muscle mass decrease due to catabolism.
- Weight may increase despite of catabolism is due to expansion of the intracellular fluid space.

SOME IMPORTANT QUESTIONS

Q1. First to be maintained in:

a. Hypotension
b. Dehydration
c. Airway
d. Cardiac status

Ans. c

Q2. Back examination of a polytrauma patient is known as:

a. Log roll
b. Barrel role
c. Chin lift
d. None

Ans. a

Q3. In trauma transfusion, a ratio of red blood cells (RBCs), fresh frozen plasma (FFP), and platelets is:

a. 1:1:3
b. 1:1:1
c. 1:1:2
d. 1:1:4

Ans. b

Q4. Trauma and injury severity score (TRISS) includes:

a. Glasgow Coma Scale (GCS) + blood pressure (BP) + respiratory rate (RR)
b. Revised Trauma Score (RTS) + Injury Severity Score (ISS) + age
c. RTS + ISS + GCS
d. RTS + GCS + BP

Ans. b

Q5. Mangled Extremity Severity Score (MESS) includes all of the following, *except:*

a. Shock
b. Ischemia
c. Neurogenic injury
d. Energy of injury

Ans. c

Q6. Best assessment score in trauma patients:

a. Modified trauma score
b. Revised trauma score
c. Injury severity score
d. Mangled extremity severity score

Ans. b

Q7. The triage system is used for:

a. Burn
b. Earthquake
c. Polytrauma
d. Floods

Ans. c

Q8. Skull base fracture is associated with all of the following, *except:*

a. Raccoon eyes
b. Hemiparesis
c. Cerebrospinal fluid (CSF) rhino-otorrhea
d. Battle sign

Ans. b

Q9. SDH is caused by injury of:

a. Middle meningeal artery
b. Cortical veins
c. Superficial temporal artery
d. None

Ans. b

Q10. During surgery, both the femoral artery and the femoral vein were injured. The next best step:

a. Ligate the femoral vein and repair the femoral artery
b. Ligate the femoral vein and femoral artery
c. Ligate the femoral artery and repair the femoral vein
d. None of the above

Ans. a

Q11. Seat belt causes injury to:

a. Duodenum
b. Head injury due to the windscreen
c. Thorax
d. All

Ans. a

Q12. Which one of the following is not a principle followed in the management of missile injuries?

a. Excision of all dead muscles
b. Removal of foreign bodies
c. Removal of fragments of bone
d. Leaving the wound open

Ans. c

MULTIPLE CHOICE QUESTIONS

Grade I	Simple

Q1. The most important technical consideration at the time of doing below-knee amputation is: (AIIMS Nov 2000)

a. Posterior flap should be longer than the anterior flap
b. Stump should be long
c. Stump should be short
d. The anterior flap should be longer than the posterior flap

Q2. A patient developed respiratory distress and hypoxemia after central venous catheterization through the internal jugular vein. The reason for this is: (AIIMS Nov 2000)
a. Pneumothorax
b. Hypovolemia
c. Septicemia
d. Cardiac tamponade

Q3. All can commonly occur in a patient who suffered decelerating injury in which the pituitary stalk was damaged, *except* one: (AIIMS Nov 2000)
a. Diabetes mellitus
b. Thyroid insufficiency
c. Adrenocortical insufficiency
d. Diabetes insipidus

Q4. In a preop patient surgical check list-which of the following is not needed? (AIIMS Nov 2017)
a. Oral consent
b. Doctor's signature
c. Site marking
d. Confirming the patient's identity

Q5. Which of the following is commonest for bag and mask ventilation? (AIIMS June 2000)
a. Septicemia
b. Tracheoesophageal fistula
c. Meconium aspiration
d. Diaphragmatic hernia

Q6. Ligation of which nerve will lead to paresthesia and pain on the dorsum of the foot during venesection of the great saphenous vein? (AIIMS June 2000)
a. Sural nerve
b. Geniculate
c. Saphenous nerve
d. Deep peroneal nerve

Q7. From the index finger infection goes to: (AIIMS Nov 1996)
a. Thenar space
b. Hypothenar space
c. Mid palmar space
d. Space of parona

Grade II — Difficult

Q1. The total score in the Glasgow Coma Scale of a conscious person is: (AII India 2006)
a. 8
b. 3
c. 15
d. 10

Q2. The most common cause of rupture of the tendon is: (AII India 2000)
a. Overuse
b. Trauma
c. Congenital defect
d. Fall from height

Q3. The most common artery for cannulation is: (PGI June 1997)
a. Radial
b. Ulnar
c. Brachial
d. Cubital

Q4. Which of the following is a nonabsorbable suture? (AII India 2008)
a. Polypropylene
b. Vicryl
c. Catgut
d. Polydioxanone

Q5. In which of the following conditions burst abdomen is commonly associated? (PGI Dec 2005)
a. Drainage coming out through the wound
b. Nonabsorbable sutures
c. Interrupted sutures
d. Median incision is at higher risk (as compared to transverse incision)
e. Transverse incision is better than paramedian incision

Q6. A patient with immune thrombocytopenic purpura (ITP) is being planned for splenectomy. What is the best time for platelet infusion in this patient? (AII India 2008)
a. 2 hours before surgery
b. At the time of skin incision
c. After ligation, the splenic artery
d. Immediately after the removal of the spleen

Q7. Popliteal artery pulsations are difficult to feel, because: (AII India 2009)
a. It is not superficial.
b. It does not cross a prominent bone.
c. It is not superficial and does not cross a prominent bone.
d. Its pulsations are weak.

Grade III — Most difficult

Q1. Fogarty's catheter is used for: (AIIMS Nov 2010)
a. Urethral catheterization
b. Removal of blood clots from the arteries
c. Bladder drainage
d. Total parenteral nutrition (TPN)

Q2. True about celiac plexus block is: (AIIMS May 2013)
a. Is given for lower abdominal malignancies
b. The ganglia are located in the retroperitoneal space along L3 vertebra

c. Diarrhea and hypotension are the common side effects
d. It is generally done unilaterally

Q3. Suture length for midline abdominal incision: (AIIMS Nov 2016)
a. Same as incision
b. Two times
c. Three times
d. Four times

Q4. The presence of trifluoracetic acid (TFA) in urine indicates that the volatile anesthetic agent used was: (AIIMS 1987)
a. Halothane
b. Methoxyflurane
c. Trichloroethylene
d. None of the above

Q5. Pyrexia due to wound infection commonly occurs after: (PGI 1981)
a. Third postoperation day
b. Fifth postoperation day
c. Seventh postoperation day
d. Second postoperation day

Q6. Least likely to regress spontaneously is: (AIIMS 1996)
a. Osteosarcoma
b. Retinoblastoma
c. Choriocarcinoma
d. Malignant melanoma

Q7. Stereotactic radiosurgery is done for: (JIPMER 2002)
a. Glioblastoma multiforme
b. Medulloblastoma spinal cord
c. Ependymoma
d. Arteriovenous (AV) malformation of the brain

ANSWERS

Grade I: 1. a (Schwartz 7/e p993-995); 2. a (Sabiston 17/e p410); 3. a; 4. b (Bailey 27/e p183); 5. d; 6. c (Bailey 26/e p912); 7. a

Grade II: 1. c; 2. a; 3. a; 4. a (Sabiston 19/e p233); 5. a, d, e (Bailey 26/e p280); 6. c (Bailey 26/e p1092); 7. a

Grade III: 1. b (Bailey 26/e p889); 2. c; 3. d; 4. a; 5. b (Sabiston 17/e p300); 6. a; 7. d (Schwartz 7/e p1908)

MODEL QUESTIONS

Q1. The coordinated physiological process that maintains most of the steady states of the organism, is about what?
a. Response to injury
b. Systemic inflammatory response syndrome (SIRS)
c. Homeostasis
d. Multiple organ dysfunction syndrome (MODS)

Ans. c

Q2. The foundation of normal physiology is:
a. Wound healing
b. Regeneration
c. Reengineering
d. Homeostasis

Ans. d

Q3. Resuscitation, surgical intervention, and critical care can return the severely injured person to a situation in which it becomes possible once again. What word is missing?
a. Physiology
b. Vitals
c. Homeostasis
d. Disease

Ans. c

Q4. Compensatory anti-inflammatory response syndrome (CARS) is:
a. Suppressed immunity and diminished resistance to infection
b. Increased immunity and increased resistance to infection
c. State of low immune response
d. State of the equilibrium

Ans. a

Q5. The more severe the injury, the greater the response is. What type of response?
a. Normal response to injury
b. Immune response
c. Graded response
d. Hypermetabolic response

Ans. c

Q6. What are counter-regulatory hormones?
a. Adrenaline
b. Noradrenaline
c. Cortisol
d. Glucagon, glucocorticoids, and catecholamines

Ans. d

Q7. Adrenocorticotropic hormone (ACTH) acts on the adrenals to increase the secretion of:

a. Glucagon
b. Insulin
c. Corticotropin-releasing factor (CRF)
d. Cortisol

Ans. d

Q8. Adaptive immune system cells are:

a. Reticulocytes
b. Red blood cells (RBCs)
c. T-cells and B-cells
d. Inflammatory cells

Ans. c

Q9. As a response to injury, proinflammatory cytokines, IL-1, and tumor necrosis factor alpha (TNF-α) act directly on the hypothalamus to produce:

a. Hypotension
b. Hypertension
c. Pyrexia
d. Hypoglycemia

Ans. c

Q10. SIRS, if prolonged, leads to:

a. Counter-inflammatory response syndrome
b. MODS
c. Hypertension
d. Hypotension
e. Shock

Ans. a

Q11. Natural response to injury includes:

a. Leukocytosis
b. Reticulocytosis
c. Immobility, rest, anorexia, and catabolism
d. Anabolism

Ans. c

Q12. Hypermetabolism following injury is mainly caused by:

a. Leukocytes
b. Lymphocytes
c. TNF
d. Acceleration of energy-dependent metabolic cycles

Ans. d

SUGGESTED READING

1. Bailey & Love's - Short Practice of Surgery, 27th edition.
2. Schwartz's Principles of Surgery, 18th edition.
3. Textbook of Surgery by David Sabiston, 21st edition.

CHAPTER 10

Tissue Repair and Regeneration

"You can increase your body's ability to repair injured tissue and increase the regeneration process by changing your lifestyle and habits."

– Vinod Kumar Nigam

INTRODUCTION

Tissue repair and regeneration are different for different cells of various organ systems. All organ systems do not have the ability to regenerate as the skeletal system does. Certain comorbidities, such as diabetes mellitus, immunodeficiency, obesity, lack of exercise, excessive alcohol, and smoking, can hamper the body's potency to repair tissues.

The tissue engineering uses a combination of cells, engineering, materials methods, and suitable biochemical and physicochemical factors to restore, maintain, improve, or replace different types of biological tissues. Tissue engineering commonly uses tissue scaffolds.

Nowadays, tissues are created by other tissues even in laboratories to neutralize in diseases of respective organ systems when required, i.e., bone, cartilage, skin, intestine, cardiac muscles, etc. These tissues are very helpful in testing the efficacy and toxicity of drugs. Stem cells **(Fig. 1)** and somatic cells are generally used for tissue engineering and regenerative research. *Somatic stem cells (SSCs) and induced pluripotent stem cells (iPSCs), and human embryonic stem cells (hESCs)* are nowadays increasingly used for tissue engineering.

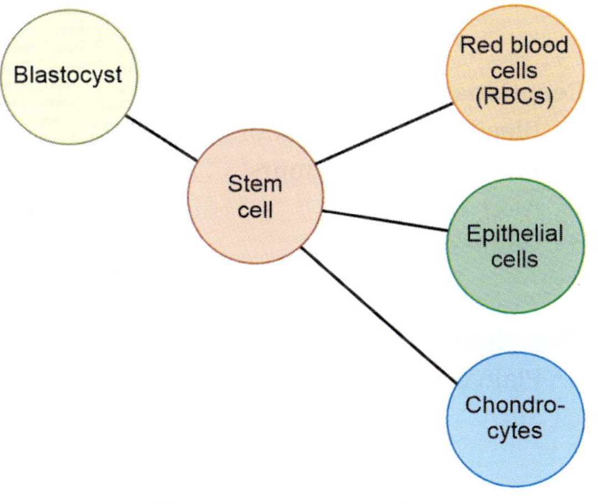

Fig. 1: Various stem cells.

> *Embryonic stem cells are pluripotent stem cells derived from blastocysts.* Stem cells have special properties of making more cells like themselves, in other words, self-renewal and differentiating into other cells also. *Almost all body organs have stem cells.* They continuously divide and renew. Stem cells are blood stem cells, epithelial stem cells, neural stem cells, and mesenchymal stem cells. The main purpose of stem cells is to repair and regenerate damaged tissue.

Scaffolds are used in tissue engineering and regeneration which provide support for cells, allow cells to attach, and help in cell migration and proliferation. The scaffold also gives shape to the tissue. *Natural scaffolds* are obtained by treating tissues with various processes to remove the resident cells leaving behind the matrix. *Artificial scaffolds* are made from natural materials, bioactive ceramics, and products.

Implantation of laboratory-made engineered tissue can also harm and cause tumor formation, transmission of infection, reduced or loss of function, and even rejection.

ELEMENTS OF TISSUE ENGINEERING (FIG. 2)

Uses of tissue engineering and regenerative therapies:

- *Treatment of diseases* (diabetes, heart failure, burns, congenital and degenerative disease, etc.)
- *In surgical treatment*
- *Models* to test therapeutic efficacy and toxicity

Scaffolds required during tissue engineering should provide structural support to the cells, allow cells to

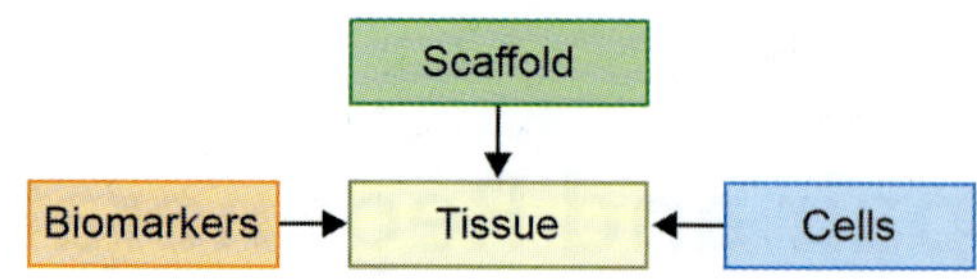

Fig. 2: Elements of tissue engineering.

attach, migrate, and proliferation, give access to oxygen and nutrients to cells, and should be biocompatible and biodegradable. Scaffolds can be:

- *Natural Scaffold*—can be prepared for natural tissue by removal of cells by detergents and extracellular materials.
- *Regenerative Scaffold*—provide scaffold growth and degeneration of cells
- *Synthetic polymers,* bioactive ceramics, or glasses

How do seeding cells attach into the Scaffold?

- Static cell seeding
- Dynamic cell seeding
- Magnetic cell seeding
  - Pressure and vacuum seeding
  - Photopolymerized hydrogels
  - Bioreactor perfusion systems

Risks of cell-based therapy:

Mn = TIGRIP

T = Tumor formation

I = Infection

G = Genetic abnormalities

R = Rejection

I = Immunosuppressor side affects

P = Poor viability

SOME IMPORTANT QUESTIONS

Q1. Postdural puncture headache is typically:

a. A result of leakage of blood into the epidural space

b. Worse when lying down than in sitting position

c. Bifrontal or occipital

d. Seen within 4 hours of dural puncture

Ans. c

Q2. Which of the following abdominal structures will be responsible for sharp pain while doing abdominal surgery?

a. Parietal peritoneum

b. Liver parenchyma

c. Small intestine

d. Colon

Ans. a

Q3. What will be the diagnosis of the child with pulsatile swelling on the medial side of the nose?

a. Ureterosigmoidostomy

b. Diarrhea

c. Vomiting

d. Ileoplasty

Ans. a

Q4. In a patient with head injury, eye opening is seen with a painful stimulus, localizes the pain, and there is an inappropriate verbal response. What would be the score on the Glasgow Coma Scale?

a. 8 b. 9

c. 10 d. 11

Ans. c

Q5. All are true about the Glasgow Coma Scale, *except*:

a. Score between 3 and 15

b. Obeying the motor command is given the maximum score

c. Consists of eye-opening, motor, and verbal responses

d. An increased score indicates a poor prognosis

Ans. d

Q6. Which gas is most commonly used in laparoscopy?

a. CO_2 b. N_2O

c. O_2 d. N_2

Ans. a

Q7. Pseudoclaudication is due to the compression of:

a. Femoral artery b. Femoral nerve

c. Cauda equina d. Popliteal artery

Ans. c

Q8. Reactionary hemorrhage:

a. Bleeding within 24 hours

b. Bleeding after 24 hours

c. After 10 days

d. While surgery is on

Ans. a

Q9. Most tissue reaction is seen with:

a. Plain catgut b. Polydioxanone

c. Silk d. Chromic catgut

Ans. c

Q10. Layers that are penetrated with trochar and canula in the production of pneumoperitoneum are:

a. Skin and superficial fascia
b. Deep fascia
c. Rectus abdominis
d. Transverse abdominis
e. Rectus sheath

Ans. a and b

Q11. Referred pain from all of the following conditions may be felt along the inner side of the right thigh, *except*:

a. Inflamed pelvic appendix
b. Inflamed ovaries
c. Stone in the pelvic ureter
d. Pelvic abscess

Ans. d

Q12. Ways to prevent a highly infectious disease transmitted by aerosol; precautions used:

a. Isolation ward
b. Facemask
c. Keep isolated in a room with positive pressure
d. Keep isolated in a room with negative pressure
e. Cohort nursing

Ans. a, b, and d

Q13. Double bubble sign is seen with:

a. Pyloric stenosis
b. Duodenal atresia
c. Ileal atresia
d. Esophageal atresia

Ans. b

Q14. Allopurinol is used in organ preservation as:

a. Antioxidant
b. Preservative
c. Free radical scavenger
d. Precursor for energy metabolism

Ans. c

MULTIPLE CHOICE QUESTIONS

Grade I	Simple

Q1. In the immediate postoperative period, the common cause of respiratory insufficiency could be because of the following, *except*: **(AIIMS June 2003)**

a. Residual effect of muscle relaxant
b. Overdose of narcotic analgesic
c. Mild hypovolemia
d. Myocardial infarction

Q2. A patient undergoing surgery suddenly develops hypotension. The monitor shows that the end tidal CO_2 has decreased abruptly by 155 mm Hg. What is the probable diagnosis? **(AIIMS June 2003)**

a. Hypothermia
b. Pulmonary embolism
c. Massive fluid deficit
d. Myocardial depression due to an anesthetic agent

Q3. A patient had undergone a renal transplantation 2 months back and now presented with difficulty breathing. The X-ray showed bilateral diffuse interstitial pneumonia. The probable etiologic agent would be: **(AIIMS June 2002)**

a. *Cytomegalovirus (CMV)*
b. *Histoplasma*
c. *Candida*
d. *Pneumocystis carinii*

Q4. In a surgical postoperative ward, a patient developed a wound infection. Subsequently, three other patients developed a similar infection in the ward. What is the most effective way of preventing the spread of infection? **(AIIMS Nov 2001)**

a. Give IV antibiotics to all patients in the ward
b. Proper handwashing of all ward personnel
c. Fumigation of the ward
d. Wash operation theater (OT) instruments with 1% perchlorate

Q5. The physiological changes seen in laparoscopy are all, *except*: **(AIIMS May 2015)**

a. Increased pH
b. Decreased functional residual capacity (FRC)
c. Increased central venous pressure (CVP)
d. Increased intracranial pressure (ICP)

Grade II	Difficult

Q1. An elective surgery is to be done in a patient taking heavy doses of Aspirin. Management consists of: **(All India 2000)**

a. Proceed with surgery
b. Stopping aspirin for 7 days and then doing surgery
c. Preoperative platelet transfusion
d. Intraoperative platelet transfusion

CHAPTER 11

Surgical Infections

"Wise and humane management of the patient is the best safeguard against infection."

– Florence Nightingale

INTRODUCTION

Acharya Sushruta, an ancient Indian Surgeon approximately 600 BC, emphasized on the importance of cleanliness, sanitation, and sterilization in surgical procedures. He recommended fumigation with herbs. He also stressed the importance of using high-quality sterile instruments. Infection and post-traumatic infection were known to ancient Egyptians. *Hippocrates (Greek Physician, the Father of Medicine, 460–375 BC)* also mentioned in his writings about infections and irrigation of wounds to treat infection. *Galen wrote about wound infection and drainage (Roman Physician, 130-200). Koch's postulates were written in 1882 by Robert Koch, a German Bacteriologist, 1843–1910.* According to Koch's postulate, an organism must be found in every case of such infection, could be isolated from the patient, could be cultured, and produce the disease if injected. *Ambroise Pare (Ambroise Pare, 1510–1590, French Military Surgery)* and *Guy de Chauliac (Guy de Chauliac, 1298-1368, French Physician)* noticed that clean wounds, closed primarily, could heal without infection or suppuration.

> *Louis Pasteur (French Bacteriologist, 1822–1895)* gave the "germ theory" that microorganisms infect humans and cause disease. *Joseph Lister (English Surgeon, 1827–1912)* worked on an aseptic surgical technique to avoid the chances of infection by killing the bacteria. *Alexander Fleming (1881–1955, English Bacteriologist) discovered penicillin in 1928. Florey (Howard Walter Florey, 1898-1968, British Pathologist) and Chain (Sir Ernest Boris Chain, British biochemist) isolated it in 1941. They were awarded the Nobel Prize for Physiology or Medicine in 1945.*

Streptococci are the most common gram-positive, in chains of bacteria inhabiting in the pharynx. β-hemolytic *Streptococcus* and *Streptococcus pyogenes* are commonly found bacteria. Staphylococci are gram-positive and found in clumps and are commonly found in the nasopharynx. *Methicillin-resistant Staphylococcus aureus (MRSA)* is difficult to treat if it infects a wound. *Staphylococcus* infections commonly form abscesses. *Clostridium* are gram-positive and obligate anaerobes and are spore-bearing. *Clostridium tetani* causes tetanus and *Clostridium perfringens* causes gas gangrene. Aerobic gram-negative bacilli such as *Escherichia coli* and *Klebsiella* are common bacilli. *E. coli* is the main cause of urinary tract infection. *Pseudomonas* is a bacteria difficult to eradicate.

Wound infection can be endogenously caused by contamination of the wound from inside, such as perforated appendix, and exogenously caused by infection from other sources, such as trauma or operation **(Fig. 1)**.

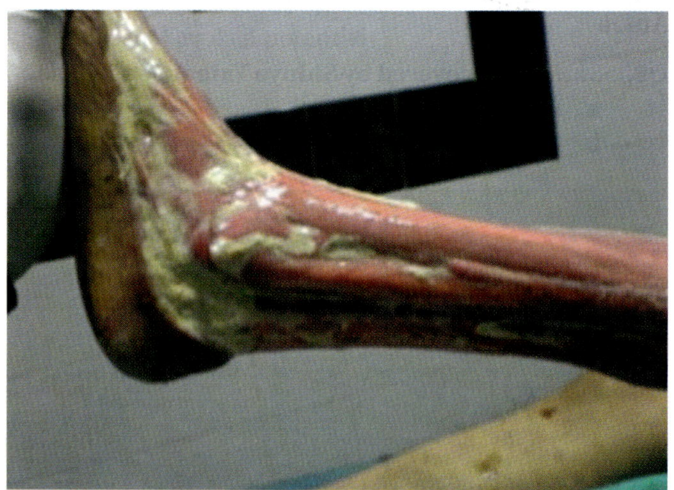

Fig. 1: Infected wound.

Risk factors for increasing wound infection:
Mn: M2P2IC
- *M* = Malnutrition
- *M* = Metabolic disease
- *P* = Poor surgical technique
- *P* = Poor perfusion
- *I* = Immunosuppression
- *C* = Colonization

SOUTHAMPTON WOUND GRADING SYSTEM

It divides the wounds by appearance in 0, I, Ia, Ib, Ic, II, IIa, IIb, IIc, IId, III, IIIa, IIIb, IIIc, IIId, and IV, IVa, IVb, and V by complications.

ASEPSIS WOUND SCORE

It divides the wound according to the status: A = Additional treatment, i.e., antibiotic and drainage, S = Serous discharge, E = Erythema, P = Purulent, S = Separation of tissues, I = Isolation of bacteria from an infected wound, S = Stay as inpatient.

Celsus (Aulus Aurelius Cornelius Celsus, 25 BC–50 AD, Roman Surgeon and Author of De Re Medico Libri Octo) was the first medical person who described the signs of localized inflammation. These are Rubor (redness), tumor (swelling), Calore (heat), Dolore means pain, and Functio laesa (loss of function) **(Fig. 2)**.

CELLULITIS

Cellulitis is an infection of soft tissue without pus formation and is poorly localized. Usually, caused by streptococci and staphylococci. A small cut or abrasion can cause cellulitis due to bacteria residing in the skin. There is swelling in the cellulitis.

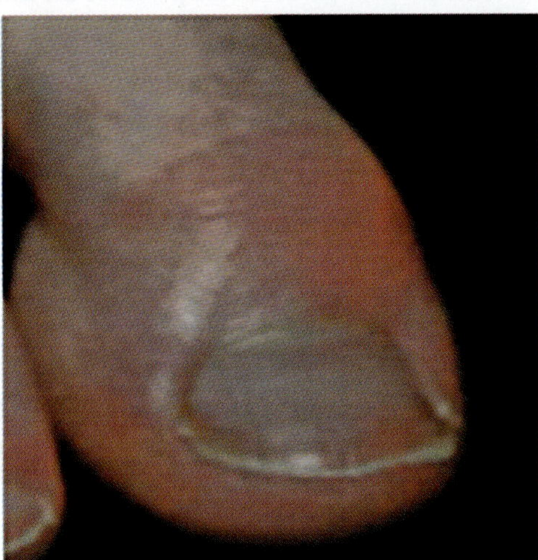

Fig. 2: Signs of inflammation.

LYMPHANGITIS

Lymphangitis is also an infectious process affecting the lymphatics, which drain the infection site. Lymphangitis has red streaks and lines along the lymphatics, which are painful.

Points not to Forget

- *The most common technique of sterilization of surgical instruments is by steam at 121°C for 15 minutes.*
- Endoscopes to be sterilized by glutaraldehyde solution.
- Hospital-acquired infection (HAI) is most common of urinary tracts (UTIs)—approximately 40% of admitted patients, commonly by catheterization.
- Wound dehiscence (burst abdomen) occurs commonly between the fifth and eighth postoperative day. Common causes of wound adhesions are wrong technique, midline incisions, diabetes mellitus, old age, obesity, and immunosuppression.
- *Erysipelas is a clearly demarcated streptococcal infection of the skin, which can be differentiated from cellulitis by its raised edges.*
- In gas gangrene, gas may enter the liver (foaming liver).

Microbiology

- *Streptococci-Gram (Hans Christian Joachim Gram, 1853–1938, Danish pharmacologist and physician, described this method of staining bacteria in 1884),* positive cocci in chains, the most important is the β-hemolytic streptococcus, which lives in the pharynx. According to *Lancefield (Rebecca Graighill Lancefield, 1895–1981, American bacteriologist, classified streptococci in 1933), classification.* It is group A streptococci that is most pathogenic. It is an infection that usually spreads as cellulitis due to the release of tissue destroying enzymes, i.e., streptolysin, streptokinase, and streptodornase.
- *Staphylococci—form* gram-positive clumps. The most common is *Staphylococcus aureus.* Methicillin-resistant *Staphylococcus aureus (MRSA)* strains are difficult to treat.

- *Clostridia*—these are gram-positive, obligate anaerobes and produce resistant spores. Clostridium perfringens causes gas gangrene, *Clostridium tetani* causes tetanus, and *Clostridium difficile* causes pseudomembranous colitis.

Aerobic gram-negative bacilli: Common organisms are:

- *Escherichia (Theodor Escherich, 1857–1911, Austrian Pediatrician, described bacterium coli commune in 1886) coli*—found in the large bowel, lactose fermenting, mainly causes urinary tract infection (UTI). *Extended spectrum β-lactamase (ESBLs)* are resistant to many antibiotics, and the strain is increasing.
- *Klebsiella (Theodor Albrecst Edwin Klebs, 1834–1913, Czechoslovakian pathologist)* is found in the large bowel and is lactose fermenting.
- *Proteus*—nonlactose fermenting.
- *Pseudomonas*—found usually in burns, tracheostomy, wards, and ICUs. Difficult to treat.
- *Bacteroids*—nonsporebearing, anaerobic, found in large bowel, vagina, and oropharynx. Bacteroides Fragilis is the most common organism, it causes SSIs in synergy with aerobic gram-negative bacilli.

GAS GANGRENE

It is caused by *C. perfringens* and has gas in the layers of the infected wound with a characteristic smell. This infection is usually related to trauma and surgery. *Nowadays, gas gangrene after clean surgery is not seen.* It is commonly seen in patients with diabetes mellitus, immunosuppression, any debilitating disease, and cancer. *Severe pain and crepitus are almost diagnostic.* An X-ray of the involved part may show gas in between tissues.

Characteristic features of gas gangrene:

- *Caused by Clostridium perfringens.*
- Smell is typical.
- *The presence of gas is diagnostic.*
- Prophylactic antibiotics are essential during the surgery for the removal of necrotic tissue.
- Immunosuppressed patients are at the highest risk.

CLOSTRIDIUM TETANI

It is an anaerobic infection of a wound. The spores of tetanus are commonly found in soil. Tetanus organisms release exotoxin tetanospasmin, affecting the anterior horn cells of the spinal cord, leading to tetanus. Tetanus is almost fatal. *The tetanus vaccine is an attenuated vaccine that is given in three separate doses at 5-year intervals.* Nowadays, tetanus is extremely rare. Tetanus causes muscle spasms, which can lead to death. It has no cure. Vaccination is the only hope to be hoped. Tetanus causes painful muscle contractions, especially in the jaw and neck. It causes a locked jaw. *Risus sardonicus is a characteristic sign of tetanus due to sustained spasms of the muscles of the upper throat and face.*

FOURNIER'S (JEAN ALFRED FOURNIER, 1832–1915, FRENCH SYPHILOLOGIST) GANGRENE (NECROTIZING FASCIITIS AND SYNERGISTIC SPREADING GANGRENE)

It is a serious mixed infection of streptococci, staphylococci, clostridia, etc. It is an infection caused by both aerobic and anaerobic bacteria. *Meleney's (Frank Lamont Meleney 1889–1963, American Surgeon)* synergistic gangrene is gangrene of abdominal wall. It is common in patients with diabetes mellitus and immunosuppression. It usually occurs after an injury or operation near the perineum. Treatment is extensive debridement of dead tissue with skin grafting if required.

Do not Forget

- Computed tomography (CT) scan is the most important investigation to diagnose psoas abscess.
- Yaws is an infection caused by *Treponema pallidum* by direct contact and has primary and secondary lesions in the skin.
- Leprosy most commonly affects the ulnar nerve.
- Anthrax is caused by *Bacillus anthracis* with cutaneous and gastrointestinal forms.
- Antibioma is formed as a lump when an abscess is treated by antibiotics and not by drainage.

SYSTEMIC INFLAMMATORY RESPONSE SYNDROME (FIG. 3)

It is a systemic infection seen in sepsis and may lead to multiple organ failure. It may be seen after major trauma,

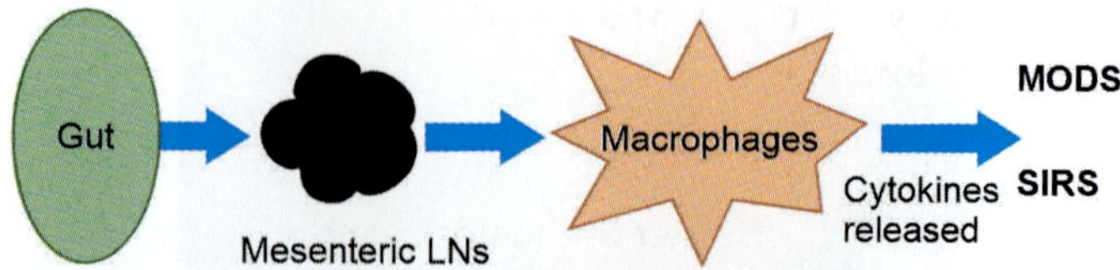

Fig. 3: Systemic inflammatory response syndrome stages. (SIRS: systemic inflammatory response syndrome; LNs: lymph nodes; MODS: multiple organ dysfunction syndrome)

burns, and pancreatitis. Surgical site infection (SSI) is the infection of a wound and deeper tissues.

HUMAN IMMUNODEFICIENCY VIRUS–TYPE I VIRUS

It is an important infection usually transmitted by body fluids, blood, and also through sexual transmission. It is gradually increasing all over the globe. This condition cannot be cured, but treatment can be helpful. It can last for years or throughout life. Initially, it causes flu-like symptoms, fever, and sore throat, etc., and gradually over time, it progresses to acquired immunodeficiency syndrome (AIDS). Treatment is an antiretroviral regimen.

Precautions to be Taken while Operating on a Human Immunodeficiency Virus Patient

- Use a full mask
- Use a fully waterproof disposable gown and drapes
- Double gloving
- Use boots
- Avoid unnecessary presence and movement in the operating theater
- Slow and meticulous dissection to minimize bleeding

HEPATITIS

Hepatitis B and C are blood-borne infections, so they can be transmitted by the surgeon to the patient and vice versa by a needle prick or cut. Transmission of hepatitis C is rare.

Some Important Points

- Antibiotics can treat infection, but cannot make pus disappear.
- Antibiotics should be used cautiously, especially after sensitivity in systemic infections.
- Hollow needle injury carries the maximum risk of disease transmission.
- Clean surgery usually does not require antibiotics.
- Pus culture is required before starting antibiotic therapy.
- Heavily contaminated wounds should be left open and closed later on.

Source of infection in surgery:

- *Endogenous*—present in the host or contamination, as in a perforated appendix.
- *Exogenous*—from outside or acquired, as in the operating theater or ward, or ICU.

The body's mechanisms to control infection:

- *Chemical*—low gastric pH
- *Humoral*—antibodies, complement, and opsonins
- *Cellular*—macrophages, phagocytic cells, polymorphonuclear cells, and killer lymphocytes

How to control infection in surgery?

- Aseptic operation theater technique.
- Antibiotics
- Delayed primary or secondary closure in a contaminated wound

Systemic inflammatory response syndrome (SIRS): When are two of these findings are present?

- Hyperthermia (>38°C) or hypothermia (<36°C)
- Tachycardia (>90/min) or tachypnea (>20/min)
- WBC count (>20,000/mm^3)

Severe sepsis or sepsis syndrome: Sepsis with one or more organ failures.

SOME IMPORTANT QUESTIONS

Q1. Cellulitis is most commonly caused by:

a. Clostridia
b. Staphylococci
c. Streptococci
d. Influenza

Ans. c

Q2. A carbuncle is treated by:

a. Incision and drainage
b. Cruciate incision and deroofing
c. Antibiotics alone
d. Wide excision

Ans. a and d

Q3. Which of the following is not true about gas gangrene?

a. Caused by *Clostridium tetani*
b. Immunocompromised patients are most at risk
c. Gas and smell are characteristic
d. Antibiotic prophylaxis is essential when performing amputations to remove dead tissue

Ans. a

Q4. The best way to prevent gas gangrene is:

a. Immunoglobulins
b. Hyperbaric oxygen
c. Proper wound debridement
d. Antigas gangrene serum

Ans. c

Q5. A 10-year-old child with pain and mass in the right lumbar region with no fever, with the right hip flexed, and an X-ray shows spine changes. The most probable diagnosis is:

a. Psoas abscess
b. Pyonephrosis
c. Retrocecal appendicitis
d. Torsion of the right undescended testis

Ans. a

Q6. A mentally retraded child aged 12 years has multiple, painful, discharging shiny white lesions around the anus. Which of the following is the most probable diagnosis?

a. Lupus vulgaris
b. Carcinoma
c. Syphilitic condyloma
d. Hemorrhoids

Ans. c

Q7. The high-risk groups for transmission of the human immunodeficiency virus (HIV) virus include the following, *except*:

a. Homosexuals
b. Hemophiliacs
c. Children of HIV mothers
d. Healthcare workers

Ans. d

Q8. Most common hand infection is due to:

a. *E. coli*
b. *S. aureus*
c. *Streptococcus*
a. *Pseudomonas*

Ans. b

Q9. Pulp space infection is known as:

a. Felon
b. Paronychia
c. Paronychia
d. Onychonychia

Ans. a

Q10. In which of the following conditions burst abdomen is commonly associated?

a. Drainage coming out through the wound
b. Nonabsorbable sutures
c. Interrupted sutures
d. The medial incision is riskier (as compared to a transverse incision)
e. Transverse incision is better than paramedian incision

Ans. a, d, and e

Q11. In a surgical patient, the causes of nonsurgical infection:

a. Lower respiratory tract infection (RTI)
b. Wound infection
c. *Clostridium difficile* diarrhea
d. Urinary tract infection (UTI)

Ans. a, c, and d

Q12. Hilton's method is used in:

a. To minimize the scar
b. To prevent injury to vital structures
c. To have complete drainage
d. To drain large abscesses

Ans. b

Q13. Multiple fistula-in-ano commonly occurs in:

a. Tuberculosis (TB)
b. Gonococcal proctocolitis
c. Lymphogranuloma venereum (LGV)
d. Colloid carcinoma of the rectum

Ans. a and c

Q14. True about surgical wounds:

a. No antibiotics required in clean surgery
b. Incision of the abscess is done in a contaminated wound
c. Spillage of stomach content converts a clean/contaminated case to a contaminated case
d. In clean/contaminated wounds infection rate is 10%
e. Hernia repair is a contaminated wound

Ans. a, c, and d

Q15. All of the following statements about necrotizing fasciitis are true, *except*:

a. Infection on the fascia and subcutaneous tissue.
b. Most commonly caused by group A beta-hemolytic streptococci.
c. The most common site is the perineum, followed by the trunk and extremities.
d. Surgical debridement is mandatory

Ans. c

Q16. A chronic thick-walled pyogenic abscess may be due to the following, *except*:

a. Presence of a foreign body
b. Prolonged antibiotic therapy
c. Virulent strains of organism
d. Inadequate drainage

Ans. c

Q17. A boil is due to a staphylococcal infection of:

a. Hair follicle
b. Sweat gland
c. Subcutaneous tissue
d. Epidermis

Ans. a

Q18. Gas gangrene is caused by:
a. *Clostridium botulinum*
b. *C. difficile*
c. *C. perfringens*
d. *C. tetani*

Ans. c

Q19. Hyperbaric oxygen is useful in:
a. Tetanus
b. Gas gangrene
c. Frostbite
d. Vincent's angina

Ans. b and c

Q20. The following may be premonitory symptoms of tetanus, *except*:
a. Sleeplessness
b. Anxious expression
c. Urinary incontinence
d. Headache

Ans. c

Q21. Painless effusion in joints in congenital syphilis is called:
a. Clutton's joints
b. Banton's joints
c. Charcot's joint
d. Synovitis

Ans. a

Q22. In acquired immunodeficiency syndrome (AIDS), lymphadenopathy is most often due to:
a. TB
b. Lymphoma
c. Nonspecific enlargement of lymph node
d. Kaposi's sarcoma

Ans. c

Q23. Which of the following should not be treated with surgery?
a. Felon
b. Acute paronychia
c. Herpetic whitlow
d. Chronic paronychia

Ans. c

Q24. Most common nosocomial infection:
a. SSI
b. RTI
c. Urinary tract infection
d. Skin and soft tissue infection

Ans. c

Q25. Follman's balanitis is caused by:
a. *Trichomonas*
b. *Candida*
c. *Haemophilus ducreyi*
d. None

Ans. d

Q26. Anaerobic infection is precipitated by:
a. Trauma
b. Impaired circulation
c. Tissue necrosis
d. All of the above

Ans. d

MULTIPLE CHOICE QUESTIONS

Grade I	*Simple*

Q1. Ways to prevent a highly infectious disease transmitted by aerosol; precautions used: **(PGI Dec 2007)**
a. Isolation ward
b. Facemask
c. Keep isolated in a room with positive pressure
d. Keep isolated in a room with negative pressure
e. Cohort nursing

Q2. All the following are sporicidal agents, *except*: **(JIPMER 2010)**
a. Ethylene oxide
b. Phenol
c. Ozone
d. Glutaraldehyde

Q3. Blood spills in operation theatre (OT) are cleaned with: **(AIIMS Nov 2017)**
a. Phenol
b. Alcohol
c. Quaternary ammonium compound
d. Chloride compounds

Q4. Sterile OT zone is: **(PGI May 2018)**
a. Changing room
b. Scrub room
c. Set up room
d. Cleaner room and stores
e. Anesthesia inducing room

Q5. Erysipelas is caused by: **(PGI 1988)**
a. *S. aureus*
b. *Staphylococcus albus*
c. *S. pyogenes*
d. *Haemophilus*

Q6. Best management of a contaminated wound with necrotic material: **(AIIMS Nov 2013)**
a. Debridement
b. Tetanus toxoid
c. Gas gangrene serum
d. Broad spectrum antibiotics

Q7. True about the treatment of gas gangrene after a contaminated road traffic accident: **(PGI Nov 2011)**
a. IV administration of antigas gangrene serum
b. Penicillin

c. Immediate suturing
d. Surgical debridement
e. Irrigation of antigas gangrene serum

Q8. In a postoperative intensive care unit, five patients developed postoperative wound infections on the same wound. The best method to prevent cross-infection from occurring in other patients in the same ward is to: (All India 2003)
a. Give antibiotics to all other patients in the ward
b. Fumigate the ward
c. Disinfect the ward with sodium hypochlorite
d. Practice proper hand washing

Q9. Orthobaric oxygen is used in: (All India 1997)
a. CO poisoning
b. Ventilation failure
c. Anerobic infection
d. Gangrene

Q10. Which is not true of carbuncle? (JIPMER 1986)
a. Infective gangrene of subcutaneous tissue
b. Caused by *Staphylococcus*
c. Diabetics are more prone
d. Caused by *Streptococcus*
e. Penicillin and excision of necrotic tissue are the treatment of choice

Grade II	**Difficult**

Q1. In a postoperative intensive care unit, five patients developed postoperative wound infections on the same wound. The best method to prevent cross-infection from occurring in other patients in the same ward is to: (All India 2003)
a. Give antibiotics to all over patients in the ward
b. Fumigate the ward
c. Disinfect the ward with sodium hypochlorite
d. Practice proper hand washing

Q2. A surgeon decides to operate on a patient with carcinoma cecum and perform a right hemicolectomy through a midline laparotomy approach. You have been instructed to prepare the parts of the patient for surgery. What will you do? (AIIMS May 2016)
a. Clean and drape from the level of the nipple to midthigh
b. Clean and drape from the umbilicus to the midthigh
c. Clean and drape from the chin to the knee
d. Clean and drape from the rib cage to the inguinal regions

Q3. True about the management of necrotizing soft tissue infection: (PGI Nov 2011)
a. Broad-spectrum antibiotics should be started
b. Penicillin is not usually effective due to resistant strains
c. Immediate debridement + intravenous (IV) antibiotic has the main role in treatment
d. Hyperbaric O_2 is useful
e. Amputation always indicated

Q4. The following is true of erysipelas, *except*: (AIIMS 1984)
a. Streptococcal infection
b. Contagious and infectious
c. Margins are raised
d. Common in tropics

Q5. Unlike cellulitis, erysipelas has features of: (PGI Nov 2017)
a. Clearly demarcated margin
b. Elevated edge
c. More deeper skin involvement
d. More generalized spread
e. More abrupt onset

Q6. Most common cause of cellulitis is: (PGI 1988)
a. *Staphylococcus*
b. *Streptococcus*
c. *E. coli*
d. *Haemophilus*

Q7. Most common form of anthrax is: (PGI 1988)
a. Wool sorters disease
b. Alimentary type
c. Cutaneous type
d. None of the above

Q8. Actinomycosis is sensitive to: (PGI 1988)
a. Streptomycin
b. Nystatin
c. Penicillin
d. Idoxuridine

Q9. Which of the following parts of the body is not affected by leprosy? (PGI 1988)
a. Testes
b. Ovary
c. Nasal mucosa
d. Axilla

Q10. Leonine facies is seen in .... leprosy: (PGI 1988)
a. Tuberculoid
b. Borderline
c. Lepromatous
d. Borderline tuberculoid

Grade III	Most difficult

Q1. A chest physician performs a bronchoscopy in the procedure room of the outpatient department. To make the instrument safe for use in the next patient waiting outside, the most appropriate method to disinfect the endoscope is by: (All India 2003)

a. 70% alcohol for 5 minutes
b. 2% glutaraldehyde for 20 minutes
c. 2% formaldehyde for 10 minutes
d. 1% sodium hypochlorite for 15 minutes

Q2. The best disinfectant for an endoscope is: (JIPMER 2014)

a. Hypochlorite
b. Formaldehyde
c. Glutaraldehyde
d. Chlorhexidine

Q3. Regarding antibiotics true statement: (PGI June 2006)

a. No prophylaxis for clean contaminated surgery
b. No prophylaxis for gastric ulcer surgery
c. Prophylaxis for colorectal surgery
d. Local irrigation with antibiotic

Q4. Preferred time for prophylactic antibiotic: (PGI June 2009)

a. 1 day before surgery
b. At the time of induction of anesthesia
c. IV during surgery
d. Intramuscular (IM) before 6 hours
e. Orally given

Q5. In a surgical postoperative ward, a patient developed a wound infection. Subsequently, three other patients developed similar infections in the ward. What is the most effective way to prevent the spread of infection? (AIIMS Nov 2001)

a. Give IV antibiotics to all patients in the ward
b. Proper hand washing of all ward personnel
c. Fumigation of the ward
d. Wash OT instruments with 1% perchlorate

Q6. Steps taken to prevent postoperative incised wound infection are: (PGI May 2018)

a. Start antibiotics at least 1 day preoperatively
b. Shaving of hair
c. One dose of antibiotic just before the incision
d. Shower preoperatively using an antiseptic
e. Prevent intraoperative hypothermia

Q7. Quick sequential organ failure assessment (qSOFA) score includes: (PGI May 2018)

a. Pulse rate
b. Respiratory rate
c. Systolic blood pressure
d. Altered mental status
e. Mean arterial pressure

Q8. What is false about cellulitis? (PGI Nov 2010)

a. Caused by *S. pyogenes*
b. Causes SIRS
c. Localized infection
d. Abscess if any, should be managed conservatively
e. I and D (incision and drainage) of abscess should be done

Q9. Universal (standard) precautions to be observed by surgeons for the prevention of hospital-acquired HIV infection include the following, *except*:

a. Wearing gloves and other barrier precautions
b. Washing hands on contamination
c. Handling sharp instruments with care
d. Preoperative screening of all patients with HIV

Q10. From the index finger infection goes to: (AIIMS Nov 1996)

a. Thenar space
b. Hypothenar space
c. Midpalmar space
d. Space of Parona

ANSWERS

Grade I: 1. a, b, d; 2. b, c, d; 3. d; 4. b, c, e; 5. c; 6. a; 7. a, b, d; 8. d (Harrison 17/e p836); 9. a; 10. d (Harrison 17/e p875)

Grade II: 1. d; 2. a; 3. a, c, d; 4. b; 5. a, b, e; 6. b (Bailey 26/e p55); 7. c (Bailey 23/e p110); 8. c (Bailey 26/e p65); 9. b (Harrison 17/e p1023); 10. c (Bailey 26/e p78)

Grade III: 1. b; 2. c; 3. c; 4. b; 5. b; 6. c, d, e; 7. b, c, d; 8. c, d; 9. d; 10. a

MODEL QUESTIONS

Q1. When do we have to start antibiotics to prevent postoperative infection?

a. 2 days before surgery
b. After surgery
c. 1 week before surgery
d. 1 hour before surgery, and continue after surgery

Ans. d

Q2. The optional timing of administration of prophylactic antibiotics for surgical patients is:

a. At the induction of anesthesia
b. Any time during the surgical procedure
c. 1 hour after induction
d. 1 hour before induction of anesthesia

Ans. a

Q3. The most effective method of reduction of incidence of institutional pediatric *Staphylococcus aureus* infection is:

a. Mask and gown use with each suspected patient
b. Meticulous hand washing before and after contact with patients
c. Treatment of all culture-positive patients with vancomycin
d. Routine isolation of culture-positive patients

Ans. b

Q4. Characteristics of systemic inflammatory response syndrome (SIRS) include all of the following, *except*:

a. Leukocytosis
b. Thrombocytopenia
c. Infectious or noninfectious caused
d. Oral temperature >38°C

Ans. b

Q5. Extensive surgical debridement, decompression, or amputation may be indicated in the following clinical setting, *except*:

a. Progressive synergistic gangrene
b. Acute thrombophlebitis
c. Acute hemolytic streptococcal cellulitis
d. Acute rhabdomyolysis

Ans. b

Q6. Treatment of spreading streptococcal cellulitis is:

a. Erythromycin
b. Penicillin
c. Tetracycline
d. Chloramphenicol

Ans. b

Q7. Which of the following is not true of gas gangrene?

a. It is caused by *Clostridium perfringens*
b. *C. perfringens* is a germ-negative spore-bearing bacillus.
c. Gas gangrene is characterized by severe local pain, crepitus, and signs of toxemia
d. High-dose penicillin and aggressive debridement of affected tissue are the treatment of established infection.

Ans. b

Q8. The most common cause of acute lymphadenitis in India:

a. Barefoot walking
b. Tuberculosis (TB)
c. Staphylococcal skin infection
d. Lymphoma

Ans. c

Q9. All are features of gummatous ulcer, *except*:

a. Punched out edges
b. syphilitic in nature
c. Wash leather slough
d. Erythematous base

Ans. d

Q10. The human immunodeficiency virus (HIV) can be transmitted by the following routes, *except*:

a. Homosexual contact
b. Intact skin
c. Maternofetal
d. Needle prick

Ans. b

Q11. Malignant pustule occurs in:

a. Melanoma
b. Gas gangrene
c. Ovarian tumor
d. Anthrax

Ans. d

Q12. Felon is:

a. Midpalmer space infection.
b. Terminal pulp space infection
c. Infection of ulnar bursa
d. Infection or radial bursa

Ans. b

Q13. Subphrenic abscess, not seen is:

a. Air fluid level
b. Leukopenia
c. More common on the right side
d. Associated with shoulder pain

Ans. b

Q14. All of the following favor postoperative wound dehiscence, *except*:

a. Malignancy
b. Vitamin B complex deficiency
c. Hypoproteinemia
d. Jaundice

Ans. b

Q15. Hilton's method of treatment of an axillary abscess is advised because it:

a. Protects vital structure
b. Ensures adequate drainage
c. Hinders the spread of infection
d. Allows local instillation of antibiotics

Ans. a

Q16. Mycotic abscesses are due to:

a. Bacterial infection
b. Fungal infection
c. Viral infection
d. Mixed infection

Ans. b

Q17. Antibioma is best treated by:

a. Partial resection
b. Complete resection
c. Aspiration
d. Administration of antibiotics

Ans. b

Q18. Which of these scoring systems is helpful in assessing the severity of wound infection and is used for research and surveillance?

a. Southampton grading scale
b. American Society of Anesthesiologists (ASA) classification
c. Glasgow score
d. Apgar

Ans. a

Q19. Use of all the following significantly decreases airborne infection in the operating room, *except*:

a. Laminar air flow
b. Air-conditioning
c. Ultraviolet light
d. Microfilters

Ans. b

Q20. Flexible endoscopes are best sterilized with:

a. Formaldehyde
b. Ethylene oxide
c. Gamma irradiation
d. Peracetic acid

Ans. d

Q21. What is the best time to give prophylactic antibiotics?

a. 1 day before surgery
b. At the time of skin incision
c. At the time of induction
d. 2 days before to 3 days after surgery

Ans. c

Q22. Ideally, when should antibiotics be given during surgery?

a. At the time of induction
b. At the time, incision
c. After the surgery is over
d. A couple of days before surgery.

Ans. a

Q23. A 60-year-old lady underwent abdominal surgery, and on the fourth postoperative day, she was diagnosed with SIRS. What are the features of SIRS?

a. Normal body temperature and normal respiratory rate
b. White blood cell (WBC) >12 × 10^9/L or <4 × 10^9/L
c. Respiratory rate >24 breaths/min and heart rate >90 beats/min
d. Respiratory rate < 10 breaths/min

Ans. b and c

Q24. Infection of all the following structures can be because of a psoas abscess, *except*:

a. Vertebrae
b. Appendix
c. Hip joint
d. Ribs

Ans. d

Q25. Chronic burrowing ulcer is caused by:

a. Microaerophilic streptococci
b. Peptostreptococcus
c. *Streptococcus viridans*
d. *S. pyogenes*

Ans. a

SUGGESTED READING

1. Harrison's Principles of Internal Medicine, 15th edition.
2. Schwartz's Principles of Surgery, 18th edition.
3. SRB's Manual of Surgery, 4th edition.

CHAPTER 12

Basic Surgical Skills

"A true surgeon is never fearless. He fears for his patients, he fears for his shortcomings, his own mistakes, but he never fears for himself or his professional reputation."

– Samuel J Mixter

INTRODUCTION

In surgical procedures, both sharp and blunt dissection are required as per the procedure.

The incision should be made with a sharp blade (scalpel) by holding firmly and pressing correct along the line of the incision. The scalpel should be straight and not oblique. Scalpels should always be kept in a kidney dish and given to the surgeon by a nurse in the same way to avoid injury. Commonly used scalpel blades are number 11, 15, and 22 **(Fig. 1)**. Skin incision should be applied along *Langer's (Karl Ritter Von Langer, 1847–1888, Austrian Anatomist)* line to get a good scar **(Fig. 2)**.

The scalpel is fixed with a Bard–Parker handle so as to give stability and firmness to the blade **(Fig. 3)**. Incision should avoid pressure points of bony prominences and should give adequate exposure. *Incision when made, a surgeon should also have cosmetic factors in mind.*
Sometimes in an incision that is making an elliptical wound, the closure may cause an elevated end called a "dog ear." Dog ears should be excised to achieve good cosmetic results.

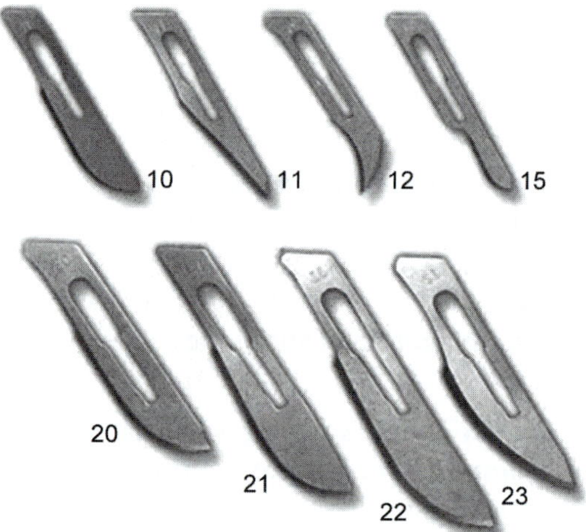

Fig. 1: Various scalpels.

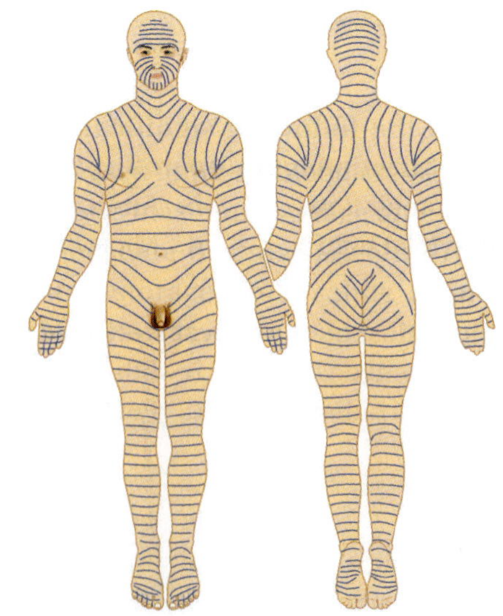

Fig. 2: Langer's line.

FACTORS IMPORTANT FOR AN INCISION

Mn = SACA

S = Skin tension line Langer lines—incision should be along these lines to get good scar.

A = Anatomical structure—avoid bones, nerves, and vessels.

C = Cosmetic factor—to get good cosmetic results.

A = Adequate access—should give good access and exposure to the organ to be operated on.

LAPAROSCOPIC PROCEDURES

Nowadays, minimal access surgery or laparoscopic surgery is commonly done due to its benefits of cosmesis, less pain,

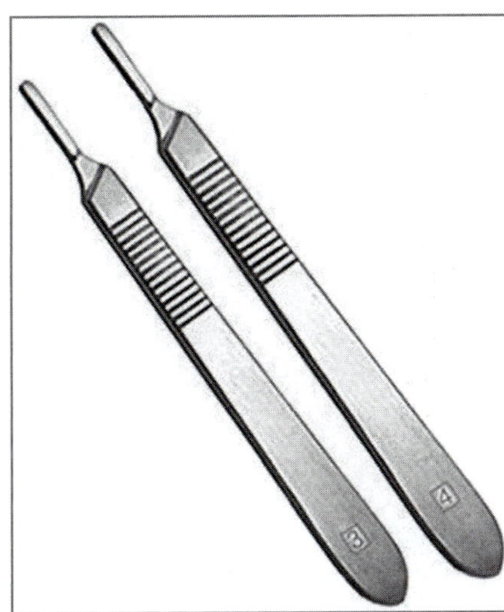

Fig. 3: Bard–Parker (BP) handle.

short hospital stay, and early return to work. The umbilicus is chosen as a point of introduction of the primary port due to the least thickness of the abdominal wall here, as the skin is fused with the peritoneum here. A primary trocar is inserted blindly, so it must be introduced with utmost precautions. Secondary trocars are always introduced under vision and should also be removed under vision. Trocars should be introduced at a right angle to the abdominal wall.

A port >5 mm in size should be closed along with the fascia.

Pneumoperitoneum is established by carbon dioxide gas at a pressure of 12 mm Hg, gas flow of 20 L/min, and 1–2 L/min gas flow.

Benefits of Laparoscopic Surgery

Mn = BLEED
B = Better cosmetics
L = Less postoperative pain
E = Early return to physiological functions
E = Early return to normal activities
D = Early discharge from the hospital, so a shorter hospital stay

Surgical Suture

Suturing of tissues is an art that should unite the tissues without pressure, but not loose. It is a matter of experience that one should learn quickly. There is no ideal way of wound closure. *Alexis Carrel, 1873-1944, French Surgeon, was given the Nobel Prize in Physiology or Medicine in 1912 for his work on vascular suture and the transplantation of blood vessels and organs.*

Suture material should be soft, easy to handle, with good tensile strength, sterile, making a secure knot, with the least tissue reaction, nonallergic, noncarcinogenic, noncapillary, and nonshrinkable. *The sizes of suture materials usually used are 2, 1, 0, 2-0, 3-0, 4-0, and 5-0.*

The main characteristics of suture should be:

- *Biological behavior:* Synthetic polymer sutures are used more progressively now than biological or natural sutures, such as catgut, as they disintegrate by proteolysis.
- *Physical structure:* Suture may be monofilament or multifilament, braided. The braided suture material is easier for the application of a knot.
- *Strength of the suture:* Strong suture material is good as it does not break easily.
- *Tensile strength:* Tensile strength of the suture is the amount of force required to break it. The memory of synthetic sutures keeps them bending and curling as they were placed in the package. A sharp pull and stretch on the suture material reduced this property of memory.
- *Absorbability:* A suture material may be absorbable or nonabsorbable—absorbable sutures are used where staying long of suture may lead to some risk, as in biliary and urinary surgery.

> *Types of sutures* ***(Figs. 4 to 7)****:*
> - *Continuous sutures:* There should not be too much or too little tension.
> - *Interrupted sutures:* The distance between sutures should be approximately twice than the depth of the sutures.
> - *Mattress sutures:* These may be applied vertically or horizontally.
> - *Subcuticular suture:* It is applied for good cosmetic result.

Needles Used to Suture

Nowadays, needles are "eyeless" or "atraumatic" with embedded suture material **(Fig. 8)**. The suture needle has the following parts:

- *Shank*
- *Body*
- *Point*

The body of the needle is either round or triangular or flattened. The triangular body has a cutting edge along all three sides. A needle should be held by a needle holder at a point one-third to one-half from the rear point of the needle.

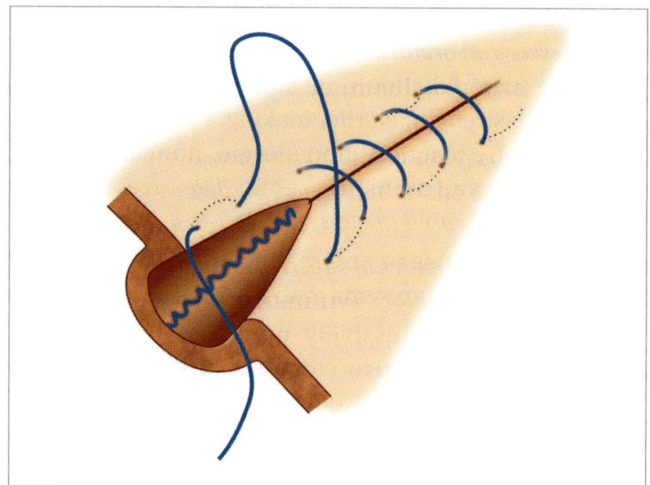

Fig. 4: Continuous suture.

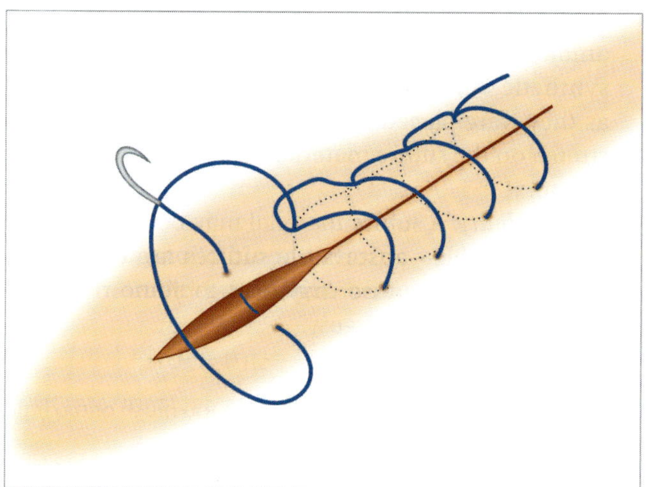

Fig. 5: Interrupted sutures.

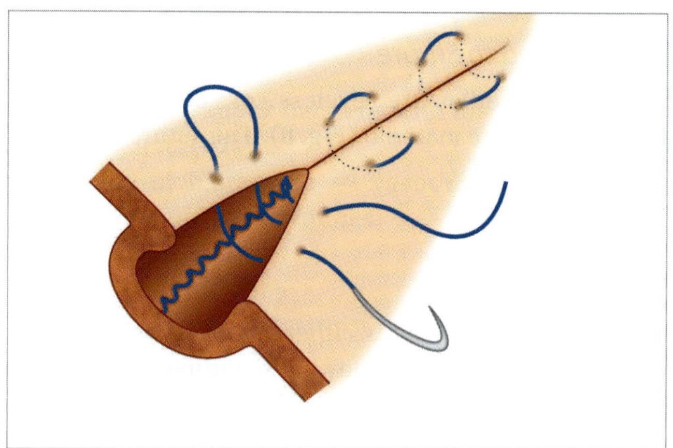

Fig. 6: Mattress sutures.

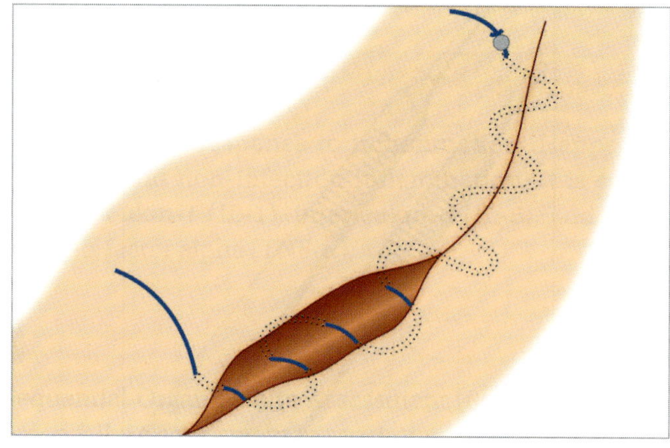

Fig. 7: Subcuticular suture.

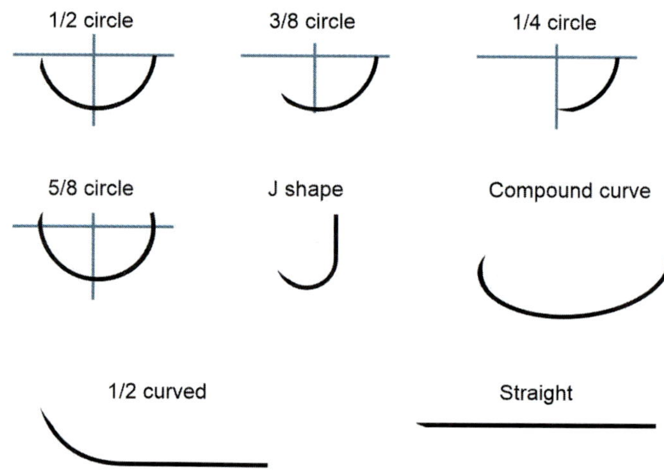

Fig. 8: Various types of needles.

Knots

Various types of knots are used to tie the suture material for closure **(Fig. 9)**. The following are commonly used knots:

- Simple knot
- Granny knot—good for application of the right tension.
- Reef knot—the third throw is used for security.
- Surgeon's knot
- When using a continuous suture, an Aberdeen knot is applied at the end.

Glue

It is a solution of n-butyl-2-cyanoacrylate. When applied leads to adhesion and hemostasis without tension.

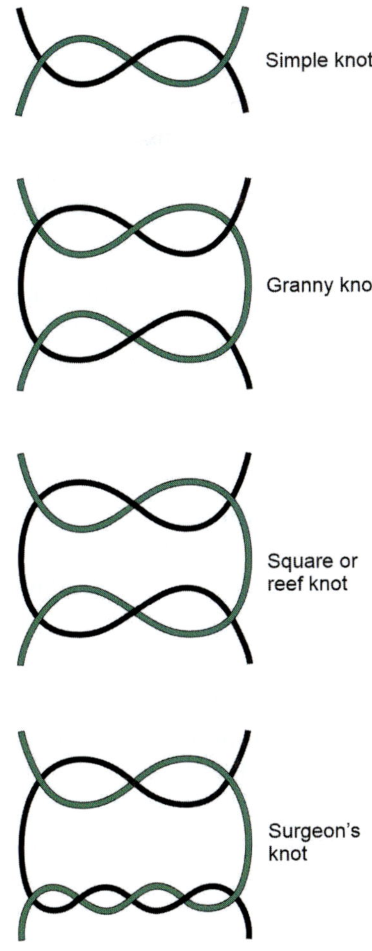

Fig. 9: Various types of knots.

Stapling

Staples are used in skin and various hollow organ anastomoses.

BOWEL ANASTOMOSES

The word anastomosis is derived from two Greek words, ana (without) and stoma (a mouth). Anastomoses are end-to-end or end-to-side, or side-to-side, depending upon the requirement. *Lambert (Antoine Lambert, 1802–1851, French Surgeon) described a seromuscular suture for intestinal anastomoses in 1826. Halsted (William Stewart Halsted, MD, September 23, 1852 to September 7, 1922) was an American surgeon* who advised one layer of extra-mucosal closure, which is even now popular. Vascular anastomoses are done with nonabsorbable monofilament suture material. It should have a smooth intimal suture line.

Drains

Drains are the articles used at the operation site or in a wound to drain the collected or continuously formed fluid. They can be used for prophylactic or therapeutic purposes. A drain may be open or closed. A closed drain system is usually used for suction.

Use of Drain

- Removes collected fluid
- Acts as indicator
- Reduces intra-abdominal abscesses

Some researchers believe that the use of drains may increase wound infections, increase hospital stay, and decrease lung function.

Diathermy

It is mostly used to secure hemostasis during surgery by coagulation of bleeding points. *Diathermy is used both for coagulation and cutting.* One should be aware of accidental burns by negligent use of diathermy.

Nowadays, two types of diathermies are in use, monopolar and bipolar. In monopolar diathermy, the current passes through the patient's body and returns to a passive electrode to earth. In bipolar diathermy, two elective electrodes are used, and the current flows between these two points.

A harmonic scalpel nowadays is in use, which cuts the tissues and at the same time seals them.

SOME IMPORTANT QUESTIONS

Q1. Which of the following is a nonabsorbable suture?

a. Polypropylene
b. Vicryl
c. Catgut
d. Polydioxanone

Ans. a

Q2. Surgically used suture material, polydioxanone suture (PDS):

a. A nonabsorbable and remains encapsulated
b. Undergoes hydrolysis and complete absorption
c. Undergoes phagocytosis and enzymatic degradation
d. It is specifically used for the heart valves of synthetic grafts

Ans. b

Q3. Catgut is prepared from the submucosal layer of the intestine of:

a. Cat b. Sheep
c. Human being d. Rabbit

Ans. b

Q4. Suture material used for laparoscopic choledochotomy repair:

a. Silk b. Catgut
c. Polyethylene d. Vicryl

Ans. d

Q5. Catgut is preserved in:

a. Glutaraldehyde b. Isopropyl alcohol
c. Iodine d. Cetrimide

Ans. b

Q6. The raw material used in nylon suture is:

a. Polyethylene terephthalate
b. Polyamide polymer
c. Polybutylene terephthalate
d. Polyester polymer

Ans. b

Q7. Which of the following sutures has maximum tensile strength and minimum tissue reaction?

a. Poliglecaprone b. Polypropylene
c. Polyglactin d. Polydioxanone

Ans. b

Q8. Disparity of the bowel ends during end-to-end anastomosis is corrected by:

a. Cheatle's maneuver b. Connell's suture
c. Lambert's suture d. Czerny technique

Ans. a

Q9. In abdominal surgery, Lembert suture refers to:

a. Single-layer suturing
b. Seromuscular sutures
c. All coat intestinal suturing
d. Skin suturing

Ans. b

Q10. Colonic anastomosis is most likely to rupture on which postoperative day?

a. 1–2 days b. 3–4 days
c. After 7 days d. After 14 days

Ans. c

Q11. Regarding vascular surgery distal to the popliteal artery, which of the following is true?

a. Suture with polypropylene
b. 6-0 suture used
c. Needle passes from within outward
d. All the above

Ans. d

Q12. Tissue suturing glue contains:

a. Cyanoacrylate b. Ethanolamine oleate
c. Methacrylate d. Polychloroprene

Ans. a

Q13. Vicryl, the commonly used suture material, is a:

a. Homopolymer of polydioxanone
b. Copolymer of glycolide and lactide
c. Homopolymer of glycolide
d. Homopolymer of lactide

Ans. b

Q14. PDS is absorbed within:

a. 7 days b. 21 days
c. 100 days d. 225 days

Ans. d

Q15. Surgically used suture material PDS:

a. Is nonabsorbable and remains encapsulated.
b. Undergoes hydrolysis and complete absorption.
c. Undergoes phagocytosis and enzymatic degradation.
d. It is specifically used for the heart valves of synthetic grafts.

Ans. b

Q16. The surgeon who introduced catgut in surgery was:

a. Astley Cooper b. Lord Lister
c. John Hunter d. Syme

Ans. c

Q17. Which of the following is the preferred suture material for vascular anastomosis?

a. Nonabsorbable, elastic
b. Nonabsorbable, nonelastic
c. Absorbable, elastic
d. Absorbable, nonelastic

Ans. b

MULTIPLE CHOICE QUESTIONS

Grade I	*Simple*

Q1. Absorbable sutures are: **(PGI 2004)**

a. Catgut b. Silk
c. Polypropylene d. Polyglycolic acid
e. Vicryl

Q2. Which of the following is a non-absorbable suture? (All India 2008)

a. Polypropylene
b. Vicryl
c. Catgut
d. Polydioxanone

Q3. Which one of the following is used as a preservative for packing catgut suture? (AIIMS Nov 2002)

a. Isopropyl alcohol
b. Colloidal iodine
c. Glutaraldehyde
d. Hydrogen peroxide

Q4. After a midline laparotomy, you have been asked to suture the incision. What length of suture will you choose? (AIIMS Nov 2016)

a. 2× incision length
b. 4× incision length
c. 6× incision length
d. 8× incision length

Q5. A woman presents with complete wound dehiscence 4 days after a laparotomy. After prescribing antibiotics for the infection, the surgeon decides to suture the wound. Which of these suture materials should he use? (AIIMS Nov 2016)

a. Vicryl
b. Mersilk
c. Catgut
d. Ethilon

Grade II	Difficult

Q1. A surgical attending has completed a modified radical mastectomy for a breast carcinoma patient. You have to suture the wound using subcuticular sutures. Which of these sutures will you choose? (AIIMS May 2016)

a. Monocryl
b. Vicryl
c. Ethicon
d. Chromic

Q2. The best dressing is: (PGI 1988)

a. Opsite
b. Amnion
c. Tulle grass
d. Skin

Q3. Skin graft for facial wounds is taken from: (AIIMS 1992)

a. Medial aspect of thigh
b. Cubital fossa
c. Groin
d. Post auricular region

Q4. What does "Take in" mean in the case of skin grafting: (AIIMS June 1997)

a. Revascularization of the graft
b. Return of the sensation
c. When the graft becomes adherent to the recipient site
d. Nonadherent graft is shed off

Q5. In a hand injury first structure to be repaired should be: (All India 1998)

a. Skin
b. Nerve
c. Muscle
d. Bone

Grade III	Most difficult

Q1. Which one of the following is used as a preservative for packing catgut suture? (AIIMS Nov 2002)

a. Isopropyl alcohol
b. Colloidal iodine
c. Glutaraldehyde
d. Hydrogen peroxide

Q2. True regarding 10-0 sutures is? (PGI May 2018)

a. Thicker than 1-0 sutures
b. Synthetic sutures
c. Diameter is 0.9 mm
d. Stronger than 1-0
e. All of the above

Q3. Intestinal anastomosis strength is provided by: (JIPMER 2015)

a. Mucosa
b. Submucosa
c. Serosa
d. Muscularis mucosa

Q4. All of the following are true, *except*: (PGI Nov 2017)

a. Surgical blade direction should be downward and away from the surgeon.
b. During bowel anastomosis, hemostatic forceps are used to grasp the intestine.
c. Needle-holding forceps damage sutures as it is a crushing in nature.
d. Toothed forceps are used to grasp skin, subcutaneous tissue, muscles, and sheaths.
e. The handle of the surgical blade is held with the thumb and index finger.

Q5. Salmon patch usually disappears by age: (PGI 1980)

a. One month
b. One year
c. Puberty
d. None of the above

CHAPTER 13

Surgical Instruments and Machines

"It is better to open and see than to wait and see."

– Sidney C Wallace

ALLIS FORCEPS (OSCAR HUNTINGTON ALLIS, 1836–1921, AMERICAN SURGEON)

It is used for holding firm tissues while causing minimal or no damage. It is useful for firm tissues **(Fig. 1)**.

- *Spencer Wells forceps (Thomas Spencer Wells, 1818–1897, British Surgeon):* It is used for clamping **(Fig. 2)**.
- *DeBakey forceps (Michael Ellis DeBakey, 1908–2008, American Heart Surgeon):* It is used for grasping tissues firmly without damage as it is toothless **(Fig. 3)**.
- *Gillies forceps (Harold Gillies, 1882–1960, British Plastic Surgeon):* It is a tooth forceps for holding tough tissues, such as skin **(Fig. 4)**.

- *McIndoe scissors (Archibald Hector McIndoe, 1900–1960, British Plastic Surgeon):* Use for tissue division without risk of damage to other structures **(Fig. 5)**.
- *Czerny retractor (Vincenz Czerny, 1842–1915, German Surgeon):* Double-ended retractor, one end has a blade while the other end has two prongs. It is used for the retraction of tissues and also to retract at the end of an incision **(Fig. 6)**.

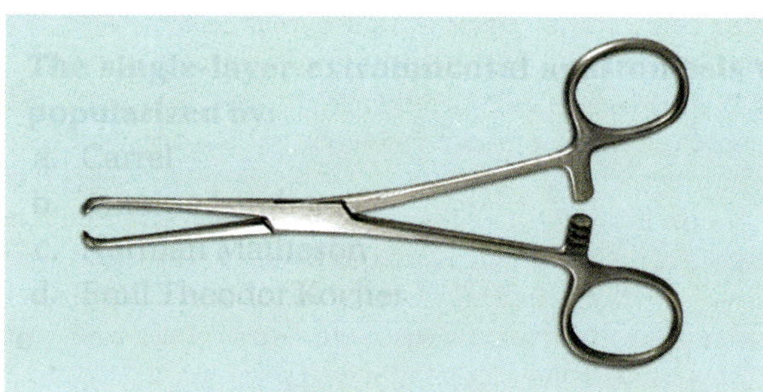

Fig. 1: Allis forceps.

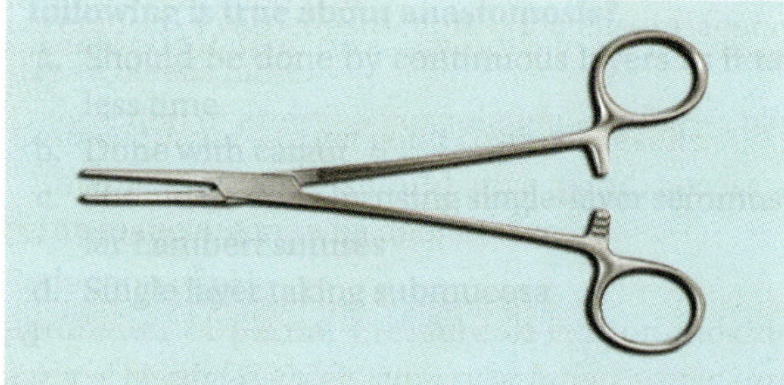

Fig. 2: Spencer Wells forceps.

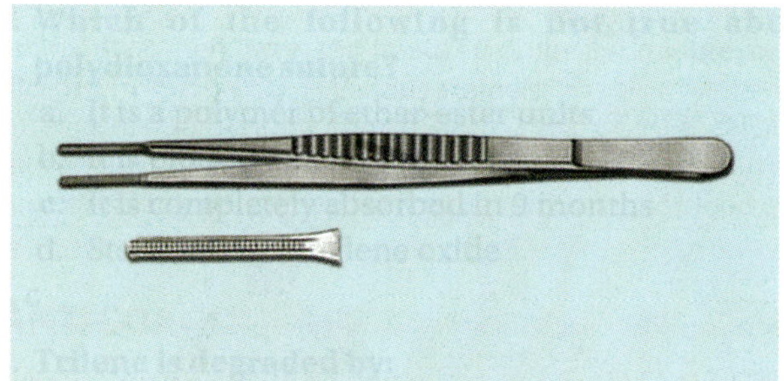

Fig. 3: DeBakey forceps.

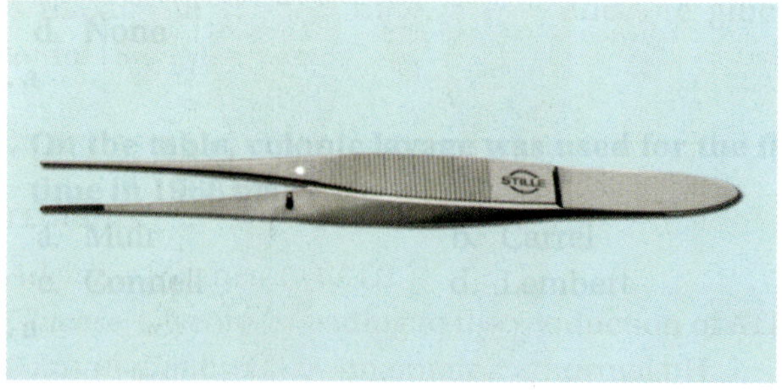

Fig. 4: Gillies forceps.

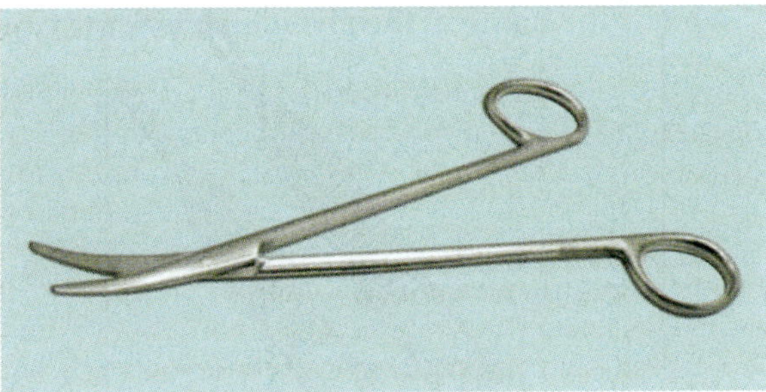

Fig. 5: McIndoe scissors.

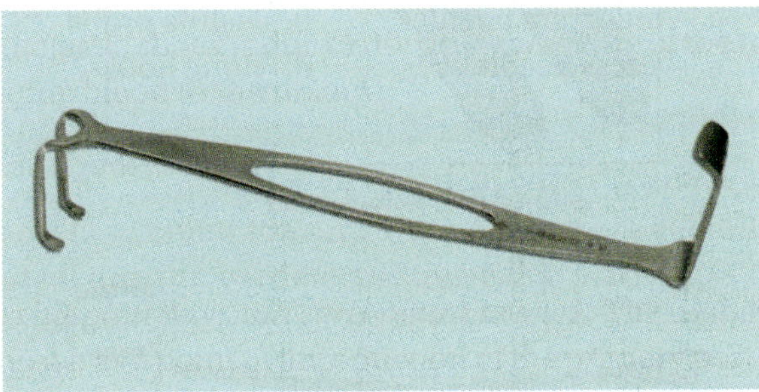

Fig. 6: Czerny retractor.

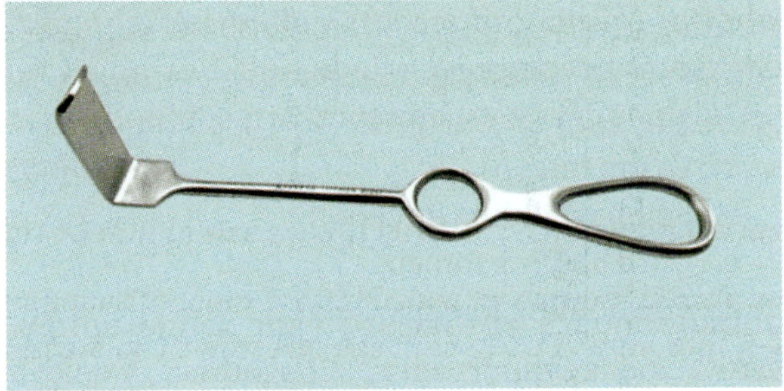

Fig. 7: Langenbeck retractor.

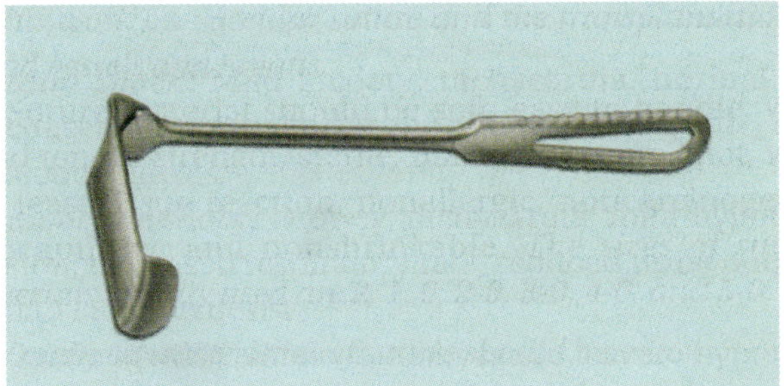

Fig. 8: Morris retractor

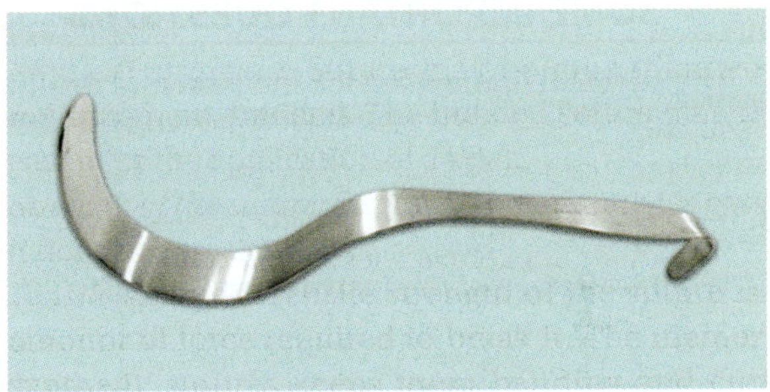

Fig. 9: Deaver retractor.

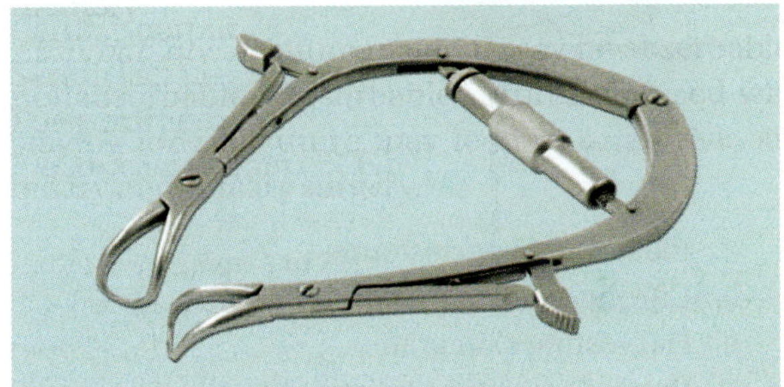

Fig. 10: Joll retractor.

- *Langenbeck retractor (Bernhard Rudolf Konrad von Langenbeck, 1810–1887, German Surgeon):* It is a small retractor that can be used in pairs **(Fig. 7)**.
- Morris retractor (Sir Henry Morris, 1844–1926, British Surgeon): It is a big-size retractor for giving maximum exposure as required in abdominal surgery **(Fig. 8)**.
- *Deaver retractor (John Blair Deaver, 1855–1931, American Surgeon):* Used for retracting the liver while performing open cholecystectomy. The liver is protected by an abdominal swab to avoid injury to the liver **(Fig. 9)**.

- *Joll retractor (Cicil Augustus Joll, 1886–1945, British Surgeon):* Self retaining retractor used in thyroidectomy **(Fig. 10)**.
- *Golligher retractor (John Cedric Golligher, 1912–1998, British Surgeon):* A self-retaining retractor used in laparotomy for operations on sigmoid colon and rectum **(Fig. 11)**.

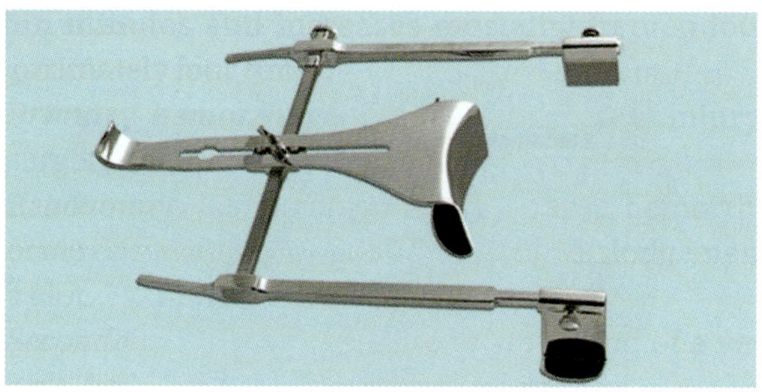

Fig. 11: Golligher retractor.

SOME IMPORTANT QUESTIONS

Q1. The surgical blade used for incision and drainage:

a. 10 b. 11
c. 15 d. 23

Ans. b

Q2. What is the use of the instrument below?

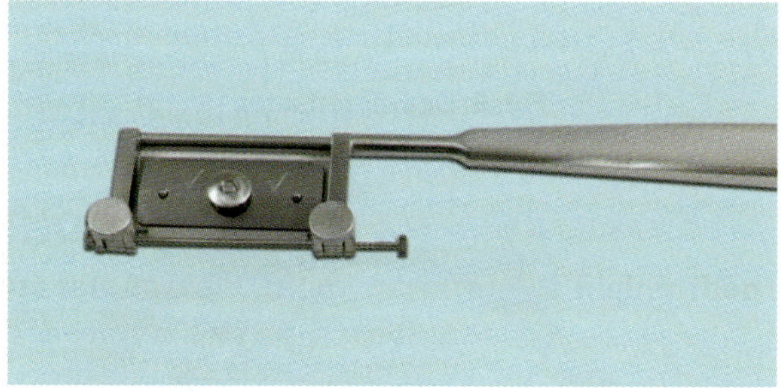

a. Elevation of periosteum
b. Cutting the bone
c. Harvesting skin graft
d. Retraction of the abdominal wall

Ans. c

Q3. The following instrument is used for the diagnosis of:

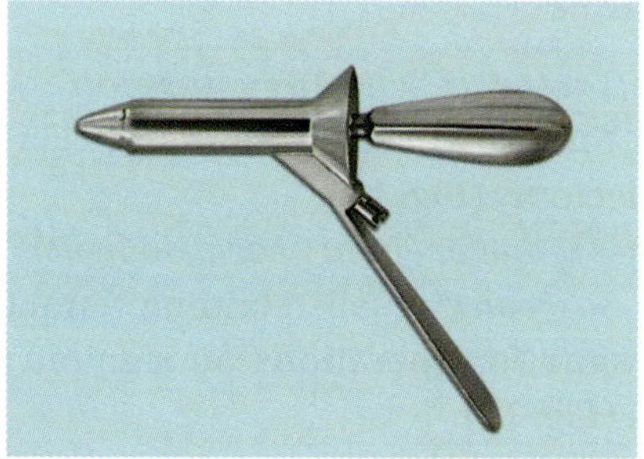

a. Hemorrhoids b. Fissure-in-ano
c. Pilonidal sinus d. All of the above

Ans. a

Q4. What is the name of the given instrument?

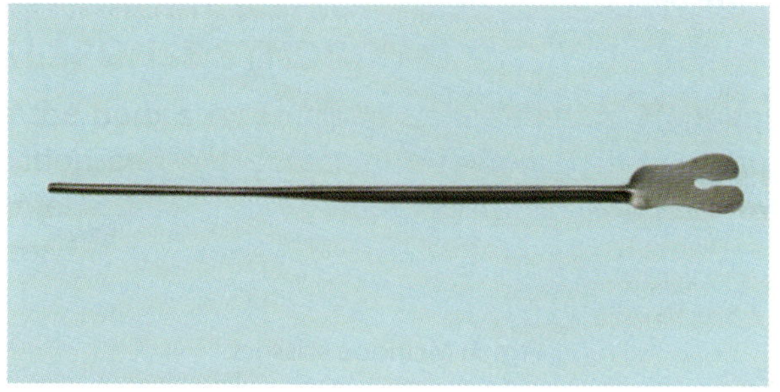

a. Aneurysm needle b. Fistula probe
c. Veress needle d. Bone hook

Ans. b

Q5. Recognize the instrument below:

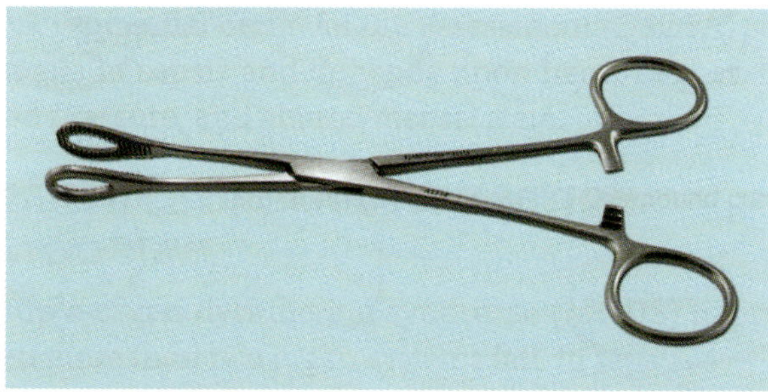

a. Ovum forceps
b. Sponge holding forceps
c. Cord holding forceps
d. Pile holding forceps

Ans. b

Q6. Name the instrument given below:

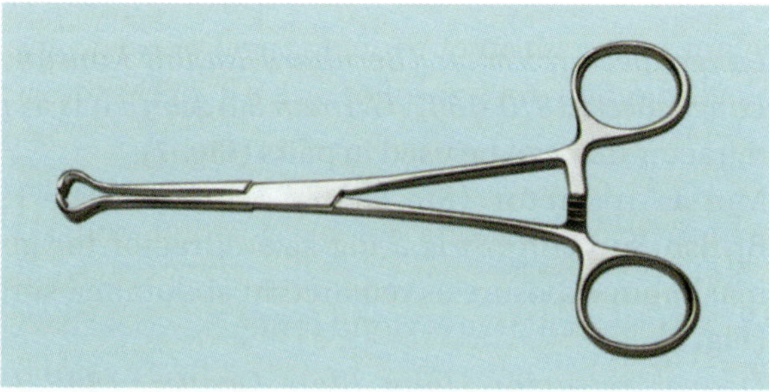

a. Lister's sinus forceps
b. Kocher's hemostatic forceps
c. Babcock's tissue forceps
d. Lane's tissue forceps

Ans. c

Q7. Identify the instruments shown here and choose the best combination:

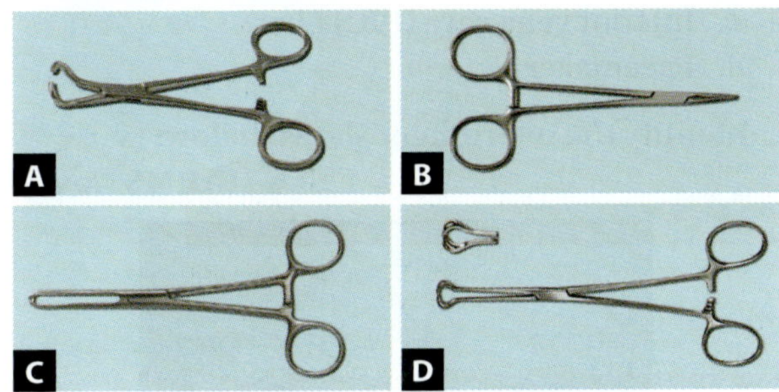

a. A = Dunhill's forceps. B = Halstead mosquito forceps. C = Allis forceps. D = Crile's hemostatic forceps.
b. A = Crile's hemostatic forceps. B = Allis intestinal forceps. C = Schnidt tonsil forceps. D = Babcock intestinal forceps.
c. A = Backhaus towel clamp. B = Halstead mosquito forceps. C = Allis forceps. D = Babcock intestinal forceps.
d. A = Backhaus towel clamp. B = Foerster sponge forceps. C = Dunhill's forceps. D = DeBakey forceps.

Ans. c

Q8. What is the name of the given instrument?

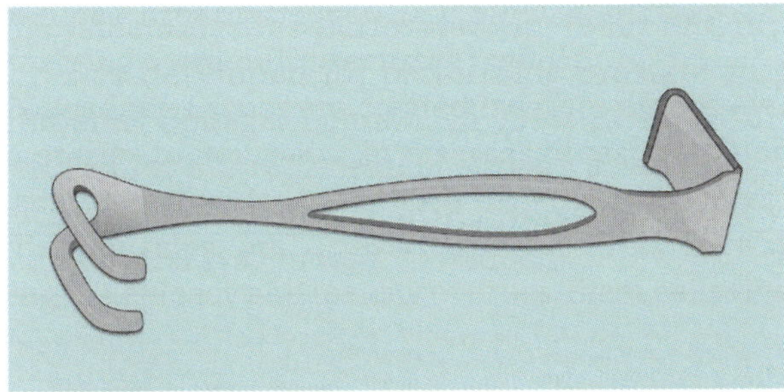

a. Morris's retractor
b. Doyen's retractor
c. Czerney's retractor
d. Deaver's retractor

Ans. c

MULTIPLE CHOICE QUESTIONS

Grade I	Simple

Q1. Blood spilled on the operation table (OT) is cleaned with: (AIIMS 2017)

a. Phenol
b. Alcohol
c. Quaternary ammonium compound
d. Chloride compounds

Q2. The best disinfectant for an endoscope is: (JIPMER 2014)

a. Hypochlorite
b. Formaldehyde
c. Glutaraldehyde
d. Chlorhexidine

Q3. Name this procedure: (AIIMS Nov 2018)

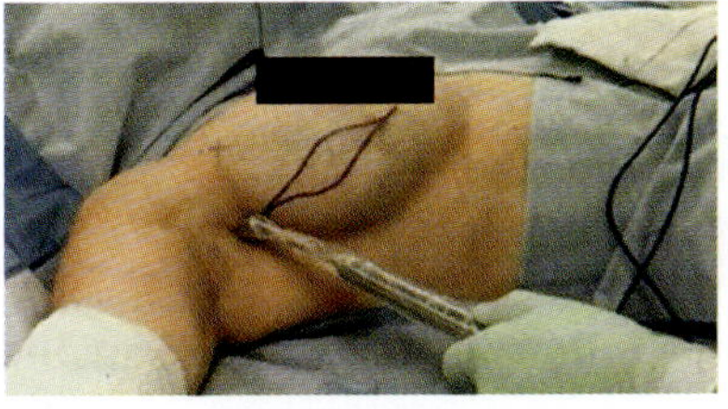

a. Sentinel lymph node biopsy
b. Ultrasound (USG)
c. Lateral pectoral nerve block
d. Brachytherapy

Grade II	Difficult

Q1. Ways to prevent highly infectious diseases transmitted by aerosol; precautions used: (PGI 2007)

a. Isolation ward
b. Facemask
c. Keep isolated in a room with positive pressure
d. Keep isolated in a room with negative pressure
e. Cohort nursing

Q2. The patient came with an ulcer on the face, as shown. What is the diagnosis? (AIIMS Nov 2017)

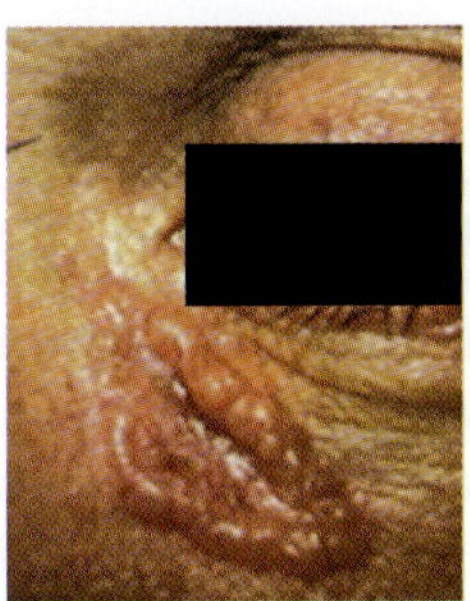

a. Squamous cell carcinoma
b. Basal cell carcinoma
c. Marjolin's ulcer
d. Nevus

Q3. The device given below is used for: **(AIIMS Nov 2018)**

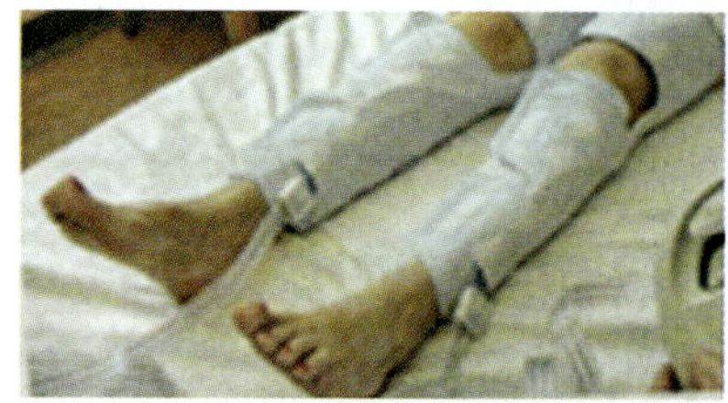

a. Prevention of deep vein thrombosis (DVT)
b. Varicose vein
c. Hypothermia
d. Cellulites

Grade III	*Most difficult*

Q1. All of the following are spiritual agents, *except*: **(JIPMER 2010)**

a. Ethylene oxide
b. Phenol
c. Ozone
d. Glutaraldehyde

Q2. Name of the given instrument: **(AIIMS Nov 2018)**

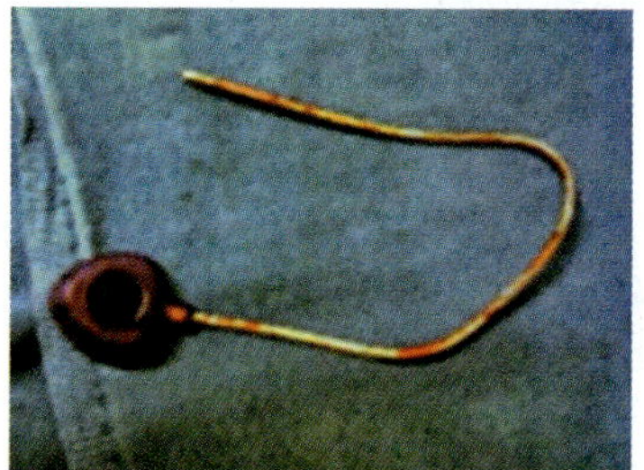

a. Gamma camera
b. Chemoport
c. Inferior vena cava (IVC) filter
d. Pacemaker

Q3. Identify the instrument shown below: **(AIIMS Nov 2016)**

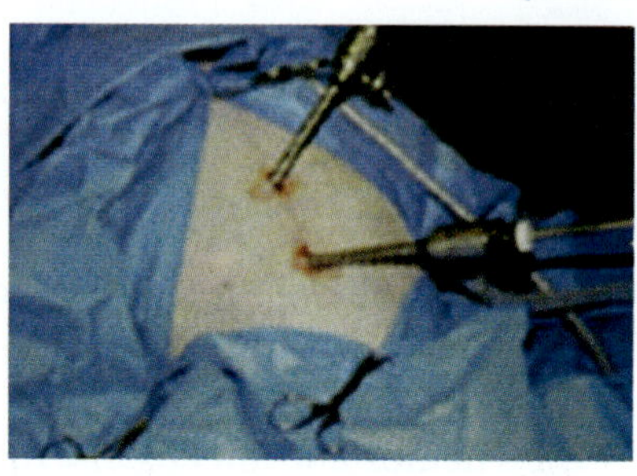

a. Diagnostic peritoneal lavage (DPL) catheter
b. Laparoscopic port trocar
c. Peritoneal dialysis catheter
d. Endoscopic ultrasound probe

ANSWERS

Grade I: 1. d; 2. c; 3. a

Grade II: 1. a; b, d; 2. b; 3. a

Grade III: 1. b; 2. b; 3. b

MODEL QUESTIONS

Q1. Use of all the following significantly decreases airborne infection in OT, *except*:

a. Laminar air flow
b. Air conditioning
c. Ultraviolet light
d. Microfilters

Ans. b

Q2. Flexible endoscopes are best sterilized with:

a. Formaldehyde
b. Ethylene oxide
c. Gamma irradiation
d. Peracetic acid

Ans. d

Q3. Name the instrument.

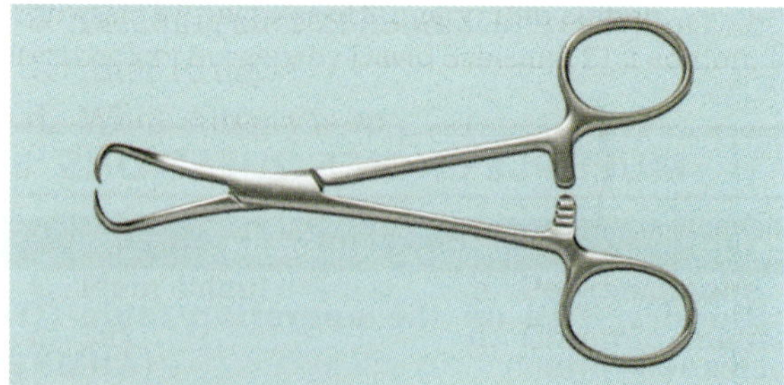

a. Doyen's towel clip
b. Mayo's towel clip

c. Moynihan's tetra towel clip
d. Kocher's forceps

Ans. b

Q4. What is the use of given instrument?

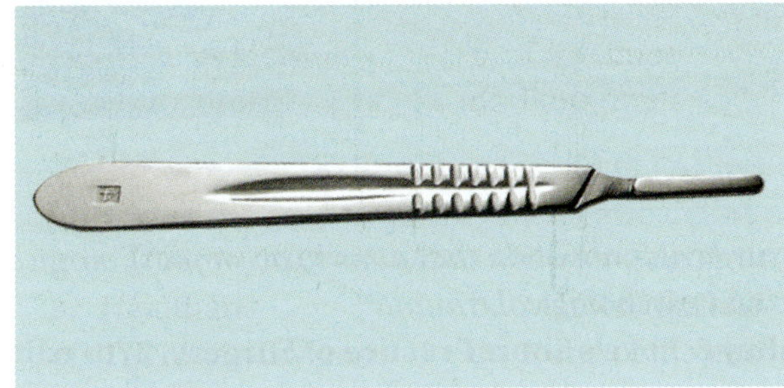

a. Jack knife
b. Elevation of periosteum
c. Suturing
d. Used with blade for skin incision

Ans. d

Q5. What is the name of given tube?

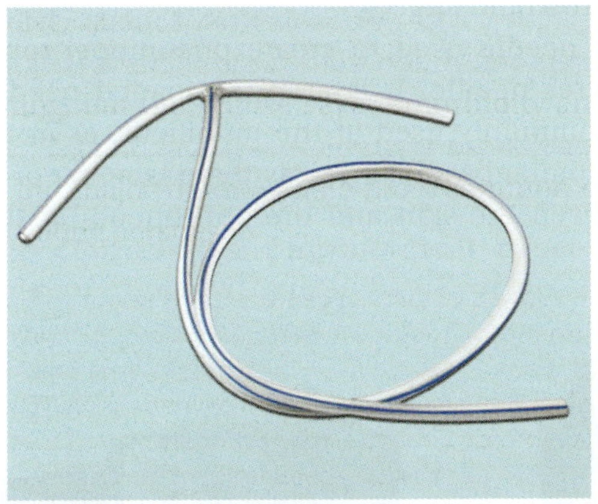

a. Kocher's T-tube
b. Kehr's T-tube
c. Nelaton's catheter
d. Mayo's T-tube

Ans. b

Q6. What is the name of the given stapler?

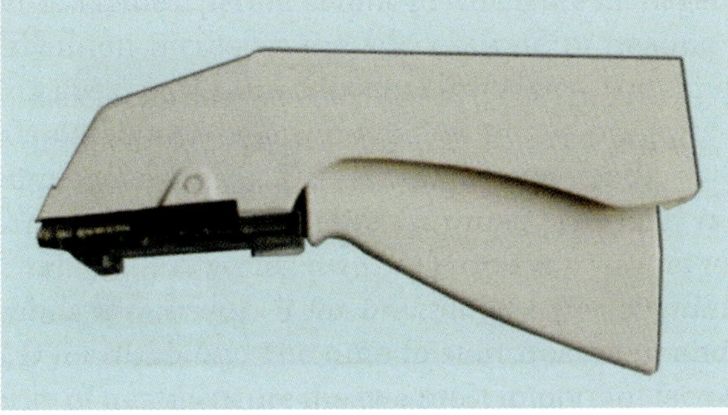

a. Skin stapler
b. Linear cutting stapler
c. Linear stapler
d. Intraluminal stapler

Ans. a

Q7. What is the name of given tube?

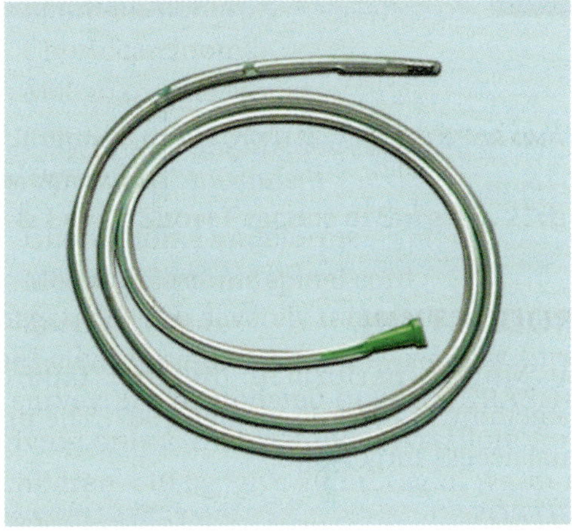

a. Kehr's T-tube
b. Flatus tube
c. Ryle's tube
d. Infant feeding tube

Ans. c

Q8. What is the name of given catheter?

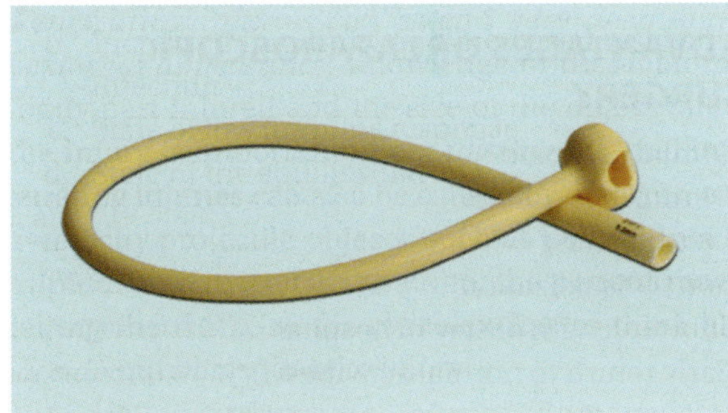

a. Nelaton's catheter
b. Fogarty catheter
c. Foley's catheter
d. Malecot's catheter

Ans. d

SUGGESTED READING

1. Bailey & Love's - Short Practice of Surgery, 27th edition.
2. Schwartz's Principles of Surgery, 18th edition.
3. Textbook of Surgery by David Sabiston, 21st edition.

CHAPTER 14

Laparoscopic Surgery

"Minimal access surgery is a product of modern technology and surgical innovation that aims to accomplish surgical therapeutic goals with minimal somatic and psychological trauma."

– Bailey & Love's Short Practice of Surgery, 27th edition

INTRODUCTION

Philippe Mouret performed the first laparoscopic cholecystectomy in Lyon, France, in 1987. The principles of minimal access surgery are:

Mn—I-VITROS:

- *I* = *Insufflate* to create space
- *V* = *Visualize*—landmarks and surgical environment
- *I* = *Identify*—structures for surgery
- *T* = *Triangulate*—surgical instruments
- *R* = *Retract*—to improve access
- *O* = *Operate*
- *S* = *Seal*/hemostasis

ADVANTAGES OF LAPAROSCOPIC SURGERY

- Diminishes pain
- Diminishes trauma
- Less bleeding
- Better visualization
- Shorter length of stay in hospital
- Early return to normal activities

DISADVANTAGES OF LAPAROSCOPIC SURGERY

- No tactile sensation
- Sometimes difficult to control bleeding
- Difficult to remove big chunks of tissue

In open surgery, trauma is caused by retraction with instruments like retractors. The force applied by the assistant to retract tissues sometimes causes serious injury. In laparoscopic surgery, this type of trauma is avoided by the establishment of pneumoperitoneum. In the case of laparotomy, manual handling of internal organs, especially loops of intestine, leads to serosal injury, which may later on cause adhesions, which is not the case in laparoscopic surgery. Handling of loops of the intestine may also cause intestinal ileus. **Figures 1 to 3** depict the essential instruments and the common setup for laparoscopic surgery.

The needle used to create pneumoperitoneum is the Verres needle. It is a spring-loaded needle. It is most commonly used at the umbilicus, as at this site the abdominal wall is thin, as there is no fat or muscle in between the skin and the peritoneum at this site.

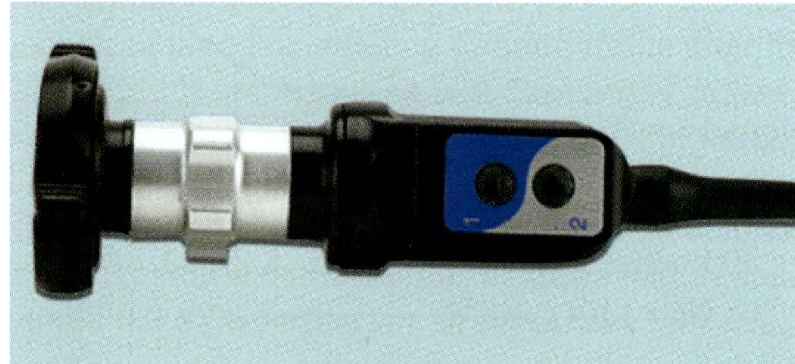

Fig. 1: Camera

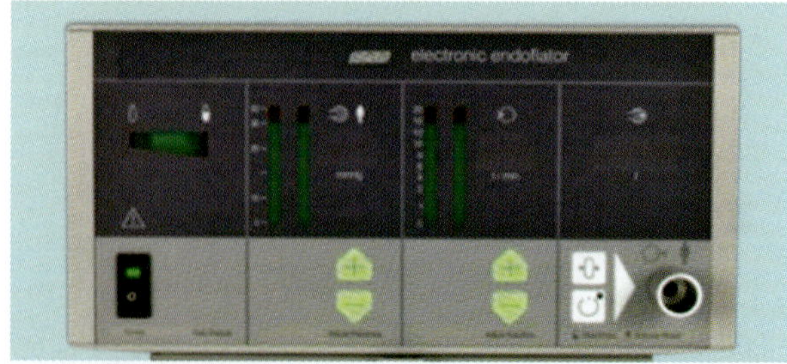

Fig. 2: Carbon dioxide insufflator.

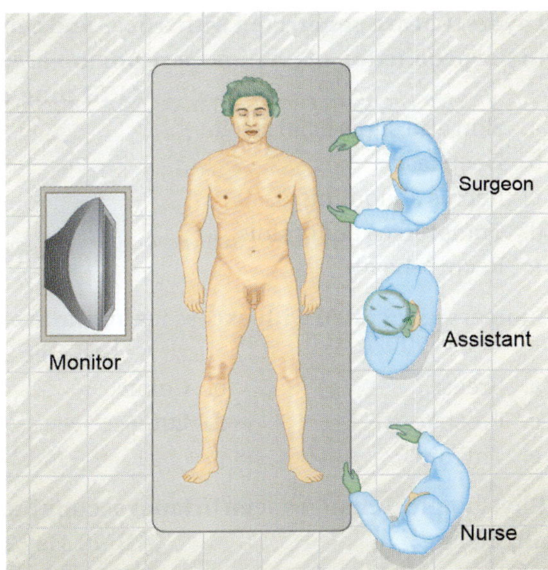

Fig. 3: Laparoscopic setup for appendectomy.

We hear two clicks as we perforate the fascia and then the peritoneum.

Generally, carbon dioxide is used for pneumoperitoneum as it has much higher solubility than air (22 times more). After finishing the laparoscopic procedure, CO_2 remains for 2–3 days. Postlaparoscopy shoulder pain is due to irritation of the diaphragm by carbon dioxide retention through the phrenic nerve, and it is a referred pain. Flow of CO_2—1 L/min.

Pneumoperitoneum can be created by the open method *[Hasson (Harrith Hasson, American Gynecologist) method]* with a low risk of major vessel injury or the closed method *[Verres (Janos Verres, 1903–1979, Hungarian Physician) needle]* to avoid bowel injury.

Physiological effects of laparoscopy:

- *Central venous system (CVS):* Increased central venous pressure (CVP), increased pulmonary capillary venous pressure (PCVP), increased systemic vascular resistance (SVR), and increased mean arterial pressure (MAP).
- *Lungs:* Decreased functional residual capacity (FRC) and increased respiratory rate.
- *Renal:* Decreased renal flow, decreased ejection fraction (EFR), and decreased urine output.

SUGGESTED READING

1. Williams NS, O'Connell PR, McCaskie AW. Bailey & Love's Short Practice of Surgery, 27th edition. New Delhi: CRC Press; 2018. p. 105.

SOME IMPORTANT QUESTIONS

Q1. The intra-abdominal pressure during laparoscopy should be set between:

a. 5 and 8 mm Hg
b. 10 and 15 mm Hg
c. 20 and 25 mm Hg
d. 30 and 35 mm Hg

Ans. b

Q2. Which gas is used in laparoscopy?

a. CO_2
b. N_2O
c. O_2
d. N_2

Ans. a

Q3. Shoulder pain postlaparoscopy is due to:

a. Subphrenic abscess
b. CO_2 retention
c. Positioning of the patient
d. Compression of the lung

Ans. b

Q4. Bariatric surgical procedures include all, *except*:

a. Gastric banding
b. Gastric bypass
c. Biliopancreatic diversion
d. Ileal transposition

Ans. d

Q5. All of the following are primarily restrictive operations for morbid obesity, *except*:

a. Vertical band gastroplasty
b. Duodenal switch operation
c. Roux-en-Y operation
d. Laparoscopic adjustable gastric banding

Ans. b

Q6. The most commonly performed and acceptable method of bariatric surgery is:

a. Biliopancreatic diversion
b. Biliopancreatic diversion with ileostomy
c. Laparoscopic gastric banding
d. Roux-en-Y gastric bypass

Ans. d

Q7. A lady presented in the emergency department with a stab injury to the left side of the abdomen. She was hemodynamically stable, and a contrast-enhanced computed tomography (CT) scan revealed a laceration in the spleen. Laparoscopy was planned, however, the patient's partial pressure of oxygen (pO_2) suddenly dropped as

soon as the pneumoperitoneum was created. What is the most likely cause?

a. Gaseous embolism through splenic vessels
b. Injury to the left lobe of the diaphragm
c. Inferior vena cava compression
d. Injury to the colon

Ans. a

Q8. Daycare surgery can be done in:

a. Lateral sphincterotomy
b. Rhinoplasty
c. Orchidectomy
d. Total thyroidectomy
e. Subcutaneous mastectomy

Ans. a, b, c, and e

Q9. Which of the following is an advantage of minimal access surgery?

a. Increase in heat loss
b. Better hemostasis control
c. Improved vision
d. Decrease in wound pain

Ans. c and d

Q10. Advantages of minimally invasive surgery over open surgery are all, *except*:

a. Wide/better field of vision
b. Less operative time
c. Less postoperative time
d. Lest postoperative morbidity

Ans. b

Q11. Minimal invasive surgery includes all, *except*:

a. Functional endoscopic sinus surgery (FESS)
b. Lap cholecystectomy
c. Endoscopic sclerotherapy
d. Percutaneous nephrolithotomy (PCNL)

Ans. d

Q12. Morbid obesity is a body mass index (BMI) greater than:

a. 25 b. 30
c. 45 d. 45

Ans. c

MULTIPLE CHOICE QUESTIONS

Grade I	Simple

Q1. Gases for pneumoperitoneum: (PGI June 2007)

a. CO_2 b. N_2
c. Room air d. N_2O

Q2. Layers that are penetrated with trocar and cannula in the production of pneumoperitoneum are: (PGI June 2005)

a. Skin and superficial fascia
b. Deep fascia
c. Rectus abdominis
d. Transversus abdominis
e. Rectus sheath

Q3. Cancers associated with excess fat intake are/is: (PGI Dec 2000)

a. Breast b. Colon
c. Prostate d. Lung
e. Thyroid

Q4. Physiological changes seen in laparoscopy include all, *except*: (AIIMS May 2015)

a. Increased intracranial pressure (ICP)
b. Decreased functional residual capacity (FRC)
c. Increased central venous pressure (CVP)
d. Increased pH

Q5. Absorbable sutures are: (PGI 2004)

a. Catgut b. Silk
c. Polypropylene d. Polyglycolic acid
e. Vicryl

Grade II	Difficult

Q1. Complications of obesity is/are: (PGI Nov 2010)

a. Venous ulcer
b. Pulmonary embolism
c. Increase in mortality
d. Prostate cancer
e. Pulmonary hypertension

Q2. After a midline laparotomy, you have been asked to suture the incision. What length of suture will you choose? (AIIMS Nov 2016)

a. 2 × incision length
b. 4 × incision length
c. 6 × incision length
d. 8 × incision length

Q3. A woman presents with complete wound dehiscence 4 days after a laparotomy. After prescribing antibiotics for the infection, the surgeon decides to suture the wound. Which of these suture materials should he use? (AIIMS Nov 2016)

a. Vicryl b. Mersilk
c. Catgut d. Ethilon

Q4. Vicryl, the commonly used suture material, is a: (UPCS 2000)
a. Homopolymer of polydioxanone (PDS)
b. Copolymer of glycolide and lactide
c. Homopolymer of glycolide
d. Homopolymer of lactide

Q5. PDS is absorbed within: (WBPG 2012)
a. 7 days
b. 21 days
c. 100 days
d. 225 days

Grade III ***Most difficult***

Q1. Surgically used suture material PDS: (WBPG 2012)
a. Is nonabsorbable and remains encapsulated
b. Undergoes hydrolysis and complete absorption
c. Undergoes phagocytosis and enzymatic degradation
d. It is specifically used for the heart valves of synthetic grafts

Q2. Which one of the following is used as a preservative for packing catgut suture? (AIIMS Nov 2002)
a. Isopropyl alcohol
b. Colloidal iodine
c. Glutaraldehyde
d. Hydrogen peroxide

Q3. Which of the following is not true about the PDS suture? (APPG 2015)
a. It is a polymer of ether-ester units
b. It is biodegradable suture
c. It is completely absorbed in 9 months
d. Sterilized by ethylene oxide

Q4. True regarding 10-0 sutures is? (PGI May 2018)
a. Thicker than 1-0 sutures
b. Synthetic sutures
c. Diameter is 0.9 mm
d. Stronger than 1-0
e. All of the above

Q5. Intestinal anastomosis strength is provided by: (JIPMER 2015)
a. Mucosa
b. Submucosa
c. Serosa
d. Muscularis mucosa

ANSWERS

Grade I: 1. a, c, d; 2. a; 3. a, b, c; 4. d; 5. a, d, e

Grade II: 1. a, b, c, d, e; 2. b; 3. d; 4. b; 5. d

Grade III: 1. b; 2. a; 3. c; 4. b; 5. b

MODEL QUESTIONS

Q1. Irrespective of comorbidity, bariatric surgeries should be done when the body mass index (BMI) is greater than:
a. 35
b. 40
c. 45
d. 50

Ans. b

Q2. The most effective bariatric surgery with treatment in the form of weight loss for morbid obesity is:
a. Roux-en-Y surgery
b. Biliopancreatic diversion
c. Vertical banded gastroplasty
d. Any of the above

Ans. b

Q3. Bariatric surgery with maximum benefits and comorbidity reduction:
a. Roux-en-Y gastric bypass
b. Laparoscopic sleeve gastrectomy
c. Biliopancreatic diversion
d. Laparoscopic adjustable gastric banding

Ans. a

Q4. During laparoscopy, the intra-abdominal pressure is:
a. 5–10 mm Hg
b. 12–15 mm Hg
c. 15–20 mm Hg
d. 20–25 mm Hg

Ans. b

Q5. The instrument used to create artificial pneumoperitoneum in laparoscopy:
a. Maryland forceps
b. Veress needle
c. Trocar
d. All of the above

Ans. b

Q6. Complications of laparoscopy:
a. Diaphragmatic rupture
b. Vascular injury
c. Pneumothorax
d. All of the above

Ans. d

Q3. A robot was used for the first time for hip replacement in 1992. Name the robot:

a. PUMA 560 b. Da Vinci
c. Robodoc d. Probot

Ans. c

MULTIPLE CHOICE QUESTIONS

Grade I | *Simple*

Q1. The intra-abdominal pressure during laparoscopy should be set between: (AIIMS Nov 2003)?

a. 5 and 8 mm Hg b. 10 and 15 mm Hg
c. 20 and 25 mm Hg d. 30 and 35 mm Hg

Q2. Gases for pneumoperitoneum: (PGI June 2007)

a. CO_2 b. N_2
c. Room air d. N_2O

Grade II | *Difficult*

Q1. Which gas is used in laparoscopy? (AIIMS June 1994)

a. CO_2 b. N_2O
c. O_2 d. N_2

Q2. Layers that are penetrated with a trocar and a cannula in the production of pneumoperitoneum are: (PGI June 2005)

a. Skin and superficial fascia
b. Deep fascia
c. Rectus abdominis
d. Transversus abdominis

Grade III | *Most difficult*

Q1. Shoulder pain postlaparoscopy is due to: (AIIMS Nov 2007)

a. Subphrenic abscess
b. CO_2 retention
c. Positioning of the patient
d. Compression of the lung

Q2. Day care surgery can be done in: (PGI Nov 2010)

a. Lateral sphincterotomy
b. Rhinoplasty
c. Orchidectomy
d. Total thyroidectomy
e. Subcutaneous mastectomy

ANSWERS

Grade I: 1. b (Sabiston 20/e p394-396); 2. a, c, d (Schwartz 10/e p417-419)

Grade II: 1. a; 2. a

Grade III: 1. b; 2. a, b, c, e (Bailey 27/e p301)

MODEL QUESTIONS

Q1. In 1985, a robot was used for brain biopsy for the first time. Name the robot.

a. Da Vinci b. Robodoc
c. PUMA 560 d. Time robot

Ans. c

Q2. In 1988, a robot was used for the first time to do a prostatectomy. Name the robot.

a. Da Vinci b. Robodoc
c. Probot d. PUMA 560

Ans. c

Q3. The Da Vinci robot works on what principle?

a. Master-slave b. Mand-eye
c. Hand-instrument d. Eye-instrument

Ans. a

SUGGESTED READING

1. Bailey & Love's - Short Practice of Surgery, 27th edition.
2. Schwartz's Principles of Surgery, 18th edition.
3. Textbook of Surgery by David Sabiston, 21st edition.

Trauma

"Trauma originates from the Greek word meaning "wound." It implies that a physical force exerted on a person has led to a physical injury."

– Bailey & Love's Short Practice of Surgery, 27th edition

INTRODUCTION

The most common trauma happens in a war or a road traffic accident (RTA). The abbreviated injury scale (AIS) and injury severity score (ISS) explain the details about a trauma and its severity, and also categorize various injuries. Major trauma, which has injury severity scores >15, involves about 15% of all traumas.

Though the major proportion of injuries are not life-threatening, but they cause severe morbidity and man-hour loss. A moderate severity trauma can kill an elderly patient, but major trauma is the most common cause of death in young persons.

> *TRIAGE (The process was described in 1792 by Baron Dominique Jean Larrey, Surgeon in Chief to Napoleon's Imperial Guard, motto—"most for the most").*
> The word TRIAGE is derived from the French word "trier," meaning "to sort out." Triage categories can be divided according to color:
> 1 = Red—immediate medical need—critical
> 2 = Yellow—urgent—critical
> 3 = Green—nonurgent—stable
> 0 = Black—unsalvageable—no medical care can help

MANAGEMENT OF TRAUMA

There is a critical period of time in which the management intervention increases the success rate of healing and saving lives, this is the *"timeline principle."* The timeline principle also gives an indication about progress and requirements for improvement of management.

Advanced trauma life support (ATLS) is an internationally accepted way of treatment priorities where A stands for airway, B for breathing, C for circulation, and D for disability. The time to start treatment and the priority of treatment are the two most important factors in the management of a severely traumatized patient. ATLS guidelines advise primary survey, secondary survey, and tertiary survey. It was updated in 2018 (CRASH-2 Trial) with 1 giving only 1 L of isotonic crystalloid for adults, and in children <40 kg, give 20 mL/kg of warm isotonic crystalloid.

> *Mechanism of injury in obvious and concealed trauma is associated with time can help assess injuries and can improve survival in severe trauma cases.* A trauma mechanically can be a blunt injury caused by direct or indirect means, or it can be a penetrating injury caused by a sharp object. Sometimes, covert injuries are missed, such as splenic rupture and a duodenal rupture, due to a hurried examination and concentrating only on obvious injuries.

Penetrating injuries can extend very deep without any external appearance. Knowledge of the anatomy of the body part injured and the size of the object inflicted on the injury is important in not missing internal injury. Penetrating injuries can also be caused by firearms, called high-velocity projectile objects, such as bullets. In a case of criminal activity causing trauma, the patient may not be telling the truth, so the clinician has to think about *nonaccidental injury (NAI).*

In case of orthopedic injury, *"damage control orthopedic (DCO)"* is followed:

- *Resuscitation—control of bleeding—decompression—splintage.*

Unnecessary delay in starting the treatment is an important part of timeline management.

TRIMODAL MORTALITY MODEL FOR TRAUMA

- *Immediate death*—within minutes—declared dead or shortly after arriving at the hospital.

- *Early death*—within hours after arrival at the hospital. Due to internal or intracranial hemorrhage/tension pneumothorax/cardiac tamponade.
- *Late death*—within days to weeks after trauma—multiple organic failure syndrome (MOFS)/sepsis.

SURVEYS AFTER TRAUMA

Primary survey—immediately, simultaneously, the survey and treatment of life-threatening trauma is done. ABCDE

Secondary survey—head to toe survey with history of *AMPLE (A = Allergies, M = Medication, P = Past illness, L = Last meal, E = Events related to injury)*

Tertiary survey—usually done after 24 hours, includes physical examination and imaging [X-ray/computed tomography (CT)].

Always remember that timeline philosophy is essential for the patient's fate in cases of major trauma.
Always look and search for hidden trauma, such as penetrating injuries and concealed hematomas, without wasting much time. Rapidly survey, identify, and treat life-threatening injuries fast to save lives.

The risk of mortality from bleeding in major trauma cases can be reduced by quick assessment, arresting hemorrhage, and giving *tranexamic acid*. It is given as 1 gm IV over 10 minutes, then 1 g is given at every 8 hours. It is better to give *tranexamic acid* in every case of moderate or major trauma within a period of 3 hours. *Tranexamic acid* diminishes mortality after severe trauma.

Whole body computed tomography (WBCT) scan is an important investigation in a major trauma case, especially in blunt injury. It covers the body from head to pelvis and is the gold standard investigation of severely traumatized patients. *WBCT should be done as soon as possible in case of major trauma.*

Trauma care has changed a lot in the present decade. It is now abbreviated as *cABCDE:*

- *c* = Control of massive external hemorrhage
- *A* = Airway
- *B* = Breathing
- *C* = Circulation
- *D* = Disability
- *E* = Exposure

Nowadays management of an injured patient must cover in first 36 hours, the damage control surgery having simultaneous resuscitation and life-limb saving procedure. The investigations which may take time such as CT scan can be postponed. Log roll and pelvic binder must be used during transfer of a severely injured patient.

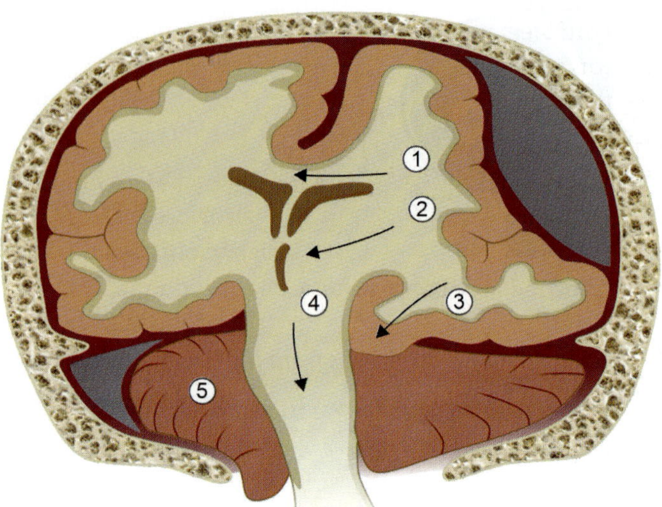

Fig. 1: Brain herniation. 1. Subfalcine herniation: Cingulate gyrus displacement under the falx cerebri; 2. Midline shift: Displacement of brain structures away from the central axis; 3. Uncal herniation: Herniation of the uncus of the temporal lobe, compressing the ipsilateral third cranial nerve; 4. Central herniation: Displacement of brain structures toward the brainstem, causing compression; and 5. Tonsillar herniation: Herniation of cerebellar tonsils, applying pressure to brainstem structures.

In head injuries, cerebral perfusion is the most important factor. Increased *intracranial pressure (ICP)* can interfere with cerebral perfusion, leading to secondary cerebral injury. Cranium is a bony cage with having the brain, fluids [*cerebrospinal fluid (CSF)*], and blood. Collection of blood or swelling of brain tissue after injury to the cranium can increase ICP. Prolonged raised ICP can cause herniation **(Fig. 1)** of part of the cerebrum and cerebellum (uncus of the temporal lobe), cerebellar tonsil, leading to pressure on vasomotor and respiratory centers, causing a combination of three features called *Cushing's triad (hypertension, bradycardia, and irregular respiration).*

GLASGOW COMA SCALE (GCS)

It was started in 1974. *Glasgow coma scale (GCS)* scale depends upon the *best eye response (E), best verbal response (V), and best motor response (M),* the best eye response score is 1-4, best verbal response score is 1-5 and best motor response score is 1-6. *Best eye response* 1—no eye opening, 2—eye opening in response to pain, 3—eye opening in response to speech, 4—spontaneously opening eyes. *Best verbal response* 1—none, 2—incomprehensible sounds, 3—inappropriate words,

4—confused, 5—oriented. *Best motor response* 1—no motor response, 2—extension in response to pain, 3—flexion in response to pain, 4—withdrawal of limb from pain, 5—localizes the site of pain, 6—obeys all commands. In 2014 revised GCS was given.

Layers of the scalp:
Mn = SCALP

- *S* = Skin
- *C* = Connected tissue
- *A*= Aponeurosis
- *L* = Loose areolar tissue
- *P* = Periosteum

FRACTURES OF SKULL

- Nondepressed
- Depressed

Noncontrast computed tomography (NCCT) is a must for scalp injuries. Elevation and fixation of the depressed fracture bone are required if there is a neurological science.

Fractures of the base of the skull can be divided into anterior (cribriform plate), middle (petrous part of the temporal bone), and posterior (occipital bone) according to the site of fracture. Significant signs clinically localized the site of injury as anterior fractures usually have a black eye, middle fractures have a battle sign, CSF otorrhea, and temporal lobe contusions, and posterior injuries have visual problems due to occipital lobe injury.

PRIMARY BRAIN INJURY

It can be a mild injury, concussion, or a severe type of injury, diffuse axonal injury (DAI). Concussion is usually caused by injuries during sports and DAI is caused by high velocity injuries. NCCT differentiates these injuries. Craniotomy is indicated if the clot size due to intracranial hemorrhage is >30 cc or there is >5 mm midline shift or >1.5 cm is the thickness of the blood clot.

CLASSIFICATION OF HEAD INJURY ACCORDING TO GLASGOW COMA SCALE

Glasgow coma scale scoring can divide the severity of head injury into four categories. (1) GCS 3-8—severe head injury, (2) GCS 9-13—moderate head injury, (3) GCS 14-15—with loss of consciousness (LOC)-mild head injury, and (4) GCS 15 without LOC—minor head injury.

KERNOHAN WOLTMAN NOTCH PHENOMENON

It is a supratentorial brain lesion causing pressure on the contralateral cerebral peduncle against the free edge of the tentorium of the cerebellum. There are neurological signs of ipsilateral localization.

SECONDARY BRAIN INJURY

It is caused by a rise in intracranial tension (ICT). *Mean arterial pressure (MAP)* and ICP are increasing, causing high systolic blood pressure (BP) with a reduction in heart rate (*Cushing's reflex*). Cushing's ulcers, and stress ulcers in acid-producing areas of the stomach also develop.

Oxygenation, adequate perfusion, IV mannitol, and elevation of the head are required. Dextrose solution should be avoided as it increases cerebral edema. Steroids have no role as they increase ICT.

BATTLE'S (WILLIAM HENRY BATTLE, 1855–1936, BRITISH SURGEON) SIGN

There is bruising over the region of the mastoid process of the temporal bone on the side of the fracture of the base of the skull. Battle's sign indicates a fracture of the base of the skull.

Severity Scores

- *I*njury severity score (ISS)
- *R*evised trauma score (RTS)
- *T*rauma score and injury severity score (TRISS)
- *M*angled extremity severity score (MESS)

EXTRADURAL HEMATOMA

It happens in a head injury case with a probable skull fracture leading to the rupture of an artery, vein, or venous sinus. It can follow after a minor trauma. There is a lucid period in which the patient may complain of headache and talk, but later on, *LOC* develops as the intracranial hematoma enlarges. CT scan of the brain shows a lentiform lesion.

ACUTE SUBDURAL HEMATOMA

It happens due to high-energy injury of the brain, leading to rapid LOC and increased ICP. It is commonly seen in elderly patients. It is an emergency and requires rapid and urgent surgery for evacuation of the hematoma (craniotomy).

CHRONIC SUBDURAL HEMATOMA

It is a common problem in elderly patients. It causes neurological deterioration suddenly. Hematoma gradually increases and raises ICP. It commonly happens in patients who have blood thinners and have a recent history of injury. It is treated by Burr hole drainage. Secondary brain injury can raise ICP, which interferes with cerebral perfusion.

SPINAL CORD INJURY

The Asia neurological impairment scale is used for assessment of spinal cord injury (ABCDE, A = Complete spinal cord injury, whereas E = Normal function).

HANGMAN'S FRACTURE (TRAUMATIC SPONDYLOLISTHESIS OF AXIS)

This happens between the C2 and C3 vertebrae.

MAXILLARY FRACTURES

Rene Le Fort (Rene Le Fort, 1869–1951, French Surgeon by dropping heavy objects on the face of cadavers) described maxillary fractures into three types, Le Fort 1 (lower level), Le Fort 2 (midlevel) and Le Fort 3 (upper level).

NECK TRAUMA

The neck is divided into three zones **(Fig. 2)**:

1. *Zone I:* From the thoracic inlet to the cricoid cartilage.
2. *Zone II:* Cricoid cartilage to angle of mandible.
3. *Zone III:* Angle of the mandible to the base of the skull.

Zone I injuries have a maximum mortality rate. Surgical intervention is required if air is coming out of the wound or there is emphysema or the neck hematoma is expanding.

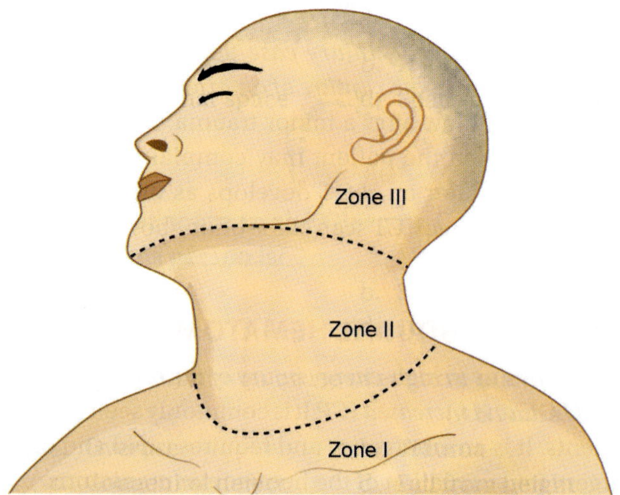

Fig. 2: Zones of the neck.

LEMON ASSESSMENT

Lemon assessment is used in the case of a difficult airway for assessment for intubation.

- *L* = Look externally
- *E* = Elevate—3-3-2 rule (three fingers in mouth, three fingers between hyoid bone and chin, and two fingers between thyroid notch and floor of mouth)
- *M* = Mallampati classification
- *O* = Look for obstruction
- *N* = Neck, spine tenderness

The Mallampati score is named after an Indian anesthesiologist, Seshagiri Mallampati. It is used to predict the ease of endotracheal intubation.

Deadly triad:
In the case of major trauma, a triad of the following features can lead to increased mortality:
- Hypothermia
- Acidosis
- Coagulopathy

PERICARDIAL TAMPONADE

It happens due to a penetrating injury of the chest. Clinically simulates tension pneumothorax by causing cyanosis and tachycardia.

TENSION PNEUMOTHORAX

It is usually caused by a penetrating wound on the chest wall or a big lung injury causing an air leak. It develops tachypnea, tachycardia, high *jugular venous pressure (JVP)*, low cardiac output, and low systolic BP **(Fig. 3)**. It is treated with needle insertion in the fifth intercostals space in the midaxillary line during an emergency. Ultimately, a chest tube in a triangle of safety is introduced **(Fig. 4)**.

FLAIL CHEST

When severe blunt injury to the chest causes multiple fractures in the ribs, with three or more ribs fractured in two or more places, there happens a paradoxical movement of the chest wall of the injured area. There is almost always an underlying lung contusion. On inspiration, the fractured part of the chest moves in, and on expiration, moves out (paradoxical respiration). Surgery to stabilize the injured chest wall is not always required.

CARDIAC TAMPONADE

It usually follows a penetrating trauma, which leads to a collection of blood in the pericardial cavity. Its clinical features are similar to the clinical features of tension

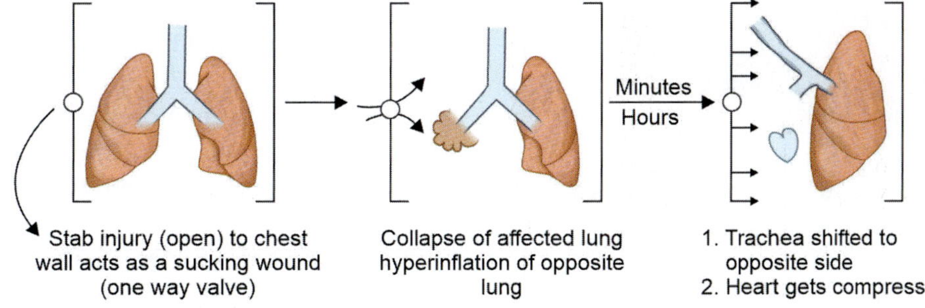

Fig. 3: Mechanism of tension pneumothorax.

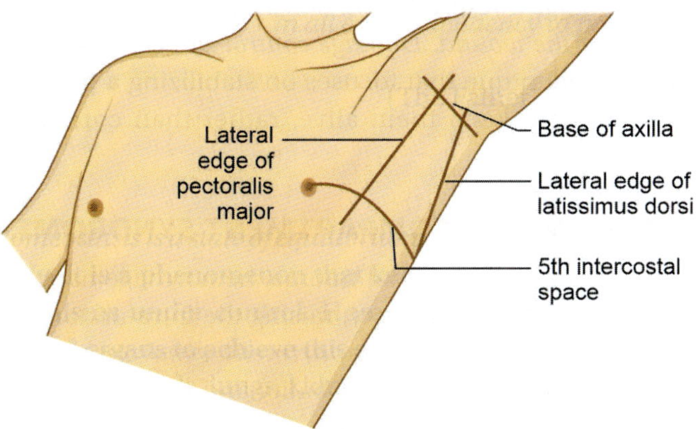

Fig. 4: Triangle of safety.

pneumothorax. Beck's triad is a term given to three clinical signs associated with acute cardiac tamponade. *The triad was first described by Claude Beck, an American Cardiothoracic surgeon, in 1935.* The triad includes low BP, distention of the jugular veins, and muffled or diminished heart sounds on cardiac auscultation.

DIAPHRAGMATIC INJURIES

These injuries are more common in penetrating trauma more than in blunt trauma. The right side of the diaphragm has less chance of injury due to the presence of the liver. Repair of the diaphragm with the introduction of a chest tube is the treatment.

FOCUSED ABDOMINAL SONAR FOR TRAUMA (FAST)

It is used to detect the presence of free fluid in a cavity, such as the peritoneal chest and pericardium. eFAST is a rapid fast that can be performed bedside of the patient. It cannot detect free fluid measuring <100 mL. It usually cannot identify hollow organ injury. The FAST should check the epigastrium, *right upper quadrant (RUQ), left upper quadrant (LUQ)*, and suprapubic region in an abdominal injury case.

Diagnostic Peritoneal Lavage

A needle with a syringe is inserted in all the quadrants of the abdomen; if blood is aspirated, it is called positive *diagnostic peritoneal lavage (DPL)*. If no aspirant is found, introduced Ringer's lactate solution 1 L through the same needle and then aspirate again. If RBCs > 100,000/mm^3, then it is positive DPL. Treatment of positive DPL is midline laparotomy. Criteria for positive DPL are blood aspiration, presence of fecal content in the aspirant, serum amylase >175 IU/L, >500 WBC/mm^3, and RBC 100,000/mm^3.

Liver injuries:
Liver trauma can be classified into five grades:
1. *Grade I:* Hematoma, subcapsular, and laceration.
2. *Grade II:* Subcapsular hematoma 10–50% of surface area. Laceration 1–3 cm depth.
3. *Grade III:* Hematoma >50% surface area. Laceration >3 cm depth.
4. *Grade IV:* Laceration 25–75% liver lobe involved. Active bleeding due to blood vessel injury.
5. *Grade V:* Laceration >75% surface area, liver lobe involved. Major venous injury.

Liver injuries cause severe bleeding. The 4Ps are remembered: (1) Push, (2) plug, (3) pack, and (4) Pringle maneuver.

Pringle (James Hogarth Pringle, 1863–1941, Australian-born British Surgeon) maneuver
Liver bleeding can be quickly controlled in a case of trauma or an elective open surgery. Either Pringle's maneuver uses fingers in open surgery or a vascular plan. A finger or one jaw of the vascular clamp is inserted into the foramen of Winslow, and the vascular pedicle containing the bile duct, hepatic artery, and portal vein are pressed **(Fig. 5)**. Compression is done for 10–20 minutes with 5 minutes release.

In a case of major liver trauma, the hepatic artery can be ligated but portal vein cannot be ligated, it should be treated by placing a stent. After major liver trauma peritoneal cavity must always be drained by putting a closed suction drainage. *American Association for the Surgery of Trauma (AAST) Organ Injury Scale (OIS)* gives guidelines to grade and manage the liver trauma.

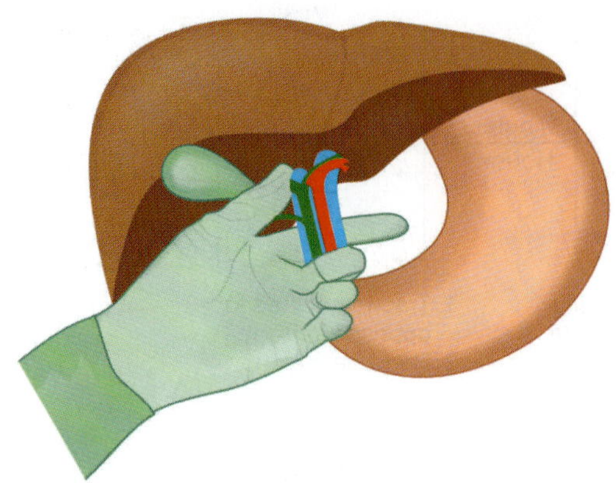

Fig. 5: The index finger is in the foramen of Winslow and the Thumb is ready to pinch the porta hepatis against the index finger.

Severe liver trauma to be resuscitated → unstable → operation → remains stable → discharge

INJURY TO THE MESENTERY

Usually, the mesenteric injury is caused by severe trauma to the abdomen or a severe jolt in RTA. It can be a longitudinal tear or a transverse tear involving many vessels.

DUODENAL INJURY

Duodenal injury can be only a hematoma or a duodenal perforation. It is a common injury in seat belt syndrome. These should be treated accordingly by conservative surgical treatment.

PANCREATIC INJURY

It is usually caused by a penetrating trauma or a major blunt trauma to the abdomen. Treat conservatively if the main pancreatic duct is not injured. If the body and tail of the pancreas are injured, then distal removal of the pancreas is advised. *Beger's procedure (preservation of the duodenum with the removal of the head of the pancreas) is advised in case of injury to the head and neck of the pancreas.*

COLON AND RECTUM INJURY

In case of perforation, peritonitis develops, which requires laparotomy and may lead to a Hartmann procedure or a colostomy.

RETROPERITONEAL INJURY

It is usually gets neglected in a severely injured person as it is difficult to diagnose and the attention of the clinician is directed toward visible injuries. The retroperitoneal injuries can be divided into three zones: Zone 1—central, Zone 2—lateral, and Zone 3—pelvic. Retroperitoneal injuries should be explored only if the hematoma is expanding and is pulsatile. *Zone 4 is the least well-defined zone, and it contains great vessels.*

DAMAGE CONTROL SURGERY

It is a process that is done in various stages. *Stage 1 selection of patient, stage 2 bleeding control and contamination control. Stage 3 resuscitation, Stage 4 surgery, and Stage 5 closure of the wound. Damage control surgery (DCS)* is a surgical technique that focuses on stabilizing a patient's physiology to keep them alive, rather than correcting anatomy.

ABDOMINAL COMPARTMENT SYNDROME

When in major abdominal trauma, hemorrhage happens inside the abdominal cavity, raising the intra-abdominal pressure, *abdominal compartment syndrome (ACS)* develops. ACS increases morbidity and mortality unless urgent intervention is not done.

DEBRIDEMENT

Debridement, meaning in French, means to unleash or cut open. Wounds of war and RTA are usually contaminated, so the basics of debridement are:

- Remove contaminants
- Remove dead tissues
- Repair major vessels
- Identify tendons and nerves that are severed, to be labeled.
- Do not close the wound with loose dressings and limb elevation.

CRUSH SYNDROME

Crush syndrome is usually associated with crush injury of tissues, lysis of skeletal muscles, and acute renal trauma that leads to kidney failure.

COMPARTMENT SYNDROME

It is produced when a compartment of muscle has injured and bleeding, with swelling of tissues increasing the pressure in that compartment, leading to pressure on the surrounding structure. Fasciotomy is performed earliest.

FROST BITE

It is also called Trench's foot. It is a variety of cold burns. It is produced by continuous exposure to extreme cold. It is like a burn. Slow warning softly and gently can protect the limb.

Rapid surveys to be done to find out the cause of the life-threatening hemorrhage. There are five major sites to search:

- Extreme hemorrhage
- Thorax
- Abdomen
- Retroperitoneal area
- Multiple long bone fractures

SPLENIC TRAUMA

Management

- *Unstable patient:* Focused Assessment with Sonography for Trauma (FAST)-Exploratory laparotomy
- *Stable patient:* FAST-CT-Grade I, II, III (observe), IV, V (exploratory laparotomy and splenectomy)

Management of Splenic Trauma

Spleen organ injury scale:

- *Grade I:* Hematoma subcapsular tear <10%, laceration capsular tear <1 cm.
- *Grade II:* Hematoma subcapsular tear 10–50%, laceration capsular tear 1–3 cm.
- *Grade III:* Hematoma subcapsular tear >50%, laceration capsular tear >3 cm.
- *Grade IV:* Laceration capsular tear >25% spleen.
- *Grade V:* Hematoma—completely shattered. Laceration—hilar vascular injury.

Penetrating Abdominal Trauma

- Gunshot—exploratory laparotomy—shock/peritonitis
- *Stab:*
    - Shock/peritonitis
    - Explore locally and repair. If the peritoneum is open, then an exploratory laparotomy is required.

Blunt Trauma Abdomen

- *Patient unstable:* FAST—exploratory laparotomy
- *Patient stable:* FAST-CECT
    - Hollow viscus injury—exploratory laparotomy
    - Solid organ injury—query exploratory laparotomy

Moore's Classification of Liver Trauma

- *Grade I:* Hematoma <10% of surface area, laceration <1 cm in parenchyma.
- *Grade II:* Hematoma 10–50% of surface, laceration 1–3 cm
- *Grade III:* Hematoma >50% of surface, laceration >3 cm
- *Grade IV:* Laceration 25–75% of hepatic lobe
- *Grade V:* Laceration >75% of hepatic lobe—Juxta hepatic venous injuries
- *Grade VI:* Vascular—hepatic avulsions

Liver Trauma

- *Unstable patient:* FAST—exploratory laparotomy
- *Stable patient:* FAST-CT—Grade I, II (observe), III, IV, V, and VI (exploratory laparotomy)

Important Points to be Remembered in Major Trauma

- X-rays of two important sites to be done, i.e., chest and pelvis.
- The best indicator for tissue perfusion is urine output.
- The best indicator for fluid requirement is CVP.
- Tranexamic acid is to be given in a hypotensive trauma patient. 1 g IV over 10 minutes, then 1 g 8 hourly. It should begin within 3 hours of trauma.
- For a log roll, ideally, five persons are required.
- Trauma society systems are Reviewed Trans Score (RTS), Trauma and Injury Severity Score (TRISS), and Mangled Extremity Severity Score (MESS).
- The most common organs injured in blunt trauma of the abdomen are splenic/liver.
- The most common organs injured in penetrating trauma are the liver/stomach, small intestine.
- The most common organ injured in seat belt syndrome is the mesentery
- The first investigation in blunt trauma abdomen is FAST.
- FAST-USG performed within 2–4 minutes, 4P to see: Pericardial sac/perihepatic/perisplenic/pelvis.

SUGGESTED READING

1. Mallampati SR, Gatt SP, Gugino LD, Desai SP, Waraksa B, Freiberger D, Liu PL. A clinical sign to predict difficult tracheal intubation: A prospective study. Can Anesth Soc J. 1985;32(4):429-34.

SOME IMPORTANT QUESTIONS

Q1. An initial fluid of choice in the treatment of hypovolemia in patients presenting after trauma is:

a. Colloid
b. Blood
c. Plasma expanders
d. Crystalloid

Ans. d

Q2. Which one of the following veins should be avoided for intravenous (IV) infusion in the management of abdominal trauma?

a. Cubital
b. Cephalic
c. Long saphenous
d. External jugular

Ans. c

Q3. With blunt trauma all over the body, the amount of N2 and nitrogen end products lost/day:

a. 35 g
b. 55 g
c. 75 g
d. 15 g

Ans. a

Q4. A 30-year-old patient person met with a road traffic accident (RTA). On admission, his pulse rate was 120/min, BP 100/60 mm Hg. Ultrasonography examination revealed laceration of the lower pole of the spleen and hemoperitoneum. He was resuscitated with blood and fluid. 2 hours later, his pulse was 84/min and BP was 120/70 mm Hg. The most appropriate course of management in this case would be:

a. Exploring the patient followed by splenectomy
b. Exploring the patient, followed by excision of the lower pole of the spleen
c. Splenorrhaphy
d. Continuation of conservative treatment under a close monitoring system and subsequent surgery if further indicated

Ans. d

Q5. FAST stands for:

a. Focused abdominal sonography for trauma
b. Fast assessment with sonography for trauma
c. Focused assessment with sonography for trauma
d. Fast abdominal sonography for trauma

Ans. c

Q6. Treatment of choice for stab injury cecum:

a. Cecostomy
b. Ileotransverse anastomosis
c. Transverse colostomy
d. Sigmoid colostomy

Ans. b

Q7. A 17-year-old boy is admitted to the hospital after an RTA. Per abdomen examination is normal. After adequate resuscitation, his pulse rate is 80/min and his BP is 110/70 mm Hg. Abdominal computed tomography (CT) reveals a 1 cm deep laceration in the left lobe of the liver extending from the dome more than halfway through the parenchyma. Appropriate management at this time would be:

a. Conservative treatment
b. Abdominal exploration and packing of hepatic wounds
c. Abdominal exploration and ligation of the left hepatic artery
d. Left hepatectomy

Ans. b

Q8. Abdominal compartment syndrome (ACS) is characterized by the following, *except*:

a. Hypercarbia and respiratory acidosis
b. Hypoxia due to increased peak inspiratory pressure
c. Hypotension due to a decrease in venous return
d. Oliguria due to ureter obstruction

Ans. d

Q9. All of the following are indications of a CT scan in a head-injured patient, *except*?

a. Glasgow Coma Scale (GCS) <13
b. Vomiting 1 episode
c. Focal neurological deficit
d. Head injury in patients aged >65 years.

Ans. b

Q10. Protein metabolism after trauma is characterized by the following, *except*:

a. Increased liver gluconeogenesis
b. Inhibition of skeletal muscle breakdown by interleukin 1 and tumor necrosis factor
c. Increased urinary nitrogen loss
d. Hepatic synthesis of acute-phase reactants

Ans. b

MULTIPLE CHOICE QUESTIONS

Grade I	Simple

Q1. To carry traumatized and conscious patients, all the following are done, *except*: (AIIMS Nov 2017)

a. In a lateral lying position
b. Talk to a patient while he is on board
c. Rolling without moving the spine
d. On a hard board with head/spine stabilized

Q2. The first step was taken in case of multiple injuries of the face and neck: (AIIMS June 1995)

a. Blood transfusion
b. Intravenous (IV) fluids
c. Reconstruction
d. Maintenance of the airway

Q3. In a trauma patient with neck pain who is hemodynamically stable with normal vitals, which of the following is the best statement regarding neck imaging? (AIIMS May 2017)

a. The doctor should order a cervical X-ray and accompany and transfer the patient himself.
b. Send the patient for an X-ray on the same trolley with neck collar support and stabilization.
c. The patient should not be shifted for an X-ray.
d. X-ray cervical spine anteroposterior (AP) and lateral view is required.

Q4. In surgical stress, all hormones are increased, *except*: (PGI June 2009)

a. Adrenaline
b. Adrenocorticotropic hormone (ACTH)
c. Epinephrine
d. Cortisol
e. Insulin

Q5. A school bus with children meets with an accident. You rush to the accident site. Which one will you attend first and give priority to? (AIIMS Nov 2017)

a. Airway obstruction child
b. Boy who has shock
c. Falil chest child
d. Severe head injury

Q6. Which color of triage is given the highest priority? (AIIMS Nov 2013)

a. Green
b. Black
c. Yellow
d. Red

Q7. Which of the following triage categories are correctly matched? (AIIMS 2017)

a. RED—deceased/dead
b. BLACK—minor injuries
c. GREEN—immediate intervention needed
d. YELLOW—serious patient

Q8. Trauma and injury severity score (TRISS) includes: (All India 2010)

a. GCS +BP+ RR
b. RTS + ISS + AGE
c. RTS + ISS + GCS
d. RTS +GCS + Age

Q9. Blunt injury abdomen, the patient was hemodynamically stable, next investigations: (AIIMS Nov 2009)

a. X-ray abdomen
b. Barium swallow
c. Focused assessment with sonography for trauma (FAST)
d. Diagnostic peritoneal lavage (DPL)

Q10. A male patient with blunt trauma abdomen is hemodynamically stable. What is the next line of management? (All India 2008)

a. Observation
b. Further imaging of the abdomen
c. Exploratory laparotomy
d. Laparoscopy

Q11. Indications of celiotomy in blunt trauma: (PGI June 2009)

a. Grade I spleen damage
b. Grade II Liver damage
c. Peritoneal air om imaging
d. Positive DPL
e. Severe hypotension

Q12. A case of blunt trauma is brought to the emergency, in a state of shock; he is not responding to IV crystalloids. The next step in his management would be: (All India 2001)

a. Immediate laparotomy
b. Blood transfusion
c. Albumin transfusion
d. Abdominal compression

Q13. The preferred incision for abdominal exploration in blunt injury abdomen is: (All India 2007)

a. Always midline incision
b. Depending upon the organ

c. Transverse incision
d. Paramedian

Q14. A child presents in the casualty in stable condition after a blunt abdominal trauma associated with splenic trauma. Treatment of choice: (AIIMS Nov 2000)

a. Observation
b. Splenectomy
c. Arterial embolization
d. Splenorrhaphy

Q15. A 30-year-old gentleman after sustaining an RTA present in an emergency with BP of 100/60 mm Hg, pulse 120/min, and CT shows splenic laceration at the inferior border, after 2 units of blood transfusion, the patient's condition are BP 120/70 mm Hg and pulse 84/min; next line of management is: (PGI June 2003)

a. Laparotomy
b. Splenorrhaphy
c. Continue the conservative treatment and take subsequent measures on monitoring the patient
d. Splenectomy
e. X-ray abdomen and aspiration

Q16. A 27-year-old patient presented with left-sided abdominal pain 6 hours after RTA. He was hemodynamically stable and FAST positive. The CT scan showed grade III splenic injury. What will be the appropriate treatment? (All India 2010)

a. Splenectomy
b. Splenorrhaphy
c. Splenic artery embolization
d. Conservative management

Q17. Management of grade III splenic trauma in a stable child: (PGI Nov 2010)

a. Embolization
b. Conservative
c. Partial splenectomy
d. Total splenectomy

Q18. A 27-year-old patient presented with left-sided abdominal pain 6 hours after RTA. He was hemodynamically stable and FAST positive. CT scan showed grade III splenic injury with contrast blush. What will be the appropriate treatment? (All India 2010)

a. Splenectomy
b. Splenorrhaphy
c. Splenic artery embolization
d. Conservative management

Q19. Following a major trauma, a patient presented 54 hours later with raised jugular venous pressure (JVP) and central venous pressure (CVP) of 16 mm Hg and persistent hypertension. The most probable diagnosis is: (PGI Dec 2000)

a. Tension pneumothorax
b. Cardiac tamponade
c. Head injury
d. Splenic trauma
e. Air embolism

Q20. The physical finding most likely to differentiate cardiac tamponade from tension pneumothorax is: (AIIMS Nov 2018)

a. Absent breath sounds
b. Raised JVP
c. Increased heart rate
d. Hypotension

Q21. Sitaram, a 40-year-old man, met with an accident and came to the emergency department with engorged neck veins, pallor, rapid pulse, and chest pain. Diagnosis is: (AIIMS June 1999)

a. Pulmonary laceration
b. Cardiac tamponade
c. Hemothorax
d. Splenic rupture

Q22. Treatment of acutely developing massive left-sided hemothorax in a young male after an accident is: (AIIMS Nov 1993)

a. Strapping off chest
b. Tube thoracostomy
c. Endotracheal intubation + intermittent positive pressure ventilation (IPPV) + pleural fluid aspiration
d. Conservative, wait, and watch

Q23. Which of the following is true about the rupture of the diaphragm? (PGI Dec 2008)

a. Chest X-ray
b. DPL
c. Repair by laparotomy
d. Laparoscopy

Q24. Aim of abbreviated laparotomy: (PGI June 2005)

a. Decreased chance of infection
b. Early ambulation
c. Early wound healing

Q25. Abbreviated laparotomy was done for: (PGI Dec 2007)

a. Coagulopathy
b. Hypotension
c. Early wound healing
d. Early ambulation
e. Hemostasis

Q26. The second phase of damage control surgery is done at: (AIIMS May 2018)

a. Prehospital setting
b. In emergency bay
c. In the intensive care unit (ICU)
d. In the operation theatre

Q27. The aim of damage control laparotomy are: (PGI June 2009)

a. Arrest hemorrhage
b. Prevent coagulopathy
c. Control contamination
d. Provide fascial closure
e. Prevent infection

Q28. Which of the following is true about damage control surgery? (AIIMS May 2013)

a. Steps done to control damage during surgery
b. Corrective surgery for iatrogenic injuries
c. Complete repair of injuries done after initial resuscitation in trauma patients
d. Minimal intervention was done to stabilize the patient and do the definitive surgery later

Q29. A fractured mandible with an edentulous Jaw is best treated with: (UPPG 2004)

a. External fixator
b. Minerva plaster
c. Interdental wiring
d. Intermaxillary elastic traction

Q30. The best view for mandible is: (UPPG 2007)

a. Antero posterior b. Lateral
c. Oblique d. Orthopantomogram

Q31. A patient of a motor vehicle accident was admitted to the casualty department. His eyes are closed but open to pain. He does not speak but moans every now and then. His right limb is not moving, but he localizes toward a painful stimulus with the left limb; both limbs are in extended posture. What will be the GCS score? (AIIMS May 2017)

a. 9 b. 11
c. 5 d. 7

Grade II	Difficult

Q1. In severe injury, the first to be maintained is: (PGI JUNE 1997)

a. Hypotension b. Dehydration
c. Airway d. Cardiac status

Q2. A patient presents in an emergency with a cervical spine fracture. The first thing to do is: (AIIMS Nov 1999)

a. Locate the fracture by shifting the patient side to side
b. X-ray of spine
c. Clear the airway and intubate him
d. Immobilize the cervical spine

Q3. A man with a blunt injury abdomen after a roadside accident has a blood pressure (BP) of 100/80 mm Hg and a pulse rate of 120 beats/min. The airway has been established, and respiration has been stabilized. The next best step in management is. (All India 2009)

a. Immediate blood transfusion
b. Blood for the cross-matching and IV fluids
c. Ventilate the patient
d. Rush the patient to the operation table (OT)

Q4. A patient is brought to the casualty with severe hypotension following an RTA. No external injury is evident. The cause of hypotension is: (AIIMS June 2001)

a. Fracture rib
b. Intrathoracic and abdominal bleed
c. Iatrogenic shock
d. Intracranial bleed

Q5. The early stage of trauma is characterized by: (All India 2003)

a. Catabolism b. Anabolism
c. Glycogenesis d. Lipogenesis

Q6. Mangled Extremity Severity Score (MESS) includes all of the following, *except*? (AIIMS May 2011)

a. Shock
b. Ischemia
c. Neurogenic injury
d. Energy of injury

Q7. Which one of the following is not a part of the revised trauma score: (UPSC 2001)

a. Glasgow coma scale b. Systolic BP
c. Pulse rate d. Respiratory rate

Q8. The best prognostic factor for head injury is: (AIIMS May 2010)

a. Glasgow coma scale b. Age
c. Mode of injury d. CT

Q9. MC (Most Common) abdominal organ injured in blunt trauma to the abdomen is: (PGI Dec 1999)

a. Spleen
b. Liver
c. Pancreas
d. Stomach

Q10. Commonly injured in blunt abdominal injury is/are: (PGI June 2006)

a. Midileum
b. Proximal jejunum
c. Mid jejunum
d. Distal ileum
e. Ileocecal junction

Q11. The organ most commonly damaged in a penetrating injury of the abdomen is: (AIIMS Nov 1995)

a. Liver
b. Small intestine
c. Large intestine
d. Duodenum

Q12. A man comes to the emergency department with a stab injury to the left flank. He has stable vitals. What would be the next step in management? (AIIMS Nov 2008)

a. Contrast-enhanced computed tomography (CECT)
b. DPL
c. Laparotomy
d. Laparoscopy

Q13. Which of the following statements related to gastric injury is not true? (All India 2007)

a. Mostly related to penetrating trauma
b. Treatment is simple debridement and suturing
c. Blood in the stomach is always related to gastric injury
d. Heals well and fast

Q14. A young patient presents with a massive injury to the proximal duodenum, head of the pancreas, and distal common bile duct. The procedure of choice for this patient should be: (All India 2008)

a. Roux-en-Y anastomosis
b. Pancreaticoduodenectomy (Whipple's operation)
c. Lateral tube jejunostomy
d. Retrograde jejunostomy

Q15. A man presented with features of the 4th–10th ribs and respiratory distress after an RTA. He is diagnosed to have a flail chest and an arterial partial pressure of oxygen (PaO_2) of <60%. Management is: (AIIMS June 2001)

a. Tracheostomy
b. Intermittent positive pressure ventilation (IPPV) with oral intubation
c. Fixation of ribs
d. Strapping of the chest

Q16. A man is brought to the casualty department who met with an RTA. He sustained multiple rib fractures with paradoxical movement of the chest. Management is: (PGI June 2006)

a. Tracheostomy
b. Consult a cardiothoracic surgeon
c. Strapping
d. Intermittent positive pressure ventilation
e. No intervention required

Q17. Which of the following is considered balanced resuscitation? (AIIMS Nov 2017)

a. Giving colloids any crystalloids ratio of 1:1
b. Maintaining pH by ensuring acid–base are balanced
c. Maintaining permissible hypotension to avoid bleeding
d. Maintaining airway, breathing, and circulation

Q18. True about intra-ACS: (PGI June 2004)

a. Intra-abdominal pressure >15 cmH_2O
b. Pneumoperitoneum can produce it
c. Increase in renal blood flow
d. Decrease in venous return
e. Increase in central blood volume

Q19. Increased intra-abdominal pressure is/are associated with: (PGI June 2004)

a. Increase in pulmonary capillary wedge pressure
b. Increase in venous return
c. Increase in Pulmonary inspiratory pressure
d. Increase in renal blood flow
e. Increase in cardiac output

Q20. True about ACS: (PGI June 2004)

a. Decrease in cardiac output
b. Decrease in pulmonary capillary wedge pressure
c. Decrease in venous return
d. Decrease in systemic vascular resistance
e. Urine output

Q21. After 4 weeks of head trauma, the patient presents with features of irritability and altered sensorium. The most common cause will be: (AIIMS Nov 2000)

a. Chronic subdural hematoma (SDH)

b. Extradural hematoma
c. Intraparenchymal bleed
d. Electrolyte imbalance

Q22. After a head injury, a biconvex, lenticular-shaped hematoma in a CT scan is characteristic of which of the following? (AIIMS June 1999)
a. Extradural hemorrhage
b. Subdural hemorrhage
c. Intracerebral hematoma
d. Diffuse-axonal injury

Q23. Which of the following is the most common source of extradural hemorrhage? (AIIMS Nov 1998)
a. Middle meningeal artery
b. Subdural venous sinus
c. Charcot's artery
d. Middle cerebral artery

Q24. A male was brought unconscious to the hospital with external injuries. CT brain showed no midline shift, but basal cisterns were compressed with multiple small hemorrhages. What is the diagnosis? (AIIMS May 2010)
a. Cortical contusion
b. Cerebral laceration
c. Multiple infarcts
d. Diffuse axonal injuries

Q25. Due to decelerations, the aorta can be ruptured at places where it is fixed, *except*: (AIIMS May 2012)
a. At ligamentum arteriosum
b. Behind the esophagus
c. Behind the crura of the diaphragm
d. Aortic valve

Q26. In traumatic transection of the femoral artery and vein, which among the following should be done? (PGI Dec 2001)
a. Femoral artery repair with vein ligation
b. Repair of artery and vein
c. Ligation of the femoral artery
d. Below-knee amputation
e. Repair of an artery with contralateral sympathectomy

Q27. In traumatic injury of the common femoral vein and external femoral artery, which among the following should be done? (PGI Dec 2003)
a. Ligation of both artery and vein
b. Repair of artery and vein
c. Below-knee amputation
d. Repair of an artery and contralateral sympathectomy
e. Sclerotherapy

Q28. Limb salvage can be done in all, *except*: (AIIMS Feb 1997)
a. Nerve injury
b. Vascular injury
c. Bone injury
d. Muscle injury

Q29. Which of the following is used to define penetrating neck injury? (AIIMS May 2009)
a. 2 cm depth of wound
b. Injury to vital structures
c. Breach of platysma
d. Through and through wound

Q30. A patient was intubated, opened an eye, and moved all four limbs in response to speech. His GCS is: (AIIMS Nov 2018)
a. 8
b. 9
c. 10
d. 11

Grade III | **Most difficult**

Q1. A patient with a massive hemorrhage presents to the emergency room (ER) after RTA. What is not to be done? (AIIMS Nov 2018)
a. Check coagulation with thromboelastography, if available.
b. IV crystalloid 2 L within a few minutes
c. Early tranexamic acid recommended
d. Massive transfusion

Q2. All the following are true about imaging is a primary survey of a trauma patient, *except*: (AIIMS May 2017)
a. Cervical X-ray is not mandatory.
b. Chest X-rays and pelvic X-rays are taken as part of the primary survey.
c. Hemodynamically stable patients should not be sent for a CT scan.
d. The patient should be shifted with neck support and cervical spine stabilization only.

Q3. A patient, after sustaining RTA, developed # (Fracture) left shaft of femur with guarding and rigidity in the abdomen. The following is to be done: (PGI Dec 2003)
a. X-ray of left lower limb and ultrasound (USG) abdomen

b. Start in vitro fertilization (IVF), Ryle's tube, and catheterization
c. Stabilize the # (Fracture) and monitor the patient, and do surgery if necessary later on
d. Grouping and cross-matching of two units of blood stabilizes the # (Fracture) only

Q4. In trauma, which of the following is increased: (PGI Dec 2001)
a. Epinephrine
b. Adrenocorticotropic hormone (ACTH)
c. Glucagon
d. Parathormone
e. Insulin

Q5. Babu is brought to the emergency department as a case of an RTA. He is hypotensive. The most likely ruptured organ is: (All India 2001)
a. Spleen
b. Mesentery
c. Kidney
d. Rectum

Q6. Investigation of choice for blunt trauma abdomen in unstable patient: (PGI Dec 2000)
a. X-ray abdomen
b. USG
c. DPL
d. MRI
e. CT scan

Q7. A patient developed hemoperitoneum following RTA, with BP 90/60 and pulse 140/min. Which of the following is to be done? (PGI Dec 2003)
a. DPL to be done
b. Liver is the MC (Most Common) organ or rupture
c. USG is better than CT scan
d. X-ray to be taken in a supine position
e. Urgent surgery to be done

Q8. The best diagnostic aid in blunt trauma abdomen is: (AIIMS 1987)
a. CT scan
b. Four-quadrant aspiration
c. Peritoneal lavage
d. Ultrasound

Q9. A driver wearing a seat belt suddenly applies the brakes to avoid a collision. Which of the following body parts is most likely to be injured? (AIIMS May 2013)
a. Spleen
b. Mesentery
c. Liver
d. Abdominal aorta

Q10. True about blunt abdominal trauma with splenic rupture: (PGI June 2008)
a. Kehr's sign-discoloration around the umbilicus
b. Spleen is the most common organ to be involved
c. Splenectomy is the treatment of choice for splenic rupture
d. Cullen's sign is seen

Q11. A 30-year-old female comes in with hypovolemic shock after blunt trauma of the abdomen. An emergency USG of the abdomen shows a splenic tear. Which of the following is to be done? (PGI Dec 2001)
a. CECT of the abdomen
b. Diagnostic lavage of the peritoneal cavity before proceeding
c. Monitor patient to assess for progression
d. Immediate surgery
e. Chest X-ray

Q12. Treatment of rib fracture: (PGI Dec 2002)
a. Immediate thoracotomy
b. IPPV
c. Analgesics
d. Strapping
e. Intercostal water seal drainage (ICWSD)

Q13. True about chest trauma: (PGI June 2008)
a. Electrocardiogram (ECG) done in all cases associated with sternal fracture
b. Underwater seal drainage if associated with pneumothorax
c. X-ray chest investigation of choice
d. Urgent surgery is needed in all cases

Q14. The most common cause of death in penetrating injury of the chest: (AIIMS June 2000)
a. Tracheobronchial injury
b. Esophageal rupture
c. Pulmonary laceration
d. Chylothorax

Q15. A 40-year-old male was brought to the emergency room with a stab injury to the chest. On examination, the patient is found to be hemodynamically stable. The neck veins are engorged, and the heart sounds are muffled. The following statements are not true for this patient, *except*: (AIIMS Nov 2002)
a. Cardiac tamponade is likely to be present.
b. Immediate emergency room thoracotomy should be done

c. Echocardiogram should be done to confirm pericardial blood
d. The entry wound should be sealed with an occlusive dressing

Q16. A patient after an RTA presents with respiratory distress, hypotension, and dilated, bulging neck veins. On examination, absent breath sounds and contralateral tracheal shift are found. What would be the first line of management? (AIIMS Nov 2013)

a. Emergency thoracotomy
b. Immediate chest X-ray
c. CT scan
d. Insert a wide-bone needle in the second intercostal space

Q17. Which of the following is MC (Most Common) cause of hypotension in fractured ribs? (T10–T12) (AIIMS Nov 1999)

a. Abdominal solid visceral organ injury
b. Injury to the aorta
c. Intercostal artery damage
d. Pulmonary contusion

Q18. In a blast injury, which of the following organs is least vulnerable to the blast wave? (AIIMS Jun 2003)

a. Gastrointestinal (GI) tract
b. Lungs
c. Liver
d. Ear drum

Q19. The most common organ injured in blast injury is: (AIIMS May 2010)

a. Lung b. Liver
c. Spleen d. Pancreas

Q20. Clinical features of fracture of the zygomatic bone include all of the following, *except*: (All India 1997)

a. Diplopia
b. Trismus
c. Bleeding
d. Cerebrospinal fluid (CSF) rhinorrhea

Q21. Mandible is commonly fractured: (JIPMER 1987)

a. At the neck of the condyle
b. Through the angle
c. Through the canine fossa
d. At the middle

Q22. LeFort II facial fracture implies: (AIIMS 1984)

a. Fracture running through the alveolar ridge.
b. Fracture running through the midline of the palate and zygomaticomaxillary suture.
c. Fracture running through the zygomatic process of the maxilla, floor of the orbit, and root of the nose on one side only.
d. Similar to C but on both sides

Q23. A 20-year-old man is hit in the eye with a ball. On examination, there is restriction of lateral and upward gaze and diplopia. There is no obvious visible sign of injury to the eyeball, but there is some enophthalmos. The likely diagnosis is: (AIIMS 1985)

a. Zygoma fracture
b. Maxillary the fracture
c. Blow-out fracture of the orbit
d. Injury to the lateral rectus

Q24. The best treatment of this condition will be: (AIIMS 1985)

a. Do nothing and assurance
b. Explore the orbit
c. Ophthalmic exercise to correct diplopia
d. Reinsertion of the lateral rectus muscle

Q25. CSF otorrhea is caused by: (AIIMS Nov 1998)

a. Fracture of cribriform plate
b. Fracture of parietal bone
c. Fracture of petrous temporal bone
d. Fracture of tympanic membrane

Q26. Management of CSF rhinorrhea is: (AIIMS Feb 1997)

a. Plain X-ray and packing of the nose
b. Nasal packing only
c. Antibiotics and observation
d. Immediate surgery

Q27. The term post-traumatic epilepsy refers to seizures occurring: (AIIMS Nov 2002)

a. Within moments of head injury
b. Within 7 days of head injury
c. Within several weeks to months after head injury
d. Many years after head injury

Q28. After rupture of the middle meningeal artery bleeding occurs in which region: (AIIMS Feb 1997)

a. Subdural bleed b. Extradural bleed
c. Intracerebral bleed d. Subarachnoid bleed

Q29. Hemostasis in scalp wounds is best achieved by: (PGI 1985)

a. Direct pressure over the wound
b. Catching and crushing the bleeders by hemostasis
c. Eversion of galea aponeurotica
d. Coagulation of bleeders

Q30. During reconstruction of an amputated limb which of the following is done first? (AIIMS Nov 2010)

a. Arterial repair
b. Venous repair
c. Fixation of the bone
d. Nerve anastomoses

Q31. The most serious complication of a pelvic fracture is: (AIIMS May 2013)

a. Rupture urinary bladder
b. Neurogenic shock
c. Hypovolemic shock
d. Malunion

ANSWERS

Grade I: 1. a; 2. d; 3. b; 4. e; 5. a; 6. d; 7. d; 8. b; 9. c; 10. b; 11. c, d, e; 12. a; 13. a; 14. a; 15. c; 16. d; 17. a, b; 18. c; 19. a, b; 20. a; 21. b; 22. b; 23. a, d; 24. d; 25. a, e; 26. c; 27. a, b, c; 28. d; 29. a; 30. d; 31. a

Grade II: 1. c; 2. d; 3. b; 4. b; 5. a; 6. c; 7. c; 8. a; 9. a; 10. b, e; 11. b; 12. a; 13. c; 14. b; 15. b; 16. d; 17. c; 18. a, b, d; 19. a, c; 20. a, e; 21. a; 22. a; 23. a; 24. d; 25. b; 26. a, b; 27. b; 28. b; 29. c; 30. b

Grade III: 1. b; 2. c; 3. a, b, d; 4. a, c; 5. a; 6. b; 7. c, e; 8. a; 9. b; 10. b, d; 11. d; 12. b, c; 13. a, b, c; 14. a; 15. b; 16. d; 17. a; 18. c; 19. a; 20. d; 21. a; 22. d; 23. c; 24. b; 25. c; 26. c; 27. c; 28. b; 29. a; 30. c; 31. c

MODEL QUESTIONS

Q1. Seat belt causes injury to:

a. Duodenum
b. Head injury due to the windscreen
c. Thorax
d. All

Ans. a

Q2. The first treatment of flail chest is:

a. O_2 administration and analgesia
b. Mechanical ventilation
c. Surgical stabilization
d. Intrapleural analgesia

Ans. a

Q3. The following are indications for performing a thoracotomy after a blunt injury of the chest, *except*:

a. 1,000 mL drainage after placing intercostals tube
b. Continuous bleeding through intercostals tube of >200 mL/h for three or more hours
c. Cardiac tamponade
d. Rib fracture

Ans. d

Q4. Which one of the following is not a principle followed in the management of missile injuries?

a. Excision of all dead muscles
b. Removal of foreign bodies
c. Removal of fragments of bone
d. Leaving the wound open

Ans. c

Q5. A person has been brought in casualty with a history of road accidents. He had lost consciousness transiently and then gained consciousness, but again became unconscious. Most likely, he is having a brain hemorrhage:

a. Intracerebral
b. Subarachnoid
c. Subdural
d. Extradural

Ans. d

Q6. The prognosis in head injury is best given by:

a. Glassgow Coma Scale
b. Age of patient
c. Mode of injury
d. CT head

Ans. a

Q7. A patient is brought to the emergency as a case of a head injury following a head injury, following a head-on collision, or an RTA. His BP is 90/60 mm Hg. Tachycardia is present. The most likely diagnosis is:

a. EDH
b. Subdural hematoma (SDH)
c. Intracerebral hemorrhage
d. Intra-abdominal bleed

Ans. d

Q8. Which of the following is true regarding nerve injury?

a. In all cases of open wounds with clinical signs of nerve injury, nerve exploration should always be done
b. Nerve conduction velocity is the best predictor within 48 hours of injury
c. Traction nerve injury should be repaired immediately
d. Positive Tinel's sign indicates the accurate location of the lesion

Ans. a

Q9. Hypotension in acute spinal injury is due to:

a. Loss of sympathetic tone
b. Loss of parasympathetic tone
c. Orthostatic hypotension
d. Vasovagal attack

Ans. a

Q10. True about aortic transaction:

a. Most commonly due to deceleration injury
b. High mortality
c. Surgery definitive treatment
d. Aortography gold standard

Ans. a, b, c, and d

SUGGESTED READING

1. Bailey & Love's - Short Practice of Surgery, 27th edition.
2. Schwartz's Principles of Surgery, 18th edition.
3. Trauma Handbook of The Massachusetts General Hospital, 1st edition.

Q5. Hyponatremia in multiple myeloma is:

a. True
b. Relative
c. Absolute
d. Pseudo

Ans. d

Q6. Body water content in percentage of body weight is lowest in:

a. Well-built man
b. Fat woman
c. Well-nourished child
d. Fat man

Ans. b

Q7. Critical pH in Mendelson syndrome:

a. 2.5
b. 3.0
c. 3.5
d. 4.0

Ans. a

Q8. The ideal colloidal solution is:

a. Dextran
b. Plasma
c. Albumin
d. Hydroxyethyl starch

Ans. c

Q9. Skin fold thickness (for assessment of nutritional status) can be measured at all the following, *except*:

a. Biceps
b. Triceps
c. Suprailiac region
d. None

Ans. d

Q10. Best vein for TPN is:

a. Subclavian vein
b. Femoral vein
c. Brachial vein
d. Saphenous vein

Ans. a

Q11. The sodium content of one liter of isotonic saline is:

a. 140 mEq
b. 154 mEq
c. 40 mEq
d. 70 mEq

Ans. b

SUGGESTED READING

1. Harrison's Principles of Internal Medicine, 15th edition.
2. Schwartz's Principles of Surgery, 18th edition.
3. Textbook of Surgery by David Sabiston, 21st edition.

SECTION 3

Surgical Diseases of Skin and Subcutaneous Tissue

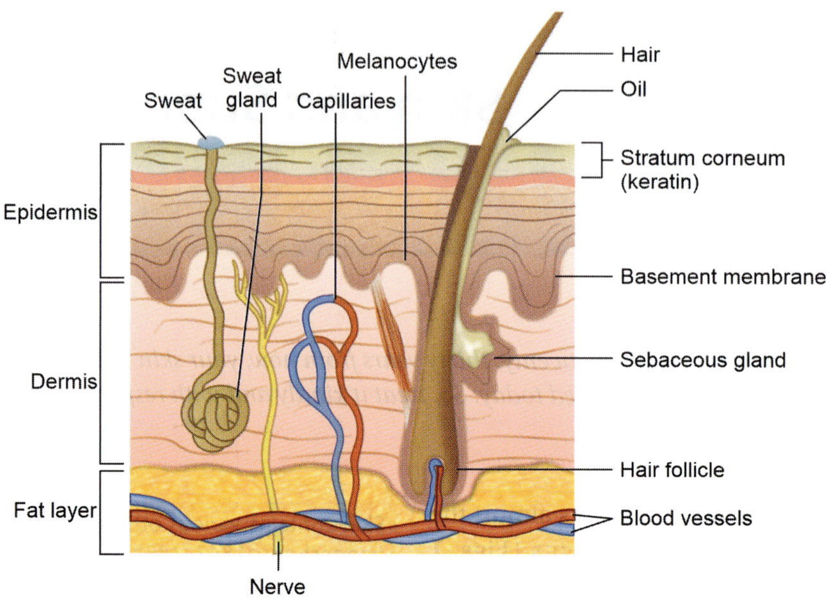

Fig. 2: Structure of skin.

NEUROFIBROMATOSIS

These are caused by genetic (chromosomal) features. *Von Recklinghausen's (Friedrich Von Recklinghausen, 1833–1910, German pathologist)* disease, which has multiple lumps, is the most common type of neurofibromatosis.

GORLINS (ROBERT J GORLIN, 1923–2006, AMERICAN DENTIST) SYNDROME

It is caused by an abnormal tumor suppressor gene on chromosome 5, 9q22.31. It has specific features such as broad nasal roots and overdeveloped supraorbital ridges.

XERODERMA PIGMENTOSUM

It is caused by an abnormality in the gene, chromosome 9q. It causes a tremendous skin cancer risk, 2,000-fold, and 60% mortality by 20 years of age.

GARDNER'S (ELDON J GARDNER, 1909-1989, AMERICAN GENETICIST DESCRIBED IN 1951) SYNDROME

It is an autosomal dominant disease caused by a gene on chromosome 5. It causes multiple epidermoid cysts and lipomas.

HIDRADENITIS SUPPURATIVA

It is caused by *Staphylococcus aureus*. It leads to suppuration and even abscess formation. One should stop smoking and reduce weight with antibiotic therapy.

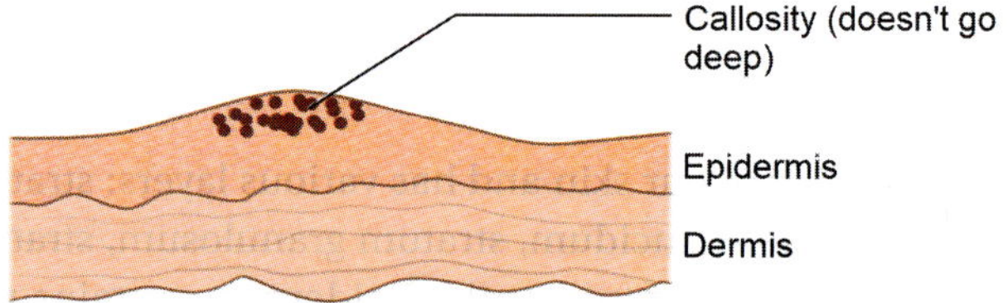

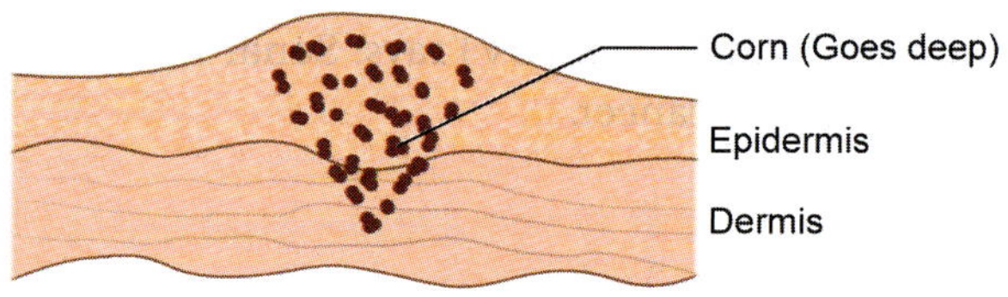

Fig. 3: Callosity and corn.

IMPETIGO

It is a superficial infection of the skin caused by staphylococci and streptococci.

EPIDERMAL CYSTS

These cysts can occur at any part of the body. These should be removed by surgery.

CALLOSITIES AND CORNS

These are caused by excessive friction or pressure over the skin with hyperkeratosis and are commonly found on the feet. Callosity is a localized painless condition of the epidermis, whereas corn is also a localized lesion, but it goes deep in the dermis, whereas callosity does not **(Fig. 3)**.

WARTS

These are associated with human papillomavirus (HPV). It has hypertrophy of horny and spinus layers of skin. Various types of warts are: *verruca vulgaris* (common wart—on fingers and toes) and *verruca plantaris* (plantar wart—soles of the foot). Few warts do not require any treatment as they disappear automatically, while others require surgical removal.

LIPOMA

It is a commonly seen benign tumor that grows slowly. It is a painless swelling that slips under the finger on examination. Dercum's disease is a lipoma at multiple sites. Lipomas are common in the trunk. They do not require removal unless growing or for cosmetic reasons.

TURBAN TUMOR

It is known as cylindroma.

Premalignant conditions of skin:
- Leukoplakia
- Radiation dermatitis
- Bowen's (John T Bowen, 1857–1940, American dermatologist) disease.
- Erythroplasia of Queyrat (Auguste Queyrat, 1856–1933, French dermatologist, described in 1911).
- Senile keratosis
- Lupus vulgaris

BASAL CELL CARCINOMA

It is a locally invasive carcinoma of the basal layer of the epidermis. It grows slowly, 90% are nodular, and UV radiation from sunlight is the risk factor. It is a low-grade malignancy and also called a rodent ulcer. It usually appears on the face above a line from the lobule of the ear to the corner of the mouth. It is of *four varieties: (1) nodular, (2) pigmented, (3) cystic, and (4) superficial.* It spreads by local invasion. Excision is the treatment.

Important Points

- Basal cell carcinoma (BCC) is a slow-growing lesion.
- UV radiation is a risk factor.
- 90% are nodular.
- High and low risk lesions.
- 95% occur between the ages of 40 and 80 years.
- 33% occur in the unexposed area of the body.
- White men are more affected.
- BCC metastasis is extremely rare.
- Types—local (nodular) and generalized (multifocal or spreading lesion).

Treatment

Mohs' (Frederic E Mohs, 1910–2002, American Surgeon developed in 1938) micrographic surgery.

SQUAMOUS CELL CARCINOMA

It is a malignant tumor originating from the stratum basalis of the epidermis. It is commonly seen after UV radiation or chemical exposure. It metastasizes in 2% of cases.

Classification of Squamous Cell Carcinoma

Tumor, node, and metastasis (TNM) classification has TX (primary tumor cannot be assessed), T0 (No evidence of primary tumor), Tis (In situ), T1 (<2 cm), T2 (>2 cm), T3 (Invasion of facial bone), T4 (Invasion of muscles and bones), NX (Nodal involvement cannot be assessed), N0 (No regional nodes), N1 (One ipsilateral LN, <3 cm), N2a (3–6 cm), N2b (>1 LN, not bigger than 6 cm), N2c (Contralateral nodes, but none >6 cm), N3 (spread to any node), M0 (No metastasis), M1 (Metastasis).

Stages

Stage 0 (Tis, N0, M0), stage 1 (T1, N0, M0), stage 2 (T2, N0, M0), stage 3 (T3, N0, M0), and stage 4 (T1-T3, N2, M0).

It is the second most common cancer of the skin and commonly seen in dark individuals who are exposed to sunlight. It metastasizes via blood and lymphatics. It has raised rolled out everted edges. Treatment is done by removal of the tumor with a 1 cm margin. *Mohs (micrographically oriented histographic surgery) surgery* is also advised, which is a precise removal of high-risk skin cancer tissue with preservation of healthy tissue.

Important Points

- It is also called *epithelioma* with rolled-out margins.
- Bowen's disease (John T Bowen, 1857–1940, American dermatologist) is a squamous cell carcinoma (SCC) in situ.
- Erythroplasia of Queyrat (August Queyret, 1856–1933, French dermatologist, described in 1911) on glans penis.

MULTIPLE CHOICE QUESTIONS

Grade I | **Simple**

Q1. A most common type of malignant melanoma is: (JIPMER 2014)

a. Superficial spreading
b. Lentigo maligna melanoma
c. Nodular
d. Acral lentiginous

Q2. The most common site of lentigo malignant melanoma is: (AIIMS Nov 2001)

a. Face b. Legs
c. Trunks d. Soles

Q3. The most malignant form of malignant melanoma is: (PGI June 1999)

a. Nodular
b. Hutchinson's melanotic freckle
c. Acral lentiginous type
d. Superficial spreading

Q4. True about malignant melanoma: (PGI June 2008)

a. Lymphatic spread
b. Lymph node biopsy is always done
c. Block dissection is to be done when the sentinel node is involved.
d. Microsatellitism

Q5. The worst prognosis in melanoma is seen in the subtype: (Kerala PG 2001)

a. Superficial spreading
b. Nodular melanoma
c. Lentigo malignant melanoma
d. Amelanotic melanoma

Q6. Which one of the following is not included in the treatment of malignant melanoma? (UPSC 2005)

a. Radiation b. Surgical excision
c. Chemotherapy d. Immunotherapy

Q7. Which of the following is true about malignant melanoma? (PGI 2005)

a. Excisional biopsy must be done.
b. Wide local excision need not be performed if a biopsy is positive.
c. Exposure to sunlight is not a risk factor.
d. Congenital giant naevi cannot transform into malignant melanoma

Q8. The most common site of a rodent ulcer is: (All India 1994)

a. Limbs b. Face
c. Abdomen d. Trunk

Q9. What of the following is true? (PGI June 2002)

a. Viral warts spontaneously resolve
b. Plantar warts should not be excised.
c. Callosity is formed occupationally.
d. Corns are viral in etiology.

Q10. True about congenital hemangioma: (PGI June 2007)

a. It stops growing after birth
b. It is fully mature at birth
c. Noninvoluting congenital hemangioma (NICH) variety persists
d. Rapidly involuting congenital hemangioma (RICH) variety involutes
e. Calcification can occur.

Grade II | **Difficult**

Q1. Prognosis of melanoma depends on: (PGI June 1998)

a. Stage
b. Depth of melanoma of biopsy
c. Duration of growth
d. Site

Q2. All of the following statements about malignant melanoma are true, *except*: (All India 1997)

a. Prognosis is better in females than in males.
b. Acral lentiginous melanoma carries a good prognosis
c. Stage II A shows satellite deposits
d. The most common type is superficial spreading melanoma

Q3. True about Marjolin's ulcer is: (PGI June 2007)

a. Ulcer over scar b. Rapid growth
c. Rodent ulcer d. Painful

Q4. Characteristic of basal cell carcinoma (BCC) is: (AIIMS May 2012)

a. Keratin pearls b. Foam cells
c. Nuclear palisading d. Psammoma bodies

Q5. In pigmented BCC, the treatment of choice is: (PGI 1998)

a. Chemotherapy b. Radiotherapy
c. Cryosurgery d. Excision

Q6. Boil can occur at all sites, *except*: **(TNPG 1995)**
a. Pinna
b. Skin
c. Scalp
d. Palm

Q7. The best treatment of strawberry angioma is: **(JIPMER 1995)**
a. Antibiotics
b. Corticosteroids
c. Masterly inactivity
d. Excision

Q8. Which one of the following is true about epidermoid cysts? **(PGI Dec 2005)**
a. Punctum is present.
b. Keratin is present.
c. Sebaceous material is present.
d. Autosomal inheritance
e. May turn malignant

Q9. Frostbite is treated by: **(AIIMS 2000)**
a. Rapid rewarming
b. Slow rewarming
c. Intravenous (IV) pentoxifylline
d. Amputation

Grade III	*Most difficult*

Q1. The most common origin of melanoma is from: **(AIIMS Nov 2001)**
a. Junctional melanocytes
b. Epidermal cells
c. Basal cells
d. Follicular cells

Q2. Biopsy from a mole on the foot shows cytologic atypia of melanocytes and diffuse epidermal infiltration by anaplastic cells, which are also present in the papillary and reticular dermis. The most likely diagnosis is: **(All India 2004)**
a. Melanoma, Clark level IV
b. Congenital melanocytic nevus
c. Dysplastic nevus
d. Melanoma, Clark level III

Q3. A 40-year-old man presented with a flat 1 × 1 cm scaly, itchy black mole on the front of his thigh. Examination did not reveal any inguinal lymphadenopathy. The best course of management would be: **(UPSC 2007)**
a. Fine-needle aspiration cytology (FNAC) of the lesion
b. Incision biopsy
c. Excisional biopsy
d. Wide excision with inguinal lymphadenectomy

Q4. Which of the following is true about melanoma? **(PGI Dec 2005)**
a. Amelanotic melanoma is associated with the worst prognosis.
b. Complete excisional biopsy is the management.
c. Thinner melanoma has a good prognosis.
d. Back is the most common site in females.
e. Congenital giant nevus is associated with minimal risk of malignancy.

Q5. Cock's peculiar tumor is: **(MCI Sept 2007)**
a. An infected sebaceous cyst
b. A malignant tumor of the scalp
c. A metastatic lesion of the scalp
d. An indicator of underlying osteomyelitis

Q6. Bedsore is an example of: **(All India 1999)**
a. Tropical ulcer
b. Trophic ulcer
c. Venous ulcer
d. Post-thrombotic ulcer

Q7. Spontaneous regression is seen in: **(All India 1993)**
a. Port-wine hemangioma
b. Strawberry hemangioma
c. Cavernous hemangioma
d. Port-wine stain

Q8. Which of the following cutaneous malignancies do not metastasize through the lymphatics? **(All India 1994)**
a. Squamous cell carcinoma
b. Basal cell carcinoma
c. Melanoma
d. Kaposi's sarcoma

Q9. Trophic ulcers are caused by: **(PGI June 2004)**
a. Leprosy
b. Buerger's disease
c. Syringomyelia
d. Deep vein thrombosis (DVT)
e. Varicose veins

Q10. Which of these do not change or remain the same throughout life? **(AIIMS Nov 2001)**
a. Salmon patch
b. Strawberry angiomas
c. Port-wine stain
d. Capillary hemangiomas

ANSWERS

Grade I: 1. a; 2. a; 3. a; 4. a, c, d; 5. d; 6. c; 7. a; 8. b; 9. a, c; 10. All

Grade II: 1. a, b, d; 2. b, c; 3. a; 4. c; 5. d; 6. d; 7. c; 8. a, b, e; 9. b

Grade III: 1. a; 2. a; 3. c; 4. a, b, c; 5. a; 6. b; 7. d; 8. b; 9. a; 10. c

MODEL QUESTIONS

Q1. Basal cell carcinoma spreads by:

a. Lymphatics
b. Hematogenous
c. Direct spread
d. None of the above

Ans. c

Q2. Diagnostic procedure for basal cell carcinoma:

a. Wedge biopsy
b. Shave
c. Incisional biopsy
d. Punch biopsy

Ans. a

Q3. Moh's micrographic excision for basal cell carcinoma (BCC) is used for all of the following, *except*:

a. Recurrent tumor
b. Tumor <2 cm in diameter
c. Tumors with aggressive histology
d. Tumors with perineural invasion

Ans. b

Q4. All of the following statements about necrotizing fasciitis are true, *except*:

a. Infection of fascia and subcutaneous tissue
b. Most commonly caused by group A β-hemolytic streptococci
c. The most common site is the perineum, followed by the trunk and extremities.
d. Surgical debridement is mandatory.

Ans. c

Q5. Which one of the following is true about apocrine glands?

a. Modified sweat glands
b. Modified sebaceous glands
c. Present in axilla and groin
d. Hidradenitis suppurativa is an infection of apocrine glands.

Ans. a, c, and d

Q6. Hidradenitis suppurativa is found to occur in:

a. Axilla
b. Circumanal
c. Scalp
d. Groin
e. All

Ans. e

Q7. The causes of persistence of a sinus or fistulae include:

a. Foreign body
b. Nondependent drainage
c. Unrelieved obstruction
d. Presence of malignancy
e. All of the above

Ans. e

Q8. A 35-year-old premenopausal patient has recently developed a 1.5 cm-sized pigmented lesion on her back. Which of the following forms of tissue diagnosis will you recommend for her?

a. Needle biopsy
b. Tru-cut biopsy
c. Excision biopsy
d. Incisional biopsy

Ans. c

Q9. Which of the following is False about malignant melanoma?

a. Radiosensitive
b. Surgery is the treatment of choice.
c. Acral lentiginous has the worst prognosis.
d. Treatment is wide local excision.

Ans. d

Q10. Dercum's disease is most common in the:

a. Face
b. Arm
c. Back
d. Thigh

Ans. c

Q11. Which is not true about Sturge–Weber syndrome?

a. Port-wine stain
b. Calcification in brain
c. Cortical atrophy
d. Intracranial hamartoma

Ans. d

Q12. Salmon patch usually disappears by age:

a. 1 month
b. 1 year
c. Puberty
d. None of the above

Ans. b

Q13. Kaposi's sarcoma is seen in:

a. Leukemia
b. Lymphoma
c. Acquired immunodeficiency syndrome (AIDS)
d. Cytomegalovirus infection

Ans. c

Q14. A chronically lymphedematous limb is predisposed to all of the following, *except*:

a. Thickening of the skin
b. Recurrent soft-tissue infections
c. Marjolin's ulcer
d. Sarcoma

Ans. c

SUGGESTED READING

1. Cecil Textbook of Medicine, 22nd edition.
2. Schwartz's Principles of Surgery, 18th edition.
3. Textbook of Surgery by David Sabiston, 21st edition.

CHAPTER 19

Burns

"Pour water on the burn."

– A slogan from the Burn Association

INTRODUCTION

As our industrial work is increasing, so is the incidence of burn injuries. Burns are painful, with high morbidity and mortality, and expensive to treat. During the last few decades, various new methods of treatment for burns have emerged, which have reduced the rate of mortality. Respiratory burns are one of the main causes of death. It can be from smoke, hot gases, steam, and inhaled chemicals, leading to laryngeal edema and even respiratory failure.

> Burn injuries lead shock as it causes inflammatory reaction which leads to vascular permeability resulting in movement of water and other important constituents from intra- to extravascular space. The fluid loss in burn is almost directly proportional to the area of burn.

PATHOPHYSIOLOGY OF BURN INJURIES

Burn injury leads to three zones of injury **(Fig. 1)**:

1. *Zone of coagulation:* It is at the center of the wound. It is irreversibly damaged.
2. *Zone of stasis:* It is outside the zone of coagulation. Vascular damage and vascular leak are present. It is salvageable.
3. *Zone of hyperemia:* It is beyond the zone of stasis. It has minimal tissue injury.

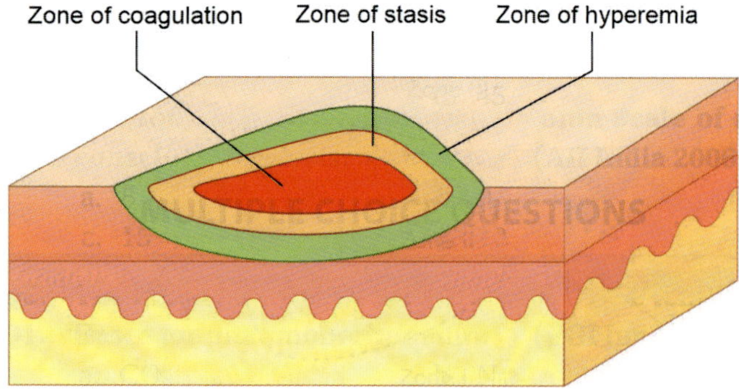

Fig. 1: Zones of burn injury.

DEPTH OF BURN (FIG. 2)

- *First-degree burn:* It involves only the epidermis, no blisters, redness due to vasodilatation, blanches to touch, and is quite painful without scar development.
- *Second-degree burn (partial-thickness burn):* It involves epidermis and partial dermis.
  - *Superficial (superficial partial-thickness burn)* involves epidermis and upper layers of dermis. Blisters are present.
  - *Deep (deep partial-thickness burn)* involves up to the reticular layer of dermis. Blisters may or may not be seen, mottled pink and white color, blanching absent, and there is no pain.
- *Third-degree burn (full-thickness burn):* It involves all layers of dermis—hard, leathery, eschar, and painless.
- *Fourth-degree burn:* It involves all layers of skin and deeper tissues.

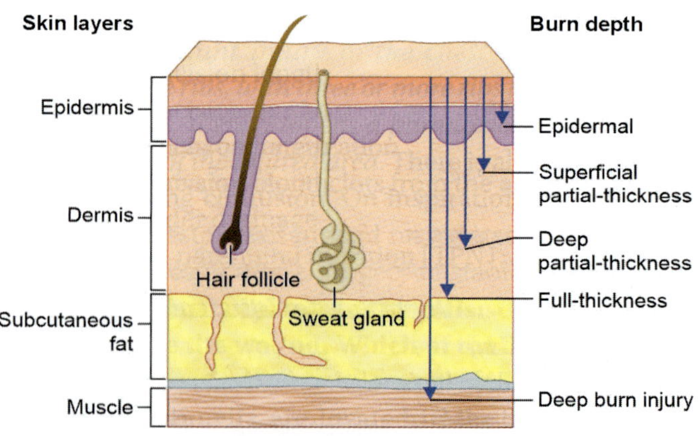

Fig. 2: Depth of burn.

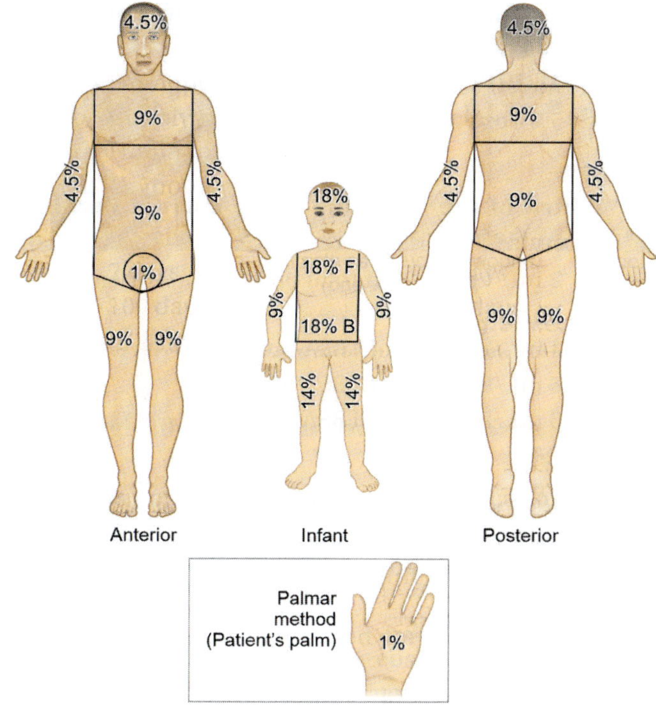

Fig. 3: Rule of nine.

How to calculate total burn surface area (TBSA)?

- *Rule of nines [Wallace (Alexander B. Wallace, British Plastic surgeon, described in 1951) rule of nines]:* It is 9% of TBSA for the upper extremity and head and neck. 18% for each lower extremity, anterior surface of trunk, and posterior surface of trunk. Perineum is 1% **(Fig. 3)**.
- *Palm method: One palm surface area without fingers on the burn area is equal to 0.5% TBSA, with fingers accounting for 1%.*
- *Lund-Browder chart:* It is considered as most accurate way of calculating TBSA, but it requires the chart, photos to be with your site, and is not like the rule of nines.

Not to forget:
- Scald burns are caused by moist heat.
- Electric burn has a burn at the point of entry and exit of the current.
- Electric burn causes less damage to skin and more to deeper tissues.
- TBSA and mortality from burns are directly proportional.
- Children have more TBSA in the head and neck as compared to the body.
- Fluid resuscitation is the most important factor in burns.
- The best fluid is Ringer's lactate in the first 24 hours of burn.
- Urine output is the best monitor.

- *Pseudomonas* is the most common organism causing infection in burns.
- The open method of burn wound management is a risk factor for infection.
- The closed method is the preferred method for body burn, except head and face.
- The most common causes of mortality in burn patients are sepsis, shock, and asphyxia.

What determines the prognosis in burns?

- Area of the burn
- Depth of the burn
- Respiratory injuries

MANAGEMENT OF THE BURN

Mn = *ABCDEF*
A = Airway control
B = Breathing
C = Circulation
D = Disability
E = Exposure
F = Fluid resuscitation

Tracheal intubation should be considered early and elective, as delay will make it difficult due to laryngeal edema.

CRITERIA OF ADMISSION TO THE HOSPITAL

- 15% burn in an adult or 10% burn in a child
- Burn injury to the respiratory tract
- Burn of hand, face, feet, and perineal
- Extreme age burn

Full-thickness burns have no sensation, whereas superficial burns have. In an adult, a 15% TBSA, and in a child, a 10% TBSA requires intravenous fluid administration. When oral liquids are allowed, salt is added. Urine output is the monitoring factor in burn cases.

Intravenous fluids are to be given in the burn:

- *Crystalloid solutions:* Ringer's lactate is the most commonly used fluid. Hartmann's (Alexis Frank Hartmann, 1898–1964, American pediatrician) solution is a routinely used solution. In children, dextrose saline is commonly given as 100 mL/kg for 24 hours for the first 10 kg and 50 mL for the next 10 kg.
- *Colloid solutions:* Human albumin solution (HAS) is a commonly used colloid solution. It improves oncotic pressure.

Muir and Barclay's (Ian Fraser Kerr Muir, 1921–2008, British plastic surgeon, Thomas Laird Barclay, British plastic surgeon) formula was given for the calculation of colloid fluid administration: 0.5 × % TBSA × weight = one portion. One portion is given in periods as 4/4/4, 6/6, and 12 hours.

Parkland formula: TBSA × weight in kg × 4 is = volume in mL, half the volume is given in the first 8 hours, and the rest is half the volume in the next 16 hours.

Important points to remember:
- When at home, examine for injuries other than burns also.
- Transfer the patient from home to hospital in a sitting position to avoid complications.
- Burns around the mouth and neck may also cause respiratory tract injuries.
- Dressing of burn wounds should be done with 1% silver sulfadiazine cream. It acts as an antibacterial agent.
- All burn cases must have antibiotic therapy as infection is common in burn cases due to immunocompromisation in burns.
- Swabs from burn wounds should be taken frequently and regularly.
- Hypertrophic scar is treated by pressure garments.
- Chlorhexidine solution is one of the best solutions for burn wound cleaning.

Burn patients need extra nutrition as they require tremendous healing. Ryle's tube feeding is advised in 15% and more of TBSA.

ESCHAROTOMY

In circumferential full-thickness burns, escharotomy is done by incising the whole length of the full-thickness burn to prevent compartment syndrome.

SOME IMPORTANT QUESTIONS

Q1. Dermoepidermal burn is a what degree of burn?
a. I
b. II
c. III
d. IV

Ans. b

Q2. The rule of nine to estimate the surface area of a burnt patient was introduced by:
a. Moritz Kaposi
b. Alexander Wallace
c. Joseph Lister
d. Thomas Barclay

Ans. b

Q3. Best fluid for resuscitation of a burnt patient:
a. Hartmann solution
b. Colloid
c. Normal saline
d. 5% dextrose

Ans. a

Q4. In cases of burn, which is the fluid of choice in the first 24 hours?
a. Ringer's lactate
b. Normal saline
c. 5% dextrose
d. Blood

Ans. a

Q5. Which of the following is the correct Parkland formula?
a. 2 mL/kg per % of total body surface area (TBSA) burn
b. 4 mL/kg per % of TBSA burn
c. 6 mL/kg per % of TBSA burn
d. 8 mL/kg per % of TBSA burn

Ans. b

Q6. An 80 kg male with bilateral upper limb, right lower limb with perineum burns third degree, the amount of fluid required in the first 8 hours is:
a. 3,920 mL
b. 4,920 mL
c. 5,920 mL
d. 6,560 mL

Ans. d

Q7. Exposure treatment is done for burns of the:
a. Upper limb
b. Lower limbs
c. Thorax
d. Abdomen
e. Head and neck

Ans. e

Q8. When does a burn patient need to be intubated?
a. Deep facial burns with singed nasal hair
b. Superficial facial burns
c. Pulse rate >100 beats/min
d. Crepitations on auscultation

Ans. a

Q9. The cold-water treatment of burns has the disadvantage that it increases the chances of:
a. Pain
b. Exudation
c. Infection
d. None of the above

Ans. c

Q10. In third-degree burns, all are seen *except*:
a. Vesicles are absent
b. Painful
c. Leathery skin
d. Reddish due to Hb infiltration

Ans. b

Q11. Which of the following is true about grade 4 burns?
- a. Involves all layers of the skin
- b. Involves the whole skin along with subcutaneous tissue
- c. Includes electric burns
- d. Involves the dermis partially

Ans. b

Q12. Blisters are seen in which type of burns?
- a. Deep first degree
- b. Superficial first-degree
- c. Superficial second-degree
- d. Third degree

Ans. c

Q13. An adult whose both lower limbs are charred along with genitalia has .... burns.
- a. 18%
- b. 19%
- c. 36%
- d. 37%

Ans. d

Q14. Head and neck involvement in burns in an infant is:
- a. 9%
- b. 18%
- c. 27%
- d. 32%

Ans. b

Q15. What is the percentage of body surface area (BSA) involved in head + face in burns?
- a. 13
- b. 15
- c. 17
- d. 09

Ans. d

Q16. Calculate the percentage of burns on the head, neck, and face in a child of 1 year:
- a. 10%
- b. 16%
- c. 13%
- d. 15%

Ans. None

Q17. Which of the following is not true about resuscitation in a burn patient?
- a. Ringer's lactate is the preferred crystalloid solution.
- b. Fluid shift from intervascular to extravascular compartment in the burnt patient is maximum in the first 24 hours.
- c. Quantity of crystalloid needed is calculated using the Parkland formula—6 mL/kg body weight per % of the TBSA burnt.
- d. Target mean arterial pressure in resuscitation is 60 mm Hg.

Ans. c

MULTIPLE CHOICE QUESTIONS

Grade I	*Simple*

Q1. A burn patient is referred when: (PGI June 2004)
- a. 10% superficial burn in a child
- b. Scald in face
- c. 25% superficial burn in adult
- d. 25% deep burn in adult
- e. Burn in palm

Q2. All require hospitalization, *except*: (All India 1991)
- a. 5% burns in children
- b. 10% scalds in children
- c. Electrocution
- d. 15% deep burns in adults

Q3. Superficial burns; true is/are: (PGI June 2001)
- a. Always requires skin grafting
- b. Dry and inelastic
- c. Blister formation
- d. Painless
- e. Can be healed within 7–10 days

Q4. Which layer is involved in blister formation in a superficial partial thickness burn? (AIIMS November 2017)
- a. Epidermis
- b. Dermis
- c. Papillary dermis
- d. Reticular dermis

Q5. True about thermal burn injury: (PGI June 2009)
- a. Zone of stasis is the innermost layer.
- b. Zone of hyperemia is the middle layer.
- c. Zone of coagulation is the outermost layer.
- d. Zone of stasis is associated with vascular damage.
- e. Hyperemia is due to vasodilatation.

Q6. The ideal temperature of water to cool the burnt surface is: (UPSC 2002)
- a. 15°
- b. 10°
- c. 8°
- d. 6°

Q7. A 5-year-old child spills boiling water accidentally over her face and trunk. Which of the following methods is the most accurate to estimate the body surface area (BSA) involved in burns? (AIIMS May 2013)
- a. Rule of palm
- b. Rule of nine
- c. Lund and Browder chart
- d. Berkow tables

Q8. A 3-year-old child suffers from burn injury with the following body parts involved: face, including scalp, both buttocks, and circumferentially around both thighs. How much is TBSA involved? (AIIMS May 2013)

a. 0.25 b. 0.26
c. 0.35 d. 0.45

Q9. What is the most important aspect of management of burn injury in the first 24 hours? (UPSC 2007)

a. Fluid resuscitation b. Dressing
c. Escharotomy d. Antibiotics

Q10. Deep skin burns are treated with: (AIIMS 1991)

a. Split-thickness graft
b. Full-thickness graft
c. Amniotic membrane
d. Synthetic skin derivatives

Grade II	Difficult

Q1. NOT a feature of deep burn is: (AIIMS November 1993)

a. Black charred skin b. White leathery skin
c. Loss of pain sensation d. Blisters

Q2. True regarding burns: (PGI December 2007)

a. Only the second and third degree is considered in the classification
b. Second-degree epidermis + papillary dermis
c. Blisters, second degree
d. Curling ulcer can occur.
e. Classified according to depth of invasion

Q3. A 2-year-old child suffers flame burns involving the face, bilateral upper limbs, and the front of the chest and abdomen. What is the BSA involved? (AIIMS May 2016)

a. 45% b. 54%
c. 40% d. 60%

Q4. True statement about burn resuscitation: (PGI December 2003)

a. Colloid preferred in the initial 24 hours
b. Colloid is preferred if a burnt area is >15% of total BSA.
c. Half of the calculated fluid is given in the initial 8 hours
d. Urine output should be maintained at 50–60 mL/h.
e. Diuretics should be given to all patients with electrical burns.

Q5. A third-degree circumferential burn in the arm and forearm region, which of the following is most important for monitoring: (UPPG 2004)

a. Blood gases
b. Carboxy-oxygen level
c. Microglobulinuria, cryoglobulinemia
d. Peripheral pulse and circulation

Q6. A 5-year-old child presents to the emergency department with burns. The burn area corresponding to the size of his palm is equal to: (All India 2011)

a. 1% BSA b. 5% BSA
c. 10% BSA d. 20%

Q7. Best method to assess burns in a 5-year-old child caused by boiling water: (AIIMS May 2013)

a. Palm method
b. Rule of 9
c. Lund and Browder chart
d. Rule of one

Q8. A child has circumferential burn of both of thighs and buttocks, face, and scalp with singeing of hairs. Calculate the percentage of burns: (AIIMS May 2013)

a. 24 b. 27
c. 37 d. 45

Q9. True statement regarding second-degree deep burn: (PGI Dec 2008)

a. Blanch on pressure
b. Erythema
c. Dry with color
d. Painless
e. Predispose to hypothermia

Q10. 2nd degree burns indicate involvement of: (JIPMER 2013)

a. Epidermis b. Dermis
c. Subcutaneous tissue d. Deep fascia

Grade III	Most difficult

Q1. Features of deep second-degree burn are: (PGI December 2008)

a. Blanching under pressure
b. Blisters
c. Hypoesthesia
d. Thrombosis of vessels at the base

Q2. Burns with vesiculation, destruction of the epidermis, and upper dermis are: (PGI June 1999)

a. First degree
b. Second degree
c. Third degree
d. Fourth degree

Q3. In third-degree burns, all are seen, *except*: (PGI December 1999)

a. Vesicles are absent
b. Painful
c. Leathery skin
d. Reddish due to hemoglobin (Hb) infiltration

Q4. Metabolic derangements in severe burns are all, *except*: (PGI June 2000)

a. Increased corticosteroid secretion
b. Hyperglycemia
c. Increased secretion of HCl
d. Neutrophil dysfunction

Q5. In excessive burns, the least useful is: (AIIMS June 1994)

a. Blood
b. Dextran
c. Ringer's lactate
d. Nasogastric intubation

Q6. Which of the following is true about burns? (PGI Dec 2005)

a. Third-generation cephalosporin is the drug of choice.
b. *Staphylococcus aureus* is most common infection of burn.
c. Toxic shock syndrome is most common in burn patients.
d. *Pseudomonas* is the most common infection in dry wounds.
e. Moist dressing is done.

Q7. Which of the following is true about burn management? (PGI Dec 2005)

a. Intravenous access fluid is done, and antibiotics are not given in children.
b. Escharotomy should be done for a peripheral circumscribed lesion.
c. Moist dressing is done
d. The Parkland formula is used with 8 mL/kg/weight.
e. Prognosis depends on the time of resuscitation of the patient

Q8. Fever in a burnt patient is caused by: (PGI June 2009)

a. Due to hypermetabolism
b. Toxin released by dead tissue
c. Infection
d. Dead tissue products

Q9. True regarding opposite dressing is: (PGI May 2018)

a. Wound can be seen
b. Vapor permeable
c. Impermeable to bacteria
d. Water permeable
e. Increased chances of maceration

Q10. Which of the following statement(s) is/are true about postburn neck contracture? (PGI June 2009)

a. Occurs because of conservative management of deep burn
b. Treated by flaps
c. Obliteration of cervicomental angle
d. Dental abnormalities may be present
e. Never develop in deep dermal burn

ANSWERS

Grade I: 1. b, d, e; 2. a; 3. e; 4. c; 5. d, e; 6. a; 7. c; 8. c; 9. a; 10. a

Grade II: 1. d; 2. b, c, d, e; 3. a; 4. c; 5. d; 6. a; 7. c (Schwartz 19/e p199-200); 8. c (Sabiston 20/e p507); 9. b, d, e; 10. b

Grade III: 1. c, d; 2. b; 3. b; 4. c; 5. a; 6. d; 7. b, e; 8. a, c; 9. a, b, c (Sabiston 20/e p517); 10. a, b, c (Schwartz 10/e p182)

MODEL QUESTIONS

Q1. Intravenous (IV) rule for burns:

a. % body surface area × weight in pounds × 4 = Volume in mL
b. % BSA × weight in kg × 4 = Volume in L
c. % BSA × weight in kg × 5 = Volume in mL
d. % BSA × weight in kg × 4 = Volume in mL

Ans. d

Q2. A woman was brought to the casualty 8 hours after sustaining burns on the abdomen, both limbs, and back. What will be the best formula to calculate the amount of fluid to replenished?

a. 4 mL/kg = TBSA in first 8 hours, followed by 2 mL/kg/hour = % TBSA in 16 hours
b. 4 mL/kg × % TBSA in next 16 hours
c. 4 mL/kg × % TBSA in next 24 hours
d. 8 mL/kg × % TBSA

Ans. b

Q3. The best guide to adequate tissue perfusion in the fluid management of patients with burns, to ensure a minimum hourly urine output of:

a. 10–30 mL
b. 30–50 mL
c. 50–70 mL
d. 70–100 mL

Ans. b

Q4. Pus in burns form in:

a. 2–3 days
b. 3–5 days
c. 2–3 weeks
d. 4 weeks

Ans. a

Q5. What should be the time required if a burn wound heals without scar formation?

a. 3 weeks
b. 2 weeks
c. 6 weeks
d. Timing is not important.

Ans. b

Q6. True about burns:

a. Hyperglycemia is seen in early burns.
b. A child with burns should have a damp dressing.
c. Chemical powder burns should be kept dry
d. Third-degree burns are painful.

Ans. a

Q7. The outcome of burns depends on:

a. Extent of burns
b. Type of resuscitation fluid
c. Maintenance of the airway
d. Skin grafting

Ans. a

Q8. All may be seen in deep burns, *except*:

a. Hyperthermia
b. Increase vascular permeability
c. Fluid loss by evaporation
d. Vasodilatation

Ans. a

Q9. In burns, heat loss is by/due to:

a. Dilatation of veins
b. Shock
c. Exposed area by evaporation
d. None of the above

Ans. c

Q10. Late deaths in burns are due to:

a. Sepsis
b. Hypovolemia
c. Contractures
d. Neurogenic

Ans. a

Q11. Which type of shock is seen in burns?

a. Cardiogenic
b. Hypovolemic
c. Both of the above
d. None of the above

Ans. b

Q12. The most common cause of death due to burns in the early period is:

a. Sepsis
b. Hypovolemic shock
c. Both
d. None

Ans. b

Q13. All of the following are causes of death in burn patients, *except*:

a. Acute respiratory distress syndrome (ARDS)
b. Shock
c. Sepsis
d. Hyperkalemia

Ans. d

Q14. A child suffers scald burns on both of his hands due to hot water treatment. The lesion is pink, oozing, and painful to the air and touch. What is the most appropriate management?

a. Observe only with silver sulfadiazine ointment application every alternate day
b. Collagen dressing
c. Debride and leave the wound open
d. Excision and grafting

Ans. a

Q15. Treatment of burns includes:

a. No bandage to head and neck
b. Immediate application of ice-cold water
c. Superficial burns without blister—no need for dressing
d. Escharotomy was done for peripheral circumscribed lesions

Ans. a, b, c, and d

Q16. In a patient with a burn wound extending into the superficial epidermis without involving the dermis would present with all of the following, *except*:

a. Healing of the wound spontaneously without scar formation
b. Anesthesia at the site of burn
c. Blister formation
d. Painful

Ans. b

Q17. Myoglobinuria is seen in which type of burns?

a. Contact burn
b. Electric burn
c. Scalded
d. Flame burn

Ans. b

SUGGESTED READING

1. Bailey & Love's - Short Practice of Surgery, 27th edition.
2. Schwartz's Principles of Surgery, 18th edition.
3. Textbook of Surgery by David Sabiston, 21st edition.

CHAPTER 20

Plastic Surgery

"I definitely believe in plastic surgery. I don't want to be an old hag. There is no fun in that."

– Scarlett Johansson

INTRODUCTION

Plastic surgery is required for cosmetic and functional needs of the body. Burn causes tissue damage, and healing causes scars, contractures, and limitation of movements, which essentially require plastic or reconstructive surgery.

> Reconstructive plastic (from the ancient Greek plassein, to mold or shape, which is also the stem of our modern use of the materials termed "plastics". India, in the sixth century BC, where Sushruta describe using the forehead flap to reconstruct a nose. Sushruta, regarded as the father of modern surgery, lived in the Indian city of Kashi (now called Banaras) in 600 BC.

SKIN GRAFTS (FIG. 1)

- *Split-thickness skin graft (STSG):* It has epidermis and part of the dermis. These are also called Thiersch (Karl Thiersch, 1822–1895, German surgeon) grafts.
- *Full-thickness skin graft (FTSG):* It has epidermis, full dermis with some underlying fat (composite graft). Also called Wolfe (John Reissberg Wolfe, 1824–1904, British ophthalmic surgeon), grafts. The composite graft may have fat or cartilage.

The skin graft survives by imbibition of plasma to start with, then inosculation happens by capillary growth and fibroblast maturation.

The principles of plastic surgery include proper debridement, good blood supply, placement to have the least scar, and clean surgery.

Meshed skin grafts are used to expand the surface area of the graft when a large area coverage is required. The drawback is high secondary contraction. Meshing ratio is 1:1.5–1:1.6.

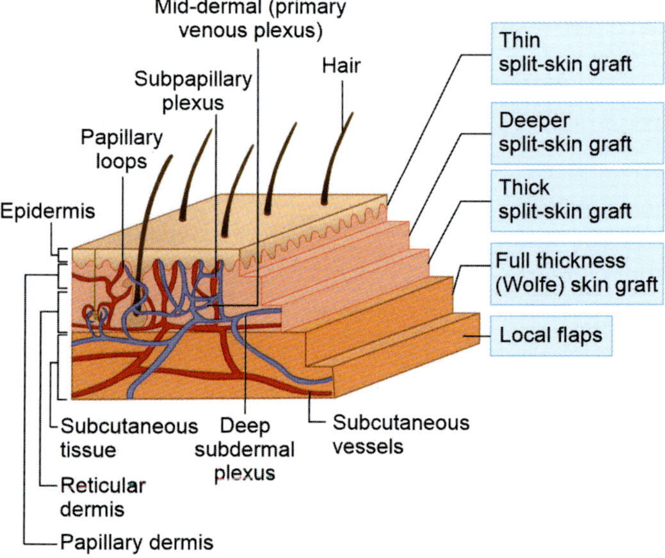

Fig. 1: Types of skin grafts.

Pedicle graft or flap: It is a completely separate segment with having own blood supply. It is used to cover exposed bones, open joints, bed sores over bony prominences, and eyelids. Flaps are of various types: random, axial, and free **(Fig. 2)**.

Random flap: It depends upon the dermal blood supply, and the best length/breadth ratio is 3:1.

It is good for postburn contractures. Examples are Z-plasty, V-Y plasty, rhomboid flap, bilobed flap, and bipedicled flap.

Axial flap: It depends upon the blood supply from the donor site. Mathes and Nahai classified axial flaps based on pedicles. Examples are *deltopectoral (DP) flap,*

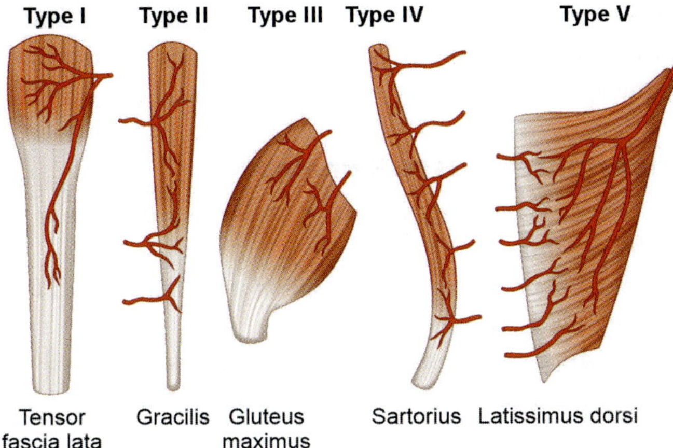

Fig. 2: Various pedicle grafts.

pectoralis major myocutaneous flap (PMMC), transverse rectus abdominis myocutaneous (TRAM) flap, and *deep inferior epigastric artery perforator (DIEP) flap.*

Free flap: It is disconnected from the original site, usually for head and neck plastic surgery. Examples are radial artery forearm flap and free fibular flap.

> *Types of grafts:*
> - *Autograft*—from the same person
> - *Isograft*—from an identical twin
> - *Allograft*—from the same species, as human to human
> - *Xenograft*—from a different species, as a pig to a man
>
> Flaps have their own blood supply, whereas grafts depend upon the recipient tissue.
>
> *Contracture of graft:*
> - *Primary contracture* is more with FTSG and less with STSG.
> - *Secondary contracture* is more with STSG and less with FTSG.

SKIN GRAFT TAKE

The body accepts a skin graft in three stages:

1. *Plasma inhibition*—first 48 hours, free absorption of nutrients into the skin graft
2. *Inosculation*—4–5 days alignment of donor and recipient capillaries
3. *Revascularization*: After 5 days graft has anterior inflow and venous outflow.

> *Marjolin's ulcer:* It is a malignant ulcer of low grade [*squamous cell carcinoma (SCC)*]. It usually arises from a chronic ulcer, a postburn scar, and a postradiation ulcer. It is a slow-growing, painless, avascular, and radioresistant. Wide local excision is the treatment of choice.

Bowen's disease: It is SCC in situ caused by chronic solar damage. It is a slow-growing epidermal lesion treated by topical 5-fluorouracil for surgical removal.

Bedsores (pressure sores): Persistent pressure on the sites of bony prominence, such as the ischium and greater trochanter. Bedsores can be divided into four stages:

1. *Stage I:* Intact skin with redness
2. *Stage II:* Loss of upper layer of skin
3. *Stage III:* Loss of full thickness of skin
4. *Stage IV:* Loss of skin and deeper tissues

Debridement, *vacuum-assisted closure (VAC)* dressing, and flap graft can be used. VAC dressing increases wound healing and simultaneously removes dead tissues. It is best used for chronic nonhealing ulcers, bedsores, and diabetic wounds.

Cleft lip and cleft palate: They occur especially when a mother uses steroids, antiepileptic drugs, and barbiturates during pregnancy. They may occur as a genetic cause, and Pierre Robin syndrome. One in 500–600 births is the incidence, with more in males. A cleft lip may be on one side or both sides. Surgery is required for speech or feeding problems and cosmetic reasons. Cleft palate can involve only the soft palate or the hard palate also.

Tissue expanders: Tissue expanders are used where the requirement of skin coverage is more than available. It causes mechanical stretching of the skin.

Basal cell carcinoma (rodent ulcer, BCC): It is a locally penetrating cancer from the basal layer of epidermis, 90% on the face, above a line drawn from the lobe of the ear to the angle of the mouth. It occurs near the inner canthus of the eye, called tear cancer. It can be of various types: nodular (most common), pigmented, cystic, and superficial. It is a localized disease without metastasis. Low-grade malignancy occurs in fair color individuals. It is treated by surgical excision **(Fig. 3)**.

> *Causes of failure of a graft:*
> - Seroma formation under the graft.
> - Hematoma formation under the graft.
> - Movement/shearing force at the recipient site.
> - Infection.
> - Granulation or fibrous tissue at the recipient site.
> - Bone or the perichondrium at the recipient site.

Squamous cell carcinoma (epithelioma, SCC): It starts from the prickle cell layer of epidermis, in dark color individuals, caused by sunlight, over the ears, cheeks, lower lip, etc. SCC is usually caused by sunlight, chronic irritation,

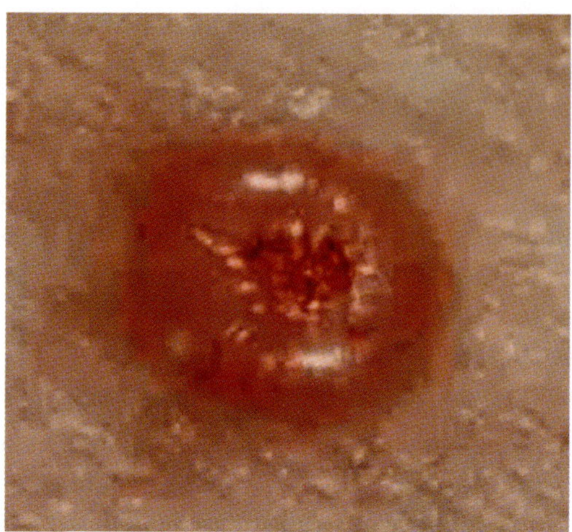

Fig. 3: Basal cell carcinoma.

and immunosuppression in old age. It is a nodular and ulcerative type of lesion. It is treated by surgical excision.

Malignant melanoma: It occurs due to malignant transformation of melanocytes over the trunk and lower extremities in fair-skinned persons with sunburns. Sunburn, UV radiation, family history of melanoma, giant melanocytic nevus, and xeroderma pigmentosum. Malignant melanoma is of several types: superficial spreading (most common), nodular, lentigo maligna (least malignant), and acral lentiginous. It is usually an asymmetrical lesion with a dark color. It metastasizes through lymphatics, commonly in the liver. It has microsatellites of 0.05 mm in tumor cells. It is a radioresistant tumor, so treated by surgical excision or chemotherapy. It is divided into five groups (Clark's levels) as I, II, III, IV, and V.

I = Epidermis, II = Papillary dermis, III = Papillary and reticular dermis, IV = Invading reticular dermis, and V = Subcutaneous tissue.

Breslow divided malignant melanoma according to thickness into four stages. *Stage I:* <0.75 mm; *Stage II:* 0.75–1.5 mm; *Stage III:* 1.6–4 mm; and *Stage IV:* >4 mm.

Prognostic factors deciding the fate of malignant melanoma depend upon depth, ulceration, metastasis, satellite lesions, and lymph node involvement.

Vascular Abnormalities in Skin

- Port-wine stain is a vascular malformation over face along fifth cranial nerve distribution at birth.
- Strawberry angiomas are capillary hemangioma appear 1–3 weeks after birth, 90% involute completely at 9 years of age.

Salmon patch: It is also known as the macular stain, present at birth, usually on the forehead, and disappears by the age of one.

Important Points to Remember

- The most common cause of skin graft failure is hematoma.
- The most common donor site of a partial skin graft is the thigh.
- The most common type of skin cancer is BCC.
- The most common type of skin cancer in darkly pigmented cases—SCC
- The most common cause of SCC—sunlight
- The most common route of metastasis in malignant lymphoma is lymphatic.
- The most common site of systemic metastasis in malignant melanoma is the liver.
- The most common subcutaneous neoplasm—lipoma.
- The most common site of lipoma is the trunk.
- Cock's (Edward Cock, 1805–1892, English Surgeon) peculiar tumor is infected/ulcerated sebaceous cyst of scalp
- *Cylindroma (turban tumor):* It is a malignant epithelial tumor.
- Pott's (Sir Percivall Pott, 1714–1788, English surgeon) puffy tumor—osteomyelitis of the frontal bone of the skull
- *Pilomatrixoma:* Benign hair follicle tumor, also known as calcifying epitheliomas of Malherbe (A Malherbe).
- The most common site of malignant melanoma in males is the back and trunk
- The most common site of malignant melanoma in females is the lower extremity
- Most commonly involved persons from malignant melanoma—Fair persons
- There is no punctum in sebaceous cysts of the scrotum on scalp sebaceous cysts.

CLARK'S CLASSIFICATION OF MALIGNANT MELANOMA

- *Level I:* Up to epiderma
- *Level II:* Invading papillary dermis
- *Level III:* Reaching the interphase of papillary and reticular dermis
- *Level IV:* Invading reticular dermis
- *Level V:* Invading subcutaneous

BRESLOW STAGING (TISSUE DEPTH BASED)

- *Stage I:* <0.75 mm
- *Stage II:* 0.75–1.5 mm
- *Stage III:* 1.6–4 mm
- *State IV:* >4 mm

SOME IMPORTANT QUESTIONS

Q1. All are advantages of split-thickness skin grafting, *except*:
a. Good uptake
b. Less contraction
c. Reusable donor site
d. Large grafts can be harvested

Ans. b

Q2. The Abbe–Estlander flap is used for:
a. Lip b. Tongue
c. Eyelid d. Ears

Ans. a

Q3. Which of the following grafts is known as Wolfe's graft?
a. Split-thickness graft
b. Full-thickness graft
c. Partial-thickness graft
d. Myocutaneous graft

Ans. b

Q4. A full-thickness graft can be obtained from all of the following, *except*:
a. Elbow b. Back of neck
c. Supraclavicular area d. Upper eyelids

Ans. b

Q5. Reconstruction of the tip of the nose after excision of basal cell carcinoma is done by:
a. Bipedicle flap b. Bilobed flap
c. Rhomboid flap d. Advancement flap

Ans. b

Q6. Bipedicle flap is used for reconstruction of:
a. Nose b. Fingertip
c. Eyelid d. Breast

Ans. c

Q7. Skin graft stored at 4°C can survive up to:
a. 1 week b. 2 weeks
c. 3 weeks d. 4 weeks

Ans. d

Q8. "Take in" of split skin graft occurs when?
a. Tight dressing is applied
b. Excessive discharge from the wound
c. β-hemolytic *Streptococcus* infection is present
d. Wound bed not vascularized

Ans. None

Q9. Thiersch graft is which type of graft?
a. Partial thickness b. Full thickness
c. Pedicle d. Patch

Ans. a

Q10. Which one of the following is not a wound closure technique? (UPSC 2008)
a. Partial thickness skin graft
b. Composite graft
c. Vascular graft
d. Musculocutaneous graft

Ans. c

Q11. Who said, "Skin is the best dressing"?
a. Joseph Lister b. John Hunter
c. James Paget d. McNeill Love

Ans. a

Q12. Within 48 hours of transplantation, the skin graft survives due to:
a. Amount of saline in graft
b. Plasma imbibition
c. New vessels growing from the donor tissue
d. Connection between donor and recipient capillaries

Ans. b

MULTIPLE CHOICE QUESTIONS

Grade I	*Simple*

Q1. The best dressing is: (PGI 1988)
a. Opsite b. Amnion
c. Tulle-gras d. Skin

Q2. The best skin graft for open wounds is: (AI 1993)
a. Isograft b. Homograft
c. Allograft d. Autograft

Q3. Within 48 hours of transplantation, skin graft survives due to: (AIIMS November 2000)
a. Amount of saline in graft
b. Plasma imbibitions
c. New vessels growing from the donor tissue
d. Connection between donor and recipient capillaries

Q4. Ideal graft for leg injury with 10 × 10 cm exposed bone: (AIIMS Nov 1999)

a. Amniotic membrane graft
b. Pedicle graft
c. Full-thickness graft
d. Split-thickness skin graft

Q5. All can take split-thickness graft, *except*: (AIIMS Sept 1996)

a. Fat
b. Muscle
c. Skull bone
d. Deep fascia

Q6. All are true about skin grafting, *except*: (All India 2000)

a. Partial-thickness graft involves epidermis and part of dermis
b. Full-thickness graft includes epidermis, dermis, without subcutaneous tissue
c. For large areas full-thickness graft is used.
d. Full-thickness graft has cosmetic value.

Q7. True statement for axial flap is: (All India 1997)

a. Carries its own vessel within it
b. Kept in limb
c. Transverse flap
d. Carries its own nerve in it

Q8. Split skin graft can be applied over: (PGI June 1999)

a. Muscle
b. Bone
c. Cartilage
d. Eyelid

Q9. A tumor arising in a burn scar is likely to be: (PGI June 2006)

a. Basal cell carcinoma
b. Squamous cell carcinoma
c. Malignant melanoma
d. Fibrosarcoma

Q10. Which of the following is true about Marjolin's ulcer?

a. Ulcer over scar
b. Rapid growth
c. Rodent ulcer
d. Painful

Grade II	*Difficult*

Q1. Best procedure to be done after an injury to the leg associated with exposure of underlying bone and skin loss: (AIIMS Nov 1998)

a. Pedicle flap
b. Split skin grafting
c. Full-thickness grafting
d. Skin flap

Q2. Full-thickness graft can be obtained from all of the following, *except*: (AIIMS 1987)

a. Axilla
b. Groin
c. Supraclavicular area
d. Elbow

Q3. Skin graft for facial wounds is taken from: (AIIMS 1992)

a. Medial aspect of thigh
b. Cubital fossa
c. Groin
d. Postauricular region

Q4. What is the most probable diagnosis based on the given image? (AIIMS Nov 2017)

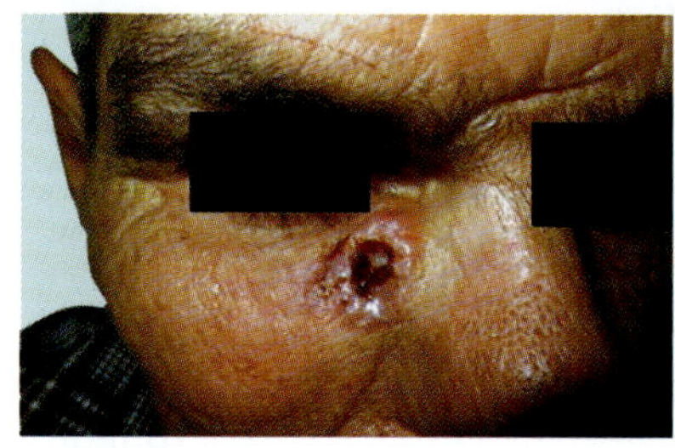

a. Basal cell carcinoma
b. Malignant melanoma
c. Squamous cell carcinoma
d. Marjolin's ulcer

Q5. True about malignant melanoma: (PGI June 2008)

a. Lymphatic spread
b. Lymph node biopsy is always done
c. Biopsy to be done when the sentinel node is involved
d. Microsatellitism

Q6. Melanoma should be excised with a margin of: (UPSC 1988)

a. 2 cm
b. 5 cm
c. 7 cm
d. 10 cm

Q7. The best results in the treatment of capillary nevus have been achieved by: (AIIMS 1984)

a. Full thickness skin graft
b. Dermabrasion
c. Tattooing
d. Argon laser treatment

Q8. An 11-month-old child presents with erythematous lesions with central clearing, which have been decreasing in size? (All India 1997)

a. Strawberry angioma
b. Nevus
c. Portwine stain
d. Cavernous hemangioma

Q9. The best cosmetic results for large capillary (port-wine) hemangiomas are achieved by: (UPSC 2005)

a. Excision and split-thickness skin
b. Laser ablation
c. Chemotherapy
d. Immunotherapy

Q10. Which is not true about Sturge-Weber syndrome? (AIIMS Sept 1996)

a. Portwine stain
b. Calcification in brain
c. Cortical atrophy
d. Intracranial hamartoma

Grade III	Most difficult

Q1. Split skin grafts in young children should be harvested from: (UPSC 2007)

a. Buttocks b. Thigh
c. Trunk d. Upper limb

Q2. Which one of the following statements about mesh skin grafts is not correct? (UPSC 2006)

a. They permit coverage of large areas
b. They allow egress of fluid collection under the graft
c. They contract to the same degree as a grafted sheet of skin
d. They "take" satisfactorily on a granulating bed

Q3. Skin grafting is absolutely C/I (contraindication) in which skin infection? (AIIMS June 1997)

a. *Staphylococcus* b. *Pseudomonas*
c. *Streptococcus* d. *Proteus*

Q4. What does "take in" mean in the case of skin grafting? (AIIMS June 1997)

a. Revascularization of the graft
b. Return of the sensation
c. When the graft becomes adherent to the recipient site
d. Nonadherent graft is shed off.

Q5. Cock's peculiar tumor is: (AIIMS Nov 2010)

a. Basal cell carcinoma
b. Squamous cell carcinoma
c. Ulcerated sebaceous cyst
d. Cylindroma

Q6. True about keratoacanthoma: (PGI 2000)

a. Benign tumor
b. Malignant skin tumor, like squamous cell carcinoma
c. Treatment same as for squamous cell carcinoma
d. Easy to differentiate from squamous cell carcinoma histologically
e. Treatment is masterly inactivity

Q7. Calcifying epithelioma is seen in: (JIPMER 1995)

a. Dermatofibroma b. Adenoma sebaceum
c. Pyogenic granuloma d. Pilomatrixoma

Q8. Which is true regarding frostbite injury? (PGI Nov 2017)

a. In first- and second-degree frostbite, the affected part shows redness and edema
b. Spontaneous recovery without any treatment is the rule
c. Extensive involvement in frostbite is called chilblain
d. Initial treatment is rewarming
e. Autoamputation may occur in severe cases

Q9. Pyogenic granuloma, true statements is/are: (PGI June 2007)

a. Vascular pathology
b. Bleeds rarely
c. Increase in pregnancy
d. Local excision
e. Recurrent and malignant

Q10. Lines of Blaschko represent: (All India 2011)

a. Lines along lymphatics
b. Lines along blood vessels
c. Lines along nerves
d. Lines of development

ANSWERS

Grade I: 1. d; 2. d; 3. b; 4. b; 5. c; 6. c; 7. a; 8. a; 9. b; 10. a
Grade II: 1. a; 2. a; 3. d; 4. a (Harrison 19/e p500); 5. a, b, c, d; 6. a; 7. d; 8. a; 9. b; 10. d (Bailey 26/e p599)
Grade III: 1. b; 2. c; 3. c; 4. a; 5. c; 6. a, e; 7. d; 8. a, d, e; 9. a, c, d; 10. d

MODEL QUESTIONS

Q1. The most commonly used myocutaneous pedicle graft for pelvis surgeries contains muscle segments from:

a. Rectus abdominis muscle
b. External oblique muscle
c. Internal oblique muscle
d. Transversus abdominis muscle

Ans. a

Q2. Z-plasty ideal angle is:

a. 30° b. 45°
c. 60° d. 90°

Ans. c

Q3. Revascularization and angiogenesis process after skin grafting is seen after how many days after the procedure?

a. 4 b. 5
c. 6 d. 7

Ans. b

Q4. How much length is increased in Z-plasty when it is done at 60°?

a. 25% b. 50%
c. 75% d. 100%

Ans. c

Q5. Longitudinal incision with Z-plasty closure is used in which of the following?

a. Hand surgery b. Breast surgery
c. Thyroid surgery d. Hernia surgery

Ans. a

Q6. The subdermal plexus forms the vascular basis for:

a. Randomized flaps
b. Axial flaps
c. Mucocutaneous flaps
d. Fasciocutaneous flap

Ans. a

Q7. In hand injury, the first structure to be repaired should be:

a. Skin b. Nerve
c. Muscle d. Bone

Ans. d

Q8. Ideal graft for leg injury with 10 × 10 cm exposed bone:

a. Amniotic membrane graft
b. Pedicle graft
c. Full thickness graft
d. Split thickness skin graft

Ans. b

Q9. Wolfe Graft is:

a. Thin split thickness graft
b. Thick split thickness skin graft
c. Medium thickness split thickness skin graft
d. Full-thickness skin graft

Ans. d

Q10. All can take split thickness graft *except*:

a. Fat b. Muscle
c. Skull bone d. Deep fascia

Ans. c

Q11. All are true about skin grafting, *except*:

a. Partial thickness graft involves epidermis and part of dermis
b. Full thickness graft includes epidermis, dermis, without subcutaneous tissue
c. For large areas, full-thickness graft is used
d. Full-thickness graft has cosmetic value

Ans. c

Q12. A split skin graft can be applied over:

a. Muscle b. Bone
c. Cartilage d. Eyelid

Ans. a

SUGGESTED READING

1. Bailey & Love's - Short Practice of Surgery, 27th edition.
2. Schwartz's Principles of Surgery, 18th edition.
3. Textbook of Surgery by David Sabiston, 21st edition.

Section 4 Head and Neck

Brain and Central Nervous System Tumors

"The brain is a wonderful organ; it starts working the moment you get up in the morning and does not stop until you get into the office."

– Robert Frost

CEREBROSPINAL FLUID

Cerebrospinal fluid (CSF) is produced by the choroid plexus of each lateral ventricle of the brain. It circulates all over the brain and flows over the surface of the brain and spinal cord into the subarachnoid space **(Figs. 1A and B)**.

CIRCULATION OF CEREBROSPINAL FLUID

Cerebrospinal fluid is produced by choroid plexus of the lateral ventricles to the third ventricle through foramen of *Monro (Alexander Monro, 1733–1817, English anatomist), then through aqueduct of Sylvius (Franciscus Salvius, 1614–1672, Dutch physician)* to the fourth ventricle, where it exits to the subarachnoid space via midline foramen of *Magendie (Francos Magendie, 1783–1855, French pathologist and physiologist)* and lateral foramina of *Luschka (Hubert von Luschka, 1820–1875, German anatomist).*

Cerebrospinal fluid performs many functions:
- Support
- Shock absorber
- Homeostasis
- Nutrition
- Immune function
- Cerebrospinal fluid, approximately 150 mL, is present in the brain.

INTRACRANIAL PRESSURE

Intracranial pressure (ICP) is important in head injuries. Continuous perfusion of the brain with oxygenated blood is important for survival. Raised ICP can affect the perfusion of the brain, causing secondary brain injury. ICP can cause high-pressure headaches that increase on straining, coughing, or bending forward. Low-pressure headache is caused by excessive loss of CSF by *lumbar puncture (LP)* drainage, and the headache is increased in an erect posture. It may be associated with nausea, vomiting, blurred vision, and other nerve compression signs. Fontanelle is tense and bulging with raised ICP in an infant. *Parinaud's syndrome is seen in children where raised ICP causes midbrain compression leading to the sunsetting sign, and loss of upgaze.*

Increased ICP can be due to a tumor, hydrocephalus, or cerebral edema. A computed tomography (CT) scan is the first line of investigation. *Magnetic resonance imaging (MRI)* is also used as an investigative tool.

HYDROCEPHALUS

Cerebrospinal fluid is produced normally about 20 mL/h. When CSF volume increases with ventricular enlargement, it is called *hydrocephalus.*

Things to remember:
- Acutely raised ICP is a neurological emergency.
- Obstructive or communicating hydrocephalus may occur due to a pathology or its treatment.
- The first line of investigation in a hydrocephalus case is a CT scan of the brain.
- Normal pressure hydrocephalus is a reversal entity.
- External ventricular drainage (EVD) can give temporary CSF diversion.
- Meningitis also appears as a complication of head injury or neurosurgery.
- Ring-enhancing lesion sign on CT brain differentiates brain abscess from brain tumor.

Obstructive Hydrocephalus

It is caused by a lesion in the ventricle or its wall. It can lead to sudden deterioration of consciousness, leading to coma and eventually death. LP is contraindicated as it can

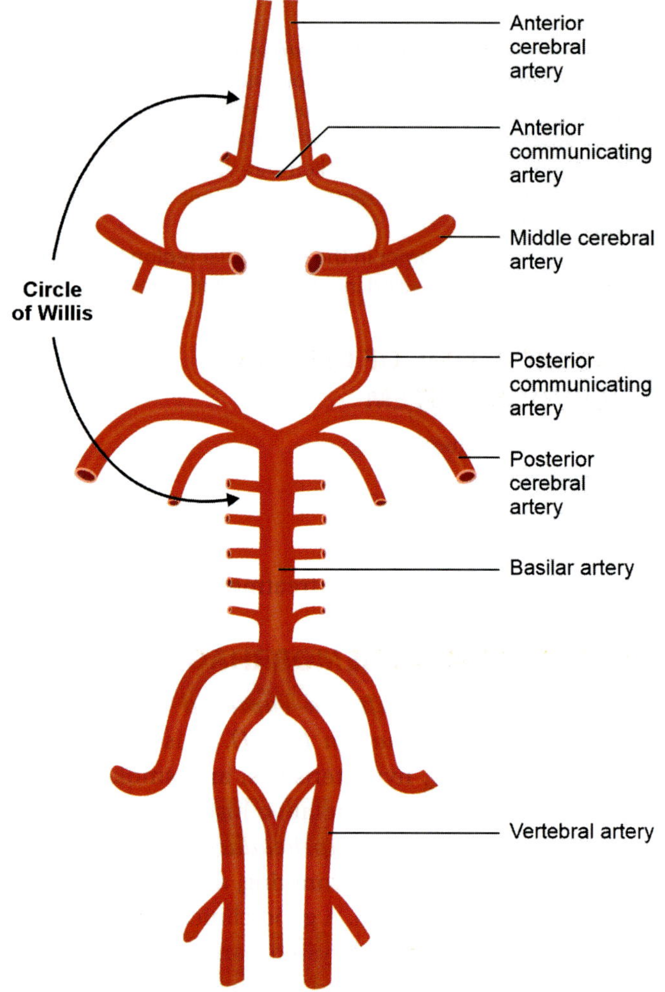

Fig. 2: Circle of Willis.

> *Not to forget:*
> - Subdural empyema on CT is shown as a typical crescentic collection with a rim.
> - Spontaneous SAH is commonly the result of a ruptured aneurysm.
> - Delayed ischemic neurological deficit (DNID) is seen 3–10 days after aneurysmal hemorrhage.
> - CT scan and LP are the initial investigations in SAH.

BRAIN TUMORS

The word brain tumor includes various entities other than tumors. One of the most common brain tumors are gliomas, which are oligodendrogliomas, astrocytomas, ependymomas, and choroid plexus tumors **(Flowchart 1)**. MRI of the brain with or without CT is a required investigation. Surgical excision is the treatment of choice. High-dose focused radiotherapy and chemotherapy as carmustine, are required in some cases.

Flowchart 1: Classification of brain tumors.

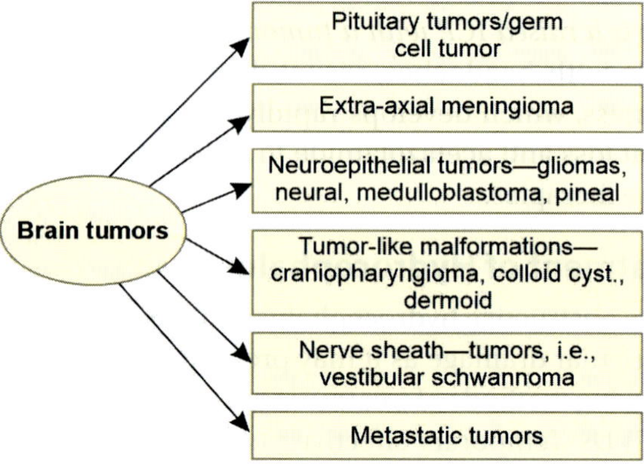

Raised ICP, worse in the morning and on straining, with nausea, vomiting, and seizures, makes a typical clinical picture. *A progressive focal deficit invites attention for a brain tumor.*

> *Mn for genetics = ReLocating Nerve Muscle Tumor Treat Very Gently*
> - *R* = Retinoblastoma
> - *L* = Ll-Fraumeni
> - *N* = NF-1&2
> - *M* = MEN1
> - *T* = Turcot's syndrome
> - *T* = Tuberous sclerosis
> - *V* = VHL syndrome
> - *G* = Gorlin syndrome

ASTROCYTOMA

It arises from astrocytes. Supratentorial and high grade in adults and infratentorial in children. They infiltrate adjacent brain tissue and are low-grade.

World Health Organization Classification of Astrocytoma

- *Grade I:* A. Pilocytic—treated in radical resection
- *Grade II:* Low grade A—radiation + Chemotherapy
- *Grade III:* Anaplastic A—cytoreductive surgery + external beam radiation therapy (EBRT)
- *Grade IV:* GBM—cytoreductive surgery + EBRT

OLIGODENDROGLIOMA

- *Characteristic features:* Histology-fluid egg cytoplasm, chicken wire vasculature, and microscopic calcification.
- *Diagnosis:* CT and MRI
- *Treatment:* Surgical resection + chemotherapy

EPENDYMOMA

Arises from the ependymal lining of the cerebral hemisphere.

- *Most common type:* Myxopapillary ependymoma
- *Diagnosis:* CT/MRI
- *Treatment:* Maximum resection + EBRT

MEDULLOBLASTOMA

- The most common malignant brain tumor of childhood.
- Highly malignant
- The most common radiosensitive tumor of the brain.
- The most common site is the vermis (75%).
- Metastasis through CSF—drop metastasis and bone, LNs, liver.

Treatment—surgical excision.

Cerebral Metastases

These are the most common brain tumors. These tumors can come from the pituitary gland, vestibular schwannoma, meningioma, lung tumor, breast tumor, prostate tumor, renal tumor, and melanoma.

MENINGIOMA

These are usually benign tumors, but malignant tumors also occur. A CT scan is the required investigation. Corticosteroids with or without surgery are required. Recurrence is noticed. Benign tumors, if resected, can give a cure.

Calcification Present

- The most common site superior sagittal sinus.
- Slow growing
- Radiology—calcification, bony hyperostosis, sun ray appearance, blistering (bone expansion with pneumatization)

Treatment—surgery.

PITUITARY TUMOR

A benign pituitary adenoma is the most common pituitary tumor. Microadenomas are smaller than 10 mm in size and macroadenomas are >10 mm in size. Malignant pituitary tumors are also found. Surgical resection by transsphenoidal root is the best.

Most pituitary adenomas develop in the anterior pituitary gland. It is the most common cause of hyperpituitarism.

Types

- *Functional*—secreting—causes symptoms due to secretion.
- *Nonfunctional*—nonsecreting—causes neurological symptoms due to pressure.
- The most common tumor is prolactinoma, which causes amenorrhea and galactorrhea.
- *Diagnosis:* MRI
- *Treatment:* Surgical research via intranasal transsphenoidal approach.

Brain Tumors in Children

Children also suffer with brain tumors:

- Teratoma
- Primitive neuroectodermal tumor (PNET)
- High-grade astrocytoma
- Choroid plexus papilloma/carcinoma
- Medulloblastoma
- Ependymoma
- Pilocytic astrocytoma

Forget me not:

- The most common tumor of the brain is metastasis.
- WHO Grade I is a benign lesion, and Grade IV is high-grade malignant.
- Triad of seizure, raised ICP, and focal neurological deficit is a common clinical feature triad in brain tumors.
- MRI is generally the best investigative modality for brain tumors.
- Harvey Williams Cushing, 1869–1939, American Neurosurgeon, is considered the father of modern neurosurgery.

Central nervous system tumors can be classified into intra-axial and extra-axial tumors:

Mn = NAL and SPM:

- *N* = Neuronal tumors
- *A* = Astrocytoma, i.e., glioma
- *L* = Lymphoma
- *S* = Schwannoma
- *P* = Pituitary tumors
- *M* = Meningioma

NEURAL TUBE DEFECTS

Failure of closure of neuro tube leads to certain defects:

- *Spina bifida occulta*—absence of spinous process without exposure of meninges or nerve tissue. It has spasticity and bladder dysfunction. There is a characteristic hair-covered area at the base of the spine.

- *Meningocele*—a sac of meningitis
- *Myelomeningocele*—herniation of meninges without skin covering, containing spinal cord or nerves or both.

Wada Test (Juhn Atsushi Wada, 1924—Japanese Neurologist)

It is a functional test to confirm language laterality. *Amobarbital* is injected into each internal carotid artery, with testing of speech and memory to localize the function.

BERRY ANEURYSMS

These are saccular, junctional, and the most common type of aneurysms. They occur in the brain and abdominal aorta. *Terson's syndrome includes SAH with vitreous hemorrhage, seen in Berry aneurysms.* Treated by clipping or coiling after cerebral angiography.

DANDY-WALKER SYNDROME

It is a cystic dilatation of the fourth ventricle. There is hypogenesis or absence of cerebellar vermis. There is hydrocephalus, occipital prominence, and macrocephaly.

Some points to be remembered:

- The most common primary brain tumor—meningioma
- The most common brain tumor—metastasis
- The most malignant brain tumor in childhood —medulloblastoma **(Fig. 3)**

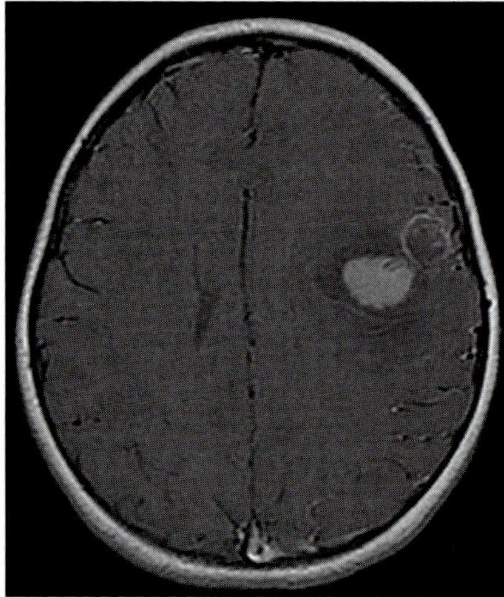

Fig. 3: Brain tumor.

- Most radiosensitive brain tumor—medulloblastoma
- Investigation of choice for brain tumor is MRI
- Most common astrocytoma in adults—glioblastoma multiforme (GBM)
- Most common astrocytoma in children—pilocytic astrocytoma
- Wada (Juhn Atsushi Wada, 1924—Japanese neurologist) test—sodium amobarbital is injected into the internal carotid arteries to confirm language laterality, so that resection on the side of the lesion will not significantly impair verbal memory function.

SOME IMPORTANT QUESTIONS

Q1. The most common extradural spinal tumor is:

a. Neurofibroma
b. Glioma
c. Meningioma
d. Metastasis

Ans. d

Q2. The nerve of Kuntz is an important landmark in:

a. Lumbar sympathectomy
b. Cervicodorsal sympathectomy
c. Obturator neurectomy
d. Splanchnicectomy
e. Herniorrhaphy

Ans. b

Q3. Neurosurgical treatment of epilepsy usually involves the removal of the epileptic focus from which lobe?

a. Frontal lobe
b. Temporal lobe
c. Occipital lobe
d. Parietal lobe

Ans. b

Q4. Which of the following brain tumors does not spread via cerebrospinal fluid (CSF)?

a. Germ cell tumor
b. Medulloblastoma
c. Central nervous system (CNS) lymphoma
d. Craniopharyngioma

Ans. d

Q5. Which is the most common childhood CNS tumor to metastasize outside the brain?

a. Ependymoma
b. Glioblastoma multiforme
c. Choroid plexus tumor
d. Medulloblastoma

Ans. d

Q6. The following are the features of raised intracranial tension, *except*:

a. Altered sensorium b. Papilledema
c. Convulsions d. Tachycardia

Ans. d

Q7. Facial nerve palsy is seen in which of the following fractures?

a. Anterior cranial fossa b. Middle cranial fossa
c. Cranial vault d. Posterior cranial fossa

Ans. b

Q8. The lowest incidence of cerebral tumors is seen in:

a. Occipital b. Frontal
c. Temporal d. Parietal

Ans. a

Q9. The most common orbital tumor causing exophthalmos is:

a. Glioma b. Meningioma
c. Hemangioma d. Neuroblastoma

Ans. a

Q10. Musculoskeletal abnormality in neurofibromatosis is:

a. Hypertrophy of the limb
b. Scoliosis
c. Café au lait spots
d. Pseudoarthrosis
e. All

Ans. e

Q11. Immediate surgery is indicated in:

a. Extradural b. Subdural
c. Intracerebral abscess d. Brain laceration

Ans. a and b

Q12. In neuroblastomas, the most common presentation is:

a. Lytic lesion in the skull with suture diastasis
b. Lung metastasis
c. Renal invasion
d. Secondaries in the brain

Ans. a

Q13. All produce carpal tunnel syndrome, *except*:

a. Colle's fracture b. Acromegaly
c. Addison's disease d. Hypothyroidism

Ans. c

Q14. The most common spinal tumor is:

a. Meningioma b. Ependymoma
c. Neurofibroma d. Neuroblastomas

Ans. c

Q15. In a patient with a head injury with rapidly increasing intracranial tension without hematoma, the drug of choice for initial management would be:

a. Lasix b. Steroids
c. 20% mannitol d. Glycine

Ans. c

Q16. Neurofibromatosis presents as all of the following, *except*:

a. Elephantiasis neuromatosa
b. Plexiform neuroma
c. Von Recklinghausen's disease
d. Lymphadenovarix

Ans. d

Q17. Mild head injury is having a Glasgow Coma Scale of:

a. 3–5 b. 5–8
c. 8–10 d. 10–15

Ans. d

Q18. Which of the following is the best treatment for subdural hematoma in a deteriorating patient?

a. By intravenous (IV) mannitol
b. Oxygenation
c. Use of steroids
d. Surgical evacuation

Ans. d

Q19. The most common neurologic abnormality that occurs with head injury is:

a. Hemiplegia b. Ocular nerve palsy
c. Altered consciousness d. Convulsion

Ans. c

Q20. Which of the following will manifest as "pachymeningitis hemorrhagica interna?"

a. Epidural hematoma
b. Subdural hematoma
c. Subarachnoid hemorrhage (SAH)
d. Brain infraction

Ans. b

Q21. Which of the following carcinomas most frequently metastasizes into the brain?

a. Small cell carcinoma of lung
b. Prostate cancer
c. Rectal carcinoma
d. Endometrial cancer

Ans. a

MULTIPLE CHOICE QUESTIONS

Grade I	Simple

Q1. The most common shunt for hydrocephalus is: (AIIMS May 2015)

a. Ventriculoperitoneal shunt
b. Ventriculoatrial shunt
c. Ventriculopleural shunt
d. Lumboperitoneal shunt

Q2. All are common sites of berry aneurysm, *except*: (AIIMS June 1993)

a. Posterior cerebral artery
b. Vertebral artery
c. Anterior cerebral artery
d. Middle cerebral artery

Q3. All of the following lower ICP, *except*: (All India 1998)

a. Mannitol
b. Furosemide
c. Corticosteroids
d. Hyperventilation

Q4. In skull fracture, the condition in which an operation is not done immediately is: (All India 1996)

a. Depressed fracture
b. Compound fracture
c. CSF leak
d. Increased size of the head

Q5. In normal pressure hydrocephalus, all are seen, *except*: (PGI Dec 1997)

a. Convulsion
b. Ataxia
c. Dementia
d. Incontinence

Q6. The most common location of hypertensive intracranial hemorrhage is: (All India 2006)

a. Subarachnoid space
b. Basal ganglia
c. Cerebellum
d. Brainstem

Q7. Which of the following brain tumors is highly vascular in nature? (AIIMS May 2016)

a. Glioblastoma
b. Meningiomas
c. Cerebellopontine angle (CP) angle epidermoid
d. Pituitary adenomas

Q8. The most preferred approach for pituitary surgery at the present time is: (All India 2006)

a. Transcranial
b. Transethmoidal
c. Transsphenoidal
d. Transcallosal

Q9. Which of the following is the most common type of glial tumor? (All India 2006)

a. Astrocytomas
b. Medulloblastomas
c. Neurofibromas
d. Ependymomas

Q10. Brain abscess in cyanotic heart disease is commonly located in: (All India 2006)

a. Cerebellar hemisphere
b. Thalamus
c. Temporal lobe
d. Parietal lobe

Q11. Plexiform neurofibromatosis commonly affects: (JIPMER 1987)

a. Facial nerve
b. Trigeminal nerve
c. Peripheral nerve
d. Glossopharyngeal nerve

Q12. Blow out carotid is characteristically seen with: (AIIMS Nov 1998)

a. Thyroidectomy
b. Radical neck dissection
c. Flap necrosis
d. Sistrunk operation

Q13. Patients with a history of falls present weeks later with headache and progressive neurological deterioration. The diagnosis is: (All India 1989)

a. Acute subdural hemorrhage
b. Extradural hemorrhage
c. Chronic subdural hemorrhage
d. Fracture skull

Q14. The most common site of meningocele is: (All India 1989)

a. Lumbosacral
b. Occipital
c. Frontal
d. Thoracic

Q15. The treatment of post-traumatic epilepsy is: (AIIMS 1984)

a. Mannitol infusion
b. Immediate corticosteroids
c. Long-term anticonvulsants
d. Long-term corticosteroids

Q16. Features of extradural hemorrhage include all, *except*: (AIIMS 1982)

a. Severe hypotension
b. Deteriorating consciousness
c. Fixed dilated pupil on the same side
d. Fracture line crossing the temporal bone

Q17. A dome-shaped skull with a high forehead in the infant with slight hydrocephalus (Olympian brow) is seen in: (JIPMER 1981)

a. Marasmus
b. Congenital syphilis
c. Rickets
d. Arnold–Chiari syndrome

Q18. After an open injury, the optimum time for nerve suture is: (PGI 1985)

a. Immediately
b. Within one month
c. 1–2 months
d. 2–4 months
e. When a wound is free from infection

Q19. Brain abscess may be due to the following: (AIIMS 1981)

a. Chronic suppurative otitis media
b. Chronic lung abscess
c. Trauma
d. Any of the above

Q20. Battle's sign is seen in: (JIPMER 1990)

a. Fracture middle cranial fossa
b. Fracture base of skull
c. Fracture anterior cranial fossa
d. All of the above

Q21. Premature filling of veins is a manifestation in cerebral angiography of: (AIIMS 1978)

a. Trauma
b. Brain tumor
c. Arteriovenous malformation (AVM)
d. Arterial occlusion

Q22. Psychiatric symptoms, true *except*: (PGI 2000)

a. More common with supra than infratentorial tumors
b. More common with slow-growing
c. More with temporal than frontal lobe tumors
d. More with brainstem lesions

Q23. All of the following conditions are known to cause diabetes insipidus, *except*: (AIIMS 2004)

a. Multiple sclerosis
b. Head injury
c. Histiocytosis
d. Viral encephalitis

Q24. All of the following hereditary conditions predispose to CNS tumors, *except*: (AIIMS 2005)

a. Neurofibromatosis 1 and 2
b. Tuberous sclerosis
c. Von Hippel–Lindau (VHL) syndrome
d. Xeroderma pigmentosum

Q25. All the following statements about neurofibromatosis are true, *except*: (ALL INDIA 2000)

a. Autosomal recessive inheritance
b. Cutaneous neurofibromas
c. Cataract
d. Scoliosis

Q26. Which of the following most common tumor associated with type 1 neurofibromatosis? (AIIMS 2007)

a. Optic nerve glioma
b. Meningioma
c. Acoustic schwannoma
d. Low-grade astrocytoma

Q27. Neurofibromatosis type 2 is associated with: (PGI 2000)

a. Bilateral acoustic schwannoma
b. Multiple café-au-lait spots
c. Chromosome 22
d. Lisch nodule
e. Posterior subcapsular lenticular cataract

Q28. Widened neural foramina is frequently seen in: (All India 2012)

a. Neurofibromatosis
b. Tuberous sclerosis
c. Sturge–Weber syndrome
d. Klippel–Feil syndrome

Q29. All of the following may be associated with VHL syndrome, *except*: (All India 2009)

a. Retinal and cerebellar hemangioblastomas
b. Gastric carcinoma
c. Pheochromocytoma
d. Renal cell carcinoma

Q30. Which of the following statements about VHL syndrome is true? (All India 2012)

a. Multiple tumors are rarely seen
b. Craniospinal hemangioblastomas are common
c. Supratentorial tumors are common
d. Tumors of Schwann cells are common

Q31. Neurofibromatosis 2 is/are associated with: (PGI 2011)

a. Meningioma
b. Schwannoma
c. Glioma
d. Lisch nodule
e. Hearing loss

ANSWERS

Grade I: 1. a; 2. b; 3. b; 4. c; 5. a; 6. b; 7. a; 8. c; 9. a (Schwartz 10/e p1733); 10. d; 11. b; 12. a (Schwartz 9/e p1344-1345); 13. c; 14. a; 15. c; 16. a; 17. b; 18. a; 19. d; 20. a,b; 21. c; 22. b, d; 23. a; 24. d (Bailey 27/e p145); 25. a; 26. a; 27. a; 28. a; 29. b (Bailey 27/e p145); 30. b; 31. a; 32. b

Grade II: 1 a, b; 2. a; 3. c; 4. a; 5. b; 6. a, b, d; 7. c; 8. a, b, d; 9. d; 10. a, b, e; 11. d (Harrison 20/e p647); 12. c (Sabiston 20/e p1913); 13. a (Bailey 27/e p664); 14. a; 15. a; 16. b; 17. a (Harrison 20/e p645); 18. a; 19. d; 20. b; 21. a; 22. a; 23. b; 24. c; 25. a; 26 a; 27. d; 28. b; 29. b; 30. c; 31. d; 32. d; 33. a

Grade III: 1. d; 2. b; 3. a; 4. d; 5. a; 6. d; 7. c; 8. a; 9. b; 10. b; 11. d; 12. None; 13. a; 14. a; 15. d; 16. c; 17. a; 18. c; 19. c; 20. a; 21. a; 22. b; 23. d; 24. a; 25. d; 26. a; 27. c; 28. a; 29. c; 30. c; 31. d (Schwartz 10/e p1749); 32. d

MODEL QUESTIONS

Q1. Most common site of brain metastasis:
a. Brainstem
b. Cerebellum
c. Cerebral cortex
d. Thalamus

Ans. c

Q2. Glioblastoma multiforme may occur in the following, *except*:
a. Cerebrum of adult
b. Brainstem of a child
c. Spinal cord of an adult
d. Adrenal medulla of a child

Ans. d

Q3. Glioblastoma multiforme is a variant of:
a. Medulloblastoma
b. Meningioma
c. Astrocytoma
d. Neuroblastoma

Ans. c

Q4. Signs of cerebral compression are all, *except*:
a. Bradycardia
b. Hypotension
c. Papilledema
d. Vomiting

Ans. b

Q5. Surgery is not useful in:
a. Cerebral edema
b. Depressed fracture
c. Extradural hemorrhage
d. Subdural hemorrhage

Ans. a

Q6. In a patient with a head injury black eye associated with subconjunctival hemorrhage occurs when there are:
a. Fracture of floor and anterior cranial fossa
b. Bleeding between the skin and galea aponeurotica
c. Hemorrhage between the galea aponeurotica and pericranium
d. Fracture of the greater wing of the sphenoid bone

Ans. a

Q7. Dumbbell tumor is seen in:
a. Meningioma
b. Neurofibroma
c. Ependymoma
d. Thymoma

Ans. b

Q8. Tinel's sign indicates:
a. Atrophy of nerves
b. Neuroma
c. Injury to nerve
d. Regeneration of nerves

Ans. d

Q9. Bilateral phrenic nerve palsy is caused by:
a. Carcinoma bronchus
b. Polio
c. Medullary carcinoma thyroid
d. Paget's disease

Ans. b

Q10. Glioblastoma multiforme may occur in the following, *except*:
a. Cerebrum of adult
b. Brainstem of a child
c. Spinal cord of an adult
d. Adrenal medulla of a child

Ans. d

Q11. The parasitic infection capable of producing spinal cord compression is/are:
a. Leishmaniasis
b. Wuchereriasis
c. Echinococcosis
d. Amoebiasis

Ans. c

Q12. The most common intramedullary spinal tumor is:
a. Secondaries
b. Neurofibroma
c. Ependymoma
d. None of the above

Ans. c

Q13. A patient presents with a sudden headache, vomiting, and unconsciousness. The diagnosis is:

a. SAH
b. Intracerebral hemorrhage
c. Subdural hemorrhage
d. Extradural hemorrhage

Ans. a

Q14. In patients with head injuries with rapidly increasing intracranial tension without hematoma, the drug of choice for initial management would be:

a. Lasix
b. Steroids
c. 20% mannitol
d. Glycine

Ans. c

Q15. The best prognosis among the following is seen in:

a. Astrocytoma
b. Oligodendroglioma
c. Meningioma
d. Medulloblastoma

Ans. c

Q16. All of the following tumors usually show psammoma bodies, *except*:

a. Papillary carcinoma of the thyroid
b. Meningioma
c. Serous cyst adenoma of the ovary
d. Hepatocellular carcinoma

Ans. d

Q17. The most common cause of a hypersecreting pituitary tumor is:

a. Pituitary adenoma
b. Pituitary carcinoma
c. Autoimmune disease of the pituitary
d. Transsection of stalk

Ans. a

Q18. The most common extradural spinal tumor is:

a. Neurofibroma
b. Glioma
c. Meningioma
d. Metastasis

Ans. d

Q19. The most common spinal tumor is:

a. Meningioma
b. Ependymoma
c. Neurofibroma
d. Neuroblastoma

Ans. c

Q20. MRI is the investigation of choice in all the following, *except*:

a. Syringomyelia
b. Brainstem tumors
c. Skull bone tumors
d. Multiple sclerosis

Ans. c

Q21. Enlargement of the pituitary tumor after adrenalectomy is called:

a. Nelson syndrome
b. Steel-Richardson syndrome
c. Hamman-Rich syndrome
d. Job's syndrome

Ans. a

SUGGESTED READING

1. Adam and Victor's Principles of Neurology, 8th edition.
2. Schwartz's Principles of Surgery, 18th edition.
3. Textbook of Surgery by David Sabiston, 21st edition.

CHAPTER 22

Cerebrovascular Diseases

"The more you use your brain, the more brain you will have to use."

– George A Dorsey

INTRODUCTION

The brain is a complex organ that is of different sizes in different species. It controls thoughts, emotions, senses, and motor functions. It is a vital organ controlling various vital processes of our body. The brain and *spinal cord (SC)* make up the *central nervous system (CNS).* It is the center of the CNS in all vertebrates and most of invertebrates. The human brain has billions of neurons or nerve cells. It is actually a biological computer.

ARNOLD–CHIARI MALFORMATION

It is a condition where brain tissue descends into the spinal canal **(Fig. 1)**. It is not common, but nowadays it is more commonly diagnosed due to better investigative methods such as *computed tomography (CT) and magnetic resonance imaging (MRI).* It happens in three types:

1. *Type I:* Symptoms occur in late childhood or in the adult state. The skull is too small. The cerebellar tonsil goes into the cervical canal. No hydrocephalus, but syringomyelia is present.
2. *Type II:* With spina bifida.
3. *Type III:* Progressive hydrocephalus with myelomeningocele is present.

Type II and Type III are present at birth, and are also known as congenital Chiari malformation.

A large number of these patients do not have any symptoms or signs, so they do not require any treatment, as it remains unknown. The symptoms that occur are pain in the neck, unsteady walking, discoordination of extremities, numbness and tingling, dizziness, hoarseness of voice, and maybe breathing trouble.

Important to remember:

- The most common site of myelomeningocele is the lumbosacral region.
- Folate is included in the risk factors and prevention factors responsible for myelomeningocele.
- Folic acid reduces the incidence of neural tube defects.
- Ischemic (85%) and hemorrhage (15%) are the causes of cerebrovascular accident (CVA).
- Smoking and hypertension are the main risk factors for Berry aneurysm.

Type III is the most serious form of the disease. It has the highest mortality. This malformation has some complications, such as hydrocephalus, spina bifida, and spinal cord stretching due to sticking of the spinal cord sticking to the spine.

- *Meningocele:* Described earlier.
- *Myelomeningocele:* Described earlier.
- *Dandy-Walker malformation:* Described earlier.
- *Berry aneurysm:* Described earlier.
- *Extradural hematoma (EDH):* Described earlier.

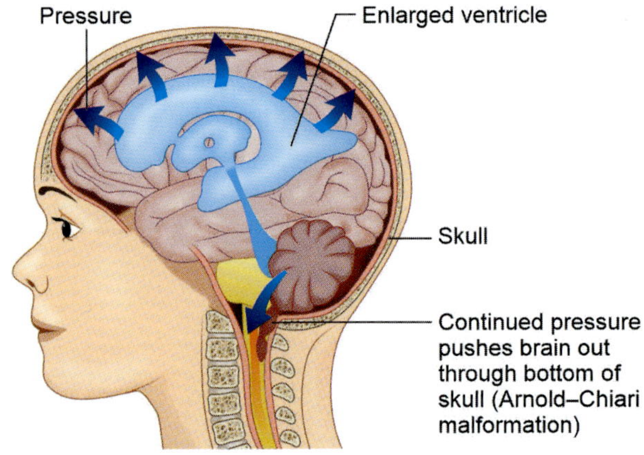

Fig. 1: Arnold–Chiari malformation.

- *Subdural hematoma (SDH):* Described earlier.
- *Subarachnoid hemorrhage:* Described earlier.

Diffuse axonal injuries (DAIs): It is a widespread axonal injury to the white matter of the brain that occurs after head injury. It can be a hemorrhagic or nonhemorrhagic injury. A coma is commonly seen. MRI is the best investigation. It carries a high mortality.

Primary brain injury: It occurs at the time of head injury, having contusions of the brainstem, cerebrum, and DAI.

Secondary brain injury: It occurs sometimes after head injury. It is caused by raised intracranial pressure (ICP), hypotension, and low brain perfusion.

Skull Base Fractures

These fractures may involve the anterior cranial fossa or the middle or posterior cranial fossa. Fractures of the anterior cranial fossa are the most common type. It can also cause periorbital hematoma (Raccoon eyes), rhinorrhea, epistaxis, etc. Middle cranial fossa fractures may cause otorrhea, Battle signs, cranial nerve injuries (seventh and eighth), and temporal lobe contusion. Posterior cranial fossa fractures can lead to visual disturbances and Vernet syndrome (involvement of 9th, 10th, and 11th cranial nerves, occipital contusion, and basilar artery injury).

CEREBROVASCULAR ACCIDENT

- *Ischemic 85%:* Embolic/thrombotic
- *Hemorrhagic 15%:* Parenchymal, epidural, subdural, and subarachnoid
  - Most common type—intracranial hemorrhage.
  - The most common cause is hypertension.

BERRY ANEURYSM

- Most common intracranial aneurysm
- 85% occur in the anterior part of the circle of Willis.
- Mostly multiple
- Predisposing factors—smoking and hypertension
- *Treatment:* Clipping or coiling

BRAIN ABSCESS

- *Cause:* Otitis media, mastoiditis, paranasal sinusitis and dental infection
- *Sites:*
  - Temporal lobe
  - Frontal lobe
  - Parietal lobe
- *Clinical features:*
  - Signs of raised ICP
  - Seizures
  - Focal sign
- *Diagnosis:* MRI
- *Treatment:* Surgical drainage.

NORMAL PRESSURE HYDROCEPHALUS

Clinical triad

A = Abnormal gait

D = Dementia (ataxic)

U = Urinary urgency or incontinence

VERTEBRAL ANOMALIES

- Spina bifida occulta
- Spina bifida aperta
  - Meningocele
  - Meningomyelocele
  - Myeloschesis

SOME IMPORTANT QUESTIONS

Q1. Battle's sign is present in:

a. Anterior cranial fossa fracture
b. Middle cranial fossa fracture
c. Posterior cranial fossa fracture
d. Fracture the lesser wing of the sphenoid

Ans. c

Q2. In a vehicular accident, extensive contusions of the brain due to acceleration and deceleration injury indicate what kind of injury?

a. Penetrating injury
b. Coup-contrecoup injury
c. Second-impact syndrome
d. Crush injury

Ans. b

Q3. The most common neurologic abnormality that occurs with a head injury is:

a. Hemiplegia
b. Ocular nerve palsy
c. Altered consciousness
d. Convulsion

Ans. c

Q4. True statements regarding the fractured base of the skull are all of the following, *except*:

a. Prophylactic antibiotics are usually not required
b. Associated with the eighth cranial nerve palsy

c. Early surgery is indicated for optimal outcome
d. May present with cerebrospinal fluid (CSF) otorrhea

Ans. c

Q5. Management of epidural abscess is:
a. Immediate surgical evaluation
b. Conservative management
c. Antibiotics
d. Aggressive debridement

Ans. a

Q6. Brain abscess may be due to the following:
a. Chronic suppurative otitis media
b. Chronic lung abscess
c. Trauma
d. Any of the above

Ans. d

Q7. The most common site of meningocele is:
a. Lumbosacral b. Occipital
c. Frontal d. Thoracic

Ans. a

Q8. Middle meningeal vessel damage results in:
a. Subdural hemorrhage
b. Subarachnoid hemorrhage
c. Intracerebral hemorrhage
d. Epidural hemorrhage

Ans. d

Q9. The common site for extradural hemorrhage is:
a. Frontal b. Temporoparietal
c. Occipital d. Brainstem

Ans. b

Q10. For chronic subdural hematoma (SDH), the duration should be more than:
a. 3 days b. 7 days
c. 15 days d. 1 month

Ans. c

Q11. Best treatment of subdural hematoma in a deteriorating patient:
a. By intravenous (IV) mannitol
b. Oxygenation
c. Use of steroids
d. Surgical evacuation

Ans. d

Q12. Chronic subdural hematoma refers to a collection present for a period of:
a. 7 days b. 6 months
c. 1 year d. 21 days

Ans. d

Q13. Tinel's sign indicates:
a. Atrophy of nerves
b. Neuroma
c. Injury of the nerve
d. Regeneration of nerves

Ans. d

MULTIPLE CHOICE QUESTIONS

Grade I | ***Simple***

Q1. The most common site of Berry aneurysm is: (All India 1994)
a. Junction of an anterior communicating artery with the anterior cerebral artery
b. Junction of the posterior communicating anterior with internal carotid artery
c. Bifurcation of the middle cerebral artery
d. Vertebral artery

Q2. All are common sites of Berry aneurysm, *except*: (AIIMS 1993)
a. Posterior cerebral artery
b. Vertebral artery
c. Anterior cerebral artery
d. Middle cerebral artery

Q3. True facts about Berry aneurysm are the following, *except*: (PGI 2000)
a. Associated with familial syndrome
b. The most common site of rupture is the apex, which causes subarachnoid hemorrhage (SAH)
c. Wall contains smooth muscle fibroblasts
d. 90% occur at the anterior part of the circulation at a branching point

Q4. The most common presentation of an intracranial aneurysm is: (PGI 1998)
a. Coarctation of the aorta
b. Systemic hypertension
c. Hypotension
d. Intracranial hemorrhage

Q5. Which is the least common site of a Berry aneurysm? (AIIMS 1995)
a. Basilar artery
b. Vertebral artery
c. Anterior cerebral artery
d. Posterior cerebral artery

Q6. The most common cause of cerebrovascular accident: (AIIMS 1996)
a. Embolism
b. Arteria thrombosis
c. Venous thrombosis
d. Hemorrhage

Q7. The most common cause of stroke among young people in India is among oral contraceptive pill (OCP) users: (PGI 1998)
a. Cortical vein thrombosis
b. Moyamoya disease
c. Atherosclerosis
d. HT

Q8. The most common cause of intracranial hemorrhage: (AIIMS 1998)
a. Subarachnoid hemorrhage
b. Intracerebral hemorrhage
c. Subdural hemorrhage
d. Extradural hemorrhage

Q9. The most common cause of intracerebral bleeding is: (All India 1995)
a. Thrombocytopenia
b. Diabetes
c. Hypotension
d. Berry aneurysm

Q10. Which among the following is not a primary brain injury? (JIPMER 2010)
a. Cortical lacerations
b. Brainstem herniation
c. Diffuse axonal injury
d. Brainstem contusion

Q11. About cranial trauma, false is: (AIIMS Nov 2010)
a. Raccoon eyes seen in subgaleal hemorrhage
b. Depressed skull fracture is associated with brain injury at the immediate area of impact
c. Caroticocavernous fistula occurs in a base skull fracture
d. Post-traumatic epilepsy is seen in 15%

Q12. Which is an ominous sign in case of severe head injury? (PGI Nov 2010)
a. Development of diabetes insipidus
b. Anisocoria
c. New focal deficit
d. Depressed skull fracture
e. Decorticate posturing

Q13. Cushing reflex is: (UPPG 2007)
a. Increase in mean arterial pressure with increased ICP
b. Increase in mean arterial pressure with decreased ICP
c. Decrease in mean arterial pressure with increased ICP
d. Decrease in mean arterial pressure with decreased ICP

Q14. Raised will cause: (MCI March 2007)
a. Tachycardia
b. Hypotension
c. Papilledema
d. Normal-looking anterior fontanelle in infants

Q15. The causes of systemic secondary insult to the injured brain include all of the following, *except*: (AIIMS May 2006)
a. Hypercapnia
b. Hypoxemia
c. Hypotension
d. Hypothermia

Q16. The total score in the Glasgow Coma Scale (GCS) of a conscious person is: (All India 2006)
a. 8
b. 3
c. 15
d. 10

Q17. Regarding the Glasgow Coma Scale, which is not true? (AIIMS Nov 1994)
a. Ranges from 6 to 12
b. Low score indicates deteriorating brain function
c. Based on the eye-opening, verbal response, and motor response
d. A score below 5 shows a poor prognosis

Q18. All are true about the Glasgow Coma Scale, *except*: (AIIMS June 1994)
a. Score between 3 and 15
b. Obeying the motor command is given the maximum score
c. Consists of eye-opening, motor, and verbal responses
d. Increased score indicates a poor prognosis

Q19. A person with inappropriate words evaluated by the Glasgow Coma Scale will have a verbal score of: (All India 2012)
a. 4
b. 3
c. 2
d. 1

Q20. What are the minimum and maximum possible values of the Glasgow Coma Score? **(AIIMS Nov 2015)**

a. Minimum = 3, Maximum = 15
b. Minimum = 0, Maximum = 13
c. Minimum = 0, Maximum = 15
d. Minimum = 3, Maximum = 18

Q21. Brain abscess in cyanotic heart disease is commonly located in: **(All India 2006)**

a. Cerebellar hemisphere
b. Thalamus
c. Temporal lobe
d. Parietal lobe

Q22. Subdural collection of pus in a head injury patient after 3 days, the responsible organism is: **(UPPG 2009)**

a. *Staphylococcus aureus*
b. Beta hemolytic *Streptococcus*
c. *Haemophilus influenzae*
d. *Pneumococcus*

Q23. A meningomyelocele patient, after being operated developed hydrocephalus due to: **(PGI Dec 1998)**

a. Arnold–Chiari malformation
b. Injury to absorptive surface
c. Central canal injury
d. Arachnoidal block

Grade II	Difficult

Q1. Which of the following is the most common location of hypertensive hemorrhage? **(AIIMS Nov 2002)**

a. Pons
b. Thalamus
c. Putamen/external capsule
d. Subcortical white matter

Q2. The most common cause of subarachnoid hemorrhage is: **(All India 1998)**

a. Rupture of the circle of Willis aneurysm
b. Rupture of vertebral artery aneurysm
c. Rupture of venecomitants of the corpus striatum
d. Rupture of dural sinuses

Q3. Which of the following is the most common cause of late neurological deterioration in the case of cerebrovascular accident? **(AIIMS Nov 2000)**

a. Rebleeding b. Vasospasm
c. Embolism d. Hydrocephalus

Q4. "Duret hemorrhages" are seen in: **(AIIMS May 2008)**

a. Brain b. Kidney
c. Heart d. Lung

Q5. Lucid interval is classically seen in: **(PGI Dec 1997)**

a. Intracerebral hematoma
b. Acute subdural hematoma
c. Chronical subdural hematoma
d. Extradural hematoma

Q6. In a patient with head injury, damage in the brain is aggravated by: **(All India 2010)**

a. Hyperglycemia b. Hypothermia
c. Hypocapnia d. Serum osmolality

Q7. The best prognostic factor for head injury is: **(All India 2007)**

a. Glasgow Coma Scale b. Age
c. Mode of injury d. CT

Q8. True regarding epidural hematoma is/are: **(PGI May 2018)**

a. Arterial bleed
b. On CT scan, it gives a biconvex lenticular hyperdense appearance
c. Located on the lateral side of hemisphere
d. Common after injury at the pterion

Q9. The earliest manifestations of increased ICP following head injury are: **(All India 2005)**

a. Ipsilateral papillary dilatation
b. Contralateral papillary dilatation
c. Altered mental status
d. Hemiparesis

Q10. False statement regarding subdural hematoma: **(JIPMER May 2018)**

a. Occurs on both sides b. Not visible on X-ray
c. Surgery can be done d. Unilateral surgery

Q11. Transtentorial uncal herniation causes all, *except*: **(AIIMS May 2001)**

a. Ipsilateral dilated pupils
b. Ipsilateral hemiplegia
c. Cheyne–Stokes respiration
d. Decorticate rigidity

Q12. Non-noxious stimuli perceived as pain is termed as: **(AIIMS May 2008)**

a. Allodynia b. Hyperalgesia
c. Hyperesthesia d. Hyperpathia

Q13. Spontaneous CSF leaks may be associated with all, *except*: **(AIIMS Nov 2008)**
a. Increased intracranial tension
b. Pseudotumor cerebri
c. Empty sella syndrome
d. Encephalocele

Q14. All of the following statements about diffuse axonal injury (DAI) are true, *except*: **(All India 2008)**
a. Caused by shearing force
b. Predominant white matter hemorrhages, in the basal ganglion and corpus callosum
c. Increased intracranial tension is seen in all cases
d. Most common at the junction of gray and white matter

Q15. All of the following lower ICP, *except*: **(All India 1998)**
a. Mannitol b. Furosemide
c. Corticosteroids d. Hyperventilation

Q16. Not true regarding Dandy-Walker cyst: **(AIIMS June 1998)**
a. Cerebellar vermis hypoplasia
b. Hydrocephalus
c. Arachnoid cyst
d. Posterior fossa cyst

Q17. What will be the diagnosis of the child with pulsatile swelling on the medial side of the nose? **(AIIMS June 98)**
a. Teratoma
b. Meningocele
c. Dermoid cyst
d. Carcinoma of the ethmoid bone

Q18. A newborn presents with swelling in the base of the spine in which the meninges herniate through a bony defect caused is? **(UPPG 2009)**
a. Defect in pedicle
b. Defect in the body
c. Defect in the fusion of vertebral arches
d. Defect in the transverse process

Q19. A newborn with meningomyelocele has been posted for surgery. The defect should be immediately covered with: **(AIIMS May 2013)**
a. Normal saline gauze
b. Povidone iodine gauze
c. Tincture benzoin gauze
d. Methylene blue gauze

Q20. In normal pressure hydrocephalus, all are seen, *except*: **(PGI Dec 1997)**
a. Convulsion b. Ataxia
c. Dementia d. Incontinence

Q21. The most commonly performed shunt for hydrocephalus is: **(AIIMS May 2015)**
a. Ventriculoperitoneal b. Ventriculopericardial
c. Ventriculopleural d. Lumboperitoneal

Q22. Carpal tunnel syndrome is due to the compression of: **(JIPMER 2011)**
a. Median nerve
b. Anterior interosseous nerve
c. Radial nerve
d. Ulnar nerve

Grade III	*Most difficult*

Q1. Extradural hematoma is associated with what % of severe trauma? **(PGI Dec 1998)**
a. 36% b. 10%
c. 77% d. 96%

Q2. Management of extradural hemorrhage is: **(AIIMS 93)**
a. Antibiotics
b. Immediate evacuation
c. Evacuation after 24 hours
d. Observation

Q3. Subdural hematoma most commonly results from: **(AIIMS May 2004)**
a. Rupture of intracranial aneurysm
b. Rupture of cerebral arteriovenous malformation (AVM)
c. Injury to cortical bridging veins
d. Hemophilia

Q4. The common cause of subarachnoid hemorrhage is: **(All India 2006)**
a. AVM
b. Cavernous angioma
c. Aneurysm
d. Hippocampus

Q5. A patient comes to the ER with a headache, describing it as the worst headache of his life. What is the next step? **(AIIMS Nov 2017)**
a. CT brain
b. MRI brain
c. Lumbar puncture
d. Observation and analgesics

Q6. A 45-year-old hypertensive male presented with a sudden onset most severe headache, vomiting, and neck stiffness. On examination, he did not have any focal neurological deficit. His CT scan showed blood in the Sylvian fissure. The probable diagnosis is: (AIIMS May 2003)

a. Meningitis
b. Ruptured aneurysm
c. Hypertensive bleed
d. Stroke

Q7. In skull fracture, the condition in which an operation is not done immediately is: (All India 1996)

a. Depressed fracture
b. Compound fracture
c. CSF leak
d. Increase the size of the head

Q8. The most important clinical finding in a case of head injury is: (JIPMER 1991)

a. Pupillary dilatation
b. Level of consciousness
c. Focal neurological deficit
d. Fracture skull

Q9. In patients of head injury with rapidly increasing intracranial tension without hematoma, the drug of choice for initial management would be: (UPSC 2000)

a. Lasix
b. Steroids
c. 20% mannitol
d. Glycine

Q10. True about Glasgow Coma Scale: (JIPMER 2011)

a. Includes verbal response
b. Includes papillary reflex
c. High score means a poor prognosis
d. Includes measurement of ICP

Q11. Peripheral nerves can withstand ischemia up to: (JIPMER 1993)

a. 30 minutes
b. 1 hour
c. 2 hours
d. 4 hours

Q12. Which of the following is the most common location of intracranial neurocysticercosis? (AIIMS Nov 2005)

a. Brain parenchyma
b. Subarachnoid space
c. Spinal cord
d. Orbit

Q13. The following are CNS findings of CO_2 narcosis: (PGI 1990)

a. Excitement
b. Increased pH of CSF
c. Decreased pH of CSF
d. Papilledema

Q14. All of the following conditions are known to cause diabetes insipidus, *except*: (AIIMS 2004)

a. Multiple sclerosis
b. Head injury
c. Histiocytosis
d. Viral encephalitis

Q15. Cells from the neural crest are involved in all, *except*: (AIIMS June 2003)

a. Hirschsprung's disease
b. Neuroblastoma
c. Primitive neuroectodermal tumor
d. Wilms' tumor

Q16. All can commonly occur in a patient who suffered a decelerating injury in which the pituitary stalk was damaged, *except* one: (AIIMS Nov 2000)

a. Diabetes mellitus
b. Thyroid insufficiency
c. Adrenocortical insufficiency
d. Diabetes insipidus

Q17. The defective migration of neural crest cells results in: (PGI June 2006)

a. Congenital megacolon
b. Albinism
c. Adrenogenital hypoplasia
d. Dentinogenesis imperfecta

Q18. Blowout fracture refers to: (JIPMER 2011)

a. Fracture of the orbit
b. Fracture of the nasal septum
c. Fracture of the base of the skull
d. Fracture of the mandible

Q19. A newborn presents with congestive heart failure. On examination has a bulging anterior fontanelle with a bruit on auscultation. Transfontanellar ultrasound (USG) shows a hypoechoic midline mass with dilated lateral ventricles. Most likely diagnosis: (AIIMS Nov 2011)

a. Medulloblastoma
b. Encephalocele
c. Vein of Galen malformation
d. Arachnoid cyst

Q20. Carpel tunnel syndrome is caused by all, *except*: (AIIMS May 2011)

a. Amyloidosis
b. Hypothyroidism
c. Addison's disease
d. Diabetes mellitus

Q21. The most common cause of carpal tunnel syndrome is: (All India 1995)

a. Malunited Colles' fracture
b. Rheumatoid arthritis involving the flexor retinaculum
c. Myxedema
d. Pregnancy

ANSWERS

Grade I: 1. a (Bailey 26/e p311); 2. b; 3. c (Harrison 19/e p1784); 4. d; 5. b; 6. a (Harrison 20/e p2560); 7. a; 8. b; 9. c; 10. b; 11. a (Schwartz 10/e p174); 12. b; 13. a; 14. c; 15. d; 16. c; 17. a; 18. d; 19. b; 20. a; 21. d; 22. a; 23. a

Grade II: 1. c; 2. a; 3. b (Harrison 20/e p2086); 4. a; 5. d; 6. a (Harrison 19/e p457); 7. a; 8. a, b, c, d; 9. c; 10. a; 11. d (Bailey 27/e p329); 12. a; 13. None; 14. c (Sabiston 20/e p1916); 15. b; 16. c; 17. b; 18. c; 19. a; 20. a; 21. a; 22. a

Grade III: 1. b (Harrison 19/e p441); 2. b; 3. c; 4. c; 5. a (Harrison 20/e p2084); 6. b; 7. c; 8. b; 9. c; 10. a (Schwartz 10/e p168); 11. d; 12. a; 13. c; 14. a; 15. d; 16. a; 17. a; 18. a; 19. c (Sabiston 19/e p1876); 20. c; 21. d

MODEL QUESTIONS

Q1. Which of the following will manifest as "pachymeningitis hemorrhagica interna?"
a. Epidural hematoma
b. Subdural hematoma
c. Subarachnoid hemorrhage
d. Brain infarction

Ans. b

Q2. Immediate surgery is indicated in:
a. Extradural hemorrhage
b. Subdural hemorrhage
c. Intracerebral hemorrhage
d. Brain laceration

Ans. a

Q3. Which of the following grading methods is used to evaluate the prognosis outcome after subarachnoid hemorrhage?
a. Glasgow Coma Scale
b. Hess and Hunt scale
c. Glasgow–Blatchford bleeding score
d. Intracerebral hemorrhage score

Ans. b

Q4. Triple H therapy for subarachnoid hemorrhage consists of all, *except*:
a. Hypertension
b. Hypervolemia
c. Hemodilution
d. Hypothermia

Ans. d

Q5. Surgery is not useful in:
a. Cerebral edema
b. Depressed fracture
c. Extradural hemorrhage
d. Subdural hemorrhage

Ans. a

Q6. In a patient with a head injury black eye associated with subconjunctival hemorrhage occurs when there is:
a. Fracture of the floor of the anterior cranial fossa
b. Bleeding between the skin and galea aponeurotica
c. Hemorrhage between the galea aponeurotica and pericranium
d. Fracture of the greater wing of the sphenoid bone

Ans. a

Q7. All of the following are indications of a CT scan in a head-injured patient, *except*:
a. Glasgow Coma Scale <13
b. Vomiting 1 episode
c. Focal neurological deficit
d. Mild head injury in patients aged >65 years

Ans. b

Q8. Minimal Glasgow Coma Scale is:
a. 0
b. 1
c. 2
d. 3

Ans. d

Q9. Mild head injury is having a Glasgow Coma Scale of:
a. 3–5
b. 5–8
c. 8–10
d. 13–15

Ans. d

Q10. Which of the following is not a component of the Glasgow Coma Scale?
a. Eye-opening
b. Motor response
c. Pupil size
d. Verbal response

Ans. c

Q11. In Erb-Duchenne paralysis, the injury is limited to the:

a. Second and third cervical nerves
b. Third and fourth cervical nerves
c. Fourth and fifth cervical nerves
d. Fifth and sixth cervical nerves

Ans. d

Q12. Neurosurgical treatment of epilepsy usually involves the removal of the epileptic focus from which lobe:

a. Frontal lobe
b. Temporal lobe
c. Occipital lobe
d. Parietal lobe

Ans. b

Q13. The "Phenomenon of Kernohan's notch" is associated with:

a. Third nerve palsy with contralateral hemiplegia
b. Subfalcine herniation
c. Transtentorial herniation
d. Foramen magnum fraction

Ans. c

Q14. Signs of the base of skull fracture are the following, *except*:

a. Raccoon eyes
b. Battle's sign
c. Constricted pupil
d. Hemotympanum

Ans. c

SUGGESTED READING

1. Bailey & Love's - Short Practice of Surgery, 27th edition.
2. Schwartz's Principles of Surgery, 18th edition.
3. Textbook of Surgery by David Sabiston, 21st edition.

CHAPTER 23

Oral Cavity

"A happy mouth is a happy body."

– World Oral Health Day Theme (2024)

INTRODUCTION

Oral cavity diseases are common in India, especially cancer of the tongue and cheek, due to tobacco chewing, betel, and betel nut chewing.

BOUNDARIES OF THE ORAL CAVITY (FIG. 1)

- *Superior*—skin—vermilion junction of the lips to the hard and soft palate junction.
- *Inferior*—line of the circumvallate papilla of the tongue.
- *Lateral*—anterior tonsillar pillars and glossotonsillar folds.

ULCERS OF THE ORAL CAVITY

- Dental ulcer
- Aphthous ulcer
- Carcinomatous ulcers
- Others—tuberculosis (TB) and syphilis

LEUKOPLAKIA

Leukoplakia are white patches on the oral mucosa. <5% transformed to cancer (speckled leukoplakia). Common in smokers. Removal of the cause cures it.

ERYTHROPLAKIA

Erythroplakia are red patches in the oral mucosa. Highly malignant transformation.

SUBMUCOSAL FIBROSIS

Fibrous bands develop under the mucosa of the oral cavity. Contraction of these bands leads to limitation of mouth opening and even tongue movement. *30% develop squamous cell carcinoma (SCC). Betel nut and pan masala chewing is a risk factors.* Treated by injection of steroids in the lesion or surgical excision.

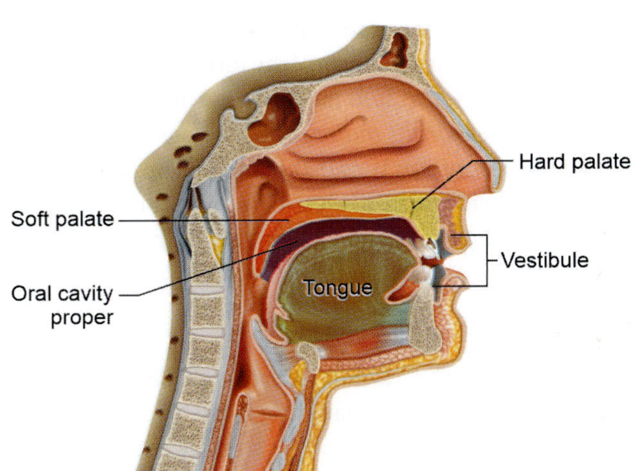

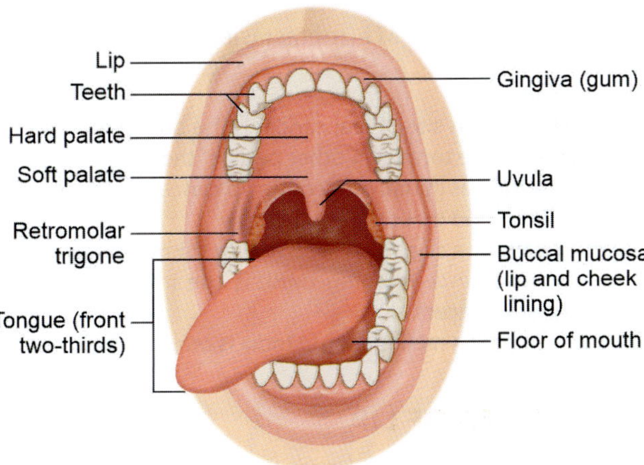

Fig. 1: Oral cavity.

ORAL CAVITY CARCINOMA

Risk factors Mn = 7S

- *S* = Smoking/tobacco/betel nut
- *S* = Spirit (Alcohol)
- *S* = Spices
- *S* = Syphilis
- *S* = Sharp tooth and ill-fitted dentures
- *S* = Sun rays [ultraviolet (UV) light]
- *S* = Syndromes (Li-Fraumeni)

PATHOLOGY

The most common is SCC (90%). *Field cancerization is due to diffuse exposure to malignant factors, synchronous (another cancer arising simultaneously within 6 months), and metachronous (cancer arising after 6 months).* It spreads by lymphatics.

TUMOR, NODE, METASTASIS STAGING (EIGHTH AICC 2017 CLASSIFICATION OF ORAL CAVITY)

T0 (no evidence), *T1* (tumor <2 cm, <5 mm depth), *T2* (2–4 cm, depth >5 mm), *T3* (>4 cm, depth >10 mm), *T4a* (Lip—involves bone, nerve, floor of mouth and skin, T4a (Oral cavity involves bone, muscles, skin and maxillary sinus), *T4b* (lip and oral involves skull base, internal carotid artery, and masticator space).

NX (unable to access), *N0* (no evidence), *N1* (metastasis single ipsilateral LN, <3 cm), *N2a* (metastasis 3–6 cm), *N2b* (multiple ipsilateral LN, >6 cm), *N2c* (bilateral or contralateral LN), *N3* (metastasis >6 cm), *N3a* (metastasis in LN more than 6 cm and ENE negative), *N3b* (metastasis in any LN ENE positive).

M0 (no metastasis), *M1* (metastasis).

Things to remember:
- The most common site of oral cancer is the buccal mucosa in India, whereas the tongue in other parts of the World.
- The best prognosis in oral cancer is in lip cancer.
- The most common oral cancer is SCC.
- The most common skip metastasis is with tongue cancer.
- Magnetic resonance imaging (MRI) is the investigation of choice for oral cancers.
- The most common malignancy in India is oral cavity cancer.

CARCINOMA OF LIP

For about 95% of the cases happen in the lower lip, occur between 40 and 70 years, metastases occur rarely, and the best prognosis in oral cancers. The most common site is vermillion of the lower lip, more common in males, and LN metastasis is rare.

Treatment

- T1 and T2: Surgery
- T3 and T4: Surgery + radiotherapy

CARCINOMA OF TONGUE

The most common in the middle one-third lateral margin.

Presents as a nonhealing ulcer, commonly Level III LN (Superior deep jugular LN) is taken for biopsy.

Treatment

- *T1:* Partial glossectomy
- *T2:* Small—hemiglossectomy level—radiotherapy
- *T3:* Total glossectomy followed by radiotherapy
- *T4:* Total glossectomy followed by radiotherapy + mandibulectomy + mandible reconstruction with a fibula free flap (MRND) + If required Laryngectomy + Postoperative radiotherapy

COMPLICATIONS OF RADIOTHERAPY

- Most common is dry mouth (xerostomia)
- Mucosal inflammation (mucositis)
- Impaired sense of taste (dysgeusia)
- Osteoradionecrosis (ORN)

MANAGEMENT OF ORAL CANCERS

- *Tongue cancer:* <2 cm excision with 2 cm margin, >2 cm *hemiglossectomy*. If the mandible is involved, then marginal or segmental resection of the mandible is required. Reconstruction of the tongue may be required by radial forearm free flap (RFFF), deltopectoral (DP) flap, and *pectoralis major myocutaneous (PMMC)* flap.
- *Carcinoma of lip:* If one-third lower lip is involved—V/W excision and closer, if more than one-third—flaps—Johansson step ladder symmetrical flaps, Fries modification of *Bernard flap, and Estlander flap.*

LUDWIG'S ANGINA

A progressive and rapidly increasing cellulitis of the submandibular space leads to airway obstruction and even death. Dental infection by streptococci is the most common cause. Treated by antibiotics, incision, and drainage.

DENTAL CYST (RADICULAR CYST)

Involves the apex of a chronically infected tooth. Common in the upper jaw, leading to expansion of the jaw. Treated by curettes and soft tissue introduction.

DENTIGEROUS CYST (FOLLICULAR ODONTOMA)

It is occurring with nonerupted permanent teeth. Commonly involves the upper or lower third molar and expands the outer wall of the jaw. Complete excision and curettage are the treatments.

EPULIS

The name in Greek means (upon the gum), swelling is on gum can originate from mucous membrane or bone. True epulis are growths and falls epulis are hyperplasia of mucous membrane. Fibrous epulis is most common and it is a true epulis.

APHTHOUS ULCERS

These are painful and superficial ulcers over the lips, buccal mucosa, tongue, and floor of the mouth. Heal within 2 weeks.

CANCRUM ORIS

It is now rarely seen in the West, but is seen in developing countries. It is a gangrenous process of the oral cavity, which destroys bones and is common in malnourished children.

Also called Noma disease or gangrenous stomatitis. It is a rapidly progressive polymicrobial infection.

Risk Factors

- Poor nutrition
- Poor oral hygiene
- Severe illness
- Malignancy

Clinical Features

- Mainly children under 12 years in poor countries of Africa.
- Ulcers and destruction of bones and soft tissue of the face and oral cavity
- High mortality

Treatment

Hygiene, nutrition, antibiotics, and reconstructive surgery.

Some important points to remember:

- Erythroplakia is a high-risk lesion for cancer.
- Submucosal fibrosis is peculiar to Asian, betel nut, and pan masala consuming populations.
- The tongue is the most common site of oral cancer.
- The *P53* gene is most commonly mutated in oral cancer.
- SCC is the most common type of oral cancer.
- The most common cancer in India is oral cancer.
- Buccal mucosa is the most common site of oral cancer.
- Most common routes of spread of oral cancer—local extension and lymphatic spread.
- The most common site of oral cancer is the LNs.
- The most common distant metastasis in oral cancer is the lung.
- Cancer of paranasal sinuses is common in hardwood furniture workers due to inhalation of nickel and chromium. The most common is the maxillary sinus.

SOME IMPORTANT QUESTIONS

Q1. Regarding premalignant oral lesions:

a. Leukoplakia should be proved by biopsy
b. Leukoplakia does not appear after cessation of smoking
c. Erythroplakia has a higher risk of malignancy
d. Oral submucosal fibrosis is seen in all parts of the world

Ans. c

Q2. The most strongly implicated premalignant condition of the oral cavity is:

a. Fordyce spots
b. Erythroplakia
c. Median rhomboid glossitis
d. Erythema multiforme

Ans. b

Q3. Treatment of erythroplakia:

a. Exclusion
b. Stoppage of alcohol and tobacco
c. Vitamin supplementation
d. Laser ablation

Ans. a

Q4. A 60-year-old nondiabetic, chronic alcoholic patient with multiple oral lesions is shown. The lesion is painful with a burning sensation. What is the diagnosis?

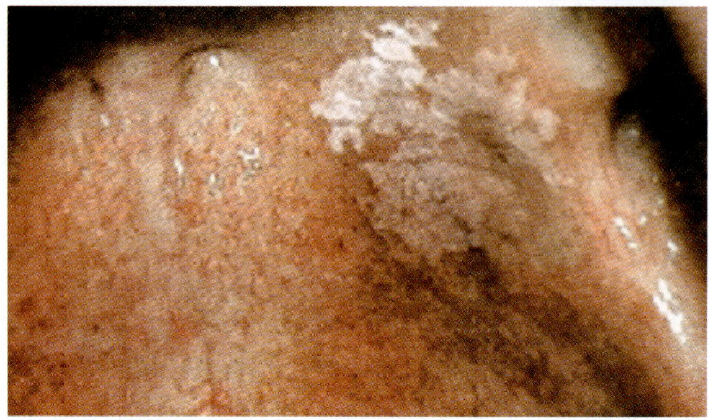

a. Erythroplakia
b. Leukoplakia
c. Submucous fibrosis
d. Melanoplakia

Ans. b

Q5. Which of the following is the cause of submucosal fibrosis?

a. Alcohol
b. Candidiasis
c. Betel nut chewing
d. Pan leaf chewing

Ans. c

Q6. Squamous cell carcinoma (SCC) in the oral cavity and lips tends to metastasize to lymph nodes (LNs) at which levels:

a. I, II, III
b. I, II, IV
c. III, IV, V
d. I, II, retropharyngeal nodes

Ans. a

Q7. Weber–Ferguson Incision is used for operating on which cancer?

a. Breast cancer
b. Hard palate cancer
c. Thyroid cancer
d. Cancer penis

Ans. b

Q8. The main disability following classical radical neck dissection is due to paralysis of which muscle?

a. Subscapularis
b. Deltoid
c. Trapezius
d. Pectoralis major

Ans. c

Q9. All of the following are precancerous lesions for carcinoma of the oral cavity, *except*:

a. Erythroplakia
b. Speckled erythroplakia
c. Discoid lupus erythematosus
d. Chronic hyperplastic candidiasis

Ans. c

Q10. Areas of carcinoma of the oral mucosa can be identified by staining with:

a. 1% zinc chloride
b. 2% silver nitrate
c. Gentian violet
d. 2% toluidine blue

Ans. d

MULTIPLE CHOICE QUESTIONS

Grade I	Simple

Q1. Treatment of leukoplakia: **(JIPMER 2011)**

a. Local excision
b. Excision and radiotherapy
c. Topical chemotherapy
d. Repositioning of ill-fitting dentures

Q2. All of the following predispose to oral cancer, *except*: **(PGI Dec 1999)**

a. Erythroplakia
b. Leukoplakia
c. Submucosal fibrosis
d. Lichen planus

Q3. Virus-causing head and neck cancer: **(PGI 2011)**

a. Epstein–Barr virus (EBV)
b. Herpes simplex virus (HSV)
c. Human papillomavirus (HPV)
d. Hepatitis B virus (HBV)
e. Hepatitis C virus (HCV)

Q4. All of the following are predisposed to SCC, *except*: **(AIIMS 1993)**

a. Lichen planus of mouth
b. Bowen's disease
c. Inverted papilloma of the nose
d. Chronic irritation of the oral mucosa by jagged teeth

Q5. The premalignant condition with the highest probability of progression to malignancy is: **(All India 2002)**

a. Dysplasia
b. Hyperplasia
c. Leukoplakia
d. Erythroleukoplakia

Q6. Correct pairing of the neck nodes: **(AIIMS Nov 2018)**

a. *Level 3:* Cricoid to clavicle
b. *Level 4:* Hyoid to clavicle
c. *Level 5:* Base of skull to cricoid
d. *Level 6:* Hyoid to clavicle

Q7. Saroj, a 32-year-old female from a rural background, presented with a history of chronic tobacco chewing since 14 years of age. Now she has difficulty in opening her mouth. On oral examination, no ulcers are seen. Most probable diagnosis is: (AIIMS June 2001)

a. Submucous oral fibrosis
b. Carcinoma of buccal mucosa
c. TM joint arthritis
d. Trigeminal nerve paralysis

Q8. An old man who is edentulous developed squamous cell carcinoma in the buccal mucosa that has infiltrated into the alveolus. The following is not indicated in treatment: (All India 2002)

a. Radiotherapy
b. Segmental mandibulectomy
c. Marginal mandibulectomy involving removal of the outer table only
d. Marginal mandibulectomy involving the removal of the upper half of the mandible

Q9. A patient presented with a 1 × 1.5 cm growth on the lateral border of the tongue. The treatment indicated would be: (AIIMS June 2002)

a. Laser ablation
b. Interstitial brachytherapy
c. External beam radiotherapy
d. Chemotherapy

Q10. Most common site of oral cancer: (Recent Question 2017)

a. Lips b. Tongue
c. Buccal mucosa d. Alveolus of teeth

Grade II | **Difficult**

Q1. The most common premalignant condition of oral cancer is: (All India 1995)

a. Leukoplakia b. Aphthous ulcer
c. Lichen planus d. Erythroleukoplakia

Q2. The second primary tumor of the head and neck is most commonly seen in malignancy of: (AIIMS 2012)

a. Oral cavity b. Larynx
c. Hypopharynx d. Paranasal sinuses

Q3. The most common site of oral cancer in the Indian population is: (All India 2004)

a. Tongue b. The floor of the mouth.
c. Alveobuccal complex d. Lip

Q4. The most common site of oral cavity carcinoma is: (All India 1996)

a. Lip b. Cheek
c. Tongue d. Palate

Q5. Abbé–Estlander flap is used for: (All India 2008)

a. Lip b. Tongue
c. Eyelid d. Ears

Q6. Abbé–Estlander flap is based on: (AIIMS 2008)

a. Lingual artery
b. Facial artery
c. Labial artery
d. Internal maxillary artery

Q7. A 70-year-old male presented with an asymptomatic white patch on the oral cavity following application of the denture. Treatment of choice is: (UPPG 2008)

a. Low-dose radiotherapy
b. Biopsy of all the tissues
c. Ascertaining that the denture is fitted properly
d. Antibiotics

Q8. A patient has carcinoma of the tongue in the right lateral aspect with a LN of 4 cm in size in level 3 on the left side of the neck. What is the stage? (AIIMS Nov 2006)

a. N0 b. N1
c. N2 d. N3

Q9. Treatment for stage T3N1 of carcinoma maxilla is: (AIIMS June 1996)

a. Radiation therapy only
b. Chemotherapy only
c. Surgery and radiation
d. Chemotherapy and radiation

Q10. The lymph is not to be involved first in maxillary carcinoma: (DNB 2007)

a. Superior deep cervical nodes
b. Jugulodigastric nodes
c. Submandibular
d. Subdigastric nodes

Grade III | **Most difficult**

Q1. Treatment of choice for carcinoma of the lip of <1 cm is: (All India 1990)

a. Radiation
b. Chemotherapy
c. Excision
d. Radiation and chemotherapy

Q2. True statement(s) about oral cancer is/are: (PGI 2004)

a. Most common in buccal mucosa
b. Metastasis is uncommon
c. Respond to radiotherapy
d. Surgery done
e. Syphilis and dental irritation predispose

Q3. Metastasis from buccal mucosa cancer goes to: (AIIMS 1996)

a. Regional LNs
b. Liver
c. Heart
d. Brain

Q4. In carcinoma cheek, what is the best drug for single-drug chemotherapy? (AIIMS 1993)

a. Vincristine
b. Cyclophosphamide
c. Cisplatin
d. Daunorubicin

Q5. All are true about carcinoma palate, *except*: (AIIMS June 1994)

a. Slow growing
b. Bilateral lymphatic spread
c. Adenocarcinoma
d. Presents with pain

Q6. A patient with CA tongue is found to have lymph nodes in the lower neck. The treatment of choice for the lymph nodes is: (All India 2005)

a. Lower cervical neck dissection
b. Suprahyoid neck dissection
c. Tele radiotherapy
d. Radical neck dissection

Q7. Tongue ulcer with everted edges is: (MHPGMCET 2005)

a. Aphthous ulcer
b. Tubercular
c. Malignant
d. Dental

Q8. A 60-year-old man presents with an ulcer on the lateral margin of the tongue also complains of ear pain. The most probable diagnosis is: (PGI 1996)

a. Dental ulcer
b. Carcinomatous ulcer
c. Tuberculosis ulcer
d. Syphilitic ulcer

Q9. An 80-year-old patient presents with a midline tumor of the lower jaw, involving the alveolar margin. He is edentulous. Treatment of choice is: (All India 2001)

a. Hemimandibulectomy
b. Commando operation
c. Segmental mandibulectomy
d. Margin mandibulectomy

Q10. All are true about cancrum oris, *except*: (PGI Dec 1997)

a. Associated with malnutrition and vitamin deficiency
b. Follows chronic infection
c. Involves jaw
d. Treatment is excision and skin grafting with tubed pedicle graft

ANSWERS

Grade I: 1. d; 2. d; 3. a; 4. a; 5. d; 6. d; 7. a (Bailey 27/e p763); 8. c; 9. b (Bailey 27/e p769); 10. b (Sabiston 20/e p796)

Grade II: 1. a; 2. a; 3. c (Bailey 26/e p709-710); 4. c; 5. a (Bailey 27/e p769); 6. c (Bailey 27/e p769); 7. c; 8. c; 9. c (Bailey 27/e p774); 10. c

Grade III: 1. c; 2. b, c, d, e (Bailey 27/e p772); 3. a; 4. c (Bailey 27/e p155); 5. d (Bailey 27/e p774); 6. d (Bailey 27/e p769); 7. c (Bailey 27/e p616); 8. b; 9. c; 10. b

MODEL QUESTIONS

Q1. The stain used to diagnose premalignant lesions of the lip is:

a. Crystal violet
b. H and E
c. Toluidine blue
d. Giemsa

Ans. c

Q2. In the reconstruction following the excision of previously irradiated cheek cancer, the flap will be:

a. Local tongue
b. Cervical
c. Forehead
d. Pectoralis major myocutaneous

Ans. d

Q3. Most common oral cancer:
a. Squamous cell carcinoma
b. Adenocarcinoma
c. Transition cell carcinoma
d. Mucoepidermoid

Ans. a

Q4. Which of the following is the most common site of malignancy in the head and neck?
a. Oral cavity
b. Nasopharynx
c. Larynx
d. Oropharynx

Ans. a

Q5. Carcinoma of the lip is characterized by the following, *except* that:
a. 90% of the lip cancers occur on the lower lip
b. The most common site of origin is the vermillion border
c. 2 × 2 cm cell carcinoma that can be treated by V-shaped excision and primary closure
d. Since lymph node metastases are common after a radical dissection of the neck is mandatory

Ans. d

Q6. Neuromuscular preserving flap in the lip:
a. Abbe flap
b. Webster flap
c. Karapandzic flap
d. Johansen flap

Ans. c

Q7. Which of the following is correct about ameloblastoma?
a. Highly malignant
b. Occurs in children <5 years
c. Most common odontogenic tumor
d. Mandible is not the most common site

Ans. c

Q8. Asymptomatic hemangioma on the ventral surface of the tongue in a 10-year-old boy is treated by:
a. Watchful expectancy
b. Surgical Excision
c. Radiotherapy
d. Laser

Ans. a

Q9. N-3 tumor, nodes, and metastasis (TNM) staging of head and neck tumors shows:
a. Metastasis in lymph nodes >2 cm
b. Metastasis in lymph nodes >5 cm
c. Metastasis in a lymph node >6 cm
d. None

Ans. c

Q10. The commando operation is:
a. Abdominoperineal resection of the rectum for carcinoma
b. Disarticulation of the hip of gas gangrene of the leg
c. Extended radical mastectomy
d. Excision of carcinoma of the jaw and lymph nodes en bloc

Ans. d

SUGGESTED READING

1. Bailey & Love's - Short Practice of Surgery, 27th edition.
2. S Das Textbook of Surgery, 3rd edition.
3. Schwartz's Principles of Surgery, 18th edition.

CHAPTER 24

Salivary Glands

"Animals have secretion in their stomach which enables them to digest food without mastication, but human beings are suppose to chew their food before they swallow it down, so chew your food and give your salivary gland a chance to work".

– Tennessee Williams

ANATOMY AND PHYSIOLOGY OF SALIVARY GLANDS

Anatomy

There are two parotid glands, two submandibular glands, two sublingual glands, and approximately 800 minor salivary glands. *The parotid gland is the largest salivary gland in the human body.* It is about 4–5 cm in size, whereas the submandibular gland is about the size of a walnut, and the sublingual gland is like an almond. Minor salivary glands are 2–3 mm in size **(Figs. 1 and 2)**.

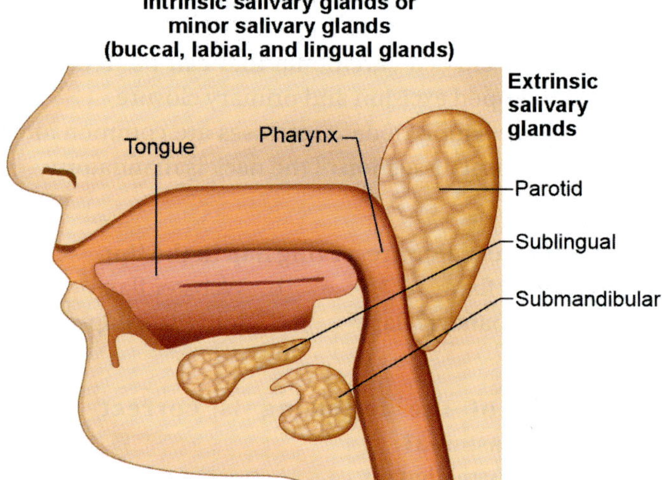

Fig. 1: The salivary glands.

Physiology

The main function of salivary glands is to produce saliva, which helps in maintaining oral health and lubricating the oral cavity and pharynx. Salivary glands produce approximately *1.5–2 L of saliva in 24 hours.* The normal *pH of saliva remains between 6.2 and 7.6. Saliva contains 99% of water, enzymes, and some buffering agents.* A few drops of saliva can display your *complete genetic makeup.*

The basic functional control of the salivary glands is by the parasympathetic nerves. *Stimulation of sympathetic or parasympathetic nerves stimulates salivary glands to secrete saliva.* Parasympathetic nerves are more active than sympathetic nerves in controlling saliva production.

Saliva has some functions:

- Lubrication helps in giving comfort to the oral cavity and pharynx.
- Lubrication helps in food to pass down during deglutition.
- Saliva contains enzymes (amylase and lipase) which help in the breakdown of certain food aliments such as starch in the food.

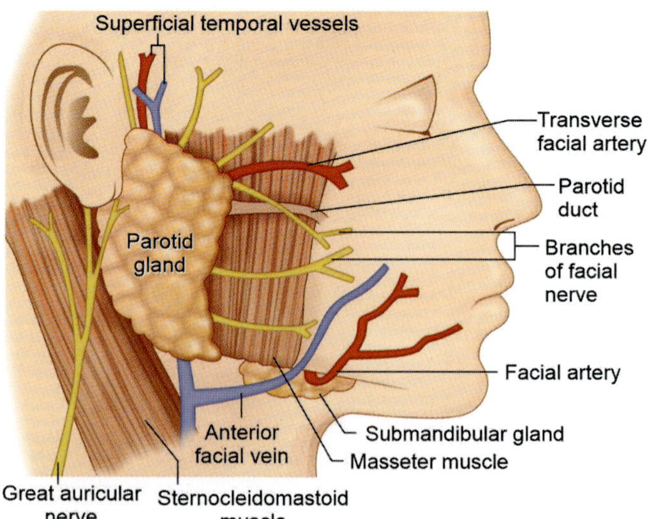

Fig. 2: Anatomy of salivary glands.

- It keeps the mouth clean and avoids the formation of cavities in the teeth and diseases of gum.
- Food particles are dissolved in saliva so that your taste buds can recognize tastes.
- Saliva also helps in avoiding the harmful effects of gastric acid by diluting it.
- Minor salivary glands are extremely small as compare to major salivary glands, but together they produce more saliva than the major salivary glands.
- Saliva is also having antimicrobial activity with the healing power of tissue repair.

HISTOLOGY OF SALIVARY GLANDS

Salivary glands are made up of acini and fat. The cells of the acini secrete saliva. The parenchyma of the salivary gland is the secretory tissue and is supported by stroma. *The parenchyma consists of acini, which secrete saliva, intercalated ducts leading to collecting ducts, and then the main duct.*

PAROTID GLAND

It lies in a space bounded by the ramus of the mandible, the mastoid process, and the base of the skull. It lies over the carotid sheath and is enveloped by deep cervical fascia. Its lower pole extends into the neck. The duct of the parotid gland *[Stensen's (Necolas Steno, also known as Niels Stensen, 1638–1686, a Danish Anatomist, described in 1660) duct]* is a tube-like structure that carries saliva from the gland to the oral cavity. It is approximately 5 cm in length **(Fig. 3)**.

The blood supply of the parotid gland is through the transverse facial artery, which is a branch of the superficial temporal artery, which is a branch of the external carotid artery. Veins are corresponding to arteries.

Superficial lobe
Deep lobe
20%
80%
ECA
Facial nerve
Retromandibular vein

Fig. 3: Lobes of the parotid gland. (ECA: external carotid artery)

The lymphatic drainage of the parotid gland is through the following lymph nodes:

- *Intraparotid lymph nodes*—80% in the superficial lobe and 20% in the deep lobe.
- Superficial parotid lymph nodes
- Deep parotid lymph nodes

The lymph nodes drain into preauricular or parotid lymph nodes, which drain into the deep cervical lymph node chain.

The parotid gland secretes saliva, and it is through the secretomotor pathway, which is as below:

Mn = IT has Lesser Options Anywhere
I = Inferior salivary nucleus
T = Tympanic branch of ninth nerve
L = Lesser petrosal nerve
O = Optic ganglion
A = *Auriculotemporal nerve*

Structures pass through the parotid gland:

- Facial nerve with its branches
- Terminal branch of external carotid artery terminating into superficial temporal artery and maxillary artery
- Retromandibular vein
- Lymph nodes
- Patey's *(David Howard Patey, 1899–1976, Surgeon, The Middlesex Hospital, London, UK)* fascio venous plane (retromandibular vein and facial nerve) divide the two lobes of parotid gland, superficial and deep lobes. The duct of parotid gland is called Stensen's duct.

Nerve Supply of Parotid Gland (Fig. 4)

- *Parasympathetic:* It is via the glossopharyngeal nerve. It causes increased saliva secretion.
- *Sympathetic:* It enhances the blood flow in the gland.

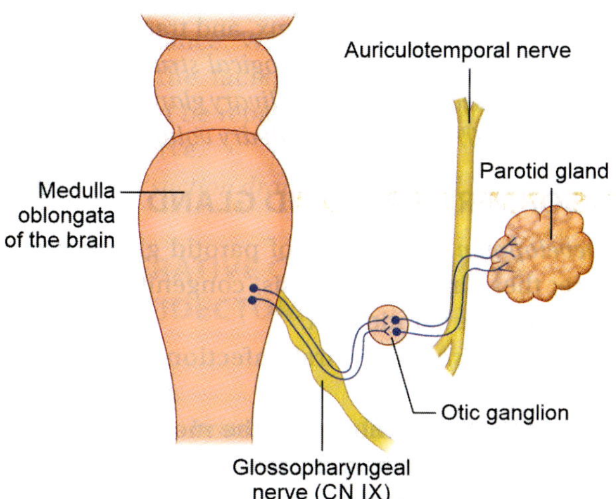

Fig. 4: Nerve supply of parotid gland.

Clinical Features

Soft cystic, fluctuant, and painless swelling in the submandibular or submental region.

Investigation

- USG
- MRI

Treatment

- Needle aspiration
- Incision and drainage
- Marsupialization
- Surgical excision

Tumors of the Sublingual Gland

Extremely rare, and 90% are malignant.

Clinical Features

- Painless rubbery swelling in the floor of the mouth
- Pain or paresthesia indicates toward malignancy

Investigation

- USG
- MRI
- True-cut or punch biopsy

Treatment

Wide excision—en bloc, with same sitting reconstruction.

DISORDERS OF MINOR SALIVARY GLANDS

Cysts are common and especially develop after trauma and are of extravasation variety, not retention. Usually, swellings are painless and translucent. *Recurrence after excision is rare.*

Tumors of Minor Salivary Glands

Tumors of minor salivary glands are usually seen at the palate, upper lip, and retromolar area.

Punch biopsy is required before surgery. Malignant tumors of minor salivary glands are rare.

NECROTIZING SIALOMETAPLASIA

It is a rare feature and mimics cancer. It is a deep, punched-out ulcer indistinguishable from a malignant lesion except by biopsy. It resolves with symptomatic treatment.

SOME IMPORTANT QUESTIONS

Q1. What is the cause of salivary gland tumors?

Ans. The following are the factors causing salivary gland tumors:

- *Genetic trisomy 5* for minor salivary gland carcinoma and polysomy 3 and 17
- *Radiotherapy*
- *Epstein-Barr virus infection* causing lymphoid carcinoma

Q2. Mention some of the most common factors in relation to the salivary gland.

Ans. The most common tumor of the salivary gland is pleomorphic adenoma.

- *Most common* site of parotid pleomorphic adenoma—tail of the parotid.
- *Most common* and best investigation for parotid lump—fine needle aspiration cytology (FNAC).
- *Most common* and best imaging test—magnetic resonance imaging (MRI)
- *Most common* malignant tumor of the salivary gland—mucoepidermoid carcinoma.
- *Most common* malignant tumor of minor salivary glands is adenoid cystic carcinoma.
- *Most common* tumor of the salivary gland in children is hemangioma.
- *Most common* malignant tumor of the salivary gland in children—mucoepidermoid carcinoma.
- *Most common* site for minor salivary glands—hard palate.

Q3. What is the incidence of malignancy in various salivary glands?

Ans. The incidence of malignancy increases with a decrease in the size of the salivary gland.

Parotid – 25%, submandibular 50%, sublingual 50%, minor submandibular glands 75%.

Q4. What are the indications of radiotherapy in the tumors of various salivary glands?

Ans. *Most salivary gland tumors are radioresistant*, but can be treated for high-grade malignant tumors, high-grade malignant tumors with bone involvement, large tumors, and positive tumor margins after excision in the specimen.

Q5. What is parotid fistula?

Ans. *It can be external or internal. Internal fistula develops inside the oral cavity. External fistula is due to rupture of the parotid gland abscess, after incision of the parotid* *abscess, trauma, or after parotidectomy.* Usually closes spontaneously, but sometimes does not and requires Newman-Seabrook operation (repair of Stensen's duct over a number of tantalum wires).

Q6. Earliest pathological finding in Sjögren's syndrome.

Ans. Periductal and perivascular lymphocytic infiltration [most important antibodies in Sjogren's syndrome are directed against SS-A (Ro) and SS-B (La)].

MULTIPLE CHOICE QUESTIONS

Grade I	*Simple*

Q1. While doing parotid surgery, the following landmarks are used to identify the facial nerve trunk, *except*: (AIIMS 2020)

a. Tragal cartilage pointer
b. Posterior belly of the digastric insertion
c. Inferior belly of the omohyoid
d. Mastoid process

Q2. Postsuperficial parotidectomy, a patient developed numbness over the cheek area. Which nerve is injured in the surgery? (AIIMS 2019)

a. Auriculotemporal nerve
b. Greater auricular nerve
c. Mandibular nerve
d. Facial nerve

Q3. A patient, after parotid surgery, on awakening, noticed lower lip paralysis. Otherwise, she is able to close her eyes normally. Which of the following nerves is most likely injured? (AIIMS 2020)

a. Cervical branch of the facial nerve
b. Facial nerve main trunk
c. Parotid duct
d. Temporal branch of the facial nerve

Q4. Best diagnostic modality for parotid swelling is: (AIIMS Nov 1994)

a. Enucleation
b. Fine-needle aspiration cytology (FNAC)
c. Superficial parotidectomy
d. Excisional biopsy

Q5. Ramavati, a 40-year-old female, presented with a progressively increasing lump in the parotid region. On oral examination, the tonsil was pushed medially, Biopsy showed it to be a pleomorphic adenoma. The appropriate treatment is: (AIIMS June 2001)

a. Superficial parotidectomy
b. Lumpectomy
c. Conservative total parotidectomy
d. Enucleation

Q6. All are true for pleomorphic adenoma, *except*: (PGI Dec 1999)

a. Arises from the parotid
b. May turn into malignant
c. Minor salivary glands are involved
d. None

Q7. Which of the following is an indication of radiotherapy in pleomorphic adenoma of the parotid? (All India 2004)

a. Involvement of deep lobe
b. Second histologically benign recurrence
c. Microscopically positive margins
d. Malignant transformation

Q8. Mucoepidermoid carcinoma of parotid arises from: (PGI June 1999)

a. Secretory cells b. Excretory cells
c. Myoepithelial cells d. Myofibril

Q9. Acinic cell carcinoma of the salivary gland arises most often in the: (All India 2006)

a. Parotid gland b. Minor salivary gland
c. Submandibular gland d. Sublingual gland

Q10. True statement(s) about salivary gland tumors: (PGI June 2004)

a. Pleomorphic adenoma can arise in submandibular gland
b. Warthin's tumor from the submandibular gland
c. Pleomorphic adenoma is the most common tumor of the submandibular gland
d. Acinic cell carcinoma is most malignant
e. Frey's syndrome is due to injury of the auriculotemporal nerve

Q11. Most of the parotid tumors are managed by: (All India 1997)

a. Total parotidectomy
b. Radical parotidectomy
c. Superficial parotidectomy
d. Radical parotidectomy and neck dissection

CHAPTER 25

Neck

"Do not ignore a lump in the neck, even if it is small and painless, as it can be a sign of a serious sickness."

– Vinod Kumar Nigam

INTRODUCTION

The neck is a very sensitive area of our body. It is divided into various parts or triangles **(Figs. 1A to C)** according to the structures contained in it. Triangles of the neck are:

- *Anterior triangle:* It can further be divided into carotid triangle, submandibular triangle (digastric triangle), submental triangle, and muscular triangle.
- *Posterior triangle:* It includes the supraclavicular and suboccipital triangles.

MIDLINE SWELLINGS IN NECK

- Ludwig's angina
- Submental lymph nodes (LNs)
- Thyroglossal cyst
- Thyroid isthmus goiter
- Subhyoid bursitis
- LN in the suprasternal space of burns

LATERAL SWELLINGS IN NECK

- *Submandibular triangle:*
  - Enlarged LNs
  - Submandibular gland
  - Sjögren's syndrome
- *Carotid triangle:*
  - Aneurysm
  - Carotid body tumor
  - Branchial cyst
  - Goiter
  - Laryngocele
  - LN enlargement

POSTERIOR TRIANGLE SWELLINGS

- Supraclavicular LNs
- Cold abscess
- Cervical rib
- Cystic hygroma
- Pharyngeal pouch

CERVICAL LYMPH NODES

There are approximately 300 LNs present in the neck.

Levels of LNs in the neck:

- *IA:* Submental
- *IB:* Submandibular
- *II:* Upper jugular
- *III:* Middle jugular
- *IV:* Lower jugular
- *V:* Posterior triangle
- *VI:* Anterior compartment or central
- *VII:* Superior mediastinal

Type I: Presence spinal accessory

Type II: Presence spinal accessory + internal jugular vein nerve

Type III: (Functional neck dissection) Presence spinal accessory nerve, the internal jugular vein, and the sternomastoid muscle.

CARCINOMA OF LARYNX

Types

- *Supraglottic cancer*
  - The most common first symptom is pain or swelling
  - Nodal metastasis early
- *Glottic cancer:* Most common site, most common symptom occurring 1st is hoarseness of voice, spreads locally to the anterior commissure.
- *Subglottic cancer:* The least common site, locally spreads, and spider is the most common and first symptom.

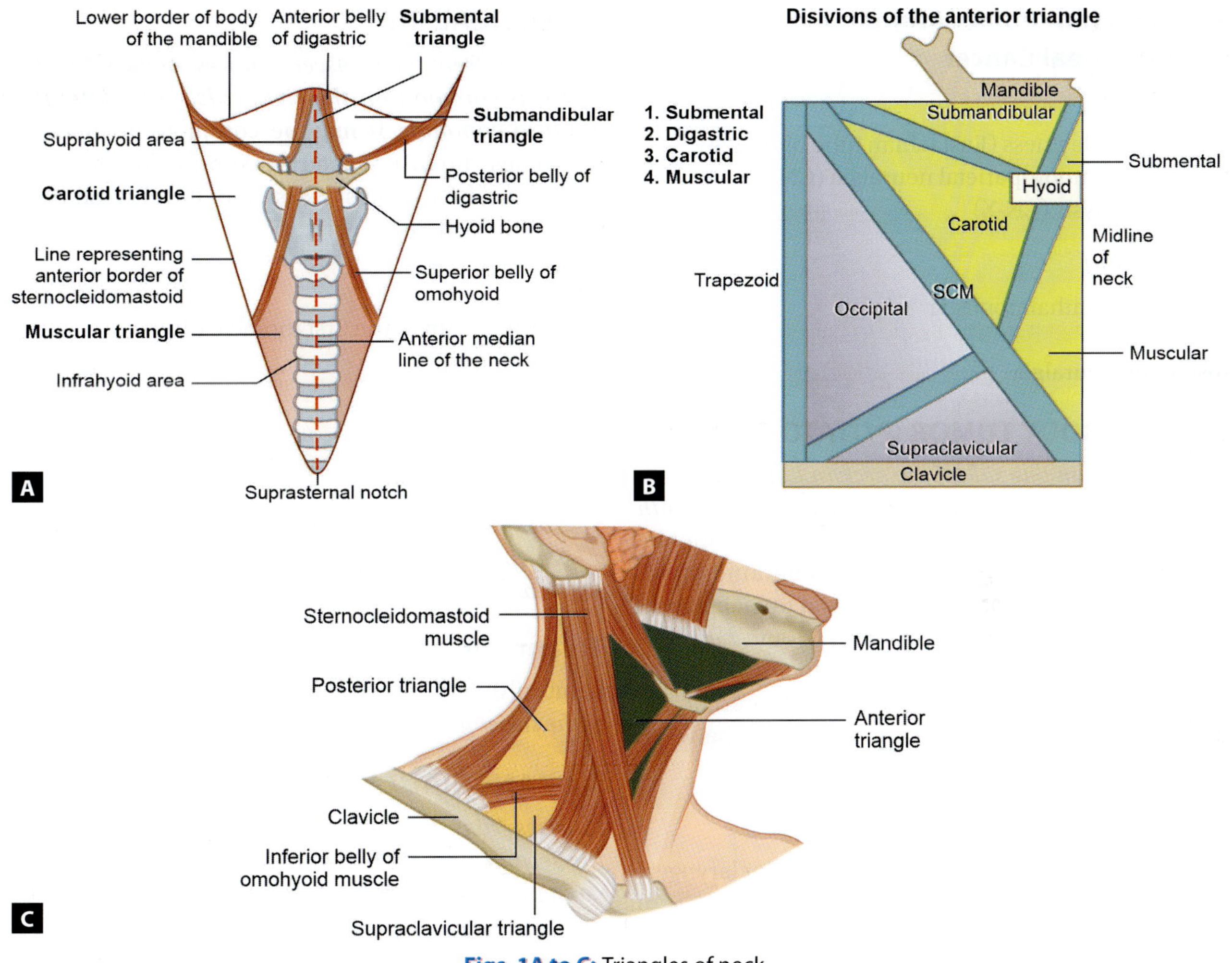

Figs. 1A to C: Triangles of neck.

Treatment

- *T1:* EBRT
- *T2:* RT in glottic and subglottic
- *T3 and T4:* Laryngectomy in supraglottic
- Total laryngectomy with neck dissection

NASOPHARYNGEAL CARCINOMA

- Common in chins and related areas.
- Secondaries in the LNs of the neck are common.

Risk Factors

- Genetic
- Epstein–Barr virus
- *Air pollution:* Burning incense and nitrosamines for dry salted fish

Histology

Squamous cell carcinoma (SCC).

Clinical Features

- Males, 40–70 years.
- The most common site is the fossa of Rosenmuller in the lateral wall of the pharynx.
- LN involvement is common and is the most common presenting symptom.
- Distant metastasis occurs in the bone, lung, and liver.

Diagnosis

Computed tomography (CT) and biopsy.

Treatment

- Radiotherapy is the treatment of choice.
- Stage III and IV may require chemotherapy also.

Some Important Points About Nasopharyngeal Cancer

Trotter's Triad

- Conductive deafness (Eustachian tube blockage)
- Ipsilateral temporoparietal neuralgia (CN V)
- Palatal paralysis (CN-X)

Jaccoud's Triad

- Ipsilateral ophthalmoplegia
- Amaurosis
- Ipsilateral neuralgia

CAROTID BODY TUMOR (POTATO TUMOR)

It usually occurs on one side of the neck in late adulthood. It is a nonchromaffin paraganglioma associated with pheochromocytoma. There is a neck mass that is mobile from side to side, but not vertically (Fontaine sign). It is pulsatile, but not expansile. It can lead to malignancy in <10% of cases, but metastasis is rare. *CT* and *magnetic resonance (MR)* angiograms are the diagnostic tests. *Lyre sign* on angiogram showing splaying of internal and external carotid arteries as the tumor appears between them.

Treatment

Surgical removal but complications, i.e., superior laryngeal nerve injury, frostbite syndrome (Pain with the start of mastication).

Shamblin classification divides it into three types: Type I (localized—25%), *Type II* (partially adherent, 50%), and *Type III* (completely adherent—25%). It is treated by excision or en-bloc removal with the *internal carotid artery (ICA). First bite syndrome* is due to sympathetic nerve damage. Pain in the neck starts with food.

THORACIC OUTLET SYNDROME

The subclavian artery is compressed at the thoracic outlet between the clavicle first rib, and the scalene muscles. The brachial plexus also gets involved. It may be congenital due to the presence of cervical rib, abnormal first rib, abnormal insertion of scalene muscle, or its hypertrophy, or it may be acquired due to fracture of clavicle, first rib, or scalene muscle injury, or tumor. It has both neurogenic and vascular symptoms such as pain, paresthesia along the ulnar nerve distribution and claudication, and cold hands with may be gangrenous tips.

Adson test, Roos test, Halstead test and Write test can be helpful in diagnosis.

CERVICAL RIB

It develops from the transverse process of the C7 vertebrae, and it is common on the right side, but bilateral cases are also common. It may be complete or incomplete. It causes mostly vascular symptoms more than neurological symptoms. Excision of the cervical rib is the treatment of choice.

Types

- Complete up to the first thoracic rib
- Bulbous end
- Tapering end
- Fibrous band

Clinical Features

- *Local symptoms* of a mass with tenderness
- *Vascular symptoms:* 3P Pain, pallor, and pulselessness
- *Neurological symptoms:* Pain/paresthesia

Treatment

Removal of cervical rib if symptoms are severe. *Scalenotomy of the scalenus anterior muscle can also help.*

BRANCHIAL CYST

It arises from a persistent cervical sinus due to fusion of the second and sixth branchial arches. It is common in young adults. There is swelling in the upper part of the neck anteriorly, and it is transluminant. Infection, sinus formation, and carcinoma are the complications. Excision of the cyst is the treatment.

BRANCHIAL SINUS

It is due to the failure of fusion of the second and sixth branchial arches. It may be congenital or acquired. External opening is typically located in the lower one-third of the neck in congenital sinus, but in acquired it is located at the upper one-third to middle one-third junction. The internal opening is usually on the lateral wall of the pharynx behind the tonsil. It is treated by excision of the fistulous tract.

CYSTIC HYGROMA

It arises as a sequestration of the jugular lymph sac. It is situated in the posterior triangle of the neck in a neonate or an infant. It is translucent, partially compressible, and a cough impulse is present. It is filled with lymph, so brilliantly translucent. Infection and respiratory difficulty due to its size are the main complications. The treatment is complete excision of all lymphatic tissues along with the cyst.

Other sites than the neck
Mn = AMIR
A= Axilla
M = Mediastinum
I = Inguinal
R = Retroperitoneal space

Treatment

Surgical excision.

LARYNGOCELE

It is a diverticulum from the herniation of laryngeal mucosa. It may be internal or external. It is common in glass blowers and wind instrument musicians. Swelling moves with deglutition. Excision is the treatment.

COLD ABSCESS IN NECK

It is usually caused by tuberculosis from a caseating LN. It usually lies in the anterior triangle. Antigravity drainage is required.

Lymph node dissection of the neck ***(Fig. 2):***
- *Radical neck dissection by Crile:* LNs level 1–5 with submandibular salivary gland, internal jugular vein, accessory nerve, lower part of parotid gland, fat, fascia, strap muscles, and sternomastoid muscle are removed en bloc.
- *Modified radical neck dissection by Bocca:* LNs level 1–5 and other structures removed as in radical neck dissection by Crile. The internal jugular vein, accessory nerve, and sternomastoid muscles are preserved.
- *Selective neck dissection:* LNs level 1–3 are removed with fat, fascia, muscles, and submandibular salivary gland.

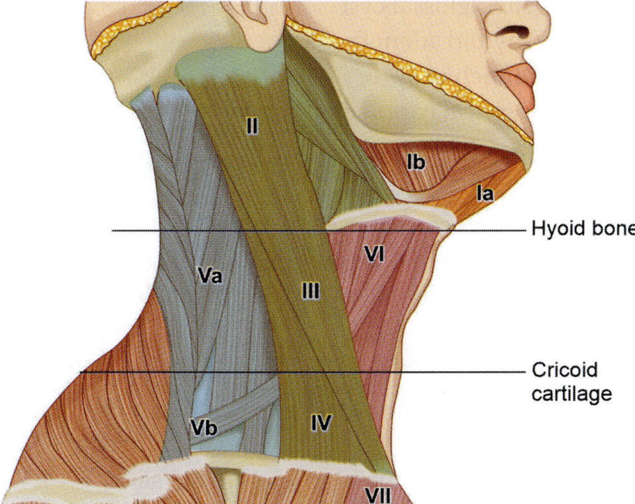

Fig. 2: Lymph node levels in the neck.

Modified radical neck dissection is also called functional neck dissection. Structures which move with deglutition are the thyroid gland, thyroglossal cyst, pre- and paratracheal LNs, and subhyoid bursa.

SOME IMPORTANT QUESTIONS

Q1. What is the swelling shown in the image?

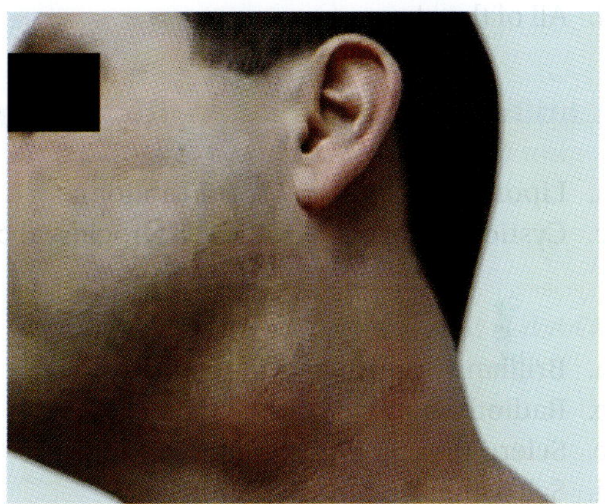

a. Branchial cyst
b. Pharyngeal pouch
c. Dermoid cyst
d. Pretracheal bursa

Ans. a

Q2. A young female presents with a swelling in the neck, which is painless. The swelling moves with deglutition and with the protrusion of the tongue. What is the diagnosis?

a. Thyroid swelling
b. Thyroglossal cyst
c. Carotid tumor
d. Branchial cyst

Ans. b

Q3. A middle-aged female with swelling in the neck with a potato-like consistency. On examination, the swelling is pulsatile. Which of the following investigations must not be done?

a. Biopsy
b. Angiography
c. Contrast-enhanced computed tomography (CECT) neck
d. MRI

Ans. a

Q4. The true about the carotid body tumor is:

a. Origin from nonchromaffin tissue
b. Most commonly seen with people who live at high altitudes
c. Family history positive

d. Fine-needle aspiration cytology (FNAC) is diagnostic
e. Painful nonmobile lump in the neck

Ans. b and c

Q5. Cystic hygroma may be associated with:
a. Turner's syndrome
b. Klinefelter's syndrome
c. Down syndrome
d. All of the above

Ans. a

Q6. A brilliantly translucent swelling in the neck region in a 2-year-old child's diagnosis is:
a. Lipoma
b. Teratoma
c. Cystic hygroma
d. Thyroglossal cyst

Ans. c

Q7. Which is incorrect about cystic hygroma?
a. Brilliantly translucent
b. Radiotherapy
c. Sclerotherapy with bleomycin
d. Sclerotherapy with actinomycin

Ans. b

Q8. All are true about cystic hygroma, *except*:
a. Pulsatile
b. May cause respiratory obstruction
c. Common in neck
d. Present in birth

Ans. a

Q9. Branchiogenic carcinoma:
a. Branchial cyst cancer
b. Carcinoma arising from the bronchus
c. Type of carcinoma lung
d. Commonly seen in young adults

Ans. a

Q10. Excision of the hyoid bone is done in:
a. Branchial cyst
b. Branchial fistula
c. Thyroglossal cyst
d. Sublingual dermoids

Ans. c

MULTIPLE CHOICE QUESTIONS

Grade I	*Simple*

Q1. Carotid body tumors: (PGI 2005)
a. Arises from the endothelial cells
b. Originates from the Schwann cells
c. Radiotherapy is the Rx of choice
d. May metastasize

Q2. True about branchial anomaly: (AIIMS 2010)
a. Cysts are more common than sinuses.
b. For sinus surgery is not always indicated
c. Cysts present with dysphagia and hoarseness of voice.
d. Most commonly due to the second branchial remnant

Q3. True about branchial cyst: (PGI 2007)
a. Seen deep to the lower one-third of the sternocleidomastoid
b. Well consists of lymphoid tissue
c. Filled with straw colored fluid with cholesterol crystals
d. Presents at birth

Q4. A young boy presented with a midline neck swelling as seen below, which moves with deglutition and protrusion of the tongue. It has been stable in size for the last 1 year. What is the likely diagnosis? (AIIMS 2017)

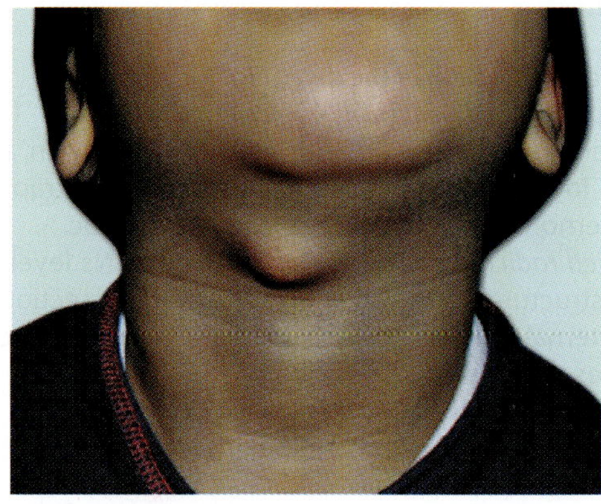

a. Thyroglossal cyst
b. Thyroid adenoma
c. Branchial cyst
d. Cervical lymphadenopathy

Q5. About congenital torticollis, all are true, *except*: (AIIMS 2010)
a. Always associated with breech extraction
b. Spontaneous resolution in most cases
c. Two-thirds of cases have a palpable neck mass at birth
d. Uncorrected cases develop plagiocephaly

Q6. Which of the following is true about a thyroglossal cyst? (AIIMS 2019)
a. Secondary infection leads to the sinus.
b. 70% contain heterotopic thyroid tissue.

c. Resolve spontaneously in 20–30% cases
d. The thyroglossal duct obliterates by the 10th week of IUL.
e. Lining epithelium is stratified squamous epithelium or ciliated columnar epithelium.

Q7. A true statement about a carotid body tumor is: (PGI June 2002)
a. Non-chromaffin paraganglioma
b. Good prognosis
c. Rarely metastasizes
d. Similar to a mixed parotid tumor

Q8. Which one is not true regarding a carotid body tumor? (AIIMS June 1997)
a. Unilateral
b. Surgical resection is the treatment
c. Nonchromaffin paraganglioma
d. The middle-aged group is affected

Q9. True regarding cystic hygroma is: (AIIMS Nov 1993)
a. Nontransilluminant
b. Lined by columnar epithelium
c. Lined by stratified squamous epithelium
d. Develops from jugular lymphatic sequestration

Q10. Structures preserved in radical neck dissection is: (All India 2000)
a. Vagus nerve
b. Submandibular gland
c. Sternocleidomastoid
d. Internal jugular vein

Grade II	*Difficult*

Q1. Treatment of cystic hygroma includes: (PGI 2011)
a. Complete excision
b. Marsupialization
c. Repeated aspiration
d. Injection of sclerosing agents
e. Observation or regular follow-up

Q2. Secondaries in the neck with no obvious primary malignancy are most often due to: (JIPMER 1993)
a. CA stomach b. CA larynx
c. CA nasopharynx d. CA thyroid

Q3. In extended supraomohyoid neck dissection, lymph node dissection is done up to: (MHSSMCET 2010)
a. 2 b. 3
c. 4 d. 5

Q4. Structures not removed in functional neck dissection is: (AIIMS Nov 1993)
a. Carotid artery, vagus nerve
b. Sternomastoid muscle, internal jugular vein
c. Spinal accessory nerve, submandibular salivary gland
d. Neck nodes

Q5. Blow out carotid is characteristically seen with: (AIIMS Nov 1998)
a. Thyroidectomy
b. Radical neck dissection
c. Flap necrosis
d. Sistrunk operation

Q6. Which of the following does not move on deglutition? (All India 1991)
a. Subligual dermoid
b. Thyroid nodule
c. Pretracheal lymph node
d. Thyroglossal cyst

Q7. Adson's test is positive in: (Kerala 1989)
a. Cervical rib
b. Cervical spondylosis
c. Cervical fracture
d. Cervical dislocation

Q8. Thyroglossal fistula develops due to: (Kerala 1991)
a. Developmental anomaly
b. Injury
c. Incomplete removal of thyroglossal cyst
d. Inflammatory disorder

Q9. Structures preserved in functional neck dissection is: (AIIMS Nov 1993)
a. Carotid artery, vagus nerve
b. Sternomastoid muscle, internal jugular vein
c. Spinal accessory nerve, submandibular salivary gland
d. Neck nodes

10. Structures not removed in radical neck dissection are: (PGI June 2007)
a. X nerve
b. X1 nerve
c. Tail of parotid
d. Parotid and postauricular nerve

Grade III | **Most difficult**

Q1. True about branchial cyst: (PGI 2007)

a. Seen deep to the lower one-third of the sternocleidomastoid.
b. The wall consists of lymphoid tissue.
c. Filled with straw colored fluid with cholesterol crystals.
d. Presents at birth

Q2. In postradical neck dissection shoulder syndrome, all are seen, *except*: (AIIMS 2008)

a. Restricted range of movement
b. Pain
c. Shoulder drooping
d. Normal electromyographic findings

Q3. Structures preserved in modified radical neck dissection: (PGI 2011)

a. Accessory nerve
b. Sternocleidomastoid muscle
c. Submandibular gland
d. Internal jugular vein
e. Omohyoid muscle

Q4. An elderly male presents with a 4 × 5 cm lump in the right neck. FNAC revealed it to be squamous cell carcinoma. No primary was found. A diagnosis of unknown primary was made. According to the American Joint Committee on Cancer (AJCC) system or classification, the tumor, nodes, and metastasis (TNM) staging of a tumor would be: (JIPMER 2014)

a. T1N2M0
b. T0N2aM1
c. T1N2cM0
d. T0N2aMx

Q5. In postradical neck dissection shoulder syndrome, all are seen, *except*: (AIIMS Nov 2008)

a. Restricted range of movement
b. Pain
c. Shoulder drooping
d. Normal electromyographic findings

Q6. Which of the following is associated with cystic hygroma? (AIIMS Nov 1997)

a. Marfan's syndrome
b. Turner's syndrome
c. Down syndrome
d. Noonan's syndrome

Q7. True about cystic hygroma: (PGI Dec 2000)

a. Congenital sequestration of lymphatics
b. Resolves spontaneously by 5 years of age
c. Common in the upper one-third of the lateral neck
d. Surgery is the treatment of choice

Q8. The commonest site of a branchial cyst is: (All India 1994)

a. Upper one-third of the sternocleidomastoid (SCM)
b. Lower one-third of the SCM
c. Upper two-thirds of the SCM
d. Lower two-thirds of the SCM

Q9. The hyoid bone is closely associated with: (All India 1998)

a. Bronchogenic cyst
b. Cystic hygroma
c. Thyroglossal cyst/fistula
d. Brachial cyst

Q10. In the management of thyroglossal cyst: (PGI Dec 2002)

a. Central portion of the hyoid excised
b. Sternothyroid muscle dissected
c. Isthmusectomy with subtotal thyroidectomy
d. Strap muscles of the neck are dissected

ANSWERS

Grade I: 1. d; 2. d (Schwartz 10/e p598); 3. b, c; 4. a; 5. a; 6. c; 7. a, b, c; 8. None; 9. d; 10. a

Grade II: 1. a, d; 2. c; 3. c (Sabiston 20/e p794); 4. a, b; 5. b; 6. a (Schwartz 9/e p1344-1345); 7. a; 8. c; 9. b (Bailey 27/e p758); 10. a, c, d

Grade III: 1. b, c; 2. d; 3. a; 4. d; 5. d; 6. b; 7. a, d; 8. a; 9. c (Bailey 27/e p755); 10. a (Sabiston 19/e p1832)

MODEL QUESTIONS

Q1. Treatment of choice for cystic hygroma:
a. Percutaneous aspiration
b. Intralesional sclerosant injection
c. En-bloc resection
d. Surgical excision
Ans. d

Q2. Cystic compressible, translucent swelling in the posterior triangle of the neck:
a. Cystic hygroma
b. Branchial cyst
c. Thyroglossal cyst
d. Dermoid cyst
Ans. a

Q3. Branchial cyst arises from which branchial cleft?
a. First
b. Second
c. Third
d. Fourth
Ans. b

Q4. Modified radical dissection of the neck, all structures are preserved, *except*:
a. Sternomastoid
b. External jugular vein
c. Internal jugular
d. Spinal accessory
Ans. b

Q5. A nerve injured in radical neck dissection leads to loss of sensation in the medial side of the arm. The nerve injured is:
a. Long thoracic nerve
b. Thoracodorsal nerve
c. Dorsal scapular nerve
d. Medial cutaneous nerve of the arm
Ans. d

Q6. In modified radical neck dissection type II (MRND type II), structures preserved are:
a. Spinal accessory nerve + SCM
b. Spinal accessory nerve + internal jugular vein
c. SCM + internal jugular vein
d. Level I–V LN + SCM
Ans. b

Q7. The main problem associated with the carotid body tumor operation is:
a. The tumor blends with the jugular vein
b. The tumor blends with a bifurcation of the carotid artery
c. Recurrence
d. Vasovagal shock
Ans. b

Q8. Cystic hygroma is known to occur in all, *except*:
a. Calf
b. Neck
c. Axilla
d. Mediastinum
Ans. a

Q9. The most frequent site of brachial cyst is at:
a. Upper third of the posterior border of the sternocleidomastoid
b. Lower third of the anterior border of the sternocleidomastoid
c. Upper third of the anteromedial border of the sternocleidomastoid
d. Supraclavicular fossa
Ans. c

Q10. Brachial cyst is lined by:
a. Columnar epithelium
b. Cuboidal epithelium
c. Squamous epithelium
d. Ciliated columnar epithelium
Ans. c

SUGGESTED READING

1. Bailey & Love's - Short Practice of Surgery, 27th edition.
2. Schwartz's Principles of Surgery, 18th edition.
3. Textbook of Surgery by David Sabiston, 21st edition.

CHAPTER 26

Face

"Injuries are our best teachers."

– Anonymous

CLEFT LIP AND CLEFT PALATE

These are one of the most common congenital abnormalities in the face. These entities are not only cosmetically bad but also functionally. Cleft lip with cleft palate occurs in about 1 in 600 births, and cleft palate only in 1 in 1,000 births. Cleft palate alone occurs in about 40% of cases, with predominance in females, and cleft lip with cleft palate is more common in males. Unilateral cleft lip is more common on the left side (60%). Cleft lip can nowadays be diagnosed by ultrasonography (USG) at 18 weeks of pregnancy. Cleft palate occurs due to failure of palatal shelves, and cleft lip due to disruption of the nasolabial and bilabial muscles. Cleft lip and cleft palate can either be incomplete or complete.

LIP, ALVEOLUS, HARD PALATE, AND SOFT PALATE

LAHSAL classification is a pictorial classification of cleft lip and cleft palate, the mouth is divided into six parts: *L*ip-right, *A*lveolus-right, *H*ard palate, *S*oft palate, *A*lveolus-left, *L*ip-left. Capital letter indicates complete cleft and small letter indicates incomplete cleft (**Figs. 1A and B**).

SYNDROMES ASSOCIATED WITH CLEFT LIP AND PALATE

- Pierre Robin (1867–1950, French dental surgeon, described in 1929) syndrome is, most common.
- Stickler's (Gunnar B Stickler, 1925–2010, Germany-born American, pediatric cardiologist) syndrome (eye and muscle disorder).
- Shprintzen's (Robert J Shprintzen, 1946, American surgeon) syndrome (cardiac disorder)
- Down (John Langdon Haydon Down, 1828–1896, British physician) syndrome.
- Apert's (Eugene Apert, 1868–1940, French physician, described in 1906) syndrome.
- Treacher–Collins' (Edward Treacher-Collins, 1862–1932, British ophthalmic surgeon, described in 1900) syndrome.

Things to remember:
- The best time to repair a cleft lip is between 3 and 6 months of age.
- The best time to repair a cleft palate is between 6 and 18 months of age.
- Cleft lip and cleft palate surgery aims to achieve good cosmetically with a minimum scar.
- Cleft lip repair technique most commonly used is the Millard technique, but others are also used, i.e., Thompson, Le Mesurier, and Tennison–Rendall.

CAUSES OF CLEFT LIP AND PALATE

- Genetic
- *Environmental:* Epilepsy to mother and drugs, i.e., diazepam, barbiturates, and corticosteroids.

MID-FACE FRACTURES

These fractures mainly involve the maxilla. They are divided as LeFort (Rene LeFort, 1869–1951, French surgeon, classified these fractures by experimenting by dropping rocks on the faces of cadavers) I, II, and III.

- *LeFort I:* Fracture line runs above and parallel to the palate.
- *LeFort II:* Pyramidal shaped, fracture line runs through root of nose, lacrimal bone, floor of orbit (always involved), maxillary sinus, and pterygoid plate.
- *LeFort III:* Complete disjunction of facial skeletal from the base of skull.

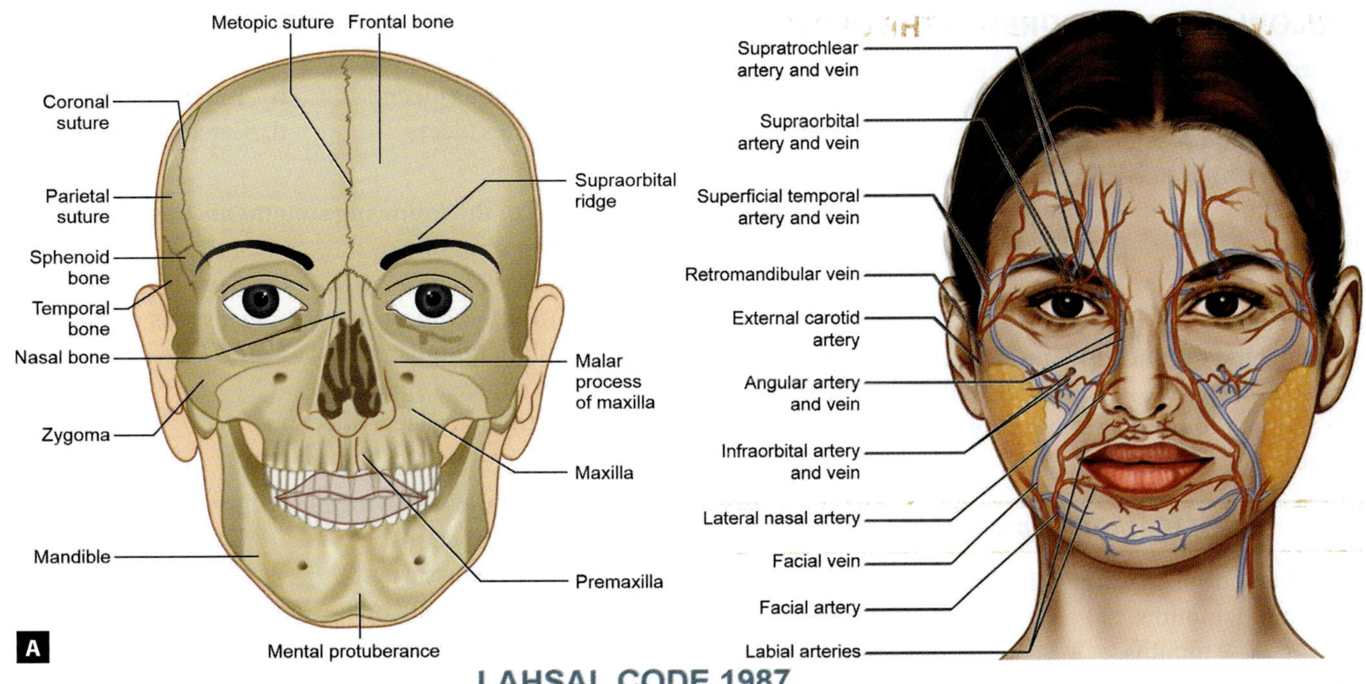

LAHSAL CODE 1987

The LAHSAL code splits the relevant parts of the mouth into six parts:

1. Right lip
2. Right alveolus
3. Hard palate
4. Soft palate
5. Left alveolus
6. Left lip

L Lip, A Alveolus, A Alveolus, L Lip; Right, Left; H Hard palate; S Soft palate

The first character is for the patient's right lip, and the last character for the patient's left lip. Example:

..HS.L:Complete cleft of hard and soft palate with left complete cleft lip

B

Figs. 1A and B: Face anatomy and LAHSAL classification.

Management

Interdental or intermaxillary fixation.

FRACTURES OF MANDIBLE

The most common site of fracture is the condylar neck. It may be direct or indirect. The fracture may be at the site of the hit or away (Guardsman fracture). When a piece of mandibular bone is separated from the mandible, it is called a "butterfly" fracture. Intermaxillary fixation and plating are required.

ZYGOMATIC BONE FRACTURE

The zygomatic bone is usually fractured at zygomatic frontal, zygomatic temporal, and infraorbital region so called *tripod fracture*. Epistaxis, diplopia, periorbital emphysema, malar prominence absence, step deformity, and loss of sensation over the area of infraorbital nerve. It is diagnosed by Warter's view X-ray and CT scan. Open reduction and internal fixation are the treatment.

BLOW-OUT FRACTURES OF THE ORBIT

A direct blow to the eye globe pushes inside the orbit. Tear-drop sign is seen with failure to rotate the eye up, diplopia, and loss of sensation over the distribution of the infraorbital nerve. Treatment should be urgent, with orbital floor exploration and replacement of displaced tissues.

RULE OF 10

Cleft lip repair should be done at 10 weeks of age, when the weight is 10 pounds and hemoglobin is 10 g%. If revision surgery is required, it should be done after the age of 2 years.

SOME IMPORTANT QUESTIONS

Q1. Ideal time for surgery in case of unilateral cleft lip:

a. <3 months b. 3–6 months
c. 6–9 months d. >12 months

Ans. b

Q2. All are to do about submucosal cleft palate, *except*:

a. Bifid uvula b. Notched hard palate
c. Lip pits d. Zona pellucida

Ans. c

Q3. Millard's "Rule of Ten" includes all, *except*:

a. 10 lbs b. 10 weeks of age
c. 10 g% of hemoglobin d. 10 months of age

Ans. d

Q4. Pierre Robin's syndrome is:

a. Cleft palate with syndactyly
b. Cleft palate with mandibular hypoplasia and respiratory obstruction
c. Cleft lip with mandibular hypoplasia
d. Cleft lip

Ans. b

Q5. Tripod fracture is seen in:

a. Zygomatic bone
b. Temporomandibular joint
c. Maxilla
d. Frontal bone

Ans. a

Q6. Gum tumor with two contralateral mobile lymph nodes in the cheek comes under:

a. T3N2M0 b. T2N2M0
c. T4N2M0 d. T3N3M0

Ans. a, b, c, and d

Q7. Multiple painful ulcers on the tongue are seen in all, *except*:

a. Aphthous ulcers b. Tuberculous ulcers
c. Herpes ulcers d. Carcinomatous ulcers

Ans. c

Q8. Which of the following statements best represents Ludwig's angina?

a. A type of coronary artery spasm
b. An infection of the cellular tissues around the submandibular salivary gland
c. Esophageal spasm
d. Retropharyngeal infection

Ans. b

Q9. Which of the following best represents "ranula?"

a. A type of epulis
b. A thyroglossal cyst
c. Cystic swelling in the floor of the mouth
d. Forked uvula

Ans. c

Q10. The most common cyst of the oral region is:

a. Dentigerous cyst b. Keratosis cyst
c. Dermoid cyst d. Periapical cyst

Ans. d

MULTIPLE CHOICE QUESTIONS

Grade I	Simple

Q1. True about cleft palate: (PGI November 2010)

a. Surgery should be done at 1 year
b. 50% recover speech after operation
c. Associated with hearing loss
d. Associated with cleft lip in 45%

Q2. Surgical correction of cleft palate primarily aims at all of the following, *except*: (MCI 2010)

a. Control of regurgitation
b. To promote normal dentition and facial growth
c. To get a normal speech
d. Normal appearance of lips, nose, and face

Q3. Ideal time for cleft lip repair surgery: (JIPMER 97)

a. 3–6 weeks b. 6–12 weeks
c. 1–1.5 years d. 3–4 years

Q4. A midline cleft lip is due to the failure of fusion between: (AIIMS May 2006)

a. Maxillary processes
b. Medial nasal processes

c. Medial and lateral nasal process
d. Medial nasal and maxillary process

Q5. Unilateral clefts are most common on: (PGI 1980)
a. Posterior displacement of alar cartilage
b. Columella elongated
c. Always cleft palate
d. Defective sucking

Q6. What is the appropriate age for repair of cleft palate? (AIIMS 1998)
a. 6 months to 1 year
b. 12–15 months
c. At puberty
d. Just after birth

Q7. The most common type of cleft lip is: (AIIMS 1991)
a. Bilateral
b. Midline
c. Combined with cleft palate
d. Unilateral

Q8. Cleft lip is due to the nonfusion of: (PGI 2001)
a. Maxillary process with lateral nasal process
b. Maxillary process with medial nasal process
c. Maxillary process with mandibular process
d. All of the above

Q9. Unilateral cleft lip is associated with: (PGI 99)
a. Posterior displacement of alar cartilage
b. Columella elongated
c. Always cleft palate
d. Defective sucking

Q10. The most common congenital anomaly of the face is: (MCI 2008)
a. Cleft lip alone
b. Isolated cleft palate
c. Cleft lip and cleft palate
d. All have equal incidence

Grade II	***Difficult***

Q1. The following is the method for operating on cleft lip, *all/except*: (AIIMS 1986)
a. Le Mesurier method
b. Tennison's method
c. Millard's method
d. Wardill's method

Q2. Which of the following is the ideal time for the repair of cleft palate? (AIIMS 2014)
a. 9–12 months
b. 18–24 months
c. 2–3 years
d. 5–6 years

Q3. Pierre Robin's sequence includes: (PGI 2008)
a. Glossoptosis
b. Airway obstruction
c. Cleft lip
d. Micrognathia
e. Heart anomaly

Q4. In a cleft lip operation, all the stitches are removed on: (AIIMS 1985)
a. Second day
b. Fourth day
c. 10th day
d. 14th day

Q5. Hynes pharyngoplasty is used to improve a child's: (JIPMER 1981)
a. Appearance
b. Teething
c. Speech
d. Feeding

Q6. Rhytidectomy operation involves: (JIPMER 1992)
a. Correction of nasal defects
b. Removal of wrinkles in the forehead
c. Straightening of curved pens
d. Correction of protruding lips

Q7. Rhinoplasty is usually done at the age (years) of—until the nose is fully grown: (AIIMS 1986)
a. 6 years
b. 12 years
c. 16 years
d. 25 years

Q8. Which one of the following is the primary defect in Pierre Robin's syndrome? (UPSC 2006)
a. Micrognathia
b. Glossoptosis
c. High-arched palate
d. cleft palate

Q9. A man sustained an injury and presented with fluid coming out through the nose. What could be the possible fracture? (MCI 2007)
a. Fracture of the base of the skull
b. Fracture of mandible
c. Fracture of maxilla
d. None of the above

Q10. Clinical features of a fracture of the zygomatic bone include all of the following, *except*: (All India 1998)
a. Diplopia
b. Trismus
c. Bleeding
d. Cerebrospinal fluid (CSF) rhinorrhea

Grade III | **Most difficult**

Q1. Fracture mandible with edentulous jaw is best treated with: (UPPG 2004)
a. External fixator
b. Minerva-plaster
c. Interdental wiring
d. Intermaxillary elastic traction

Q2. Best view for mandible is: (UPPG 2008)
a. Anteroposterior
b. Lateral
c. Oblique
d. Orthopantomogram

Q3. The most common site of oral cancer among the Indian population is: (All India 2004)
a. Tongue
b. Floor of mouth
c. Alveobuccal complex
d. Lip

Q4. Predisposing factors for the development of oral carcinoma is: (JIPMER 1988)
a. Smoking
b. Alcohol
c. Syphilis
d. All of the above

Q5. Carcinoma tongue <2 cm is treated by: (JIPMER 1987)
a. Excision
b. Radiotherapy
c. Chemotherapy
d. Excision and radiotherapy
e. Excision and chemotherapy

Q6. Metastasis of Ca buccal mucosa goes to: (AIIMS Nov 1996)
a. Regional lymph node
b. Liver
c. Heart
d. Brain

Q7. A patient has small, oval, multiple ulcers in the oral cavity with red erythematous margins. The diagnosis is: (AIIMS Nov 1993)
a. Carcinoma
b. Aphthous ulcer
c. Tubercular ulcer
d. Syphilitic ulcer

Q8. Painless ulcer of the tongue is due to: (PGI 1980)
a. Dyspepsia
b. Syphilis
c. Tuberculosis
d. None of the above

Q9. A 60-year-old man presents with an ulcer on the lateral margin of the tongue also complains of ear pain. The most probable diagnosis is: (PGI 1996)
a. Dental ulcer
b. Carcinomatous ulcer
c. Tuberculosis ulcer
d. Syphilitic ulcer

Q10. All of the following predispose to squamous cell carcinoma, *except*: (AIIMS June 1993)
a. Lichen planus of mouth
b. Bowen's disease
c. Inverted papilloma of the nose
d. Chronic irritation of the oral mucosa by jagged teeth

ANSWERS

Grade I: 1. a, c, d (Bailey 27/e p688-700); 2. d (Sabiston 20/e p1947); 3. b; 4. b; 5. a; 6. a; 7. c; 8. b; 9. a; 10. c

Grade II: 1. d (Schwartz 10/e p1840); 2. a; 3. a, b, d (Bailey 27/e p689, 691, 701); 4. b; 5. c (Bailey 27/e p695); 6. b; 7. c (Bailey 27/e p699); 8. a; 9. a (Schwartz 10/e p576); 10. d

Grade III: 1. a (Sabiston 20/e p1949); 2. d; 3. c; 4. d; 5. a (Schwartz 10/e p582); 6. a (Bailey 27/e p764); 7. b (Harrison 19/e p237, 413); 8. b (Harrison 19/e p237); 9. b (Bailey 27/e p765); 10. a (Bailey 27/e p761)

MODEL QUESTIONS

Q1. Costen's syndrome refers to neurological pain associated with:
a. Sphenopalatine ganglion
b. Temporomandibular joint
c. Glossopharyngeal nerve
d. Lingual nerve

Ans. b

Q2. Triage is defined as:
a. To classify according to severity
b. To classify according to site
c. To classify according to depth
d. To categorize the number of injuries

Ans. a

Q3. Which of the following is not included in a primary survey of a trauma patient?
a. Airway, breathing, circulation

b. Contrast-enhanced computed tomography (CECT) abdomen to look for bleeding
c. Recording BP
d. Exposure of the whole body

Ans. b

Q4. What is the diagnosis of the image shown below?

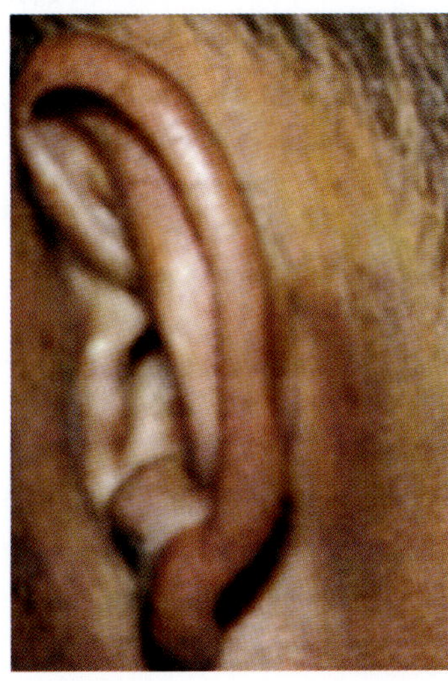

a. Battle sign
b. Milian's ear sign
c. Injury to the pinna
d. Erysipelas

Ans. a

Q5. Lucid interval is seen in:

a. Extradural hematoma
b. Subdural hematoma
c. Subarachnoid hemorrhage
d. Scalp hematoma

Ans. a

Q6. Battle's sign is seen in:

a. Bruise over mastoid
b. Bitemporal bruises
c. Bruises around the eye
d. Bruises in the neck

Ans. a

Q7. A patient presents with a head injury and increased intracranial pressure (ICP) with low blood pressure (BP). Which of the following drugs is used?

a. Mannitol
b. Prednisolone
c. Dexamethasone
d. Frusemide

Ans. a

Q8. Patient with T3N2M0 lower alveolar Ca requires:

a. Surgery
b. Surgery + radiotherapy
c. Radiotherapy
d. Chemotherapy

Ans. b

Q9. An 80-year-old patient presents with a midline tumor of the lower jaw, involving the alveolar margin. He is edentulous Rx of choice is:

a. Hemimandibulectomy
b. Commando operation
c. Segmental mandibulectomy
d. Marginal mandibulectomy

Ans. c

Q10. For cancrum oris, all are true, *except*:

a. Associated with malnutrition
b. Inflammatory swelling
c. Associated with vitamin deficiency
d. Treatment is excision and skin grafting

Ans. None

SUGGESTED READING

1. Bailey & Love's - Short Practice of Surgery, 27th edition.
2. Schwartz's Principles of Surgery, 18th edition.
3. Textbook of Surgery by David Sabiston, 21st edition.

Breast

CHAPTER 27

Breast

"With breast cancer, its all about detection. You have to educate young women and encourage them to do everything they have to do."

– Bill Rancic

ANATOMY, PHYSIOLOGY, AND BASICS

The breast is a modified sweat gland. It extends from the second to sixth rib vertically and midline to the anterior or midaxillary line horizontally. It has a small extension called "axillary tail of spence *(James Spence Scottish surgeon, President of the Royal College of Surgeons in Edinburgh in the later half of the 19th Century)* which lies in axilla by piercing' the deep fascia through foramen of Langer *(Karl Langer 1819–1887, Austrian anatomist)*. It is rudimentary in males and well developed in females after puberty. The breast is divided into four quadrants for notification of examination findings. It is an accessory organ of the female reproductive system and provides milk to the newborn as nutrition. The breast lies on the chest over the deep fascia covering the pectoral major muscle. There is loose areolar tissue between the breast and pectoral fascia called the *retromammary space*. Due to this loose areolar tissue, the normal breast is freely mobile over the pectoralis major muscle.

STRUCTURE OF THE BREAST (FIGS. 1 AND 2)

The breast has three main structures:

Skin

A conical projection called nipple is present just below the center of the breast at the fourth intercostal space.

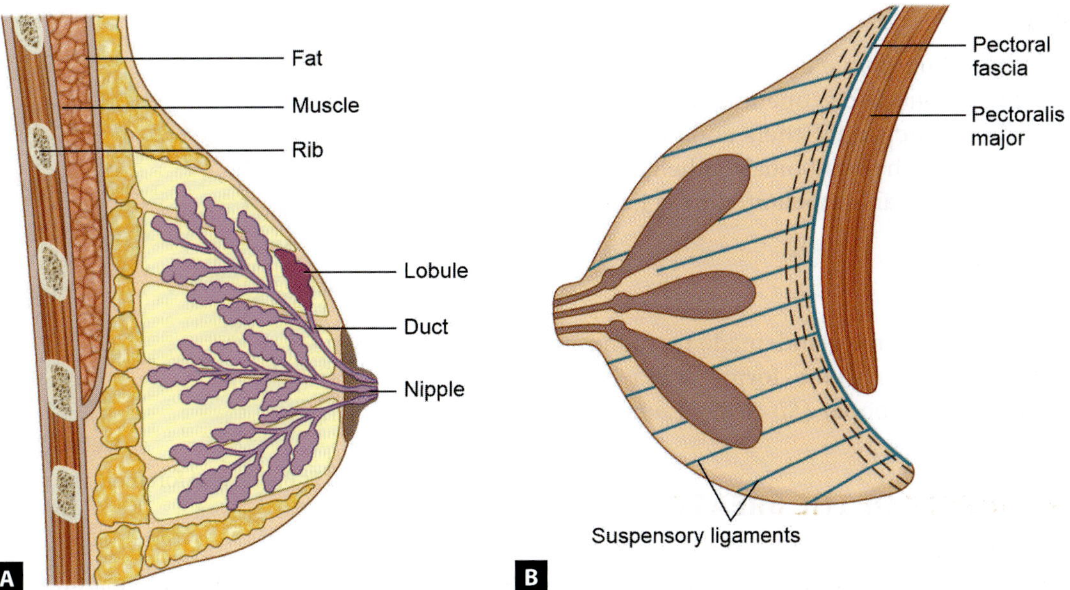

Figs. 1A and B: Structure of the breast.

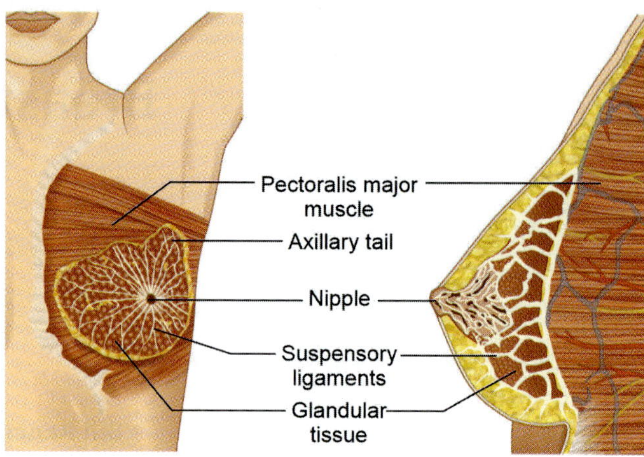

Fig. 2: Location of the breast.

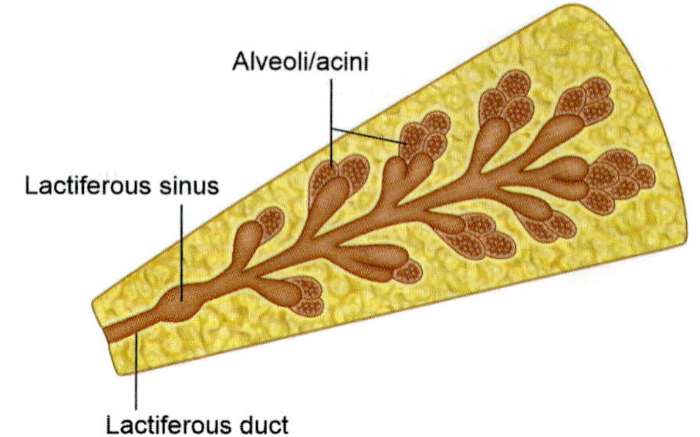

Fig. 3: Structure of a lobule.

Nipple has:

- 15–20 lactiferous ducts.
- Circular and longitudinal smooth muscle. The nipple becomes stiff and flat due to the contraction of these muscles.
- Modified sweat glands
- Sebaceous glands
- The nipple is surrounded by a pigmented area called the areola. It contains sebaceous glands which enlarge during pregnancy and lactation, then called tubercles of Montgomery (William Fetherston Montgomery, 1797–1859, obstetrician, Dublin, Ireland, described in 1837). It also contains accessory mammary glands. Nipple and areola are devoid of hair.

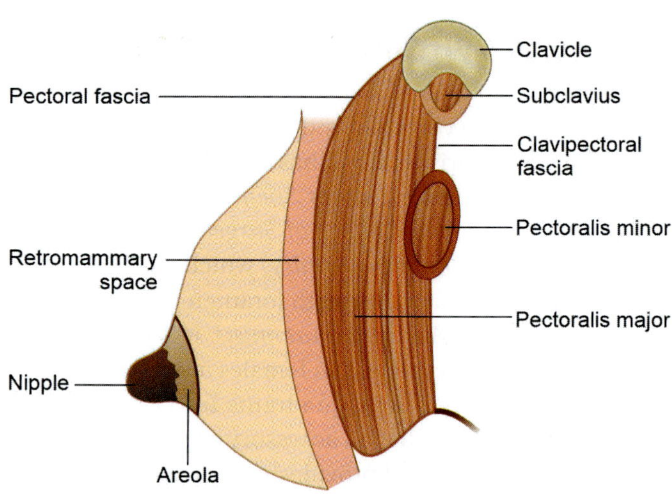

Fig. 4: Deep relations of the breast.

Parenchyma

It is made up of glandular tissue containing 15–20 lobes terminating in lactiferous ducts, opening in the nipple. A dilatation of these ducts near their ends is called a lactiferous *sinuses*. Alveoli have cuboidal epithelium in the resting phase and columnar epithelium during lactation **(Figs. 3 to 5)**.

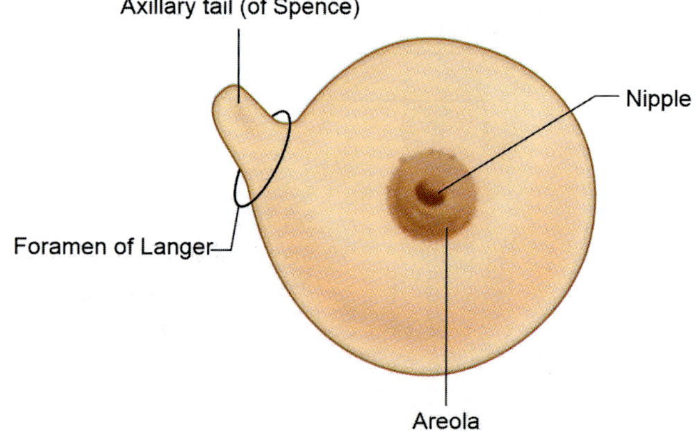

Fig. 5: Breast and foramen of Langer.

Stroma

It is a supporting tissue for the gland, made up of fibrous and fatty tissues. Fibrous tissue forms septa called suspensory ligaments of Cooper *(Sir Astley Cooper, first described in 1840)*.

ARTERIAL SUPPLY OF THE BREAST

It comes from the following arteries:

- Internal thoracic artery, a branch of the subclavian artery.
- Lateral thoracic, superior thoracic, and acromiothoracic arteries, branches of the axillary artery **(Fig. 6)**.

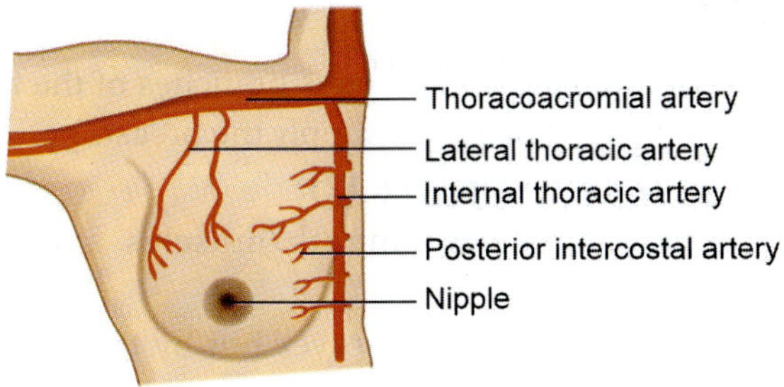

Fig. 6: Arterial supply of the breast.

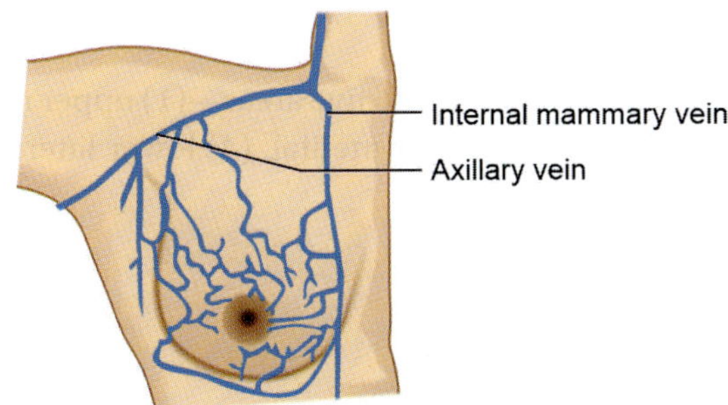

Fig. 7: Venous drainage of the breast.

VENOUS DRAINAGE OF THE BREAST

Veins of the breast follow arteries. Veins form an anastamotic circle around the nipple, and from it, veins drain blood to superficial and deep veins.

- *Superficial vein*: Internal thoracic vein and veins of the neck.
- *Deep veins*: Internal thoracic, axillary, and posterior intercostal veins **(Fig. 7)**.

LYMPHATIC DRAINAGE OF THE BREAST

- Superficial lymphatics (Breast skin, except nipples, and areola).
    - Axillary, internal mammary, supraclavicular, and cephalic lymph nodes (LNs).
- Deep lymphatics (Parenchyma, nipple, and areola).
    - Lymphatics from the deep surface of the breast pass through the pectoral major muscle and pectoral fascia to the apical LN **(Fig. 8)**.

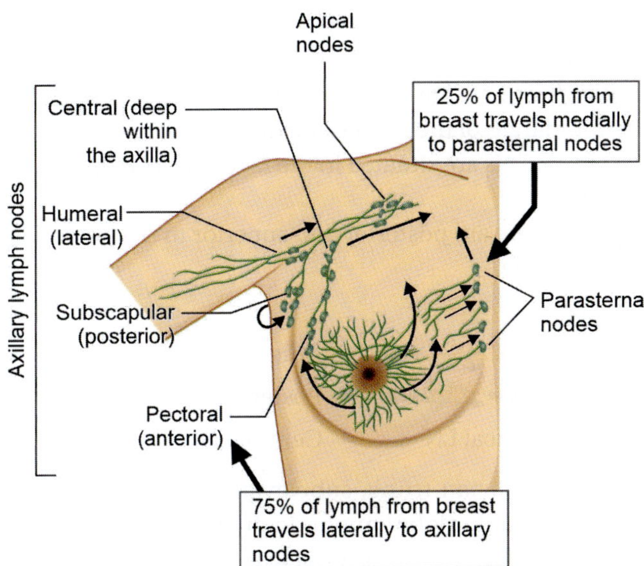

Fig. 8: Lymphatic drainage of the breast.

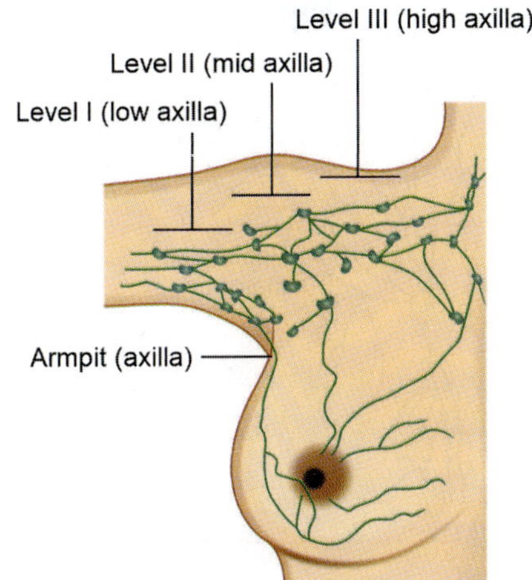

Fig. 9: Levels of axillary lymph nodes.

LEVEL OF LYMPH NODES (FIG. 9)

Surgically, LNs of the breast can be divided into different levels:

- *Level I*: LNs are lateral to the pectoralis major muscle.
- *Level II*: Posterior to the pectoralis major muscle.
- *Level III*: Medial to the pectoralis major muscle.

The LN between the pectoral major and minor muscles is called Rotter's *(Josef Rotter, 1857–1924, German Surgeon, described in the late 19th century)* node.

There are five axillary LN groups, namely the lateral (humeral), anterior (pectoral), posterior (subscapular), central, and apical nodes.

The apical nodes are the final common pathway for all of the axillary LNs.

Lateral LNs are posteromedial to the axillary vein.

Anterior LNs are at the inferior border of the pectoralis minor muscle.

Posterior LNs are on the suprascapular vessels in the inferior margin of the posterior axillary wall.

Central LNs are situated in the fat of the axilla **(Figs. 10 and 11)**.

Apical LNs are posterior and superior to the pectoralis minor muscle.

Lateral LNs:

Central LN ← Posterior LN; Central LN → Anterior LN
Apical LN ← Anterior LN; Apical LN → Posterior LN
Deep cervical LN ← Central LN

Apical: Subclavian trunk, subclavian nodes LN, jugular lymphatic trunk, right lymphatic duct (left into thoracic duct), and inferior deep cervical LNs.

NERVE SUPPLY

- Anterior and lateral cutaneous branches of the fourth to sixth intercostal nerves supply the breast.
- Sensory fibers to skin **(Fig. 12)**.
- Autonomic fibers to smooth muscles and blood vessels.
- Milk secretion is not by nerves but by the hormone prolactin.
- Damage to the long thoracic nerve of Bell *(Charles Bell, 1774–1842, Scottish surgeon)* can be damaged during trauma or mastectomy, which may lead to winging of the scapula.

The breast is divided into five areas—(1) upper medial, (2) upper lateral, (3) lower medial, (4) lower lateral, and (5) central **(Fig. 13)**.

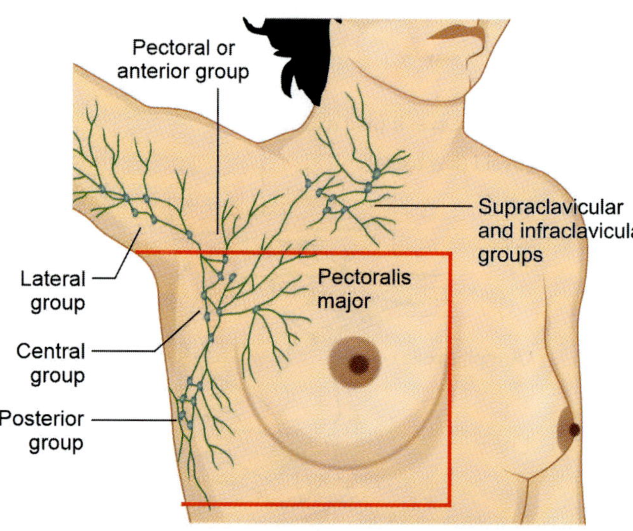

Fig. 10: Axillary lymph nodes.

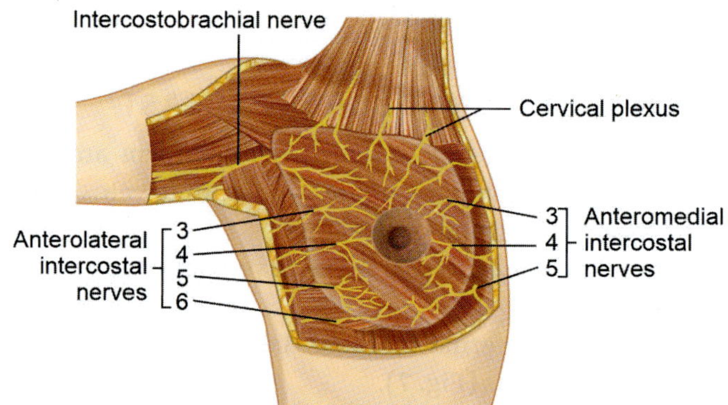

Fig. 12: Nerves supplying of breast.

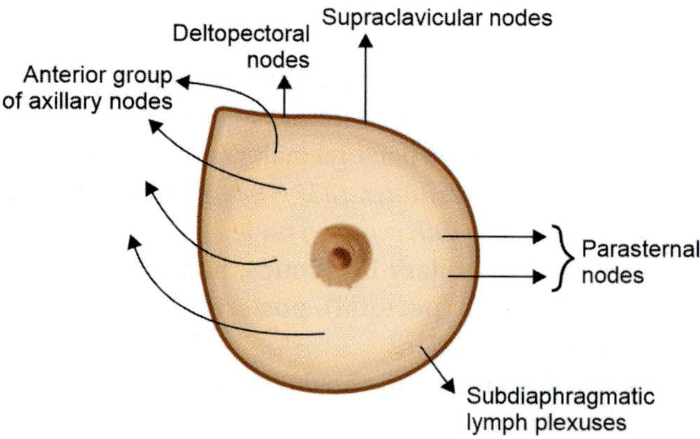

Fig. 11: Lymphatic drainage of the breast.

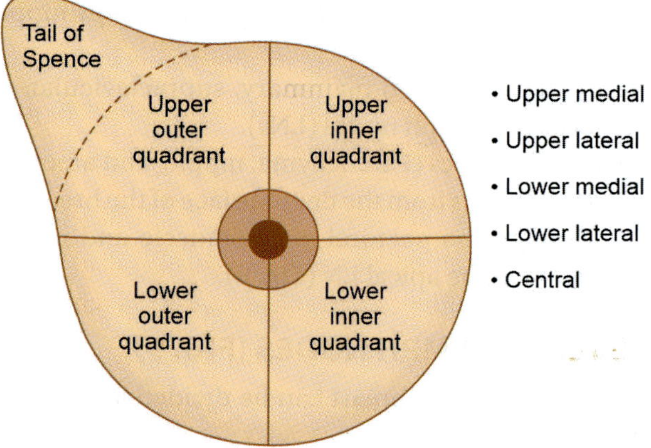

Fig. 13: Quadrants of the breast.

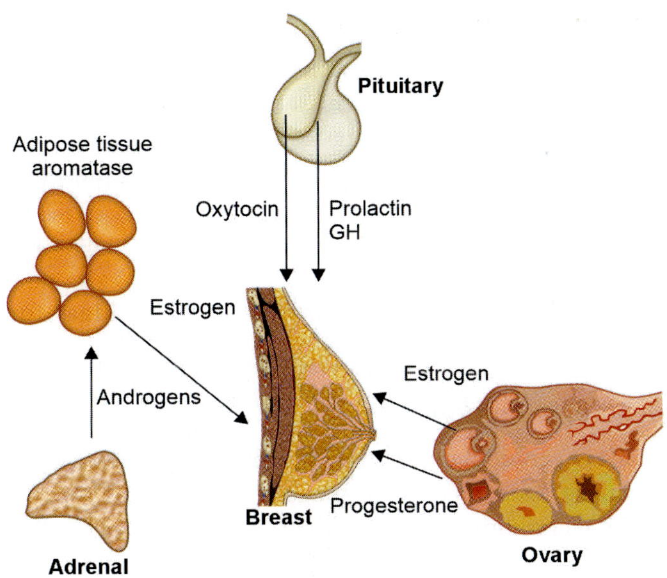

Fig. 14: Physiology of the breast.

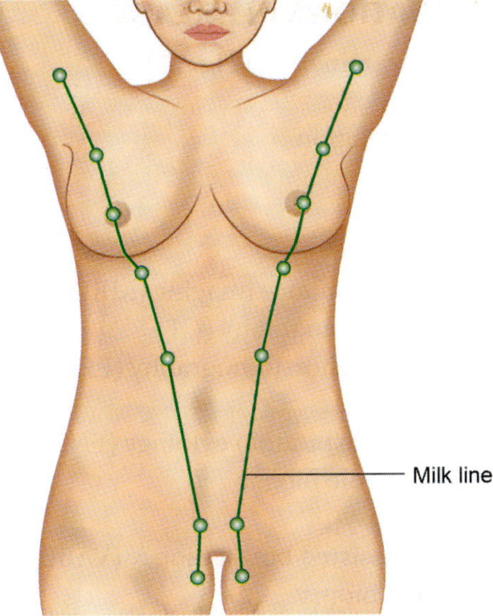

Fig. 15: Milk line of the breast.

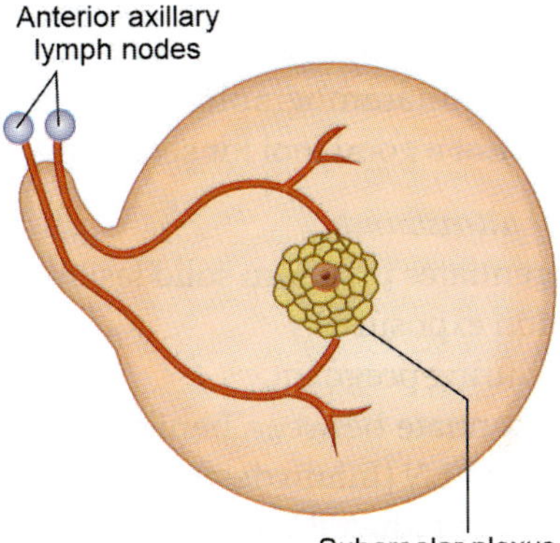

Fig. 16: Subareolar plexus (Sappey's plexus).

PHYSIOLOGY OF THE BREAST (FIG. 14)

Placental hormones stop production after childbirth, but a regular and sustained *secretion of prolactin leads to the stimulation for lactation.* The expulsion of milk is caused by the *hormone oxytocin, which causes contraction of smooth muscles.* Suckling of the nipple by the newborn stimulates the pituitary gland to secrete prolactin and oxytocin. Stimulation of the nipple is the physiologic signal for both the continued pituitary secretion of prolactin and for the acute release of oxytocin.

DEVELOPMENT OF THE BREAST

The breast develops from the mammary or milk line, or line of Schultz, or mammary or milk ridge, which is an ectodermal thickening in the fourth week of intrauterine life (IUL). The gland is ectodermal in origin. Stroma is mesodermal. Mammary glands grow at puberty due to estrogen. Secretory alveoli by progesterone and prolactin **(Fig. 15)**.

Important points:
- Halsted's ligament—also known as the costoclavicular ligament. It is taken as the medial limit for axillary dissection in breast cancer.

  Halsted costoclavicular ligament is at the apex of the axilla where the axillary vein enters the thorax and becomes the subclavian vein.

William Stewart Halsted, an American surgeon, emphasized strict aseptic technique during surgical procedures introduced Halsted's ligament and radical mastectomy for breast cancer. He, along with *William Osler (Professor of Medicine), Howard Atwood Kelly (Professor of Gynecology) and William H. Welch (Professor of pathology) were called "Big Four," founding professors at the Johns Hopkins Hospital.*

- Sappey's (Marie Philibert Constant Sappey, 1810–1896, French Anatomist, discovered in 1874) plexus—lymphatics under nipple and areola **(Fig. 16)**.
- The central lymph node is the first lymph node to which the cancer cells in carcinoma of the breast spread from the primary tumor. It is also called as Giuliano (AE Giuliano discovered in 1994) node.
- The Batson venous plexus drains the vertebrae and skull and forms anastomoses with the vein draining thoracic, abdominal, and pelvic organs and the breast. This valveless venous system serves as a pathway to transit metastatic cells to the spinal column.

INVESTIGATIONS IN BREAST

- Self-breast examination **(Fig. 17)**
- History
- Clinical examination
- Imaging:
  - USG
  - Mammography
  - Magnetic resonance imaging (MRI)
  - Computed tomography (CT)
  - Positron emission tomography (PET)
- Histopathology:
  - Fine needle aspiration cytology (FNAC)
  - Tru-cut needle biopsy
  - Punch biopsy
  - Vacuum-assisted breast biopsy (VABB)
  - Excisional biopsy

Ultrasound (Fig. 18)

Good for young females, below 40 years, with dense breasts, in whom mammography is avoided due to low sensitivity. It is not a good tool for screening.

Advantages of ultrasound:

- Well differentiates cyst from solid lesion.
- No radiation exposure.
- Preferred during pregnancy.
- It can differentiate between benign (hilum preserved) and malignant LN (hilum destroyed).
- It can detect intraductal lesions.
- It can detect the rupture of breast implant, intracapsular (stepladder pattern) or extracapsular (snowstrom pattern).

Breast Self-Exam

1. Lie on your back and put your right hand behind your head,
2. Use your left hand to press down to examine the right breast
3. Apply light, medium, and firm pressure to check all layers of your breast tissue
4. Sit up and press into your right armpit to check for lumps
5. Squeeze your nipples to check for any discharge
6. Lie back down, switch arms, and repeat

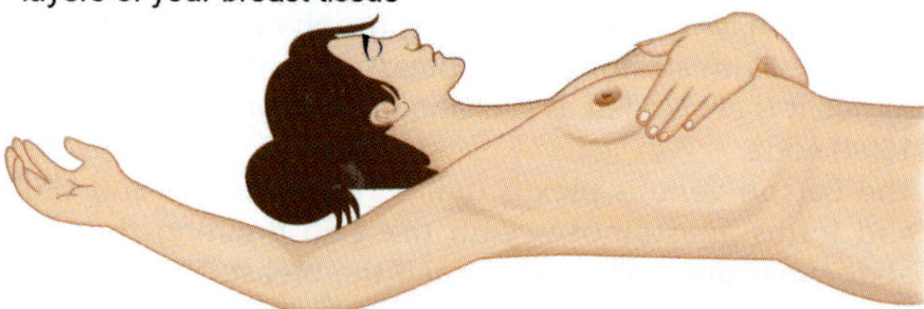

Fig. 17: Breast self examination.

Mammography (Fig. 19)

It is a radiograph of the breast with low radiation (0.1/0.2 cGY)

- 5% of breast cancers are missed in mammography.
- *Type*: Bremsstrahlung type.
- A normal mammogram does not exclude the presence of carcinoma.
- Digital mammography can manipulate images for better screening.
- Tomosynthesis mammography is more ideal for diagnosis.

Views in Mammography

- MLO—mediolateral view: It demonstrates the whole breast tissue on a single image.
- CC—craniocaudal view

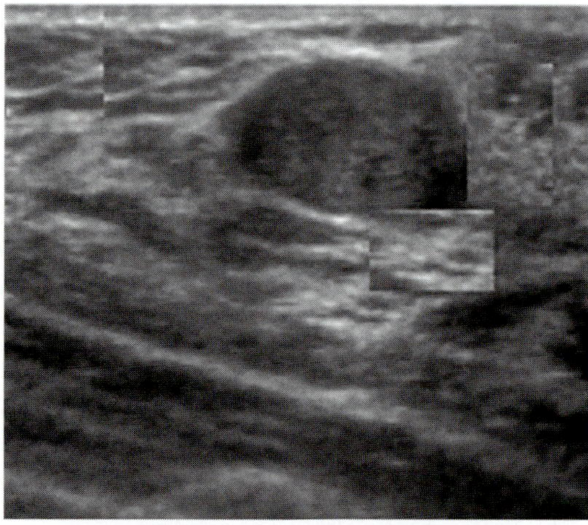

Fig. 18: Ultrasound of breast.

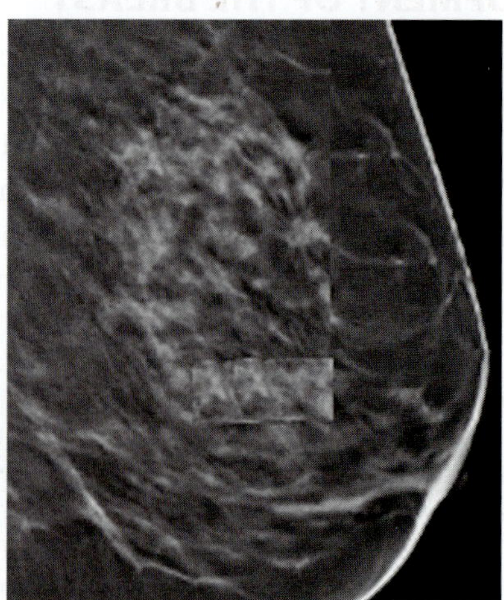

Fig. 19: Mammography.

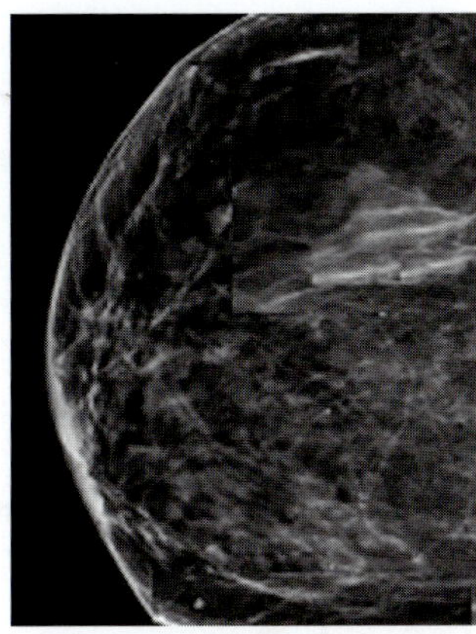

Fig. 20: Breast Imaging-Reporting and Data Systems (BI-RADS), ultrasound.

Mammography is not recommended for those younger than 30 years of age due to dense breasts. Ultrasound may be better.

Radiation risk of BC in mammography—NO

BC screening in average-risk patients—mammography

Screening in high-risk—mammography + MRI

Breast Imaging-Reporting and Data Systems ***(Fig. 20):***
- 0: Normal
- 1: Negative
- 2: Benign
- 3: Probably benign
- 4: Suspicious
- 5: Highly suspicious of malignancy
- 6: Malignant

Magnetic Resonance Imaging (Fig. 22)

A good screening tool for high-risk women with a family history of breast cancer can be a good tool to detect ductal carcinoma in situ (DCIS), can identify multiple lesions in one quadrant of the breast (multifocal), and multiple lesions in more than one quarter of the breast (multicentric) **(Table 1)**.

It can show breast implant rupture (Linguini's sign, which shows intracapsular rupture; Linguini is a type of Italian pasta).

Computed Tomography and Positron Emission Tomography

Positron emission tomography-CT is an ideal tool for staging breast cancer. It is good for metastasis, but not for brain metastasis, for which MRI is the best tool. The dye used is commonly 18-Fluorodeoxyglucose (18 FDG).

TABLE 1: Difference between benign and malignant breast lesions.

Benign breast lesion (Fig. 21)	*Malignant breast lesion*
Margin—smooth	Irregular
Density—low	High
Calcification—macro	Micro
Breast structure—normal	Distorted
Lymph nodes—hilum preserved	Rounded due to fat loss

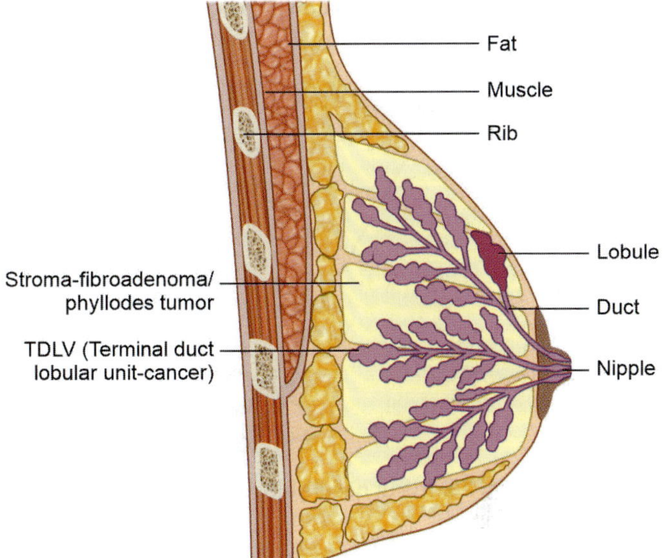

Fig. 21: Structure of breast.

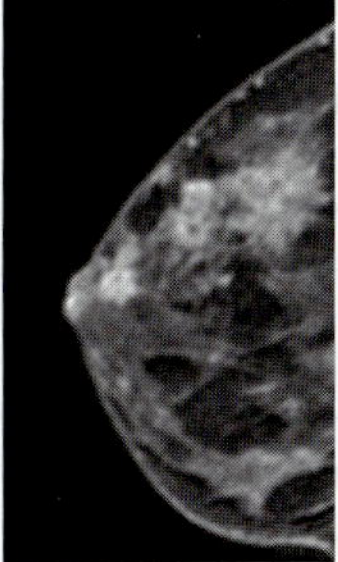

Fig. 22: Magnetic resonance imaging of breast.

Fine-needle Aspiration Cytology (Fig. 23)

- Cytology is obtained by a 21 G or 23 G needle with a 10 mL syringe
- Least invasive technique
- Good at accuracy

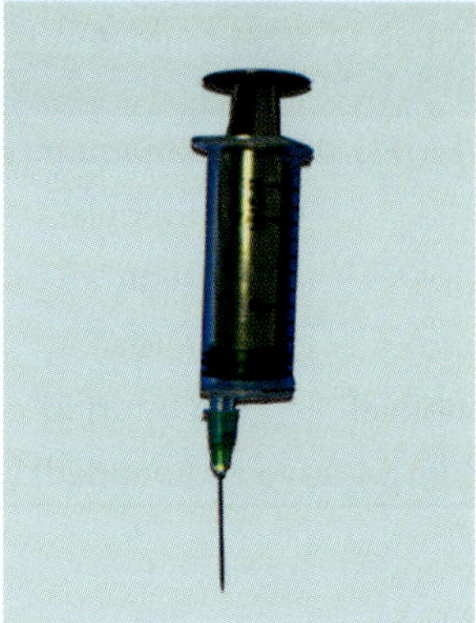

Fig. 23: Fine-needle aspiration cytology equipment.

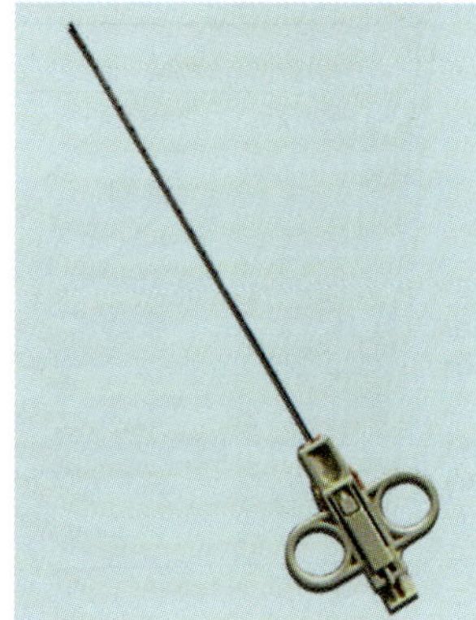

Fig. 24: Trucut needle biopsy needle.

- False negative results are present
- Cannot distinguish DCIS from invasive carcinoma of the breast
- ER/PR status cannot be detected

True Cut Needle Biopsy (Fig. 24)

It is done with a special needle of 14G caliber.

Advantages

- Gives a good amount of tissue to the pathologist.
- ER (Estrogen receptor)/PR (Progesterone receptor) status can be detected.
- A good diagnostic procedure for breast lesions.

Punch Biopsy (Fig. 25)

Punch instruments are of various sizes and used for skin lesions and Paget's disease.

Vacuum-assisted Breast Biopsy

8–11 G probe. Good for fibroadenoma breast.

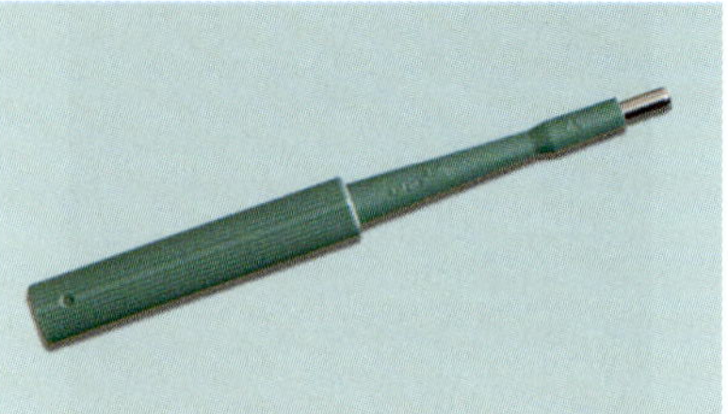

Fig. 25: Punch for punch biopsy.

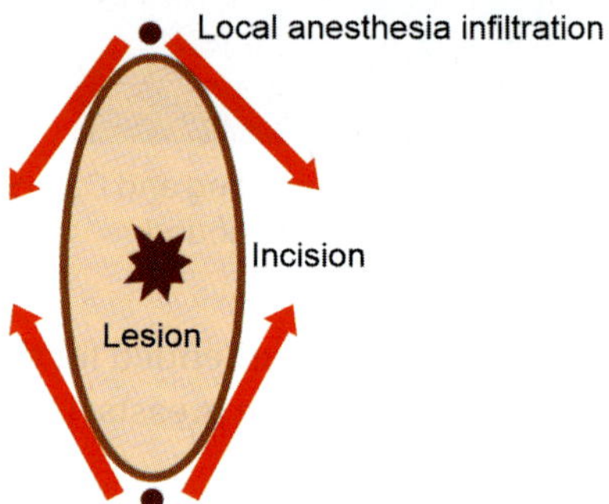

Fig. 26: Excisional biopsy.

Excisional Biopsy (Fig. 26)

Gold standard histopathology technique for breast lumps (100% accuracy). False/negative results are rare.

Breast Cancer Markers

- *ER/PR:* Nuclear receptors. The score is 0–8, it is used to determine the hormone receptor status of BC. Scores 0–2 are negative, 3–8 are positive.
- HER2 neu are membranous markers
- Ki67 is a proliferative index marker.

Immunohistochemistry Test

- *If positive:* A marker is found on the cell during biopsy. You might have inherited a genetic condition. It diagnoses cancer prediction, predicts treatment, and indicates prognosis.
- *If negative:* No gene change found.
- IHC test score is 0 to 3+
- 0 to 1+ = HER2 negative
- If 2+ = Borderline
- If 3+ = HER2 positive

Triple Assessment

Combination of clinical examination, radiological imaging and tissue sample is called triple assessment which gives *99.9% accuracy.*

AMERICAN SOCIETY OF BREAST SURGEONS

- Women >25 years undergo formal risk assessment for breast cancer.
- Women at average risk at 40 years should have a yearly mammogram.
- Benign lesions on mammogram show macrocalcifications, i.e., popcorn calcification.
- Malignant lesions show microcalcification.
- Average risk of breast cancer—yearly mammogram after 40 years.
- Higher risk of breast cancer.
  - Annual MRI after 25 years.
  - Three-dimensional (3D) mammogram yearly after 30 years.

LESIONS OF THE BREAST (AMAZIA)

- Nipple **(Fig. 27)**
- Congenital absence of nipple breast
- Supernumerary nipples occur on the milk line (polymazia).
- Retraction of nipple:
  - At puberty (simple nipple inversion), in 25% of cases, it is bilateral.
  - Disease—duct ectasia, chronic periductal mastitis (Slit-like retraction).
  - Carcinoma (circumferential retraction).
  - Treatment, if at puberty, may not be required as it may become normal during lactation.

Cracked nipple occurs during lactation and can lead to mastitis. Treatment is rest to the breast and the use of a breast pump.

Papilloma of nipple—to be excised as anywhere else.

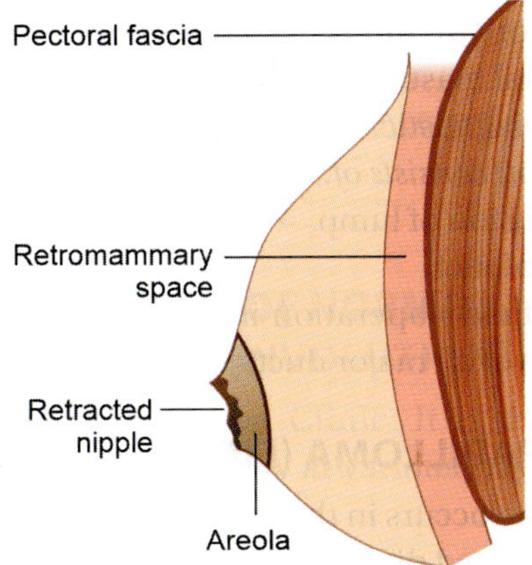

Fig. 27: Amezia.

PAGET'S DISEASE (SIR JAMES PAGET, SURGEON, ST BARTHOLOMEW'S HOSPITAL, LONDON, DESCRIBED IN 1874) (FIG. 28)

Looks like eczema, malignant cells are present in the subdermal layer, and are usually associated with carcinoma of the breast.

- Paget's disease is unilateral, whereas eczema is bilateral.
- There is destruction of nipple and areola in Paget's disease, whereas there is no destruction in eczema.
- In Paget's disease, there may be a lump in the breast, but there is no lump in eczema.

Treatment of Paget's disease (mastectomy + axillary staging) or wide excision of nipple and areola + axillary staging or lumpectomy + radiation + axillary node dissection).

DISCHARGE FROM THE NIPPLE (FIG. 29)

- A clear and serious discharge may be normal in a multiparous woman; it is physiological.
- Blood-stained discharge—duct ectasia, duct papilloma, and carcinoma.
- Black or green discharge—duct ectasia.
- Discharge from one duct—intraductal papilloma or carcinoma.
- Discharge from more than one duct—carcinoma, duct ectasia, infection, fibrocystic disease, and lactation.
- *Treatment*:
  - Exclude carcinoma
  - Reassurance
  - Microdochectomy

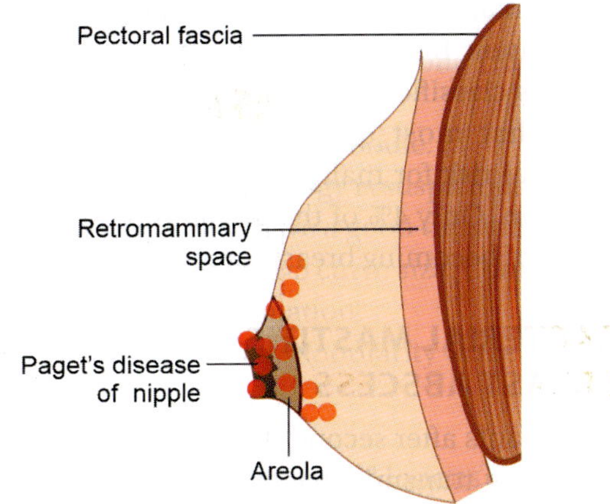

Fig. 28: Paget's disease of the breast.

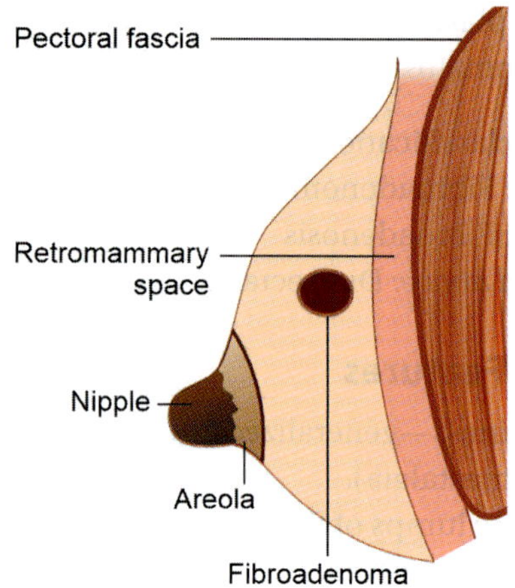

Fig. 32: Fibroadenoma.

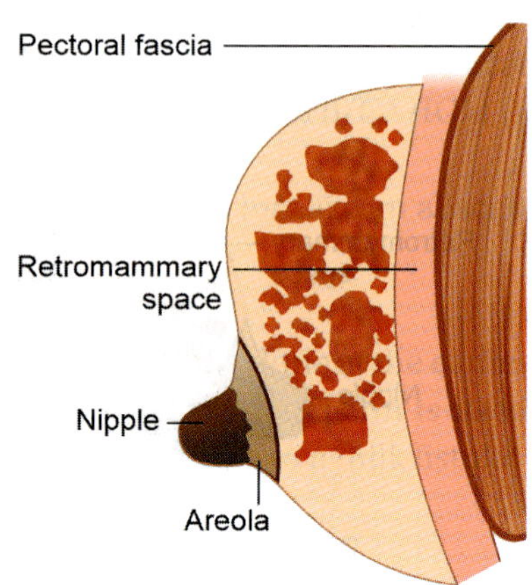

Fig. 33: Phyllodes tumor.

- True-cut needle biopsy is advised for solid lesions
- *USG*: Smooth margin, normal vascularity.
- *MRI*: Popcorn, macrocalcification
- *Staging*: BI-RADS–MC BI-RADS II, if BI-RADS IV, excisional biopsy advised.
- *Treatment*: Excision/VABB

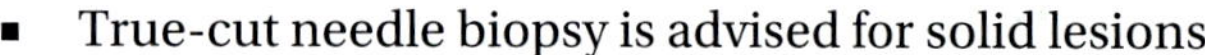

PHYLLODES TUMOR (FIG. 33)

- Earlier was known as serocystic disease of *Brodie (Sir Benjamin Collins Brodie, 1783–1862, surgeon, St. George's Hospital, London, UK, described serocystic disease of the breast in 1840)* or cystosarcoma phyllodes. Appear in women above 40 years of age. Have uneven, bosselated surface with ulcers sometimes. Rarely develops sarcoma, if so, then metastasis happen via bloodstream.
  - Stromal tumor
  - Breast size rapidly increases
  - Variegated appearance (soft/firm)
  - Lymphatic metastasis <10%
  - Most common (MC) metastasis in lungs
- *Types:* Benign/borderline/malignant
- *Investigations:* USG/True-cut needle biopsy.
- *Treatment:* Lumpectomy/simple mastectomy. Chemotherapy has no effect.

CARCINOMA OF THE BREAST

The most common cause of death in middle-aged women in Western countries. In England and Wales, 1 in 12 women will develop the disease during their lifetime.

Etiology

The following factors are considered as factors responsible for carcinoma of the breast:

- Geographical—common in Western countries.
- *Age:* 20–90 years.
- *Gender:* <0.5% of patients are male.
- Genetic—common in women with a family history of breast cancer.
- *Diet:* Low consumption of phytochemicals and alcohol consumption are considered factors that may be responsible.
- *Endocrine:* Breastfeeding acts as a protective factor, as breast cancer is found less commonly in multiparous women and more commonly in nulliparous females:
  - Obesity
  - Use of oral contraceptives does not cause breast cancer risk.
- Hormone replacement therapy (HRT)—estrogen and progesterone combination increases breast cancer risk. Only estrogen does not cause breast cancer risk.
- Previous radiation.
- Smoking doesn't cause breast cancer risk.

GENES AND BREAST CANCER (FIG. 34)

- About 10% of breast cancers are familial or hereditary. 90% are acquired. They are due to gene changes or mutations passed from a parent. The most common inherited mutation occurs in BRCA-1 (BReast CAncer gene 1) and BRCA-2 (BReast CAncer gene 2), and they are passed to offspring, increasing their risk of developing BC.
- The *MC* gene is mutated in BC.
- TNBC (Triple negative breast cancer subtype).
- It is named as three receptors in its tumor cells:
- ER/PR/HER2 are absent)—p53.
- It is most aggressive with the worst prognosis.
- The TNBC paradox conveys that it responds best to chemotherapy.
- ER/PR negative BC: P/K3CA
- Familial BC: BRCAI

(HER2: Human epidermal growth factor receptor 2)

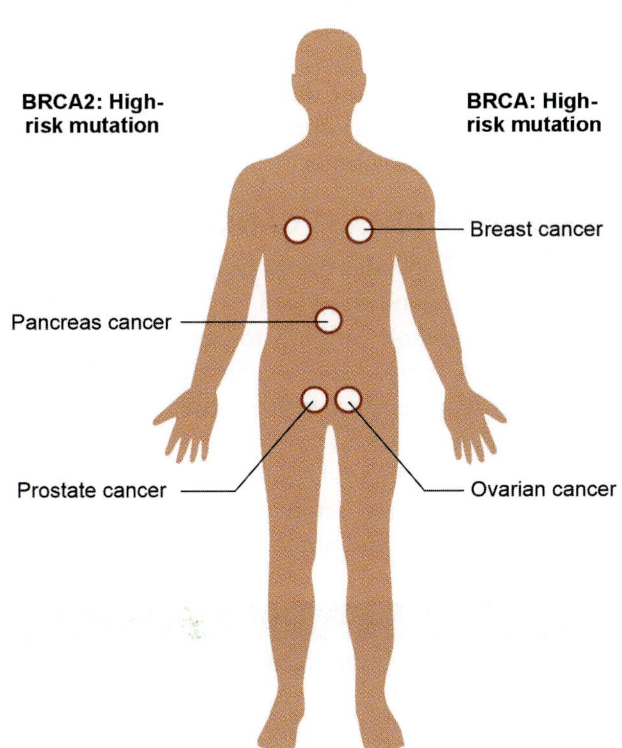

Fig. 34: Genes and breast cancer.

HBOC SYNDROME (HEREDITARY BREAST AND OVARIAN CANCER SYNDROME)

- It is a genetic condition that increases the chances of getting breast, ovarian, prostate, and some other organ cancers.
- The *BRCA1* gene is attached to 17 (especially on 17q21) chromosome, and BRCA2 to 13 (especially on 13q12.3).
- *BRCA1* is more aggressive in causing breast and ovarian cancer.
- *BRCA2* is more aggressive in causing pancreatic, prostate, and male breast cancer.
- *BRCA1* and 2 play an equal role for colorectal and peritoneal cancer.

INDICATIONS OF BRCA TESTING

It is done to predict a high risk of developing cancer. This gene test is a blood test.

- A personal history of breast cancer or ovarian cancer.
- Pancreatic or prostatic cancer
- A blood relative with a history of cancer of the breast, ovary, pancreas, and prostate.
- A blood relative who had genetic testing and was found to have a gene change that increases the risk of breast cancer.
    - Positive test—means you have changes in a gene that is associated with a high risk of cancer.
    - Negative test—no gene changes found, and you have cancer risk as anybody in the general population.

Lifestyle changes to reduce the risk of breast cancer in people with a BRCA mutation:

- Stop smoking
- Stop alcohol consumption
- Keep weight normal
- Regular physical exercise

STAGING OF BREAST CANCER

- Tumor-node-metastasis (TNM) **(Box 1 and Table 2)**
- Union for International Cancer Control (UICC)

Pathological N staging
PN1 Met: Micro/1–3 axillary LNs
PN2 Met: 4–9 axillary LNs
PN3 Met: 10 or supra or infraclavicular LNs

RISK FACTORS FOR CARCINOMA OF THE BREAST

- Advanced age
- Family history of breast cancer
- HRT
- Early menarche
- Late menopause
- Nulliparity
- Obesity—fat converts to estrogen
- Alcohol consumption
- Smoking increase risk of breast lesions.
- Ductectasia
- Mondor's disease

BOX 1: 8th American Joint Committee on Cancer (AJCC), 2017 TNM Staging for Breast Cancer.

T: Primary tumor
- *T1:* Tumor ≤2 cm[Q]
- *T2:* Tumor >2 cm and ≤5 cm[Q]
- *T3:* Tumor >5 cm[Q]
- *T4a:* Extension to chest wall, not including pectoralis muscle[Q]
- *T4b:* Edema (including peau d'orange – French for orange skin) or ulceration of skin, or satellite skin nodules confined to the same breast[Q]
- *T4c:* Both T4a and T4b[Q]
- *T4d:* Inflammatory carcinoma[Q]

N: Regional lymph nodes
- *N1:* Metastasis to movable ipsilateral level I, II axillary LNs[Q]
- *N2a:* Metastasis in ipsilateral level I, II axillary LNs fixed or matted[Q]
- *N2b:* Metastasis only in clinically apparent ipsilateral internal mammary LNs and in the absence of clinically evident axillary LNs metastasis[Q]
- *N3a:* Metastasis in ipsilateral infraclavicular LNs[Q]
- *N3b:* Metastasis in ipsilateral internal mammary LNs and axillary LNs[Q]
- *N3c:* Metastasis in ipsilateral supraclavicular LNs[Q]

M: Distant metastases
- *M0:* No distant metastasis
- *M1:* Distant metastasis

Note: Clinically apparent is defined as detected by imaging studies (excluding lymphoscintigraphy) or by clinical examination or grossly visible pathologically[Q]

TYPES OF BREAST CARCINOMA

- Ductal carcinoma
- Lobular carcinoma
- Colloid or mucinous carcinoma
- Medullary carcinoma
- Tubular carcinoma (good prognosis)
- Inflammatory carcinoma
- *In situ carcinoma*: It is a preinvasive carcinoma, no breachment of the basement membrane. It occurs in the female breast, but it can also occur in the male breast. Two types **(Table 3)**:
  1. *DCIS—ductal*: It occurs only in the female breast and is mostly multicentric. There is a risk of invasive cancer. There is distension and distortion of the terminal ducts. Malignant cells invade an Indian file pattern and look as calcifications occurring adjacent to tissue, and called neighborhood calcification, is almost a diagnostic feature. Treatment may be wait and observe or even prophylactic bilateral mastectomy.
  2. *LCIS—lobular*: Progress to invasive cancer. It can be a papillary growth pattern or a cribriform growth pattern (necrolic). It can be low-grade or high-grade type (preferably a combination). Mammographic calcifications are a diagnostic feature. Treatment depends upon the progress of the disease as lumpectomy/lumpectomy + radiotherapy methods.

SPREAD OF BREAST CANCER

- *Local spread*: Invades breast tissues, skin, pectoralis major muscle, and chest wall.
- *Lymphatic spread*: Spreads to axillary and internal mammary lymph nodes. Involvement of the supraclavicular and other side lymph nodes indicates advanced disease.
- *Blood stream spread*: Osteolytic metastases occur in lumbar vertebrae, femur, thoracic vertebrae, ribs, skull, liver, lungs, and brain.

TABLE 2: TNM staging.

Stage I	*State IIA*	*Stage IIB*	*Stage IIIA*	*Stage IIIB*	*Stage IIIC*	*Stage IV*
T1 N0M0	T0N1 M0 T1N1 M0 T2 N0M0	T2N1 M0 T3 N0M0	T0 N2 M0 T1-2 N2 M0 T3 N1-2 M0	T4 N0-2 M0	AnyT N3 M0	AnyT anyN M1

(TNM staging is also abbreviated for some factors as cTNM: clinical TNM, pTNM: pathological TNM, rTNM: recurrent TNM, mTNM: multiple tumor TNM; yTNM: After chemo/radio TNM)

TABLE 3: LCIS and DCIS differences.

	LCIS (Lobular carcinoma in situ)	*DCIS (Ductal carcinoma in situ)*
Age	Early	Late
Common	Less common	More common
Sign	No	Lump/nipple discharge
Mammography	*Micros features:* None	Micros features—calcification
Prolactin test	More cases of 50–70%	Fewer cases of 10–20%
Axillary LN involvement	1%	1–2%

DCIS (according to Van Nuys System)—can be classified as per the patient's age, type of DCIS, and microcalcification.

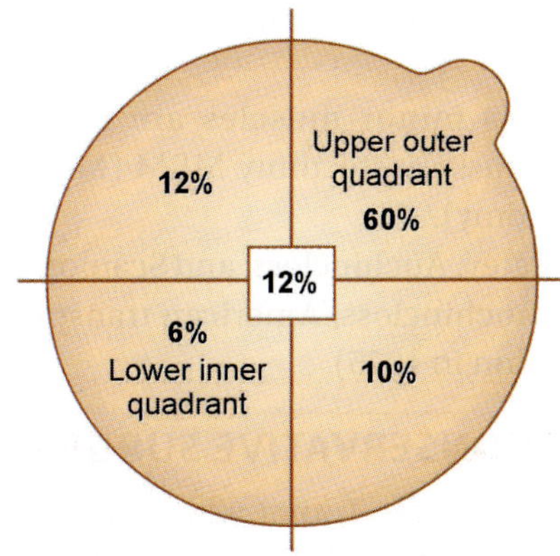

Fig. 35: Incidence of carcinoma in different quadrants of the breast.

BOX 2: Most common (MC) factors in breast cancer.

- MC factor in breast cancer
- MC cancer in females
- MC adenocarcinoma
- MC is invasive duct cancer
- MC sits in UOQ (L > R)
- MC metastasis in bones

CLINICAL PRESENTATION OF BREAST CANCER (FIG. 35 AND BOX 2)

- Most common upper outer quadrant (UOQ) and least common in the lower inner quadrant (LIQ)
- Hard lump in the breast
- Nipple retraction
- Peau d'orange
- Ulceration
- Fixation to the chest wall (Cancer-en-cuirasse)

PROGNOSTIC FACTORS FOR BREAST CANCER

- Tumor size, grade, and LN status.
- Histological grade of tumor
- Hormone receptor status
- Ki-67
- Growth factor analysis
- Oncogene

How does breast cancer metastasis reach the brain?

Cancer cells from the breast detach from the tumor and enter the posterior intercostal vein. They travel from this vein to intraspinal veins, Batson's plexus (Oscar Vivian Batson anatomist, described in 1940) to intracranial sinuses.

TREATMENT OF BREAST CANCER

Principles

- To reduce the chance of local recurrence
- To reduce the risk of brain metastatic spread

Modalities of Treatment of Breast Cancer

- Surgery
- Chemotherapy (CT)
- Radiotherapy (RT)
- Hormonal therapy (HT)

Breast Surgeries

- Simple or total mastectomy (SM)—removal of the whole breast.
- Extended simple mastectomy (ESM)—SM + Removal of level I axillary LNs.
- Halsted's Radical mastectomy (HRM) Breast + Pectoralis major and minor muscles + Level I, II, III axillary LNs.
- Modified radical mastectomy (MRM)—extended RM (ERM) RM + Internal mammary LNs.
- Super radical mastectomy—extended RM + removal of mediastinal and supraclavicular LNs (SRM).

Mastectomy

- Simple mastectomy
- Radical Halsted *(William Stewart Halsted, 1852–1922, Professor of Surgery, Johns Hopkins Medical School, Baltimore, MD, USA)* mastectomy includes excision of:
  - Breast + NAC (Nipple areola complex)
  - Axillary LNs (Level I, II, and III)
  - Pectoralis major and minor muscles
- *Not in use today due to*:
  - High morbidity
  - No survival benefits
- MRM

Structures Preserved in Modified Radical Mastectomy

- Axillary vessels
- Bell's nerve
- Cephalic vein
- Nerve to latissimus dorsi
- Pectoralis major muscle (thoracodorsal N)

Structures Preserved in Axillary Dissection

- Thoracodorsal neurovascular bundle
- Long thoracic nerve of Bell

Total 10 LNs of round is called complete axillary dissection.

Postoperative Complications of Mastectomy

- Hemorrhage
- Infection
- Nerve injury to:
  - Long thoracic—winging of the scapula.
  - Intercostobrachial—hypoesthesia in axilla.
  - Thoracodorsal affects the latissimus dorsi muscle
  - *Lateral and medial pectoral nerves:* Pectoral major and minor affected
- Flap necrosis
- *Seroma formation*: Aspirate and do a pressure dressing.
- *Lymphoedema:* MC in upper limbs.
- Local recurrence—repeat biopsy. Local recurrence can cause cancer en cuirasse (armor-like).
- *Phantom phenomenon*: The patient feels that the breast is still present.

PAIN SYNDROMES IN BREAST SURGERY

- Neuralgia—intercostobrachial nerve (PMP = post-mastectomy pain syndrome)— usually caused by nerve injury during axillary clearance surgery. Pain happens in the axilla medial part of the upper limb and chest wall.
- Phantom phenomenon
- Neuroma pain—MC after surgery, after radiotherapy.

Patey's *(David Howard Patey, 1899–1976, Surgeon, The Middlesex Hospital, London, UK)* MRM:

It removes:

- Breast + NAC
- A large portion of skin
- Fat, fascia, and axillary LNs (Level I, II and III)
- The pectoralis major and minor muscles are not removed.
  - Pectoralis minor muscles are retracted in the Auchincloss mastectomy MRM (Modified radical mastectomy).
  - Cut in Patey, Auchincloss, and Scanlon mastectomy (Hugh Auchincloss, American transplant surgeon, EF Scanlon in 1975).

BREAST CONSERVATIVE SURGERY

- *Wide local excision:* Tumor with a margin of normal breast tissue removed. Excision of a benign breast tumor called lumpectomy.
- *Quadrantectomy*: Removal of a quadrant of the breast with the tumor. These two methods can be combined with axillary clearance surgery (level II or level III lymph nodes).

Contraindications of Breast Conservative Surgery

- *Absolute*: Pregnancy/multicentric
- Relatives

Sentinel node biopsy is done after injection of patent blue dye in the subdermal plexus around the nipple to identify sentinel node. This procedure is now controversial. Cabanas first used in penile cancer. It identifies LNs draining cancer tumor which are removed and histopathology diagnoses cancer. It is also used for penile cancer, head and neck cancer and vulvar cancer.

Other than methylene blue and isosulfan blue it is also done by following methods:

- Radionucleotide technique (TC^{99} tagged sulfur colloid)
- Indocyanine green technique (ICG)
- Sentimag technique (Ferric oxide compound)

The most commonly used dye is methylene blue.

Complications:
- Skin tattooing
- Bluish discoloration of urine
- Skin necrosis
  Sentimag technique has zero radiation exposure.

Contraindications for surgery in BC:
- Pregnancy: Absolute
- H/O radiotherapy to chest wall—relative
- SLE/RA: Relative

DUPONT AND PAGE'S CLASSIFICATION OF RISK OF BC IN PRE-EXISTING LESIONS IN THE BREAST

- Nonproliferation—ANDI—PR—No risk
- Proliferative without atypia—PR 1.3
- Proliferation with atypia—PR 1.9
- Typical ductal or lobular hyperplasia
- Carcinoma in situ RP-9 - PR 2, i.e., moderate infraductal hyperplasia/intraductal papilloma/fibrosis/adenosis.
- Prior RT (Radiotherapy)
- Multiform tumor
- Large tumor
- Diffuse tumor
- Locally advanced tumor
- Collagen vascular disease as SLE/RA (Rheumatoid arthritis).

CHEMOTHERAPY

6-monthly cycle of cyclophosphamide, methotrexate, and 5-fluorouracil (CMF) gives a reduction in the rate of relapse or four cycles—AC/EC four cycles of T. CMF is not used nowadays as other agents have better results.

A: Adriamycin
C: Cyclophosphamide
T: Taxanes
E: Epirubicin

(F = 5-Fluorouracil, M = Methotrexate, C = Carboplatin, H = Herceptin, P = Pertuzumab)

New drugs Mn: LIS
L - Lapatinib - good for AC+ Taxane-resistant tumor
I - Ixabepilone - second line HER-2 treatment
S - Sunitinib - for refractory BC with metastasis

Indications of Chemotherapy

- Metastasis
- ER, PR-ve tumor
- Positive LNs on biopsy.
- Locally advanced tumor
- HER2/neu+ve

When not to give chemotherapy?
- Poor Karnofsky Score (David A Karnofsky defined the scale in 1949).
- High risk of recurrence.

Molecular testing in breast cancer has become an important factor in BC management. Common tests are Oncotype Dx (gene 21), MammaPrint (gene 70), EndoPredict (gene 12), and *PAM50* (gene 50).

Neoadjuvant Chemotherapy

It is a systemic treatment of breast cancer, especially before surgery. It can reduce the risk of recurrence.

Indications

- LABC (Locally Advanced Breast Cancer)
- TNBC
- HER-2 neu +ve
- Large tumor with BCS

Advantages

- Reduces the size of tumor.
- Reduces micrometastasis.

RECIST is considered as Gold Standard for evaluating treatment response in solid tumors.
- Complete response (CR)
- Partial response (PR)
- Progressive disease (PD)
- Stable disease (SD)

CHEMOPORT (FIG. 36)

It is a small device that can be attached to a vein to draw blood and give drugs such as chemotherapy. Usually placed below the clavicle. It prevents thrombophlebitis even in long-term use. It is an implantable device for the

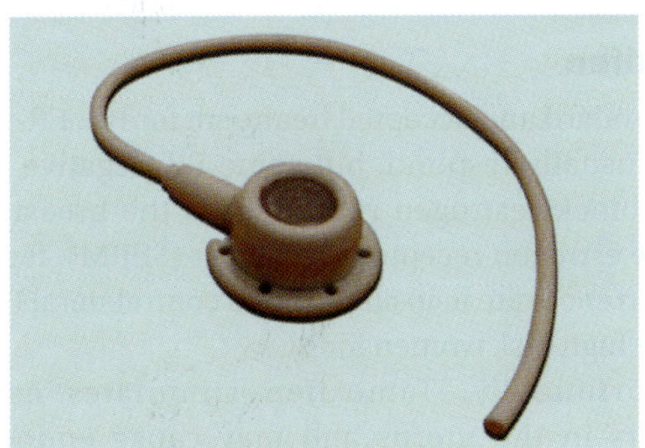

Fig. 36: Chemotherapy port.

delivery of intravenous medications and chemotherapy. It is most commonly placed below the clavicle.

RADIOTHERAPY

It uses high-energy radiation to destroy BC cells. It can be used as palliative radiotherapy or with chemotherapy, or after surgery. It can be used for target sites as whole breast irradiation (WBI), and also as accelerated partial breast irradiation (APBI).

Radiotherapy after mastectomy reduces the risk of recurrence. It is good for the following cases:

- Large tumor
- Large number of positive LNs.
- Extensive lymphovascular invasion.

Indications of Accelerated Partial Breast Irradiation

Electrodes are placed in the cavity of the tumor:

- ER/PR positive
- Unifocal
- Margins of the tumor are clear or negative
- Elderly patient—>50 years
- T1 tumor
- Lymphovascular tumor invasion is absent.

Radiotherapy is used generally for reducing the recurrence rate in LABC (Locally Advanced Breast Cancer), after mastectomy with margins involved, after BCS (Breast Cancer Surgery), and if LN metastasis are >4.

HORMONE THERAPY

- *Indications*: ER, PR +ve
- Tamoxifen reduces the rate of recurrence and the rate of death
- *Premenopause:* Tamoxifen
- *Postmenopause:* Aromatase inhibitors (letrozole and anastrozole)

Tamoxifen

It is a standard and accepted treatment for BC. ER-positive tumors usually respond, but some ER-negative tumors also. It blocks estrogen receptors on the breast. It is a selective estrogen receptor modulator (SERM). It reduces the recurrence rate in ipsilateral and contralateral BCs. It is good for high-risk women for BC.

Unfortunately, Tamoxifen stimulates estrogen receptors in the uterus and may cause endometrial hyperplasia and even cancer.

Dose: 10 mg twice a day for about 5 years.

Adverse reactions of tamoxifen:

- Hot flushes
- Menstrual irregularities
- Thromboembolism
- Cataracts
- Endometrial cancer

Clinical problems after advanced breast cancer causing lymphatic obstruction:

- Peau d'orange
- Lymphoedema
- Cancer-en-cuirasse
- Lymphangiosarcoma

MOLECULAR SUBTYPES OF BREAST CANCER

Breast cancer has four subtypes, primary molecular by hormone receptors (HR):

- Luminal A or HR+/HER 2-(HR-positive/HER2-negative)
- Lumine B or HR+/HER2 + (HR-positive/HER2-positive)
- Triple-negative or HR-HER 2-(HR/HER2)
- HER2-positive—negative.

According to the American Cancer Society in USA, the distribution is as:

- Luminal A: 73%
- Luminal B: 11%
- Triple negative: 12%
- HER-2 enriched: 4%

Luminal A:

- Breast cancer grew slowly
- Are ER + ve and PR + ve so the drugs which lower ER & PR used in treatment of this type are of BC.

Luminal B:

- Grow faster and are more aggressive.
- They are HR+ and HER-2 positive.

Triple-Negative: These are invasive tumors and begin in ducts.

They are ER -ve, PR -ve and HER negative, so cannot be treated by hormones or medications which block HER-2 such as trastuzumab. Chemotherapy and Radiation can treat such tumors.

HER-2 Positive: They are ER-ve, PR-ve and HER-2 positive. Treated by a correlation of surgery, radiation & chemotherapy.

PROTECTIVE FACTORS FOR BREAST CANCER

- Multiparous
- Breastfeeding
- Maternal age at first live birth more than equal to 20 years.
- Maintain normal weight, avoid obesity
- Be physically active. Regularly exercise.
- Limited alcohol consumption
- Do not smoke.
- Avoid birth control pills.
- Avoid hormone pills.
- MRI breast screening.

How to reduce risk of breast cancer?

- B/L (bilateral) prophylactic mastectomy (95%)
- B/L salpingophorectomy (50%)
- Drugs, i.e., tamoxifen (47%)

GYNECOMASTIA (FIG. 37)

Gynecomastia is an increase in the breast tissue, with enlargement of the breast in a male. This looks like a female breast, which is embarrassing to the boy. It is due to the hormonal imbalance, especially in the body level of estrogen and testosterone. Gynecomastia can affect one or both breasts.

Grades of Gynecomastia

- *Grade I*: Mild enlargement without skin redundancy
- *Grade IIa*: Moderate breast enlargement

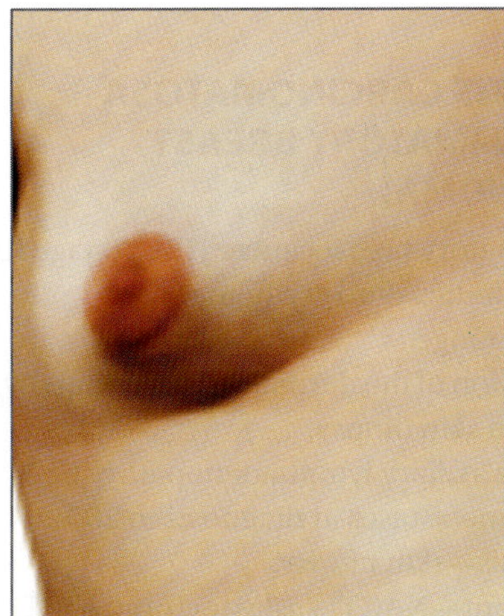

Fig. 37: Gynecomastia.

- *Grade IIb*: Moderate breast enlargement with skin redundancy
- *Grade III*: Marked breast enlargement + skin redundancy + ptosis, like female breast.

Types

- Physiological (NEWBORN, puberty, and old age).
- Pathological Mn: DIKLOP [D = Drug induced (Digoxin, steroids, cimetidine), I = idiopathic, K = Klinefelter syndrome, L = Liver diseases, O = Mumps orchitis, P = Paraneoplastic conditions (HCC/RCC)].

Causes

- *Hormonal:* Stilbestrol therapy in cancer of prostate—use of steroids in body builders—teratoma testis—bronchial carcinoma due to ectopic hormonal production.
- Leprosy due to bilateral testicular atrophy.
- Cirrhosis of the liver.
- Klinefelter's (Harry Fitch Klinefelter Jr, 1912–1990, Physician of Baltimore, MD, USA, described this syndrome in 1942) syndrome (47,XXY trisomy).

Treatment

- Reassurance
- Mastectomy with preservation of areola and nipple.

CARCINOMA OF THE MALE BREAST

- <0.5% of all cases of breast cancer.
- Infiltrating ductal carcinoma.
- Treatment is mastectomy and as in female breast cancer.

TREATMENT OF BREAST CANCER DURING PREGNANCY

- Investigation USG/core biopsy
- *Treatment*: Surgery
  - Mastectomy in the first trimmer
  - Conservative surgery in two-thirds trimester: RT after delivery.

Axillary clearance (Minimum 10 LNs are removed):

- Limits or boundaries for dissection
- *Anterior*: Pectoral muscle
- *Post*:
  - Latissimus dorsi
  - Teres major
  - Subscapularis

- *Lateral*: Axillary skin + thoracodorsal pedicle (Halsted ligament)
- *Medial*: Chest wall

The most common nerve injury in axillary clearance is the intercostobrachial nerve. It is a branch of the second intercostobrachial nerve.

All common BCs are adenocarcinoma:
- *Most common BC*: Invasive ductal CA (second most common CA is infiltrating lobular carcinoma)
- *Worst prognosis BC*: Invasive ductal CA (of no special type)
- *Best prognosis:* Tubular carcinoma
- *Comedo carcinoma:* It shows comedonecrosis, which is central necrosis of cancer cells within involved ducts. It is high-grade DCIS
- Medullary CA is common in younger patients.
- Mucinous CA is common in elderly patients.
- Almost all invasive lobular carcinomas are ER+ve.

Gail model—MC (most common) model in use
- Breast Cancer Risk Assessment Tool (BCRAT)
- *Clause model*: Based on family history and first and second degree relatives with cancer of breast.

After Dr Mitchell Gail (Dr Mitchell Gail, American physician). It calculates women's risk of developing BC in the next 5 years. It incorporates menarche age, number of breast biopsies, and number of final degree relatives who suffered with breast cancer.

Best first tissue investigation: FNAC

Best and definitive—open biopsies

How to treat advance locoregional BC (stage III)?
Neoadjuvant chemotherapy + MRM + adjuvant radiation therapy + chemotherapy + antiestrogen therapy.

How to treat BC with distant metastasis (stage IV)?
(Palliative treatment)
(Hormonal therapy + systemic chemotherapy + Bisphosphonates)

ONCOPLASTY

It is a surgical procedure that combines the removal of the breast cancer tumor with plastic surgery to improve the cosmetic appearance of the breast.

Breast Reconstruction

- Silicon implant:
  - Gel implant
  - Saline implant
- TRAM flap—most common (Transversus Rectus Abdominis Muscle). There is a risk of incisional hernia as muscle is removed.
- Latissimus dorsi myocutaneous flap
- Gluteal flap
- *DIEP*: Deep inferior epigastric artery perforative flap (Best flap surgery as muscle is not removed and less abdominal complications).

BEST PROGNOSTIC FACTORS FOR BREAST CANCER

- Stage of BC
- LN status
- HER-2 previously was called HER-2/neu

- *Zuska's disease*—or recurrent periductal mastitis—smoking is a risk factor.
- *Key features*—keratinizing squamous metaplasia of nipple.
- *Treatment*—antibiotic 1 CD if abscess forms.

Ductography: Introduction of codeine containing contrast medium in discharging ducts

Ductoscopy is done for nipple discharge.

How to examine Peau d'orange and retraction of nipple?
Arms raised above head.
Linguine sign: Floating membrane in silicon breast implant on MRI means rupture of capsule.

Poor prognostic markers in BC (expressions):
- PCNA
- Ki-67
- BCL-2
- Bax: BCL-2
- VEGF
- HER-2/neu
- EGFr

MASTITIS CARCINOMATOSA (INFLAMMATORY BREAST CARCINOMA)

- Inflammatory breast cancer (IBC) (stage IIIB)
- Brawny induration, erythema.
- Peau d'orange
- Permeation of the dermal lymph vessels by cancer cells is seen in skin biopsy.
- Palpable axillary lymphadenopathy.
- Distant metastases at diagnosis in 25%.
- Diagnosis—skin biopsy.
- Treatment—NACT + Mastectomy + RT ± hormonal therapy.

SOME IMPORTANT QUESTIONS

Q1. The best diagnostic method for a breast lump is:
a. Ultrasonography (USG)
b. Mammogram
c. Biopsy
d. Fine-needle aspiration cytology (FNAC)

Ans. c

Q2. A 26-year-old female came for the first time in the OPD with a lump in her breast. First investigation would be:
a. USG
b. Mammogram
c. Magnetic resonance imaging (MRI)
d. Positron emission tomography (PET) scan

Ans. a

Q3. A 45-year-old woman presents with a hard and mobile lump in the breast. The next investigation is:
a. FNAC
b. USG
c. Mammography
d. Excision biopsy

Ans. c

Q4. BI-RADS stands for:
a. Breast Imaging Reporting and Diagnosing System
b. Brain Imaging Reporting and Data System
c. Best Imaging Reporting and Diagnosing System
d. Breast Imaging Reporting and Data System

Ans. d

Q5. Peau d'orange appearance for the mammary skin is due to:
a. Intraepithelial cancer
b. Subepidermal cancer
c. Lymphatic permeation
d. Vascular embolization

Ans. c

Q6. The treatment of choice for duct papilloma of a breast is:
a. Simple mastectomy
b. Microdochectomy
c. Local wide excision
d. Chemotherapy

Ans. b

Q7. Gynecomastia may be seen in patients with all, *except*:
a. Cimetidine therapy
b. Cirrhosis of the liver
c. Klinefelter's syndrome
d. Turner's syndrome

Ans. d

Q8. Unilateral amastia is associated 90% of the time with the absence or hypoplasia of the following muscle:
a. Latissimus dorsi
b. Subclavian
c. Pectoral
d. Serratus anterior

Ans. c

Q9. An adolescent boy presents himself with bilateral prominence of breasts and wants the breasts to be removed. Which one of the following incisions would be ideal?
a. Radial incision
b. Incision along the areolar margin
c. Submammary incision
d. Ellipitical incision

Ans. b

Q10. The following condition has no increased risk of invasive breast carcinoma, *except*:
a. Hyperplasia atypical
b. Sclerosing adenosis
c. Apocrine metaplasia
d. Duct ectasia

Ans. a

Q11. Single file pattern is seen in breast cancer type:
a. Intraductal
b. Infiltrating lobular
c. Infiltrating ductular
d. None

Ans. b

Q12. Components of QUARTZ, *except*:
a. Quadrantectomy
b. Axillary dissection
c. Radiotherapy
d. Tamoxifen

Ans. d

Q13. Carcinoma breast is most commonly seen in which quadrant of the breast:
a. Upper outer
b. Upper inner
c. Lower inner
d. Lower outer

Ans. a

Q14. In which of the following types of breast carcinoma is, comedo growth pattern seen?
a. Ductal carcinoma in situ
b. Medullary carcinoma
c. Lobular carcinoma in situ
d. Infiltrating lobular carcinoma

Ans. a

Q15. The following are true of Paget's disease of the breast, *except*:
a. Usually bilateral
b. Associated intraductal carcinoma
c. Prognosis is good in the absence of a lump
d. Treatment was simple mastectomy with axillary clearance

Ans. a

MULTIPLE CHOICE QUESTIONS

Grade I	Simple

Q1. Triple assessment for breast cancer includes: (All India 2009)

a. History, clinical examination, and mammogram
b. History, clinical examination, and fine needle aspiration cytology (FNAC)
c. Ultrasonography (USG), mammogram, and FNAC
d. Clinical examination, mammogram, and FNAC

Q2. What is the sensitivity of axillary ultrasound in identifying axillary metastases in clinically node-negative breast carcinoma? (AIIMS May 2017)

a. 10–20%
b. 20–30%
c. 30–40%
d. 55–60%

Q3. All are risk factors for breast cancer, *except*: (AIIMS Nov 1998)

a. Ovarian malignancy
b. Family h/o breast cancer
c. Fibroadenosis
d. Multiparity

Q4. The type of fibroadenosis most likely to undergo malignant change is: (AIIMS June 1993)

a. Adenosis
b. Epitheliosis
c. Sclerosing adenosis
d. Cystic

Q5. Breast cancer is more common in: (PGI Dec 2001)

a. Those who avoid breastfeeding to the infant
b. Multiparity
c. Nulliparity
d. High fat diet
e. Family history of (H/O) breast cancer

Q6. Risk factors for breast cancer are: (PGI Nov 2010)

a. Nulliparity
b. Multiparity
c. Family history
d. Breast cancer type 1 susceptibility protein (BRCA1) mutation
e. Oral contraceptive pill (OCP)

Q7. On a mammogram, all of the following are the features of a malignant tumor, *except*: (AIIMS Nov 2003)

a. Spiculation
b. Microcalcification
c. Macrocalcification
d. Irregular mass

Q8. In patients with breast cancer, chest wall involvement means involvement of any one of the following structures, *except*: (AIIMS Nov 2005)

a. Serratus anterior
b. Pectoralis major
c. Intercoastal muscles
d. Ribs

Q9. Ipsilateral supraclavicular LNs are positive in a patient of breast cancer. Stage is: (AIIMS May 2012)

a. II
b. III B
c. III C
d. IV

Q10. The most malignant type of breast carcinoma is: (NIMHANS 1986)

a. Paget's disease
b. Anaplastic carcinoma
c. Scirrhous carcinoma
d. Atrophic scirrhous carcinoma
e. Mastitis carcinomatosa

Q11. Not true about breast cancer in India: (AIIMS June 1998)

a. Incidence is 20/100,000
b. Average age 42 years
c. Positive family history is a risk factor
d. More common in Muslims

Q12. Which of the following carcinomas is familial? (All India 1999)

a. Breast
b. Prostate
c. Cervix
d. Vaginal

Q13. BIRADS stands for: (AIIMS Nov 2012)

a. Breast Imaging Reporting and Data System
b. Best Imaging Reporting and Data System
c. Brain Imaging Reporting and Data System
d. Best Imaging Reporting and Data System

Q14. Risk factors for breast carcinoma: (PGI Nov 2011, Nov 2010)

a. Nulliparity
b. OCP
c. Family history
d. BRCA-1 mutation
e. Estrogen

Q15. Popcorn calcification in mammography is seen in: (AIIMS June 2000)

a. Fibroadenoma
b. Fat necrosis
c. Cystosarcoma phyllodes
d. Breast cancer

Q16. Ca breast stage I and II managed by: (PGI Dec 2002)

a. Total mastectomy
b. Modified radical mastectomy
c. Lumpectomy and axillary clearance
d. Lumpectomy, axillary clearance, and radiotherapy

Q17. Use of tamoxifen in carcinoma of the breast patients does not lead to the following side effects: (AIIMS June 2003)

a. Thromboembolic events
b. Endometrial carcinoma
c. Catraract
d. Cancer in the opposite breast

Q18. Breast conservation surgery is indicated in one of the following conditions: (AIIMS Nov 2003)

a. T 1 breast tumor
b. Multicentric tumor
c. Extensive in situ cancer
d. T4b breast tumor

Q19. BRCA-1 positive women have .... % increased risk of breast carcinoma. (JIPMER 2011)

a. 10
b. 20
c. 40
d. 60

Q20. In inflammatory breast cancer with metastasis to axilla treatment of choice is: (PGI Dec 1996)

a. Radical mastectomy + chemotherapy
b. Radical mastectomy + radiotherapy
c. Simple mastectomy + radiotherapy
d. Chemotherapy + radiotherapy

Q21. All of the following are used for the reconstruction of the breast, *except*: (AIIMS Nov 2000)

a. Transverse rectus abdominis myocutaneous flap
b. Latissimus dorsi myocutaneous flap
c. Pectoralis major myocutaneous flap
d. Transversus rectus abdominis free flap

Q22. Least risk of CA breast is seen in: (AIIMS Nov 2006)

a. BRCA-1
b. BRCA-2
c. Li-Fraumeni syndrome
d. Ataxia telangiectasia

Q23. LN first involved in CA breast is/are: (PGI Nov 2009)

a. Axillary LN
b. Internal mammary LN
c. Supraclavicular LN
d. Contralateral axillary LN

Q24. In breast carcinoma metastasis, prognosis depends best upon: (All India 1998)

a. Estrogen receptor status
b. Axillary LN status
c. Size of tumor
d. Site of the tumor

Q25. Breast cancer good prognostic markers are: (PGI Dec 2006)

a. ER +ve
b. Progesterone (receptors) + ve
c. HER - 2/neu (receptors) +ve
d. CD44 receptor +ve
e. *p53* gene +ve

Q26. Paget's disease of the breast are true, *except*: (PGI Dec 1997)

a. Treated by simple mastectomy
b. Represents underlying malignancy
c. Presents as eczema
d. Cytology diagnostic

Q27. In breast cancer following are expressed: (PGI Dec 2007)

a. Her-2-neu
b. p53
c. BRCA-1
d. BCL-1
e. CEA

Q28. Which is the most conspicuous sign in breast cancer? (AIIMS Nov 2018)

a. Nipple retraction
b. Peau d'orange
c. Puckering
d. Both nipple retraction and puckering

Q29. True regarding male breast cancer: (PGI June 2009)

a. MC (most common) lobular type
b. Estrogen receptor positive
c. H/O gynecomastia may be present
d. Paget's disease of the nipple is more common in males than females
e. Undescended testis is a risk factor

Q30. True about the lymphatic spread of breast cancer: (PGI June 2005)

a. Axillary nodes are most commonly involved
b. Internal mammary nodes are also involved
c. If the supraclavicular LN is involved, then it is N3
d. Axillary nodes are treated by surgical resection

Q31. In patients with breast cancer, chest wall involvement means involvement of any one of the following structures, *except*: (AIIMS Nov 2005)

a. Serratus anterior
b. Pectoralis major
c. Intercostal muscles
d. Ribs

Q32. Large breast is not seen in: (AIIMS Dec 1995)

a. Filariasis
b. Giant fibroadenoma
c. Cystosarcoma phyllodes
d. Scirrhous carcinoma

Q33. A blood-stained discharge from the nipple indicates: (AIIMS Nov 2003)

a. Breast abscess
b. Fibroadenoma
c. Duct papilloma
d. Fat necrosis of the breast

Q34. Green discharge is most commonly seen with: (AIIMS Nov 1998)

a. Duct papilloma
b. Duct ectasia
c. Retention cyst
d. Fibroadenosis

Q35. True statement(s) about nipple discharge is/are: (PGI June 2004)

a. Mammography is diagnostic
b. Cone excision done in a single intraductal tumor
c. Mammography is done when the duct papilloma is >4.5 cm
d. Red discharge indicate malignancy
e. Blue-black discharge indicate duct ectasia

Q36. Gynecomastia may be seen in all of the following conditions, *except*: (All India 1998)

a. Kilnefelter syndrome
b. Cirrhosis of the liver
c. Cryptorchidism
d. Sex cord tumor of Sertoli cells

Q37. All are true regarding gynecomastia, *except*: (AIIMS Nov 1993)

a. May be seen in Addison's disease
b. Usually unilateral in young males
c. Acini are not involved
d. Bilaterality is due to endocrinopathy

Q38. Complication of postmastectomy lymphedema is: (JIPMER 1995)

a. Metastases of cancer
b. Recurrence
c. Lymphosarcoma
d. Pain

Q39. Contraindication for radical mastectomy in breast cancer: (PGI Dec 2006)

a. Distant metastasis
b. Fixity of chest wall
c. Axillary LN involvement
d. Supraclavicular LN involvement

Q40. Pre-menstrual fullness in the breast in 21-year-old unmarried female is: (AIIMS 1998)

a. Galactocele
b. Fibroadenoma
c. Fibroadenosis
d. Breast cancer

Q41. All of the following are removed in radical mastectomy, *except*: (AIIMS 1992)

a. Pectoralis major
b. Pectoralis minor
c. Axillary LN
d. Supraclavicular LN

Q42. A 25-year-old lady presents with spontaneous nipple discharge of 3 months duration. On examination, the discharge is bloody and from a single duct. The following statements about management of this patient are true, *except*: (AIIMS Nov 2004)

a. Ultrasound can be a useful investigation
b. Radical duct excision is the operation of choice
c. Galactogram, though useful, is not essential
d. The majority of blood-stained nipple discharges are due to papillomas or other benign conditions

Q43. Aromatase inhibitors used in breast cancer are: (PGI June 2007)

a. Letrozole
b. Anastrozole
c. Exemestane
d. Tamoxifen

Q44. A 36-year-old patient underwent breast conservation therapy and chemotherapy for a 1.5 × 1.2 cm estrogen receptor (ER)-positive breast cancer with one positive axillary LN. She is now on tamoxifen. How will you follow up the patient? (AIIMS May 2017)

a. Annual bone scan
b. Assessment of tumor markers 6-monthly
c. Routine clinical examination 3 monthly in the first year with annual mammogram
d. Routine clinical examination 3 monthly and 6 monthly liver function tests

Q45. True about screening mammography: (PGI June 2004)

a. Indicated in 50–70 years of age
b. Mortality reduced by 30%

c. Radiation due to mammography can cause carcinoma
d. MRI is better than mammography
e. USG is better than mammography

Q46. A 45-year-old female presented with a H/O a painless breast lump of size 6 × 5 cm in the left upper quadrant with no axillary LNs. A true-cut biopsy was suggestive of ductal carcinoma in situ. She undergoes surgery with resection of all tumor tissue with adequate margins, and postoperative histopathological examination (HPE) shows ductal carcinoma in situ (DCIS) with high-grade necrosis with 4 mm clearance on margins. Which of the following is needed? (AIIMS May 2017)

a. Adjuvant chemotherapy
b. Adjuvant chemoradiotherapy
c. Adjuvant radiotherapy
d. No additional treatment

Q47. True regarding axillary LN dissection in breast cancer: (PGI Nov 2017)

a. Axillary dissection can be carried out through the incision for a mastectomy
b. Level I, II, and III nodes are removed in modified radical mastectomy
c. In Halsted radical mastectomy, all breast tissue and skin, the nipple, areola complex, the pectoralis major and pectoralis minor muscles, and the level I, II, and III axillary LNs are removed
d. The arm is kept abducted at 90° during axillary dissection.
e. Halsted radical mastectomy preserves the pectoralis major and the lateral pectoral nerve

Q48. A 17-year-old female underwent Fine Needle Aspiration Cytology (FNAC) for a lump in the breast, which was nontender, firm, and mobile. Which of the following features would suggest the finding of a benign breast disease? (AIIMS Nov 2014)

a. Dyscohesive ductal epithelial cells without cellular fragments
b. Tightly arranged ductal epithelial cells with dyscohesive bare nuclei
c. Stromal predominance with spindle cells
d. Polymorphism with single or arranged ductal epithelial cells

Q49. Features, which are evaluated for histological grading of breast carcinoma, include all of the following, *except*: (AIIMS Nov 2005)

a. Tumor necrosis
b. Mitotic count
c. Tubule formation
d. Nuclear pleomorphism

Q50. A lady 35-year-old lactating mother presented with a painful breast lump. The most appropriate initial investigation should be: (AIIMS Nov 2012)

a. Mammography
b. USG
c. MRI
d. X-ray

Q51. In sentinel node biopsy for breast cancer, the most commonly injured nerve is: (AIIMS May 2013)

a. Lateral pectoral nerve
b. Nerve to latissimus dorsi
c. Intercostobrachial nerve
d. Long thoracic nerve (Never to the serratus anterior)

Q52. A patient underwent a mastectomy for breast carcinoma and presents with upper limb swelling after 3 months. What is the diagnosis? (All India 2021)

a. Upper limb lymphangiosarcoma
b. Upper limb lymphedema
c. Recurrence of cancer
d. Cancer en cuirasse

Q53. A 14-week postnatal woman presents with fluctuating breast swelling. What would be the treatment? (All India 2019 Question)

a. Incision and drainage
b. Continue breastfeeding with antibiotics
c. Analgesics
d. Repeated aspirations under antibiotic cover

Q54. Molecular classification of breast cancer is based on: (AIIMS Nov 2014)

a. Serum hormone levels
b. Expression of hormone receptors (ER/PR)
c. In vitro response to chemotherapeutic agents
d. Gene expression profiling

Q55. Estrogen receptor studies in breast carcinoma is done on: (JIPMER 1987)

a. Blood
b. Urine
c. Tumor tissue
d. Ovary

Grade II | **Difficult**

Q1. The most conspicuous sign of breast cancer is: (AIIMS Nov 2018)

a. Puckering
b. Nipple retraction
c. Both puckering and nipple retraction
d. Peau d'orange

Q2. The clinician was palpating with finger pads except the thumb. He started at the 2 o'clock position, palpated at 3 points on a line joining the periphery to the nipple. Again, went to the 3 o'clock point directly and examined centripetally while palpating at 3 points again on the line joining the periphery to the nipple. Method of palpation is (In examination, this was a video-based question) (AIIMS Nov 2018)

a. Dial Clock method
b. Quadrant
c. Circular Pattern
d. Vertical strips

Q3. In the cases of carcinoma breast with Her-2-neu immunohistochemistry staining, which of the following scores needs further FISH study? (AIIMS Nov 2017)

a. 0
b. 1+
c. 2+
d. 3+

Q4. A female patient present with a hard mobile lump in her right breast. Which investigation would be most helpful in making the diagnosis? (AIIMS Nov 2001)

a. FNAC
b. Needle biopsy
c. Excision biopsy
d. Mammography

Q5. A 32-year-old lactating mother presented with a painful, palpable lump in her left breast. The most appropriate investigation to diagnose her condition would be: (AIIMS Nov 2013)

a. Mammography
b. USG
c. MRI
d. SPECT

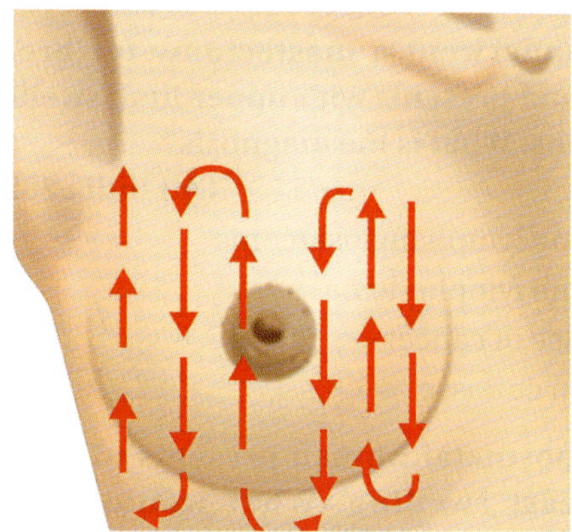

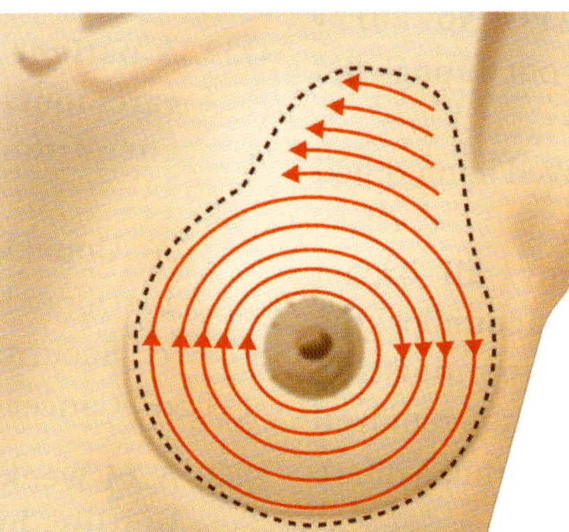

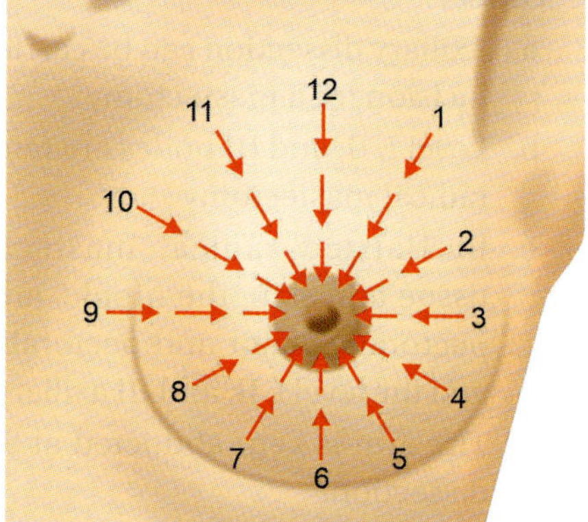

Breast palpation methods.

Q6. On a mammogram, all of the following are features of a malignant tumor, *except*: (AIIMS Nov 2003)

a. Spiculation
b. Microcalcification
c. Macrocalcification
d. Irregular mass

Q7. Popcorn calcification in mammography is seen in: (AIIMS June 2000)

a. Fibroadenoma
b. Fat necrosis
c. Cystosarcoma phyllodes
d. Breast cancer

Q8. The least risk of breast cancer is seen in: (AIIMS Nov 2006)

a. BRCA1
b. BRCA2
c. Li-Fraumeni syndrome
d. Ataxia telangiectasia

Q9. Risks for carcinoma breast are: (PGI Dec 2000)

a. First-degree relative
b. Atypical hyperplasia
c. Sclerosing adenosis
d. Increased fat intake

Q10. Breast cancer is epidemiologically common with: (PGI Dec 2001)

a. Smoking
b. Nulliparity
c. Oral contraceptives
d. Multiparity
e. First pregnancy after 30 years

Q11. In breast Ca 6 cm with fixed ipsilateral axillary LN. The TNM staging is: (PGI 1996)

a. T3N2
b. T2N2
c. T4N2
d. T1N1

Q12. 4 cm breast nodule with ipsilateral mobile LN in axilla stating: (PGI June 2000)

a. T2N1M0
b. T2N2M0
c. T1N1M0
d. T3N2M1

Q13. Ca breast stage T4b involves all, *except*: (AIIMS May 2012)

a. Nipple retraction
b. Skin ulcer over the swelling
c. Dermal edema
d. Satellite nodule

Q14. Luminal A breast cancer shows the following features: (PGI May 2018)

a. Low-grade tumor
b. HER-2-neu amplification
c. Good prognosis
d. High-grade tumor
e. ER-negative

Q15. The type of mammary ductal carcinoma in situ (DCIS) most likely to result in a palpable abnormality in the breast is: (All India 2006)

a. Apocrine DCIS
b. Neuroendocrine DCIS
c. Well-differentiated DCIS
d. Comedo DCIS

Q16. Poor prognosis of breast carcinoma is associated with: (PGI May 2018)

a. Overexpression of HER-2-neu
b. Increased estrogen and progesterone receptor expression
c. Triple negative tumor
d. Decreased percentage of cells in "S" phase of mitosis
e. Increased percentage of cells expressing the Ki-67 marker

Q17. "Peau d'orange" appearance of the mammary skin is due to: (PGI Dec 1995)

a. Intraepithelial cancer
b. Subepidermal cancer
c. Lymphatic permeation
d. Vascular embolization

Q18. Which of the following indicates breast cancer? (PGI Dec 2002)

a. Serous discharge
b. Recent retraction of nipple
c. Ulceration of nipple
d. Cracked nipple
e. Cellular atypia

Q19. True about lymphatic spread of breast cancer: (PGI June 2005)

a. Axillary nodes are most commonly involved
b. Internal mammary nodes are also involved
c. If the supraclavicular LN is involved, then it is N3
d. Axillary nodes are treated by surgical resection

Q20. In Patey's mastectomy, the step not done is: (PGI 1995)

a. Nipple and areola removed
b. The surrounding normal tissue of the tumor is removed
c. Pectoralis major removed
d. Pectoralis minor removed

Q21. Breast conservation surgery includes: (PGI Dec 2007)

a. Lumpectomy
b. Radiotherapy
c. Chemotherapy
d. Axillary LN dissection
e. Sentinel LN biopsy

Q22. Conservative surgery in breast cancer is not to be done in: (PGI Dec 2001)

a. Low socioeconomic status
b. Age >40 years
c. Multicentricity
d. LN involvement in axilla
e. Family H/O breast cancer

Q23. Absolute contraindication of conservative breast cancer therapy is: (PGI Dec 2005)

a. Large pendulous breast
b. H/O previous radiation
c. Axillary node involvement
d. Subareolar lump present
e. First trimester pregnancy

Q24. A 40-year-old female with a 2 cm nodule in the breast and a proven metastatic node in the axilla, treatment is: (PGI 1996)

a. Quadrantectomy
b. Mastectomy with local radiotherapy
c. Patey's with adjuvant chemotherapy
d. Halsted's operation with tamoxifen

Q25. In inflammatory carcinoma breast with metastasis of the axilla, the treatment of choice is: (PGI Dec 1996)

a. Radical mastectomy + chemotherapy
b. Radical mastectomy + radiotherapy
c. Simple mastectomy + radiotherapy
d. Chemotherapy + radiotherapy

Q26. Treatment of cystosarcoma phyllodes in a young woman: (JIPMER 2011)

a. Wide excision with a margin
b. Wide excision with chemotherapy
c. Wide excision with radiotherapy
d. Modified radical mastectomy (MRM)

Q27. In case of breast cancer most prognostic factor is: (AIIMS Feb 1997)

a. Size of tumor
b. LN status
c. Presence of estrogen receptor
d. Age of menopause

Q28. In breast cancer following are expressed: (PGI Dec 2007)

a. HER2/neu
b. P53
c. BRCA1
d. BCL-1
e. CEA

Q29. Features, which are evaluated for histological grading of breast carcinoma, include all of the following, *except*: (AIIMS Nov 2005)

a. Tumor necrosis
b. Mitotic count
c. Tubule formation
d. Nuclear pleomorphism

Q30. The most important prognostic factor in breast carcinoma is: (All India 2006)

a. Histological grade of the tumor
b. Stage of the tumor at the time of diagnosis
c. Status of estrogen and progesterone receptors
d. Overexpression of the p53 tumor suppressor gene

Q31. True about phyllodes tumor is: (PGI May 2018)

a. Associated with BRCA1
b. FNAC can diagnose reliability
c. Treated with mastectomy
d. Axillary LNs are commonly involved
e. Associated with BRCA2

Q32. Gynecomastia may be seen in all of the following conditions, *except*: (All India 1998)

a. Klinefelter's syndrome
b. Cirrhosis of the liver
c. Cryptorchidism
d. Sex-cord tumor of Sertoli cells

Q33. All of the following statements about gynecomastia are true, *except*: (All India 2007)

a. Subcutaneous mastectomy is the initial treatment of choice
b. Seen in liver disease
c. There may be an estrogen/testosterone imbalance
d. Can be drug-induced

Q34. True about breast carcinoma in men. (PGI June 2007)

a. Estrogen receptor positive
b. Associated with gynecomastia
c. Radiotherapy contraindicated due to close proximity to the chest wall
d. Seen in young males

Q35. Which of the following is least likely to be associated with gynecomastia? (All India 2012)

a. Prolactinoma
b. Adrenal tumors
c. Human chorionic gonadotropin (hCG) secreting tumors
d. Estrogen-secreting tumors

Q36. Paget's disease of the breast, true statements are: (PGI Nov 2009)

a. Prolactinoma
b. Adrenal tumors
c. hCG-secreting tumors
d. Estrogen-secreting tumors

Q37. A woman noticed a mass in her left breast with bloody discharge, histopathology revealed duct ectasia treatment is: (AIIMS Nov 2008)

a. Simple mastectomy
b. Microdochotomy
c. Lobectomy
d. Hadfield operation

Q38. All are true regarding gynecomastia, *except*: (AIIMS Nov 1993)

a. May be seen in Addison's disease
b. Usually unilateral in young males
c. Acini are not involved
d. Bilaterality is due to endocrinopathy

Q39. A 25-year-old female complains of discharge of blood from a single duct in her breast. The most appropriate treatment is: (All India 2008)

a. Radical excision
b. Microdochectomy
c. Radical mastectomy
d. Biopsy to rule out carcinoma

Q40. A woman noticed a mass in her left breast with bloody discharge. Histopathology revealed duct ectasia. Treatment is: (AIIMS Nov 2008)

a. Simple mastectomy
b. Microdochotomy
c. Lobectomy
d. Hadfield's operation

Q41. All of the following statements about gynecomastia are true, *except*: (All India 2007)

a. Subcutaneous mastectomy is the initial treatment of choice
b. Seen in liver disease
c. There may be an estrogen/testosterone imbalance
d. Can be drug-induced

Q42. Lymphatic drainage of breast: (PGI Dec 2003)

a. Axillary
b. Supraclavicular
c. Internal mammary
d. Mediastinal
e. Celiac

Q43. A 25-year-old female complains of discharge of blood from a single duct in her breast. The most appropriate treatment is: (All India 2008)

a. Radical excision
b. Microdochectomy
c. Radical mastectomy
d. Biopsy to rule out carcinoma

Q44. A female patient presents with a hard mobile lump in her right breast. Which investigation would be most helpful in making the diagnosis? (AIIMS Nov 2001)

a. FNAC
b. Needle biopsy
c. Excision biopsy
d. Mammography

Q45. Most sensitive imaging for DCIS of the breast is: (AIIMS Nov 2010)

a. Mammography
b. MRI
c. PET
d. USG

Q46. The type of fibroadenosis most likely to undergo malignant change is: (AIIMS June 1993)

a. Adenosis
b. Epitheliosis
c. Sclerosing adenosis
d. Cystic

Q47. Which of the following carcinomas is familial? (All India 1998)

a. Breast
b. Prostate
c. Cervix
d. Vaginal

Q48. Which of the following is an increased risk of breast cancer: (PGI Dec 2005)

a. Sclerosing adenosis
b. Atypical hyperplasia
c. Fibroadenoma
d. Florid hyperplasia

Q49. Drug used in estrogen-dependent breast cancer: (AIIMS May 2012)

a. Tamoxifen
b. Clomiphene citrate
c. Estrogen
d. Adriamycin

Q50. A 30-year-old female presented with unilateral breast cancer associated with axillary lymph node enlargement. Modified radical mastectomy was done, further treatment plan will be: (AIIMS May 2007)

a. Observation and follow-up
b. Adriamycin-based chemotherapy followed by tamoxifen, depending on estrogen/progesterone receptor status
c. Adriamycin-based chemotherapy only
d. Tamoxifen only

Q51. Postoperative radiotherapy in breast is given for: (JIPMER 1995)

a. To prevent metastasis
b. For ablation of remnants of cancer tissue
c. To prevent recurrence
d. Prevents distant metastasis

Q52. In which of the following types of breast carcinoma, would you consider biopsy of the opposite breast? (All India 2006)

a. Adenocarcinoma, poorly differentiated
b. Medullary carcinoma
c. Lobular carcinoma
d. Comedo carcinoma

Q53. The type of mammary DCIS most likely to result in a palpable abnormality in the breast is: (All India 2006)

a. Apocrine DCIS
b. Neuroendocrine DCIS
c. Well-differentiated DCIS
d. Comedo DCIS

Q54. Best prognosis amongst the following histological variants of breast carcinoma is seen with: (All India 1998)

a. Intraductal
b. Colloid (Mucinous)
c. Lobular
d. Medullary

Q55. All are true about CA breast, *except*: (AIIMS May 1993)

a. Affected sibling is a risk factor
b. Paget's disease of the nipple is an intraductal type of CA
c. Common in aged nulliparous
d. Increased incidence with prolonged breastfeeding

Q56. "Peau d'orange" is due to: (AIIMS Nov 2015)

a. Arterial obstruction
b. Blockage of subdermal lymphatics
c. Invasion of the skin with malignant cells
d. Secondary infection

Q57. The clinician was palpating with the tips of fingers, except the thumb, starting from 2 o'clock posteriorly, palpating at 3 points on the line joining the periphery to the nipple. Then again went to the 3 o'clock point directly and came back centripetally while palpating at 3 points again on the line joining the periphery and nipple. What is the method of breast examination depicted in the video? (AIIMS Nov 2018)

a. Vertical strip method
b. Concentric method
c. Dial of clock method
d. Quadrant method

Q58. Ipsilateral supraclavicular LNs are positive in a patient with CA breast. Stage is: (AIIMS Nov 2008)

a. II
b. IIIB
c. IIIC
d. IV

Q59. Breast cancer stage T4b involves all, *except*: (AIIMS May 2012)

a. Nipple retraction
b. skin ulcer over the swelling
c. Dermal edema
d. Satellite nodule

Q60. Which of the following stages of breast cancer corresponds with the following feature: Breast mass of 6 × 3 cm size with hard, mobile ipsilateral axillary lymph node and ipsilateral supraclavicular lymph node: (AIIMS June 2000)

a. T4N2M0
b. T1N0M1
c. T4N1M1
d. T3N3M0

Grade III	Most difficult

Q1. What is the sensitivity of axillary ultrasound is in identifying axillary metastases in clinically node-negative breast carcinoma? (AIIMS May 2017)

a. 55–60%
b. 30–40%
c. 20–30%
d. 10–20%

Q2. True about screening mammography. (PGI June 2004)

a. Indicated in 50–70 years of age
b. Mortality reduced by 30%
c. Radiation due to mammography can cause carcinoma
d. MRI is better than mammography
e. USG is better than mammography

Q3. All are indicators of malignancy in a mammography, *except*: (PGI Dec 1999)

a. Nodular calcification
b. Speckled margin
c. Attenuated architecture
d. Irregular mass

Q4. A 55-year-old postmenopausal woman, on hormone replacement therapy (HRT), presents with heaviness in both breasts. A screening mammogram reveals a high-density speculated mass with cluster of pleomorphic microcalcification and ipsilateral large axillary LNs. The mass described here most likely represents: (AIIMS Nov 2003)

a. Cystosarcoma phyllodes
b. Lymphoma
c. Fibroadenoma
d. Carcinoma

Q5. Breast carcinoma is seen in women who: (PGI June 2002)

a. Consume fatty food
b. Have early menopause
c. Smoke

d. Have multiple sex-partners
e. Did not breastfeed their children

Q6. Following are risk factors for breast cancer, *except*: (PGI Dec 1996)

a. Maternal grandmother had history
b. Paternal grandmother had history
c. Long term estrogen
d. Fat necrosis

Q7. BRCA-1 positive woman have _____ % increased risk of breast carcinoma: (JIPMER 2011)

a. 10 b. 20
c. 40 d. 60

Q8. Breast conservation surgery indicated in: (PGI Nov 2011)

a. Tumor size <4 cm
b. Central
c. Mobile
d. Pendulous breast
e. Diffuse microcalcification

Q9. A 43-year-old lady presents with a 5 cm lump in right breast with a 3 cm node in the supraclavicular fossa. Which of the following TNM stage she belongs to as per the latest American Joint Committee on Cancer (AJCC) stating system? (AIIMS June 2004)

a. T2N0M1 b. T1N0M1
c. T2N3M0 d. T2N2M0

Q10. Molecular classification of breast is based on: (AIIMS Nov 2014)

a. Gene expression profiling
b. Hormonal receptors and HER-2 status
c. Biochemical markers
d. Tumor size and nodal status

Q11. Breast cancer which is multicentric and bilateral: (AIIMS Feb 1997)

a. Ductal b. Lobular
c. Mucoid d. Colloid

Q12. In which of the following types of breast carcinoma, would you consider biopsy of opposite breast? (All India 2006)

a. Adenocarcinoma poorly differentiated
b. Medullary carcinoma
c. Lobular carcinoma
d. Comedo carcinoma

Q13. Use of tamoxifen for breast cancer can cause all of the following adverse effects, *except*: (AIIMS May 2011)

a. Thromboembolism
b. Endometrial carcinoma
c. Carcinoma in contralateral breast
d. Cataract

Q14. Carcinoma breast with high incidence of involving opposite breast is: (AIIMS Nov 1994)

a. Lobular carcinoma
b. Medullary carcinoma
c. Scirrhous adenocarcinoma
d. Atrophic scirrhous carcinoma

Q15. LN first involved in Ca breast is/are: (PGI Nov 2009)

a. Axillary LN
b. Internal mammary LN
c. Supraclavicular LN
d. Contralateral axillary LN

Q16. Malti, a 45-year-old female patient with a family H/O breast carcinoma, showed diffuse microcalcification on mammography. Intraductal carcinoma in situ was seen on biopsy. Most appropriate management is: (AIIMS June 2001)

a. Quadrantectomy
b. Radical mastectomy
c. Simple mastectomy
d. Chemotherapy

Q17. For breast cancer best chemotherapeutic regimen is: (PGI June 1996)

a. Cyclophosphamide, methotrexate, 5-fluorouracil
b. Methotrexate and cisplatin
c. Cisplatin, adriamycin, and steroid
d. Methotrexate, adriamycin, and steroid

Q18. A 30-year-old female presented with unilateral breast cancer associated with axillary LN enlargement. Modified radical mastectomy was done; further treatment plan will be: (AIIMS May 2007)

a. Observation and follow-up
b. Adriamycin-based chemotherapy followed by tamoxifen, depending on estrogen/progesterone receptor status
c. Adriamycin-based chemotherapy only
d. Tamoxifen only

Q19. Breast conservation surgery is not indicated: (PGI Dec 2002)

a. Large pendular breast
b. Systemic lupus erythematosus (SLE)
c. Diffuse microcalcification
d. Bilateral carcinoma
e. Family history

Q20. For breast cancer, the best chemotherapeutic regimen: (AIIMS Sep 1996)

a. Cyclophosphamide, methotrexate, 5-fluoronracil
b. Methotrexate and cisplatin
c. Cisplatin, adriamycin, and steroid
d. Methotrexate, adriamycin, and steroid

Q21. A 9-week pregnant woman comes with a 2.5 cm mass in the upper outer quadrant of the left breast. Ultrasound examination is normal. The next step in the management would be: (AIIMS May 2015)

a. Do mammography
b. Call the patient one month after delivery
c. Palpation-guided core biopsy
d. Aspiration and reassurance

Q22. A 65-year-old female presented with a H/O a painless breast lump of size 3 × 2 cm in the left upper quadrant with no palpable axillary lymph nodes. A FNAC was suggestive of ductal carcinoma in situ. A wide local excision of the tumor was done, and post-operative histopathology came out as invasive ductal carcinoma, high grade with necrosis, with 3 mm negative resection margins. What will be the adjuvant therapy required for this patient? (AIIMS May 2017)

a. Adjuvant chemotherapy
b. Adjuvant radiotherapy
c. Adjuvant radiochemotherapy
d. No additional treatment

Q23. A 36-year-old patient underwent breast conservation therapy and chemotherapy for a 1.5 × 1.2 cm ER-positive breast cancer with one positive axillary LN. She is now on tamoxifen. How will you follow up with the patient? (AIIMS May 2017)

a. Routine clinical examination 3 monthly in the first year with annual mammogram
b. Assessment of tumor markers 6-monthly
c. Annual bone scan
d. 6-monthly USG abdomen for liver metastasis.

Q24. On which of the following does the prognosis in male breast cancer depend? (AIIMS May 1995)

a. Duration of disease
b. Nipple discharge
c. Ulceration of nipple
d. LN status

Q25. The risk factors for increased incidence of relapse in stage I, carcinoma breast include all, *except*: (All India 1998)

a. Negative estrogen/progesterone receptor status
b. High "s" phase
c. Aneuploidy
d. Decreased Her-2/neu oncogene

Q26. In cases of breast cancer with HER-2 neu amplification, when will you do FISH? (AIIMS Nov 2017)

a. HER-2 neu 1+
b. HER-2 neu 2+
c. Irrespective of HER-2 neu
d. HER-2 neu 3+

Q27. The oncotype Dx test is done for the following in breast cancer: (AIIMS May 2015)

a. Hormone therapy in hormone receptor positive
b. Chemotherapy in hormone receptor positive patients
c. Chemotherapy in hormone receptor negative patients
d. Herceptin in HER2+ve

Q28. True regarding male breast cancer: (PGI June 2009)

a. Invasive lobular carcinoma in the most common type
b. Estrogen receptor positive
c. Paget's disease of the nipple is more common in men than women
d. Undescended testes are a risk factor
e. H/O gynecomastia may be present

Q29. Treatment of cystosarcoma phyllodes in a young woman: (JIPMER 2011)

a. Wide excision with a margin
b. Wide excision with chemotherapy
c. Wide excision with radiotherapy
d. MRM

Q30. Treatment of choice in duct papilloma of the breast is: (All India 1998)

a. Simple mastectomy
b. Microdochectomy
c. Local wide excision
d. Chemotherapy

Q31. A 14-year-old healthy girl of normal height and weight for age complains that her right breast has developed twice the size of her left breast since the onset of puberty at the age of 12 years. Both breasts have a similar consistency on palpation with normal nipple areolae. The most likely cause for these findings is: (AIIMS Nov 2003)

a. Cystosarcoma phyllodes
b. Virginal hypertrophy
c. Fibrocystic disease
d. Early state of carcinoma

Q32. A 25-year-old lady presents with spontaneous nipple discharge of 3 months duration. On examination, the discharge is bloody and from a single duct. The following statements about the management of this patient are true *except*: (AIIMS Nov 2004)

a. Ultrasound can be a useful investigation
b. Radical duct excision is the operation of choice
c. Galactogram, though useful, is not essential
d. Majority of blood-stained-nipple discharges are due to papillomas or other benign condition

Q33. The tumor, which may occur in the residual breast or overlying skin following wide local excision and radiotherapy for mammary carcinoma, is: (All India 2006)

a. Leiomyosarcoma
b. Squamous cell carcinoma
c. Basal cell carcinoma
d. Angiosarcoma

Q34. Not a poor prognostic factor in breast carcinoma: (PGI May 2011)

a. HER-2-neu positive
b. Progesterone receptor positive
c. Extranodal metastasis
d. Vascularity of the tumor
e. ER positive

Q35. A patient underwent sentinel node biopsy for the treatment of breast carcinoma. Which of the following nerves is likely to be injured during this procedure? (AIIMS May 2013)

a. Intercostobrachial nerve
b. Nerve to latissimus dorsi
c. Nerve to the serratus anterior
d. Lateral pectoral nerve

Q36. Retromammary abscess arises from: (JIPMER 1986)

a. Tuberculous rib
b. Infected hematoma
c. Chronic empyema
d. All of the above

Q37. True statement(s) about nipple discharge is/are: (PGI June 2004)

a. Mammography
b. Cone excision done in a single intraductal tumor
c. Mammography is done when the duct papilloma is <4.5 cm
d. Red discharge indicates malignancy
e. Blue-black discharge indicates duct ectasia

Q38. A 45-year-old woman presents with a hard and mobile lump in the breast. Next investigation is: (All India 2001)

a. FNAC
b. USG
c. Mammography
d. Excision biopsy

Q39. A 60-year-old lady comes with blood-stained discharge from the nipple with family H/O breast cancer. Next best step for her will be: (AIIMS May 2015)

a. Ductoscopy
b. Sonomammogram
c. Nipple discharge cytology
d. MRI

Q40. In case of breast cancer most important prognostic factor is: (AIIMS Nov 1996)

a. Size of tumor
b. LN status
c. Presence of estrogen receptor
d. Age of menopause

Q41. The risk factors for increased incidence of relapse in stage I carcinoma breast include all, *except*: (All India 1998)

a. Negative estrogen/progesterone receptor status
b. High "S" phase
c. Aneuploidy
d. Decreased HER-2-neu oncogene

Q42. In breast cancer following are expressed: (PGI Dec 2007)

a. Her-2-neu
b. p53
c. BRCA-1
d. BCL-1
e. CEA

Q43. The most important prognostic factor in breast carcinoma is: (All India 2006)
a. Histological grade of the tumor
b. Stage of the tumor at the time of diagnosis
c. Status of estrogen and progesterone receptors
d. Overexpression of the p53 tumor suppressor gene

Q44. All of the following are used for the reconstruction of the breast, *except*: (AIIMS Nov 2000)
a. Transverse rectus abdominis myocutaneous flap
b. Latissimus dorsi myocutaneous flap
c. Pectoralis major myocutaneous flap
d. Transversus rectus abdominis free flap

Q45. Not true about breast cancer in India: (AIIMS June 1998)
a. Incidence is 20/1,00,000
b. Average age 42 years
c. Positive family history is a risk factor
d. More common in Muslims

Q46. True regarding male breast cancer: (PGI June 2009)
a. MC (most common) lobular type
b. Estrogen receptor positive
c. H/O gynecomastia may be present
d. Paget's disease of the nipple is more common in males than females
e. Undescended testis is a risk factor

Q47. A 43-year-old lady presents with a 5 cm lump in the right breast with a 3 cm node in the supraclavicular fossa. Which of the following TNM stages does she belong to as per the latest AJCC staging system? (AIIMS June 2004)
a. T2N0M1 b. T1N0M1
c. T2N3M0 d. T2N2M0

Q48. True about the treatment of early breast cancer. (AIIMS May 2008)
a. Aromatase inhibitors are replacing tamoxifen in premenopausal women
b. Postmastectomy radiation therapy is given when four or more LNs are positive
c. Tamoxifen is not useful in postmenopausal women
d. In premenopausal women, multidrug chemotherapy is given in selected patients

Q49. A 50-year-old female has undergone a mastectomy for breast cancer. After a mastectomy patient is not able to extend, adduct, and internally rotate the arm. Now, supply to which of the following muscles is damaged? (AIIMS May 2012)
a. Pectoralis major b. Teres minor
c. Latissimus dorsi d. Long head of triceps

Q50. A 40-year-old female with a 2 cm nodule in the base and a proven metastatic node in the axilla, treatment is: (PGI 1996)
a. Quadrantectomy
b. Mastectomy with local radiotherapy
c. Patey's with adjuvant chemotherapy
d. Halsted's operation with tamoxifen

Q51. Mondor's disease is: (MCI June 2018)
a. Thrombophlebitis of the superficial veins of the breast
b. Carcinoma of the breast
c. Premalignant condition of the breast
d. Filariasis of the breast

Q52. Oncotype Dx test is done to for the following in breast cancer: (AIIMS May 2015)
a. Chemotherapy in hormone receptor-positive patients
b. Hormone therapy in hormone-positive
c. Chemotherapy in hormone receptor negative patients
d. Herceptin in HER-2-neu positive

Q53. A 50-year-old lady presented with a lump in the left breast, which had developed suddenly in weeks. Perimenstrual symptoms are present. No associated family history. On examination, the lump is well circumscribed, fluctuant, and 1.5 cm oval in shape. Most likely diagnosis: (JIPMER May 2018)
a. Breast cyst b. Galactocele
c. Fibroadenoma d. Breast cancer

Q54. Cystosarcoma phyllodes is treated by: (AIIMS May 1993)
a. Simple mastectomy
b. Radical mastectomy
c. Modified radical mastectomy
d. Antibiotic with conservative treatment

Q55. Premenstrual fullness in the breast in a 21-year-old unmarried female is: (AIIMS 1998)
a. Galactocele b. Fibroadenoma
c. Fibroadenosis d. Breast cancer

Q56. Regarding cystic disease of the breast, which one is true? (AIIMS Nov 1997)

a. Common in 25 years of age
b. Excision is the treatment
c. May turn into malignant
d. Aspiration is the treatment

Q57. Lymphatic drainage of breast: (PGI Dec 2003)

a. Axillary
b. Supraclavicular
c. Internal mammary
d. Mediastinal
e. Celiac

Q58. True about galactorrhea: (PGI Dec 2008)

a. Always bilateral
b. Found in pregnancy and lactation
c. Associated with prolactinoma and other endocrinopathies
d. Surgery is done
e. Hypothyroidism can cause galactorrhea

Q59. Large breast is not seen in: (AIIMS Dec 1995)

a. Filariasis
b. Giant fibroadenoma
c. Cystosarcoma phyllodes
d. Scirrhous carcinoma

Q60. A 14-year-old healthy girl of normal height and weight for age complains that her right breast has developed twice the size of her left breast since the onset of puberty at the age of 12. Both breasts have a similar consistency on palpation with normal nipple areolae. The most likely cause for these findings is: (AIIMS Nov 2003)

a. Cystosarcoma phyllodes
b. Virginal hypertrophy
c. Fibrocystic disease
d. Early stage of carcinoma

ANSWERS

Grade I: 1. d; 2. d (Schwartz 10/e p527); 3. d; 4. b; 5. a; 6. a, c, d; 7. c (Bailey 27/e p861, 26/e p799); 8. b; 9. c; 10. e; 11. d; 12. a; 13. a (Sabiston 20/e p831, 19/e p834); 14. a, c, d, e (Schwartz 10/e p511-512); 15. a (Robbins 9/e p1069); 16. b, d; 17. d; 18. a, c; 19. d (Schwartz 10/e p514-515); 20. None; 21. c; 22. d (Sabiston 20/e p832); 23. a, b (Bailey 27/e p873); 24. a; 25. a, b; 26. None; 27. a, b, c, e (Schwartz 9/e p438); 28. b (Bailey 27/e p873); 29. b, c, e; 30. a, b, c, d (Bailey 27/e p873); 31. b (Sabiston 20/e p843); 32. d; 33. c; 34. b; 35. a; 36. c; 37. a, b; 38. c; 39. a (Bailey 27/e p876); 40. c; 41. d (Schwartz 9/e p461); 42. b; 43. a, b, c (Sabiston 20/e p857-858); 44. c (Bailey 27/e p879); 45. a, b; 46. c (Bailey 27/e p877); 47. a, b, c, d (Schwartz 10/e p547); 48. b; 49. a (Bailey 27/e p872); 50. b; 51. c; 52. b; 53. d; 54. d (Harrison 19/e p526); 55. c (Schwartz 9/e p453)

Grade II: 1. d; 2. a; 3. c (Sabiston 20/e p840); 4. c; 5. b; 6. c; 7. a; 8. d; 9. a; 10. b, e; 11. a; 12. a; 13. a; 14. a, c (Sabiston 20/e p840); 15. d; 16. a, c, e (Schwartz 10/e p535-536); 17. c; 18. b, e; 19. All; 20. c; 21. a, b, d, e; 22. a, c; 23. b, e; 24. c; 25. (Schwartz 10/e p555); 26. a (Sabiston 20/e p841-842); 27. b; 28. a, b, c; 29. a; 30. b; 31. c (Bailey 27/e p870); 32. c (Schwartz 10/e p505-506); 33. a (Sabiston 20/e p824); 34. a, b; 35. a (Harrison 20/e 92676, 19/e p2267); 36. a, b, c (Bailey 27/e p873); 37. d; 38. a, b; 39. b; 40. d; 41. a; 42. a, b, c; 43. b; 44. b; 45. b (Grainger 5/e p1190, 1188); 46. b; 47. a; 48. b, d; 49. a; 50. b; 51. c; 52. c; 53. d; 54. b; 55. d; 56. b; 57. c; 58. c; 59. a; 60. d

Grade III: 1. a; 2. a, b; 3. a; 4. d; 5. a; 6. c, d; 7. d; 8. a, c; 9. c; 10. a; 11. b; 12. c; 13. c; 14. a; 15. a > b; 16. c; 17. a; 18. b; 19. a, b, c; 20. a; 21. c; 22. b; 23. a; 24. d; 25. d; 26. b; 27. b; 28. b; 29. a; 30. b; 31. b; 32. b; 33. d; 34. b, e; 35. a; 36 d; 37. a, b, d, e; 38. c; 39. d; 40. b; 41. d; 42. a, b, c, e; 43. b; 44. c; 45. d; 46. b, c, e; 47. c; 48. b; 49. c; 50. b; 51. a (Bailey 27/e p867); 52. a; 53. a; 54. a; 55. c (Schwartz 10/e p507); 56. d (Bailey 27/e p869); 57. a, b, c; 58. c, d, e (Harrison 20/e p2676); 59. d (Norman Brous/e p277); 60. b (CPDT 16/e p1128)

MODEL QUESTIONS

Q1. With reference to mammography, which one of the following statements is correct?

a. A baseline study should be done for all women at age 30 years
b. It uses less radiation energy than a chest X-ray
c. It should be part of the regular follow-up of a woman following therapy for unilateral breast cancer
d. It provides an effective substitute for biopsy of suspicious lesions

Ans. c

Q2. In a mammogram, all of the following are features of breast carcinoma, *except*:

a. A solid lesion with ill defined edge or stellate configuration
b. True microcalcification
c. Areas of macrocalcification
d. Increased skin thickness

Ans. c

Q3. A patient with a 1.2 cm breast lump with three lymph nodes in the axilla with no metastasis is in which stage as per AJCC?

a. T1N0M0
b. T1bN1bM0
c. T1cN1bM0
d. T2N1cM0

Ans. c

Q4. In which of the following types of breast carcinoma, comedo growth pattern is seen?

a. Ductal carcinoma in-situ
b. Medullary carcinoma
c. Lobular carcinoma in-situ
d. Infiltrating lobular carcinoma

Ans. a

Q5. Treatment of hormone-dependent fungating carcinoma of the breast with secondaries in the lung in a female patient aged 30 years is:

a. Simple mastectomy followed by oophorectomy
b. Radical mastectomy followed by oophorectomy
c. Adrenalectomy
d. Lumpectomy followed by castration

Ans. b

Q6. A 50-year-old woman complains of intermittent bleeding from the left nipple over the past 3 months. No mass is palpable, but a bead of blood can be expressed from the nipple. The ideal procedure in this case would be:

a. Cytological examination of discharge, and if no malignant cells, to be kept under careful observation.
b. Segmental excision of the breast
c. Microdochectomy
d. Simple mastectomy

Ans. c

Q7. Which one of the following familial carrier syndromes is associated with a mutation in the *BRCA* genes?

a. Hereditary nonpolyposis colorectal cancer
b. Von Hippel–Lindau disease
c. Peutz–Jeghers syndrome
d. Familial breast/ovarian cancer

Ans. d

Q8. Which of the following statements is fully true?

a. Paget's disease of the nipple is a type of breast cancer with prominent Paget cells and presence of S-100 Ag immunostaining
b. *BRCA*1 and 2 gene mutations cause breast cancer and are passed from mother to daughter by mitochondrial inheritance
c. Raloxifene is an SERM that prevents breast cancer but increases the risk of endometrial cancer
d. Lobular carcinoma in situ arises from the epithelial lining of the minor ducts, and 10% occur in males

Ans. c

Q9. True about male breast cancer is all, *except*:

a. <2% of all cases of breast cancer
b. Most commonly, it is infiltrating duct carcinoma
c. Most commonly, it is infiltrating lobular carcinoma
d. Exocrine or endocrine estrogen exposure can predispose to it

Ans. c

Q10. Mondor's disease is superficial thrombophlebitis of:

a. Axillary vein
b. Long saphenous vein
c. Veins of the breast
d. Internal mammary vein

Ans. c

Q11. Treatment of duct ectasia:

a. Hadfield's operation
b. Patey's mastectomy
c. Modified radical mastectomy
d. Radical mastectomy

Ans. a

Q12. Consider the following statements regarding Paget's disease of the breast:

1. It is a malignant disease
2. Diagnosis can be established by scrape cytology
3. Lymph node involvement is an associated clinical feature
4. The treatment of choice is a simple mastectomy

Which of the statements given above is/are correct?

a. 1, 2, and 4 only
b. 1, 2, and 3 only
c. 3 and 4 only
d. 1, 2, 3, and 4

Ans. d

Q13. Sign seen in a large duct papilloma is:

a. Nipple discharge
b. Breast mass
c. Skin excoriation
d. LN involvement

Ans. a

Q14. Which does not have an underlying malignancy?

a. Paget's disease of bone
b. Paget's disease of the nipple
c. Paget's disease of the vulva
d. Paget's disease of anal region

Ans. a

Q15. Unilateral amastia is associated 90% of the time with the absence or hypoplasia of the following muscle:

a. Latissimus doris
b. Subclavian
c. Pectoral
d. Serratus anterior

Ans. c

SUGGESTED READING

1. Bailey & Love's - Short Practice of Surgery, 27th edition.
2. Dupont WD, Rogers LW, Vander Z, Waag R, Page DL. The epidemiologic study of anatomic markers for increased risk of mammary cancer. Pathol Res Pract. 1980; 166(4):471-80.
3. Ghozale A. Breast fibrocystic change and Page's classification. Journal of Medical Sciences. 2023;55(4).
4. Gould E, Winship T, Philbin PH, Kerr HH. Observations on a "sentinel node" in cancer of the parotid cancer. 1960;13:77-8.
5. Hartmann LC, Sellers TA, Frost MH, Lingle WL, Dengnim AC, Ghosh K, et al. Benign breast disease and the risk of breast cancer. N Engl J Med. 2005;353(3):229-37.
6. In: Rinaldi RM, Sapra A, Bellin LS (Eds). Breast lymphatics. Treasure Island (FL): Statlearls Publishing; 2024.
7. In: Williams NS, O'Connell AR, McCaskie AW (Eds). Bailey and Love's Short Practice of Surgery, 27th edition. New Delhi: CRC Press; 2018. pp. 870-1.
8. Jasmen JO, David Schiff. Metastatic Disease and the nervous system. In: Jasmen JO, David Schiff (Eds). Aminoff's Neurology and General Medicine, 5th edition. Amsterdam: Elsevier; 2014.
9. Johns Hopkins Medicine: The Four Founding Professors. Archived from the original on March 10, 2015.
10. LandB, p877.
11. Pacifici S, Niknyad M, Bell D. (2023). Axillary lymph nodes. [Online] Avaialble from https://radiopaedia.org/articles/axillary-lymph-nodes-1 [Last accessed May, 2025].
12. Schwartz's Principles of Surgery, 18th edition.
13. Textbook of Surgery by David Sabiston, 21st edition.
14. The American Society of Breast Surgeons website. Position statement on screening mammography, 2019.

SECTION 6

Endocrine

CHAPTER 28

Thyroid

"I saw a woman wearing a sweatshirt with Guess on it. I said, Thyroid problem?"
- Arnold Schwarzenegger

INTRODUCTION

The thyroid gland is a butterfly-shaped gland. The thyroid gland is situated in front of the neck, weighing 20–25 g. The functioning unit is the lobule of the thyroid gland, lined with cuboidal epithelium, having thyroglobulin stored as colloid in it.

EMBRYOLOGY

The thyroglossal duct, a tubular structure, descends down from the median bud of the pharynx from the foramen caecum, starting at the junction of the anterior two-thirds and the posterior one-third of the tongue. It divides into two branches, developing thyroid lobes which unite with the structures arising from the fourth pharyngeal pouch. Parafollicular cells (c-cells) are derived from the neural crest. Parathyroid glands develop from the third and fourth pharyngeal pouches. The thymus also develops from the third pharyngeal pouch **(Figs. 1 and 2)**.

The thyroid gland is connected with the thyroglossal duct, which descends down from the cecum and later obliterates.

ANATOMY OF THE THYROID GLAND

The thyroid gland is closely related with the *parathyroid glands and recurrent laryngeal nerves (RLNs).*

The thyroid gland is a highly vascular structure. *The thyroid gland is supplied by the superior thyroid artery*

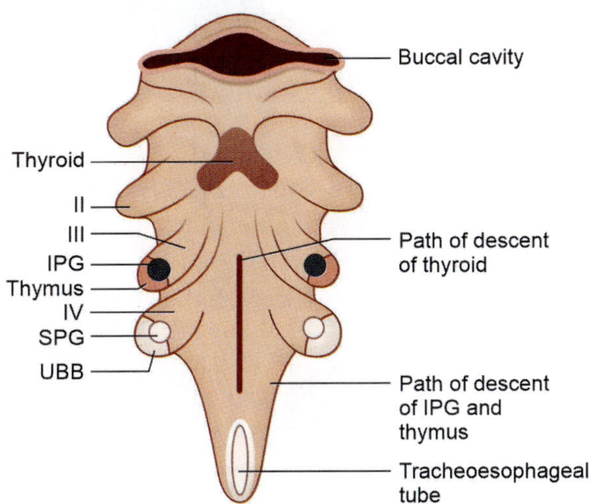

Fig. 1: Development of thyroid and parathyroid glands. (IPG: inferior parathyroid gland; SPG: superior parathyroid gland; UBB: ultimobranchial body)

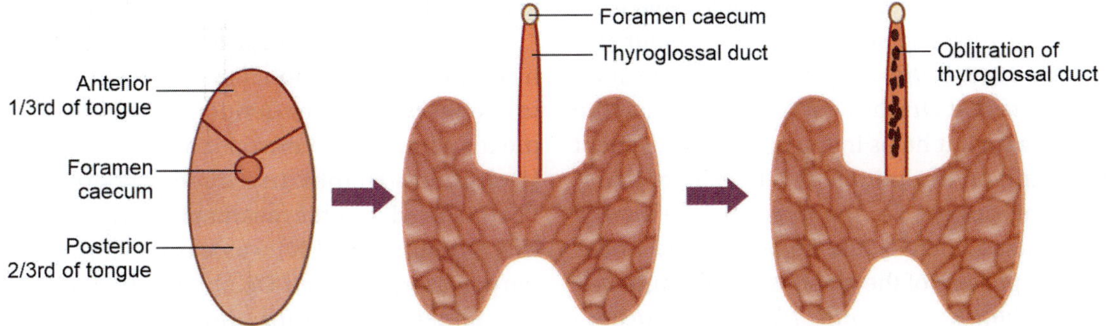

Fig. 2: Thyroglossal duct, foramen cecum and thyroid gland.

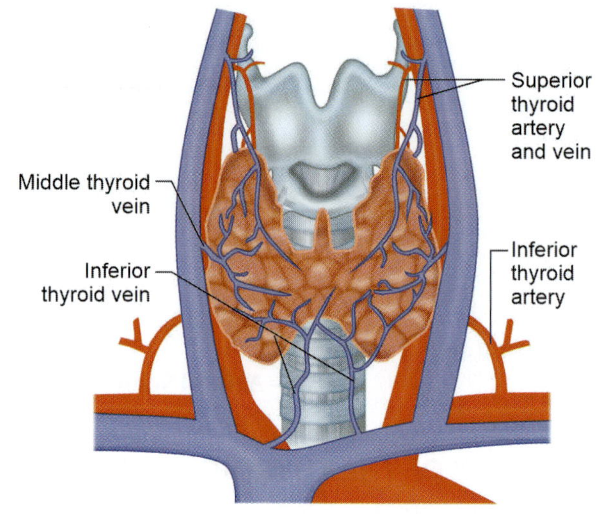

Fig. 3: Blood supply of the thyroid gland.

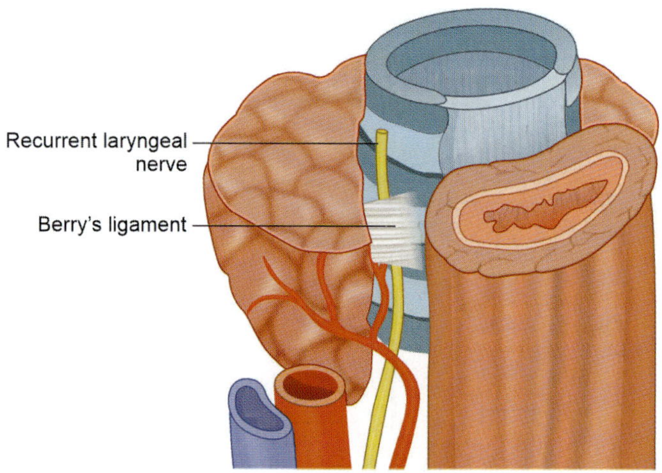

Fig. 4: Berry's ligament.

(STA), a branch of the external carotid artery, and the inferior thyroid artery (ITA), a branch of the thyrocervical trunk from the subclavian artery. ITA also supplies 4 parathyroid glands. Rarely is an *artery thyroidea ima from the arch of the aorta* is also seen. *Berry's ligament (Sir James Berry, 1860-1946, British Surgeon)* is a condensation of pretracheal fascia that attaches the thyroid gland to the trachea **(Figs. 3 and 4)**. It helps in the upward movement of the thyroid gland on deglutition. It is the site of injury to the nerve during surgery. During surgery of the thyroid lobe, when mobilized laterally, the nerve is found under the posterolateral portion of the gland called the tubercle of *Zuckerkandl (Emil Zuckerkandl, 1849-1901, Austro-Hungarian Anatomist)* **(Fig. 5)**.

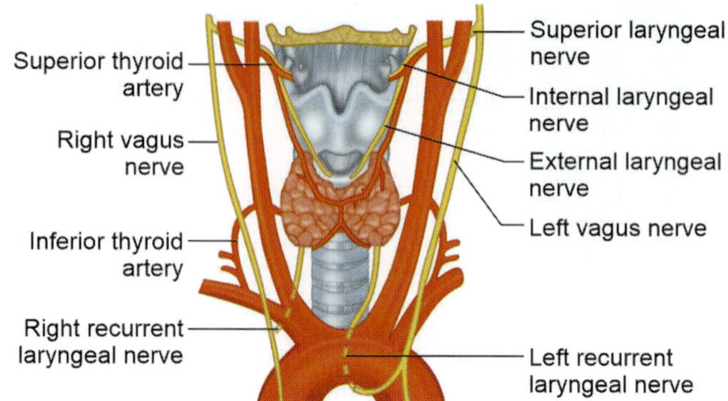

Fig. 5: Nerve supply of thyroid gland.

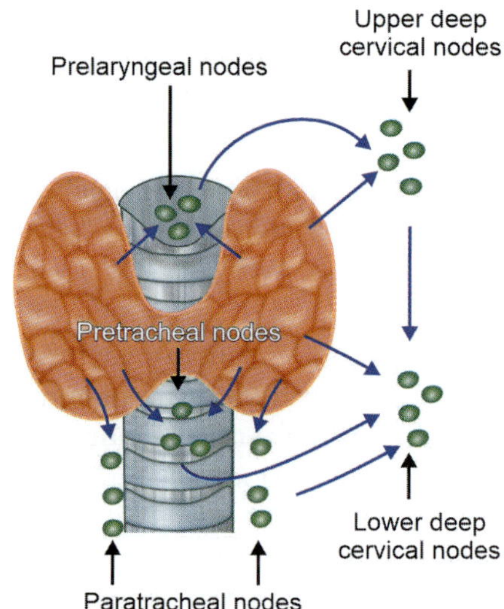

Fig. 6: Lymphatic drainage of the thyroid gland.

Superior thyroid vein (STV) drains into the *internal jugular vein (IJV). Inferior thyroid vein (ITV)* drains into the brachiocephalic vein. *The middle thyroid vein (MTV)* drains into IJV was observed in only 30% of cases. Sometimes a fourth vein, Kocher's vein drains into the IJV. It is the first vessel ligated during (surgery a lobectomy or thyroidectomy).

The lymphatic drainage of the thyroid depends upon its heavy network of lymphatics. Some lymph directly passes to deep cervical nodes *(levels II, III, IV and V)*, subcapsular plexus drains to central compartment juxtathyroid (Delphian—Delphi in Greece where snake women Phythia used to utter meaningless words to create magic, this lymph node (LN) was earlier thought of uncertain purpose and so called Delphian) and paratracheal nodes and nodes on superior and ITVs (level VI), ultimately lymph goes to mediastinal LNs (level VII) **(Fig. 6)**.

Note: Earlier it was a practice to ligate superior thyroid artery near upper pole of the gland to avoid injury to external laryngeal nerve and to ligate ITA away from gland to avoid injury to right laryngeal nerve, but nowadays it has been observed and found in various researches that if we ligate both superior thyroid artery and ITA close to thyroid gland it prevents development of hypocalcemia due to injury to parathyroid gland or its blood supply.

THYROID GLAND AND VAGUS NERVES

The right vagus nerve gives the *right recurrent laryngeal (RRL)* nerve, which hooks around the subclavian artery. The *left recurrent laryngeal (LRL)* arises from the left vagus nerve and hooks around the arch of the aorta. RRL supplies the intrinsic muscles of the larynx except the cricothyroid muscle. Its paralysis leads to hoarseness of voice if unilateral and stridor and dyspnea if bilateral. In 2% of cases, the nerves on the right are nonrecurrent. *RLN* can be found in the tracheoesophageal groove at the site of *Beahrs (Oliver H Beahrs, 1914-2006, American Surgeon) triangle (the other two sites are the carotid artery and ITA). It is also called as RLN triangle. Importance: During the operation of the thyroid gland, it helps to locate the RLN. Boundaries of Beahrs triangle—lateral—common carotid artery (CCA), superomedial—RLN, and inferomedial—ITA. Superior laryngeal* nerve, also a branch of vagus nerve, gives the *external and internal laryngeal nerves. The external laryngeal nerve* supplies the cricothyroid muscle of the vocal cord, and the *internal laryngeal nerve* supplies the mucous membrane above the vocal cord. The paralysis of the external laryngeal nerve leads to loss of timbre of voice and huskiness. Internal laryngeal nerve paralysis causes nocturnal cough and aspiration **(Figs. 7 and 8)**.

PHYSIOLOGY OF THYROID

Thyroid hormones tri-iodothyronine (T_3) and L-thyroixine (T_4) are attached with thyroglobulin and contained in colloid. The thyroid hormone complex formation happens in the following processes:

- Trapping of inorganic iodine
- Oxidation of iodide to iodine
- Binding of tyrosine with iodine to form iodotyrosine
- Coupling of mono and diiodotyrosines to form T_3 and T_4.

Whenever thyroid hormones are required the complex is broken and thyroglobulin is liberated and broken down to T_3 and T_4. Unbound free T_4 and T_3 are responsible for the metabolic effects of thyroid hormones. T_3 is more important, it is quick acting (within hours) than T_4 (4–14 days).

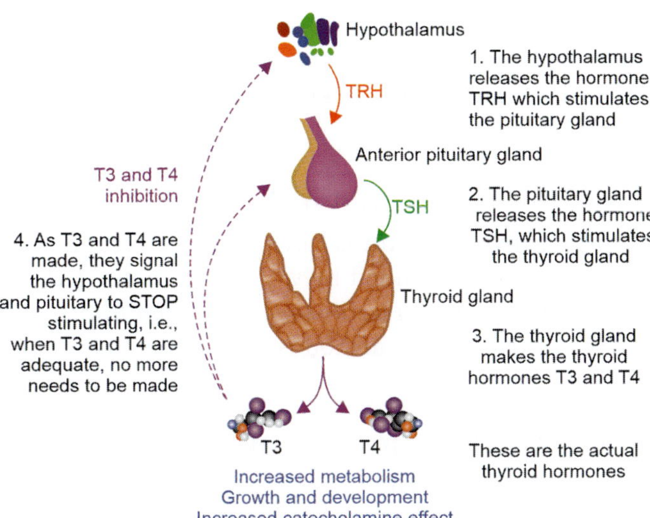

Fig. 7: Thyroid physiology. (TRH: thyrotropin-releasing hormone; TSH: thyroid-stimulating hormone)

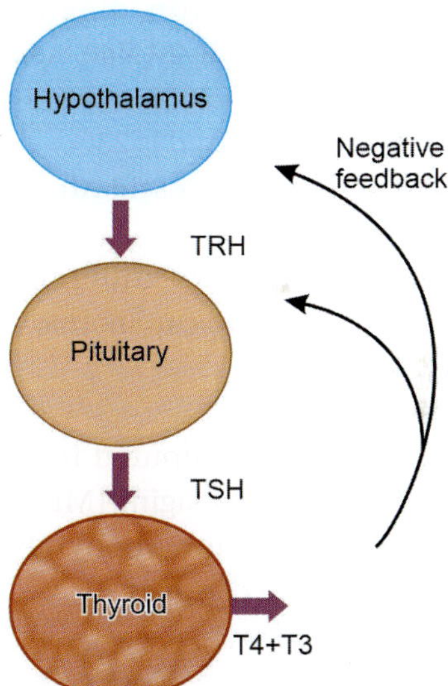

Fig. 8: Thyroid physiology, T3, T4. (TRH: thyrotropin-releasing hormone; TSH: thyroid-stimulating hormone)

CALCITONIN

Calcitonin is produced by parafollicular C-cells, which are of neuroendocrine origin.

PITUITARY-THYROID AXIS

Thyroid-stimulating hormone (TSH) controls the synthesis and release of thyroid hormones from the thyroid gland. TSH is secreted from the anterior pituitary gland. TSH secretion depends upon the amount of circulating thyroid hormones through a negative feedback. TSH secretion is controlled.

Thyrotropin-releasing hormone (TRH) is released from hypothalamus. *Thyroid antibodies are* Thyroid peroxidase antibodies (TPOAb) and Thyroglobulin antibodies (TgAb).

METHODS OF EXAMINATION

A normal thyroid gland is not palpable or cannot be seen. It can be examined by various methods, *Lahey's method (from back), Pizzillo's method (from front), and Crile's method.* Crile's method is a good way to examine nodules.

INVESTIGATIONS FOR THE THYROID GLAND

- *Thyroid function test (TFT)*—TSH, T3, and T4.
- *Fine needle aspiration cytology (FNAC) [ultrasound (USG)-guided]—Royal College of Pathology (RCP) classification:* Thy1 (Non-diagnostic), Thy1c (Nondiagnostic cystic), Thy2 (Non-neoplastic), Thy3 (Follicular), Thy4 (Suspicious of malignancy), Thy5 (Malignant). The needle used is 23G.
  - *Advantages*—best investigations for thyroid swelling
  - *Disadvantages*—cannot differentiate between follicular adenoma and carcinoma.
- Serum calcium
- Serum calcitonin
- Imaging—X-ray chest, computed tomography (CT), and magnetic resonance imaging (MRI).
- A positron emission tomography (PET) scan has limited value in thyroid diseases.
  - *Indications*
    - *Retrosternal goiter*
    - *Large malignant tumor*
- *Isotope scanning—by low-dose radio-labeled iodine (^{123}I) or technetium (^{99m}Tc). (Half life of I^{123} is 1 hour—I^{131} is 8 days, and I^{132} is 2–3 hours).*
  - *Indications*
    - Low TSH with hyperthyroidism
    - Ectopic thyroid lesion
- Ultrasonography
- It can differentiate between benign and malignant tumors **(Table 1)**.
- Laryngoscopy—preoperatively done to check vocal cord movements.
- Core biopsy—rarely done due to the risk of hemorrhage.

TABLE 1: Difference between benign and malignant lumps.

Benign	Malignant
Hyperechoic	Hypoechoic
Macrocalcification	Microcalcification
Margins not infiltrated	Infiltrated
Lymph nodes—kidney-shaped	Round
Vascularity—normal	Increased

THYROID IMAGING REPORTING AND DATA SYSTEMS SCORING

TR1 (benign), *TR2* (not suspicious), *TR3* (mildly suspicious), *TR4* (moderately suspicious), *TR5* (highly suspicious). FNAC is not required in TR1 and TR2.

It is based on Mn = MESC: M = Margin, E = Echogenicity, S = Shape, C = Composites.

THYROID GLAND SWELLINGS

Thyroid gland enlargement is called goiter (Gutter = the throat, in Latin).

- Simple goiter—diffuse, physiological in puberty and pregnancy.
- Toxic nodular goiter—diffuse, *Graves (Robert James Graves, 1796-1853, British Physician, discovered in 1835)* disease, multinodular, and adenoma.
- Neoplastic—benign and malignant
- Inflammatory thyroid gland—autoimmune [Hashimoto's (Hakaru Hashimoto, 1881-1934, Japanese physician) disease], granulomatous *[De Quervain's (Friedrich Joseph De Quervain, 1868-1940, Swiss Surgeon, described in 1902) thyroiditis], fibrosing [Riedel's (Bernhard Moritz Carl Ludwig Riedel, 1846-1916, German Surgeon, described in 1896)* thyroiditis], infective (acute) viral or bacterial or chronic (tubercular) and amyloid. A retrosternal goiter is called only when >50% of thyroid tissue is below the thoracic cage opening.

SIMPLE GOITER

It is caused by stimulation of the thyroid gland by TSH due to inappropriate secretion from a microadenoma of the anterior pituitary (rare) or in response to a longstanding low level of blood thyroid hormone. The most common cause is dietary deficiency of iodine. We require 0.1–0.15 mg of iodine per day. Endemic goiters are found in endemic areas like mountainous ranges such as the Himalayas and the Rocky Mountains. Enzymic deficiencies may cause sporadic goiters.

GOITROGENS

Certain substances are called goitrogens as they can cause goiter:

- Vegetables of the Brassica family, such as cabbage.
- Para-aminosalicylic acid
- Antithyroid drugs

How is a goiter formed?

Continuous growth stimulation of the thyroid gland causes diffuse hyperplasia, and as a result of irregular stimulation, a mixed effect occurs, leading to active and inactive lobules. Active lobules become more vascular and hyperplastic, whereas necrotic lobules unite to form nodules filled with colloid. Prolonged recurrence of this process leads to nodular goiter.

THYROGLOSSAL CYST

It is a cystic swelling in the midline that moves with deglutition and protrusion of the tongue. The thyroglossal tract is persistent. The most common site is subhyoid, but it can occur anywhere along the path of the thyroglossal duct (from the base of the tongue to the suprasternal notch).

- Investigation—FNAC
- *Treatment:* Sistrunk operation (removal of cyst + part of hyoid bone along with tract till the base of tongue).

Complications

- Infection
- Thyroglossal fistula
- Papillary thyroid cancer (PTC)

LINGUAL THYROID

It is a lump below the tongue made of undescended thyroid tissue at the foramen cecum.

Investigation

- FNAC—thyroid tissue
- USG to confirm normal thyroid gland, as lingual thyroid may be the only thyroid tissue, and its removal unknowingly may lead to permanent hypothyroidism.

Treatment

Excision

Fistula

- *Branchial fistula:* It is either congenital or acquired on the lateral side of the neck along the sternomastoid muscle.
- *Thyroglossal fistula:* It is an acquired fistula in the midline.

THYROID GLAND NEOPLASMS

- Benign follicular adenoma
- *Malignant:*
  - Primary—follicular, papillary, anaplastic, medullary (parafollicular cells), and lymphoma.
  - Secondary—metastatic and local infiltration

The most common factor responsible for thyroid cancer is radiation under the age of 5 years.

Clinical Features

It is three times more common in females than males. The incidence of papillary carcinoma is increasing due to increasing diagnostic imaging techniques. Anaplastic carcinoma has a poor prognosis. Thyroid swelling and enlarged cervical LNS are common. RLN *paralysis shows advanced cancer.*

PAPILLARY THYROID CARCINOMA

It is the most common thyroid cancer, arising from differentiated follicular epithelium. It has a large number of occult micrometastases, and a patient may live normally with an undetected disease. It is more common in males, 3:1. It has the best prognosis among thyroid cancers. Radiation exposure in childhood can cause papillary carcinoma of the thyroid gland in adult life.

- *Common age*—20–60 years
- *Risk factors*, Mn = FRO [Family history of (H/O), radiation exposure, and obesity]
- *Genes:* BRAF (M/C), glial-derived neurotrophic factor (GDNF), RET
- *Multicentric*
- *Metastasis*
  - Lymphatic (the first LN involved is the Delphian LN).
  - Hematogenous—Most common lungs

MULTIPLE ENDOCRINE NEOPLASIA SYNDROME

- *Multiple endocrine neoplasia type 1 (MEN1) (Wermer syndrome):* It is due to changes in ChII. The tumors seen with MEN1 are parathyroid adenoma, pituitary adenoma and pancreatic endocrine tumors, thymic tumors, adrenocortical tumors, and collagenoma.
- *MEN2:* It is due to Ch10, MEN2a (Sipple syndrome—parathyroid adenoma, pheochromocytoma, and megacolon) MEN2b (MEN3 syndrome—Marfanoid features, neuromas, and corneal fibers involvement and megacolon).
- *MEN4 syndrome:* Pituitary and parathyroid adenomas, regional tumors, adrenocortical tumors, and reproductive organ tumors.

Syndromes associated with thyroid cancer:
- Cowden syndrome
- Carney complex
- Batman's syndrome
- Familial PTC
- Familial nonmedullary thyroid carcinoma (non-MTC)

THYROTOXICOSIS (HYPERTHYROIDISM)

It is a condition developed by overproduction of thyroid hormone, thyroxine.

It is of the following types:
- Diffuse thyroid toxic goiter called Graves' disease.
- *Solitary:* Toxic nodule of the thyroid gland
- Toxic multinodular goiter
- Plummer's (Henry Plummer, American physician described in 1913) disease—affects many organs due to the development of hyperthyroidism.
- Factitious hyperthyroidism—due to high intake of thyroxine.
- Jod-Basedow (Carl Adolph von Jod-Basedow, German physician) phenomenon—iodine-induced hyperthyroidism.
- Pituitary adenoma—secreting TSH.
- Struma (River Struma along mountains in Bulgaria, goiter develops in people living along this river) ovarii—ectopic thyroid tissue in the ovary.

Clinical Features of Thyrotoxicosis

Mn = PITH LOAD
- *P* = Palpitation (tachycardia)
- *I* = Irritability
- *T* = Tremors
- *H* = Heat intolerance
- *L* = Loss of weight
- *O* = Oligomenorrhea
- *A* = Anxiety and nervousness
- *D* = Diarrhea

Treatment of Thyrotoxicosis

Drugs

- *Propylthiouracil (PTU):* It inhibits:
  - Iodine and peroxidase from their normal interaction with thyroglobulin to form T3 and T4, which leads to a reduction in thyroid hormone production.
  - Interferes with conversion of T4 to T3 (T3 is more potent)—reduces activity of thyroid hormones.
- *Carbimazole:*
  - It works like PTU drugs.
  - It converts into methimazole, which is the active form.
  - These drugs are safe in the first trimester of pregnancy and lactation.

Side-effects

First is a sore throat. It can also cause agranulocytosis.

RIA (Radioiodine Ablation)

Radioactive iodine is used to destroy thyroid cells. It is used in Graves' disease, toxic nodular goiter and carcinoma of thyroid.

Surgery

Antithyroid drugs to be started 6–8 weeks before surgery to make euthyroid to avoid thyroid storm.

GRAVES' DISEASE

It is an autoimmune disease and the most common cause of hyperthyroidism. Common in females. There is diffuse enlargement of the thyroid gland.
- *Cause:* TRAB (Thyroid Receptor Antibodies)
- *Clinical features:* PITH-LOAD
  - *Acropathy:* Subperiosteal bone formation
  - *Exophthalmos (upper sclera is visible)—eye signs:* Von Graefe Sign (lid lag), Dalrymple sign (lid retraction), Joffroy's Sign (absence of forehead wrinkles when patient looks up), Moebius Sign (loss of accommodation reflex, it is a sign of severe toxicity), and Stellwag Sign (infrequent blinking/staring look).

- Muller's muscle [it is also called superior tarsal muscle (STM)]. It is a part of the levator palpebrae superioris muscle (LPSM), and spasm causes lid retraction.
- *Investigations:* FNAC
- *Treatment:* Medical, drugs.
- *Surgery:* Thyroidectomy.

Thyroid Storm (Thyroid Crisis)

It is a life-threatening condition due to excessive release of thyroid hormones in an uncontrolled thyrotoxicosis.

- *Cause:* Triggered by trauma (operation), upper respiratory tract infection (URTI), and anesthetic drugs in inadequately treated patients.
- *Clinical features:* Hypertensive crisis, palpitation, arrhythmias, dehydration, and hypothermia.
- *Treatment:* Intravenous (IV) fluids, cold packs, drugs (PTU, etc.), IV steroids, beta-blockers.

Note: Do not give aspirin as it deteriorates the condition.

ANTITHYROID DRUGS

- Carbimazole
- Propylthiouracil

These drugs are used to control hyperthyroidism and maintain euthyroid status. It has the *advantage* of avoiding surgery and radioactive substances, while the *disadvantage* is a long treatment with a 50% failure rate.

RADIOIODINE THERAPY

- *It destroys cells of the thyroid gland, a sort of thyroidectomy*. It is having advantage of avoiding surgery and prolonged drug treatment while the patient is quarantined during high radiation levels, not suitable for pregnant ladies and children. It gives mainly (90%) *beta radiations,* which penetrate only 0.5 mm of thyroid tissue.
- *Indications:* Carcinoma of the thyroid with distant metastasis

THYROID SOLITARY NODULE

Generally, either a colloid nodule (60%) or a follicular adenoma (30%). Palpate the thyroid gland and nodule from the back. Hard and fixed to the surrounding structures of the neck makes it suspicious of malignancy.

History

- Family history of thyroid gland cancer
- Radiation exposure

Investigations

- *TSH level:* Most of the patients are euthyroid
- FNAC
- Thyroglobulin (Tg) level. In total, thyroidectomy patients for recurrence
- Calcitonin estimation in MTC
- USG

Treatment

Lobectomy or thyroidectomy.

Surgery

It cures rapidly with a high rate of success, but recurrence occurs in 5% of cases, RLN injury and permanent hypoparathyroidism risk.

What operations are performed for thyroid diseases?

- *Lobectomy:* Removal of a lobe
- *Subtotal lobectomy:* Removal of the lobe, leaving a part.
- *Hemithyroidectomy:* Removal of one lobe with the isthmus
- *Total thyroidectomy:* Removal of the whole thyroid gland
- *Subtotal thyroidectomy:* Removal of the whole thyroid gland, leaving a part of it (4–8 gm)
- *Near total thyroidectomy:* Removal of the whole thyroid gland, leaving a small amount in both lobes.
- *Hartley Dunhill (Sir Thomas Peel Dunhill, 1876–1957, British Surgeon) procedure:* One side hemithyroidectomy with the other side lobectomy.
- *Sternotomy:* It is usually done in the midline for retrosternal goiter and invasive cancer of the thyroid gland.

INDICATIONS OF THYROIDECTOMY

- *Neoplasia:* Benign/malignant.
- Thyrotoxicosis
- To confirm the diagnosis of a mass of the thyroid gland if FNAC is inconclusive.
- *Pressure symptoms:* Dysphagia/respiratory distress.
- Cosmetic purpose
- Recurrent cyst

STEPS OF THYROIDECTOMY

Thyroidectomy is done by placing a collar incision, then cutting the platysma and making a tunnel, splitting the strap muscles, ligation of vessels, localization of parathyroid glands, and removal of the thyroid gland with closure of the wound after placing a drain. *Minimally invasive surgery (MIT)* and *minimally invasive video-assisted surgery (MIVIT)* are also done; they have *advantages:*

- Less postoperative pain
- Faster recovery
- Small scar

Approaches

- Transaxilla
- Transoral
- Retroauricular
- Transnipple

  Transoral robotic surgery (TORS) is nowadays in use.

Position

Rose position. The neck is extended 30° (a block is kept under the shoulders).

- Incision
- Making a subplatysmal tunnel
- Strap muscles should be splitting or cutting at a higher level to avoid injury to the ansa cervicalis nerve.
- *Thyroid vessels ligation:* First ligate the middle thyroid vein, then the superior pole vessels, and then the ITA.
- *Parathyroid gland localization:* Yellowish gland in the golden sentinel pad of fat.
- Excision of the thyroid gland, part, or whole.
- Introduction of suction drain
- Closure of incision

POSTOPERATIVE COMPLICATIONS OF THYROIDECTOMY

- *Hemorrhage*
- *Respiratory distress*—MC cause is laryngeal edema and hematoma (open sutures and evacuate hematoma, and if still bleeding, ligate the bleeder).
  - Laryngomalacia, bilateral RLN injury.
- *RLN injury*—unilateral or bilateral—2–10%. Common nerves injured are ELN (hoarseness of voice), RLN (less common, hoarseness of voice)
  - RLN and ELN injuries can lead to aspiration, which is life-threatening with RLN injury.
- *Thyroid deficiency*
- *Parathyroid deficiency:* Hypoparathyroidism due to ITA ligation causes an insult to the parathyroid gland. It develops 2–3 days after surgery.
  - Clinical features—perioral numbness is the first symptom.
  - *Chvostek sign (Frantisek Chvostek, 1835–1884, Austrian Physician)* (Tapping over the facial nerve causes itching of facial muscles on the same side).
  - *Trousseau sign (Armand Trousseau, 1801–1867, French Physician)* [Carpopedal spasm when blood pressure (BP) cuff is inflated above systolic BP].
  - If serum calcium level is <8 mg/dL, then symptoms are severe (IV calcium gluconate followed by oral vitamin D and calcium). If <8 mg/dL, then mild (oral vitamin D and calcium).
  - In 1% of cases of parathyroidism, it is permanent due to the removal of parathyroid glands.
- *Thyroid storm (thyrotoxic crisis):* It is an acute exacerbation of hyperthyroidism when a patient for thyroidectomy is not prepared adequately. It requires IV fluids, carbimazole 10–20 mg 6 hourly, Lugol's iodine, and propranolol IV.
- Wound infection
- Keloid

Things to remember:
- Psammoma bodies, local features of dystrophic calcification, are seen in PTC, papillary renal cell carcinoma (RCC), meningioma, and serous cyst adenoma.
- Thyroid incidentaloma is an incidental diagnosis.
- *Lateral aberrant thyroid:* It is level VI LN enlargement.

THYROID CYST

- *Simple cyst:* Aspiration
- *Complex cysts:* Mix of cyst and solid parts
  - If aspiration fails three times
  - Cyst size is big (>4 cm)
  - Complex cyst

Done in obese and short-necked persons.

- *Pizzillo's method:* Ask the patient to place their hands on the back of their head and press the head backward, and ask to swallow, the thyroid moves with deglutition.
- *Clinical feature:* Usually asymptomatic, but can lead to symptoms by compression on the trachea (scabbard trachea)

Mn: DDERP

- *D* = Dyspnea
- *D* = Dysphagia
- *E* = Engorgement of the veins of the neck and chest

- *R* = Recurrent nerve palsy
- *P* = Pemberton's sign

Whole body iodine scan is done to find residual disease and metastasis after surgery of the thyroid gland, TSH should be >20. It is done 4–6 weeks after surgery without giving thyroxine. It has the disadvantage of making the patient hypothyroid for 4–6 weeks.

SOME IMPORTANT QUESTIONS

Q1. Most probable pathological diagnosis would be:

a. Anaplastic carcinoma
b. Follicular carcinoma
c. Medullary carcinoma
d. Papillary carcinoma

Ans. d

Q2. A 20 years old female patient presented with a thyroid swelling. Most probably, the fine needle aspiration cytology will not be diagnosed:

a. Papillary carcinoma of thyroid
b. Medullary carcinoma of thyroid
c. Non-Hodgkin's lymphoma of thyroid
d. Follicular carcinoma of thyroid

Ans. d

Q3. The fine needle aspiration cytology (FNAC) of lesion should reveal:

a. "Orphan-Annie eye" nucleus cells
b. Amyloid deposits
c. Epithelioid cells and giant cells
d. Follicular cells

Ans. a

Q4. All of the following are true for follicular carcinoma of thyroid, *except*:

a. Lymph node involvement rare
b. Vascular involvement common
c. Younger patients have good prognosis
d. Diagnosis by FNAC

Ans. d (Bailey 27/e p818)

Q5. Medullary carcinoma thyroid arises from:

a. Parafollicular cells
b. Cells lining the acini
c. Capsule of thyroid
d. Stroma of the gland

Ans. a

Q6. The ideal treatment of the above condition would be:

a. Total thyroidectomy with lymph nodal dissection of the same side
b. Radiotherapy
c. Lobectomy
d. Lobectomy with isthmusectomy

Ans. a

Q7. A 52-year-old female patient presents with symptoms of pheochromocytoma. She also has a thyroid carcinoma. Her thyroid carcinoma is of which type:

a. Anaplastic
b. Medullary
c. Follicular
d. Papillary

Ans. b

Q8. Thyroid nodule of 4 cm size, mobile but causing compressive symptoms. All are true, *except*:

a. FNAC is investigation of choice
b. FNAC cannot distinguish follicular adenoma from carcinoma
c. Managed by subtotal thyroidectomy
d. Cold nodules are diagnostic of malignancy

Ans. d

Q9. Needle biopsy of solitary thyroid nodule in a young woman with palpable cervical lymph nodes on the same sides demonstrates amyloid in stroma of lesion. The likely diagnosis is:

a. Medullary carcinoma thyroid
b. Follicular carcinoma thyroid
c. Thyroid adenoma
d. Multinodular goiter

Ans. a

Q10. Thyroid carcinoma associated with hypocalcemia is:

a. Follicular carcinoma
b. Medullary carcinoma
c. Anaplastic carcinoma
d. Papillary carcinoma

Ans. None (Sabiston 20/e p909)

MULTIPLE CHOICE QUESTIONS

Grade I	*Simple*

Q1. Which of the following would be the best treatment for a 2 cm thyroid nodule in a 50-year-old man with FNAC revealing it to be a papillary carcinoma? (AIIMS May 2011)

a. Hemithyroidectomy
b. Total thyroidectomy with left sided modified neck dissection

c. Near total thyroidectomy with radiotherapy
d. Hemithyroidectomy with modified neck dissection

Q2. A 10 years old boy presented with cervical lymph adenopathy. Needle biopsy from the nodes revealed secondaries from papillary carcinoma of thyroid. The child underwent complete removal of tumor near total thyroidectomy and radical neck dissection. What should be the immediate next line of management? (All India 2012)
a. Start thyroxine suppression therapy
b. I-131 whole body scan to assess the extent of disease
c. Bone scan to evaluate secondaries
d. Contrast-enhanced computed tomography (CECT) scan to assess any residual disease

Q3. Nerve injury will be the least during thyroid surgery: (AIIMS May 2020)
a. Ansa cervicalis
b. RLN
c. SLN
d. Marginal mandibular

Q4. Appropriate FNAC specimen in case of thyroid contains: (AIIMS May 2020)
a. 6 Follicular cell group containing 10 cells each
b. 10 Follicular cell group containing 6–8 cells each.
c. 3 Follicular cell group containing 10–12 cells each.
d. 12 Follicular cell group each containing 10–15 cells each

Q5. Occult thyroid malignancy with nodal metastasis is: (AIIMS Sept 1996)
a. Medullary carcinoma
b. Follicular carcinoma
c. Papillary carcinoma
d. Anaplastic carcinoma

Q6. A 21-year-old woman has 3 cm node in the lower deep cervical chain on the left. The biopsy is interpreted as revealing normal thyroid tissue in a lymph node. The most likely diagnosis is: (DNB 2012)
a. Subacute thyroiditis
b. Metastatic carcinoma thyroid
c. Hashimoto's disease
d. Lateral aberrant thyroid

Q7. All of the following regarding papillary carcinoma thyroid is true, *except*: (All India 1990)
a. Multicentric origin
b. Secondaries to lymph nodes
c. Slowing growing
d. Bony metastasis in early stage

Q8. Most probable pathological diagnosis would be: (COMEDK 2011)
a. Anaplastic carcinoma
b. Follicular carcinoma
c. Medullary carcinoma
d. Papillary carcinoma

Q9. The FNAC of the lesion should reveal: (COMEDK 2011)
a. "Orphan-Annie eye" nucleus cells
b. Amyloid deposits
c. Epithelioid cells and giant cells
d. Follicular cells

Q10. The ideal treatment of the above condition would be: (COMEDK 2011)
a. Total thyroidectomy with lymph nodal dissection of the same side
b. Radiotherapy
c. Lobectomy
d. Lobectomy with isthmusectomy

Q11. Most common thyroid malignancy is: (DNB 2012)
a. Anaplastic carcinoma
b. Follicular carcinoma
c. Medullary carcinoma
d. Papillary carcinoma

Q12. Psammoma bodies are seen in the following, *except*: (PGI 2002)
a. Serous cystadenoma of ovary
b. Mucinous cystadenoma of ovary
c. Meningioma
d. Papillary carcinoma of thyroid

Q13. Which type of thyroid carcinoma has the best prognosis? (DNB 2010)
a. Papillary carcinoma
b. Anaplastic carcinoma
c. Follicular carcinoma
d. Medullary carcinoma

Q14. A 27-year-old lady with 20 weeks pregnancy presented with a thyroid nodule on the right side. FNAC from the nodule was suggestive of papillary

carcinoma. Which of the following is contraindicated in her management? (AIIMS May 2017)

a. Total thyroidectomy plus neck node dissection
b. Right lobectomy
c. Radioactive iodine ablation
d. Total thyroidectomy

Q15. All of the following are true for follicular carcinoma of thyroid, *except*: (COMEDK 2006)

a. Lymph node involvement rate
b. Vascular involvement common
c. Younger patients have good prognosis
d. Diagnosis by FNAC

Q16. Thyroid carcinoma with pulsating vascular skeletal metastasis is: (All India 1995)

a. Follicular
b. Anaplastic
c. Medullary
d. Papillary

Q17. A 20-year-old female patient presented with a thyroid swelling. Most probably, the fine needle aspiration cytology will not diagnose: (AIIMS Nov 1997)

a. Papillary carcinoma of thyroid
b. Medullary carcinoma of thyroid
c. Non-Hodgkin's lymphoma of thyroid
d. Follicular carcinoma of thyroid

Q18. Hürthle cells tumor is: (WBPG 2012)

a. Papillary carcinoma thyroid
b. Follicular carcinoma thyroid
c. Medullary carcinoma thyroid
d. Anaplastic carcinoma

Q19. Screening method of medullary carcinoma thyroid is: (All India 1997)

a. Serum calcitonin
b. Serum calcium
c. Serum alkaline phosphate
d. Serum acid phosphate

Q20. Thyroid carcinoma associated with hypocalcemia is: (AIIMS Dec 1994)

a. Follicular carcinoma
b. Medullary carcinoma
c. Anaplastic carcinoma
d. Papillary carcinoma

Q21. About papillary carcinoma what is/are true? (PGI Dec 2008)

a. Often encapsulated
b. Prognosis is bad
c. Lymph node metastases is common
d. Can metastasize to lung
e. Multiple foci of tumor is seen

Q22. Variant of papillary carcinoma thyroid: (PGI June 2007)

a. Medullary
b. Warthin
c. Columnar
d. Insular
e. Diffuse sclerosing

Q23. Medullary carcinoma thyroid arises from: (AIIMS Nov 1993)

a. Parafollicular cells
b. Cells lining the acini
c. Capsule of thyroid
d. Stroma of the gland

Q24. Features of papillary carcinoma includes: (PGI May 2011)

a. FNAC easy
b. Almost always unifocal
c. Psammoma body
d. Spread of cervical LN
e. Bad prognosis

Q25. About papillary carcinoma true statement is/are: (PGI Nov 2010)

a. Radiation is a risk factor
b. Multifocal
c. Hematogenous spread is common
d. Distant metastasis is seen

Q26. Needle biopsy of solitary thyroid nodule in a young woman with palpable cervical lymph nodes on the same sides demonstrates amyloid in stroma of lesion. Likely diagnosis is: (All India 2002)

a. Medullary carcinoma thyroid
b. Follicular carcinoma thyroid
c. Thyroid adenoma
d. Multinodular goiter

Q27. A 52-year-old female patient presents with symptoms of pheochromocytoma. She also has a thyroid carcinoma. Her thyroid carcinoma is of which type: (AIIMS June 1999)

a. Anaplastic
b. Medullary
c. Follicular
d. Papillary

Q28. Multiple endocrine neoplasia type 2 (MEN-2) is seen with the following type of thyroid carcinoma: (All India 1997)

a. Papillary
b. Medullary
c. Anaplastic
d. Follicular

Q29. Compared to follicular carcinoma, papillary carcinoma of thyroid have: (PGI Dec 2007)

a. More male preponderance
b. Bilaterality
c. Local recurrence common
d. Increased lymph node metastasis
e. Increased mortality

Grade II	*Difficult*

Q1. Least malignant thyroid cancer is: (AIIMS Nov 2003)

a. Papillary carcinoma
b. Follicular carcinoma
c. Anaplastic carcinoma
d. Medullary carcinoma

Q2. Lateral aberrant thyroid refers to: (AIIMS June 2002)

a. Congenital thyroid abnormality
b. Metastatic foci form primary in thyroid
c. Struma ovarii
d. Lingual thyroid

Q3. Which of the following is used in the treatment of differentiated thyroid cancer? (All India 2006)

a. I-131 b. 99mTc
c. P-32 d. I-131 MIBG

Q4. In treatment of papillary carcinomas thyroid, radioiodine destroys the neoplastic cells predominantly by: (AIIMS Nov 2005)

a. X-rays b. Beta rays
c. Gamma rays d. Alpha particles

Q5. Follicular carcinoma of thyroid is due to mutation of: (JIPMER 2010)

a. RAS
b. Hepatocyte growth factor (HGF)
c. Rearranged during transfection (RET)
d. ABL

Q6. A well differentiated follicular carcinoma of thyroid can be best differentiated from a follicular adenoma by: (All India 2011)

a. Hürthle cell change
b. Lining of tall columnar and cuboidal cells
c. Vascular invasion
d. Nuclear features

Q7. Serum calcitonin is a marker for: (DNB 2003)

a. Anaplastic carcinoma
b. Papillary carcinoma
c. Medullary carcinoma
d. Follicular carcinoma

Q8. Treatment of choice for medullary carcinoma of thyroid is: (AIIMS May 2005)

a. Total thyroidectomy
b. Partial thyroidectomy
c. I-131 ablation
d. Hemithyroidectomy

Q9. True regarding follicular carcinoma of thyroid: (JIPMER 2014)

a. Hematogenous spread
b. Commonly multifocal
c. Readily diagnosed by face
d. Most commonly carcinoma of thyroid

Q10. Which of the following gene defects is associated with development of medullary carcinoma of thyroid? (All India 2004)

a. Ret proto-oncogene b. *FAP* gene
c. *Rb* gene d. *BRCA-1* gene

Q11. FNAC cannot detect which of the following? (AIIMS Nov 2014)

a. Follicular carcinoma
b. Papillary carcinoma
c. Colloid goiter
d. Hashimoto's thyroiditis

Q12. Treatment of medullary carcinoma thyroid: (AIIMS May 2011)

a. Surgery and radiotherapy
b. Radiotherapy and chemotherapy
c. Surgery only
d. Radioiodine ablation

Q13. False statement about feature of medullary thyroid carcinoma (MTC): (PGI Nov 2011)

a. Familial MTC may presents in second decade
b. It has characteristic of the amyloid stroma
c. Secrete serotonin
d. Take up radioiodine
e. Secrete calcitonin

Q14. Thyroid radioiodine ablation therapy is useful in all, *except*: (PGI May 2011)

a. Recurrent papillary carcinoma
b. Residual papillary carcinoma

c. Anaplastic carcinoma
d. Follicular carcinoma
e. Medullary carcinoma

Q15. The treatment of choice for anaplastic carcinoma of thyroid infiltrating trachea and sternum will be: (AIIMS Nov 2005)

a. Radical excision
b. Chemotherapy
c. Radiotherapy
d. Palliative/symptomatic treatment

Q16. A biopsy from a mass in front of the neck revealed parafollicular cells. How do you follow up? (JIPMER Nov 2017)

a. Calcitonin
b. T4
c. Thyroxine
d. Thyroglobulin

Q17. Treatment of medullary carcinoma thyroid: (AIIMS Nov 2008)

a. Surgery and radiotherapy
b. Radiotherapy and chemotherapy
c. Surgery only
d. Radioiodine ablation

Q18. Metastasis in thyroid gland come most commonly from carcinoma of: (PGI June 1998)

a. Testis
b. Prostate
c. Breast
d. Lungs

Q19. The expression of the following oncogene is associated with a high incidence of medullary carcinoma of thyroid: (AIIMS Nov 2005)

a. p53
b. Her-2-new
c. Ret proto-oncogene
d. *Rb* gene

Q20. Amyloid stroma is seen in which carcinoma thyroid? (AIIMS June 2000)

a. Papillary carcinoma
b. Medullary carcinoma
c. Anaplastic carcinoma
d. Follicular carcinoma

Q21. A patient has pituitary tumor and pheochromocytoma and a thyroid nodule. Which carcinoma is most likely to occur? (AIIMS Nov 2000)

a. Papillary carcinoma
b. Medullary carcinoma
c. Anaplastic carcinoma
d. Follicular carcinoma

Q22. Not true about anaplastic thyroid carcinoma: (PGI May 2011)

a. Local infiltration common
b. Spread by lymphatic route
c. Long term survival in patient undergoing surgery
d. Surgery is of limited value
e. Highly chemosensitive

Q23. All of the following are true about lymphoma of the thyroid, *except*: (All India 2007)

a. More common in females
b. Slow growing
c. Clinically confused with undifferentiated tumors
d. May present with respiratory distress and dysphagia

Q24. Which of the following is not a histological variant of thyroid neoplasm? (All India 2007)

a. Follicular
b. Merkel cell
c. Insular
d. Anaplastic

Q25. The most common histologic type of thyroid cancer is: (All India 2008)

a. Medullary type
b. Follicular type
c. Papillary type
d. Anaplastic type

Q26. Thyroid carcinoma causes laryngeal paralysis due to: (PGI June 1996)

a. Recurrent laryngeal nerve palsy
b. Vagus nerve palsy
c. Glossopharyngeal nerve palsy
d. Hypoglossal nerve palsy

Q27. Which of the following is used in the treatment of thyroid malignancy? (PGI June 2001)

a. I-131
b. I-125
c. Tc-99
d. P-32
e. Strontium

Q28. True about solitary thyroid nodule: (PGI Dec 2006)

a. Thyroid hormone receptor (THR)-antibody
b. Lined by columnar epithelium
c. Diffuse hyperplasia of the thyroid
d. Common in female
e. Thyroidectomy done

Q29. A case of solitary thyroid nodule, investigation of choice is: (AIIMS Nov 1997)

a. T3, T4 estimation
b. Thyroid scan
c. FNAC
d. Excision biopsy

Grade III	Most difficult

Q1. Which of the following is true? (AIIMS May 2011)
a. Colloid goiter mostly presents as hyperthyroidism
b. Thyroid storm, the clinical features are primarily due to increased thyroxine
c. Excess calcium intake can lead to hyperthyroidism
d. Goiter >5% of population is endemic goiter

Q2. A 45-year-old male presents with a 4 × 4 cm, mobile right solitary thyroid nodule of 5 months. The patient is euthyroid. The following statements about his management are true, *except*: (AIIMS Nov 2005)
a. Cold nodule on thyroid scan is diagnostic of malignancy
b. FNAC is the investigation of choice
c. The patient should undergo hemithyroidectomy if the FNAC report is inconclusive
d. Indirect laryngoscopy should be done in the preoperative period to assess the mobility of the vocal cords

Q3. The most common solitary thyroid nodule is: (AIIMS Nov 2004)
a. Follicular adenoma
b. Hürthle cell carcinoma
c. Papillary carcinoma
d. Solitary idiopathic goiter

Q4. All of the following conditions are associated with hyperthyroidism, *except*: (All India 2011)
a. Hashimoto's thyroiditis
b. Graves' disease
c. Toxic multinodular goiter
d. Struma ovary

Q5. Hyperthyroidism occurs in: (PGI Nov 2011)
a. Hashimoto's thyroiditis
b. Medullary thyroid carcinoma
c. Plummer's disease
d. Struma ovarii

Q6. Which of the following is a symptom of hypothyroidism? (JIPMER 2014)
a. Hyperactivity
b. Palpitation
c. Diarrhea
d. Hair loss

Q7. A patient underwent thyroidectomy for hyperthyroidism. Two days later, he presented with features of thyroid storm. What is the most likely cause? (AIIMS Nov 2015)
a. Poor antibiotic coverage
b. Rough handling during surgery
c. Removal of parathyroid
d. Inadequate preoperative preparation

Q8. The most common solitary thyroid nodule is: (AIIMS Nov 2004)
a. Follicular adenoma
b. Hürthle cell carcinoma
c. Papillary carcinoma
d. Solitary idiopathic goiter

Q9. In which of the following conditions can radioactive iodine (Irradiation) be used in Graves' disease? (PGI Nov 2010)
a. Recurrence
b. Age >40 years
c. Elderly
d. Pregnant
e. Presence of associated comorbidities

Q10. All of the following are true about Graves' disease, *except*: (JIPMER 2013)
a. Cardiac failure is common
b. Hypertrophy and hyperplasia or the thyroid gland are due to TSH-Rab
c. Remission and exacerbations are not infrequent
d. It is highly vascular with an audible bruit

Q11. Horner's syndrome, all are true, *except*: (AIIMS May 2011)
a. Miosis
b. Anhidrosis
c. Hyperchromatic iris
d. Apparent exophthalmos

Q12. Horner's syndrome is seen in all, *except*: (AIIMS Nov 2010)
a. Miosis
b. Anhidrosis
c. Hyperchromatic iris
d. Apparent exophthalmos

Q13. Hypoparathyroidism following thyroid surgery occurs within: (AIIMS Nov 2004)
a. 24 hours
b. 2–5 days
c. 7–14 days
d. 2–3 weeks

Q14. Complications of hemithyroidectomy include all of the following, *except*: (All India 2008)

a. Hypocalcemia
b. Wound hematoma
c. Recurrent laryngeal nerve palsy
d. External branch of the superior laryngeal nerve palsy

Q15. What is the most appropriate operation for a solitary nodule in one lobe of the thyroid? (All India 2003)

a. Lobectomy
b. Hemithyroidectomy
c. Nodule removal
d. Partial lobectomy with a 1 cm margin around the nodule

Q16. A patient with autoimmune thyroiditis presents with hypothyroidism. Which of the following is true? (JIPMER 2011)

a. Thyroid peroxidase antibodies
b. Painless enlargement of the thyroid
c. Common in men
d. No malignant risk

Q17. Hashimoto's thyroiditis, all are true, *except*: (AIIMS May 2011)

a. Follicular destruction
b. Increase in lymphocytes
c. Oncocytic metaplasia
d. Orphan Annie-eye nuclei

Q18. The laboratory investigation of a patient shows decreased T4 and increased TSH. Which of the following is the most likely diagnosis? (All India 2011)

a. Graves' disease
b. Hashimoto's disease
c. Pituitary failure
d. Hypothalamic failure

Q19. Which of the following conditions is associated with hypothyroidism? (All India 2011)

a. Hashimoto's thyroiditis
b. Graves' disease
c. Toxic multinodular goiter
d. Struma ovary

Q20. Not a feature of De Quervain's disease: (All India 2002)

a. Autoimmune in etiology
b. Increased erythrocyte sedimentation rate (ESR)
c. Tends to regress spontaneously
d. Painful and associated with the enlargement of the thyroid

Q21. A 20-year-old girl presents with a 9-month history of neck swelling with thyrotoxic symptoms. On investigation, increased T4 and decreased TSH with a palpable 2 cm nodule were found. Next investigation will be: (AIIMS May 2007)

a. Ultrasonography (USG)
b. Thyroid scan
c. Radioactive iodine uptake
d. Computed tomography (CT) scan

Q22. Indications of surgery in a case of thyroid swelling is/are: (PGI June 2004)

a. Cosmetic
b. Pressure symptoms
c. Myxedema
d. Pain
e. Swelling with symptoms

Q23. In a patient presenting with a swelling of the thyroid, the radionuclide scan showed a cold nodule, and the ultrasound showed a noncystic solid mass. The management of this patient would be: (AIIMS June 2002)

a. Lobectomy
b. Hemithyroidectomy
c. Eltroxin
d. Radioiodine therapy

Q24. Most common symptom of retrosternal goiter: (PGI June 1997)

a. Dysphagia
b. Stridor
c. Dyspnea
d. Superior vena cava syndrome

Q25. The following statements about thyroglossal cyst are true, *except*: (All India 2006)

a. Frequent cause of anterior midline neck masses in the first decade of life
b. The cyst is located within 2 cm of the midline
c. Incision and drainage is the treatment of choice
d. The swelling moves upwards on the protrusion of the tongue

Q26. The occurrence of hyperthyroidism following administration of supplemental iodine to the subject with endemic iodine deficiency goiter is known as: (All India 2012)

a. Jod-Basedow effect
b. Wolff-Chaikoff effect
c. Thyrotoxicosis factitia
d. De Quervain's thyroiditis

Q27. Which of the following most closely represents the lowest detection limit for third-generation TSH assays? (All India 2012)

a. 0.4 mIU/L
b. 0.04 mIU/L
c. 0.004 mIU/L
d. 0.0004 mIU/L

Q28. True about struma ovarii: (PGI June 2007)

a. Ectopic thyroid
b. Ectopic ovary
c. Malignancy
d. Benign lesion
e. Included in teratoma

Q29. A post-thyroidectomy patient develops signs and symptoms of tetany. The management is: (All India 2000)

a. IV calcium gluconate
b. Bicarbonate
c. Calcitonin
d. Vitamin D

ANSWERS

Grade I: 1. b; 2. a (Schwartz 10/e p1549); 3. a; 4. a; 5. c; 6. d; 7. d (Bailey 27/e p818); 8. d; 9. a; 10. a; 11. d; 12. b; 13. a; 14. c (Schwartz 10/e p1546); 15. d (Bailey 27/e p818); 16. a; 17. d; 18. b (Schwartz 10/e p1546); 19. a (Bailey 27/e p820); 20. None (Sabistan 20/e p909); 21. c, d, e; 22. c, d, e; 23. a; 24. a, c, d; 25. a, b, and d; 26. a; 27. b; 28. b; 29. b, c, d

Grade II: 1. a; 2. b; 3. a; 4. b; 5. a; 6. c; 7. c; 8. a; 9. a; 10. a; 11. a; 12. c; 13. d; 14. c, e; 15. d; 16. a; 17. c; 18. c (Schwartz 10/e p1551); 19. c; 20. b; 21. b; 22. c, e; 23. b; 24. b; 25. c; 26. a; 27. a (Bailey 27/e p819); 28. d, e (Schwartz 10/e p1537); 29. c (Schwartz 10/e p1538)

Grade III: 1. d; 2. a (Schwartz 10/e p1537); 3. a; 4. a; 5. b, d, e; 6. d; 7. d; 8. a; 9. b, c, e; 10. c; 11. d; 12. b; 13. b; 14. a; 15. b (Schwartz 10/e, p1540); 16. a; 17. d; 18. b; 19. a; 20. a; 21. b (Schwartz 10/e p1537); 22. a, b, e (Schwartz 9/e p1358); 23. b; 24. c (Bailey 27/r p810); 25. c; 26. a; 27. b; 28. d; 29. a

MODEL QUESTIONS

Q1. Site of the isthmus of the thyroid gland:

a. Hyoid bone
b. First and second tracheal cartilage
c. Second and third, and fourth tracheal cartilage
d. Third and fourth tracheal cartilage

Ans. c (Schwartz 10/e p1523)

Q2. The weight of the thyroid gland is:

a. 8–14 g
b. 14–16 g
c. 28–30 g
d. 18–20 g

Ans. d (Bailey 27/e p800)

Q3. How does dietary iodine have an affect on the weight of the thyroid gland?

a. Inversely
b. Proportionate
c. Fixed
d. Not fixed

Ans. a

Q4. The least common thyroid carcinoma is:

a. Inflammatory
b. Follicular
c. Medullary
d. Anaplastic

Ans. c (Bailey 27/e p816)

Q5. What thyroid carcinoma has the best prognosis?

a. Papillary carcinoma
b. Follicular carcinoma
c. Medullary carcinoma
d. Inflammatory carcinoma

Ans. a (Schwartz 10/e p1542)

Q6. Investigation of choice to differentiate between benign and malignant thyroid nodules:

a. USG
b. FNAC
c. Magnetic resonance imaging (MRI)
d. Biopsy

Ans. b (Bailey 27/e p805)

Q7. FNAC is not very useful in:

a. Follicular
b. Anaplastic
c. Papillary
d. Medullary

Ans. a (Bailey 27/e p808)

Q8. What is true about follicular thyroid carcinoma (FTC)?

a. Mean age 40 years
b. Nonencapsulated
c. More common in endemic area
d. Histopathology differentiates

Ans. c (Schwartz 10/e p1544)

Q9. Which of the following is true about medullary CA of the thyroid?

a. Elevated levels of serum calcitonin
b. Seen in MEN I syndrome
c. Associated MEN2A
d. Most common thyroid cancer

Ans. a (Schwartz 10/e p1549)

Q10. Not true about medullary thyroid carcinoma:

a. Type of inflammatory carcinoma

b. Associated with MEN 2A and 2B syndrome
c. Forms about 25% of the thyroid malignancies
d. Tumor cells may secrete serotonin. ACTH and VIP

Ans. c (Bailey 27/e p816)

Q11. The cause of goiter in India is commonly because of:

a. Hashimoto's thyroiditis
b. Toxic multinodular goiter
c. Papillary carcinoma
d. Diffuse endemic goiter

Ans. d (Bailey 27/e p 805)

Q12. Most dangerous thyroid cancer:

a. Anaplastic carcinoma
b. Carcinoma in situ
c. Follicular carcinoma
d. Medullary carcinoma

Ans. a (Bailey 27/e p820)

Q13. Radiation exposure can cause:

a. Papillary carcinoma
b. Medullary carcinoma
c. Lymphoma
d. Follicular carcinoma

Ans. a (Bailey 27/e p820)

Q14. Which of the following is true about subtotal thyroidectomy?

a. Excision of both lobes, leaving behind 6–8 g of tissue
b. Excision of one lobe
c. Excision of the entire thyroid
d. Excision of one lobe with the isthmus and the second lobe partially

Ans. a (Bailey 27/e, p807)

Q15. The treatment of choice for medullary carcinoma of the thyroid is:

a. Partial thyroidectomy b. Total thyroidectomy
c. I-131 ablation d. Hemithyroidectomy

Ans. b (Schwartz 10/e, p 1543)

Q16. What surgery is required in one lobe of the thyroid gland, FTC?

a. Hemithyroidectomy
b. Total thyroidectomy
c. Near total thyroidectomy
d. Enucleation

Ans. a (Bailey 27/e p821)

Q17. The thoracic extension of a cervical goiter is usually approached through:

a. Chest
b. Neck
c. Combined cervicothoracic route
d. Thoracoscope

Ans. b (Schwartz 10/e p1554)

Q18. Radioiodine therapy is preferred in:

a. 20–30 years female
b. Pregnancy
c. Recent onset of toxic goiter
d. Postsurgery for papillary thyroid cancer

Ans. d (Schwartz 10/e p1546)

Q19. What is used in the treatment of well-differentiated thyroid cancer?

a. I131 b. Radiotherapy
c. P32 d. 99m TC

Ans. a (Bailey 27/e p819)

Q20. What is the percentage of nontoxic thyroid nodules that become malignant?

a. 50% b. 15%
c. 60% d. 40%

Ans. b (Bailey 27/e p804)

Q21. Which of the following is not true about medullary thyroid carcinoma (MTC)?

a. FNAC cannot be used for diagnosis
b. Metastases to bone are osteoblastic
c. Carcinoembryonic antigen is a better predictor of prognosis compared to calcitonin
d. Medullary carcinoma of the thyroid is not hormone dependent

Ans. a (Bailey 27/e p808)

Q22. Thyroid nodule increased radioisotope uptake IOC is:

a. USG b. Thyroid scan
c. FNAC d. MRI

Ans. c (**FNAC – Warm nodule** – a warm nodule takes up isotope, and so does normal thyroid tissue around it. **Cold nodule** – it takes up no isotope).

Q23. A thyroid nodule is causing compressive symptoms. All are true, *except*:

a. MRI
b. FNAC in the investigation of choice
c. Cold nodules on thyroid scan are diagnostic of malignancy
d. Managed by sub- and total thyroidectomy

Ans. c (Bailey 27/e p804)

Q24. What treatment is required for a thyroid nodule with LNs involvement?

a. Excision of nodule
b. Chemotherapy
c. Radiation
d. Total thyroidectomy + MRND

Ans. d (Schwartz 10/e p1543)

Q25. Prophylactic thyroidectomy is indicated in:

a. MEN type 2
b. Viral thyroiditis
c. Reidel thyroiditis
d. De Quervain's thyroiditis

Ans. a

Q26. What is required before thyroidectomy?

a. Check serum calcium levels
b. Do serum parathyroid hormone (PTH) assay
c. Indirect laryngoscopy
d. Do an iodine-131 scan

Ans. c (Schwartz 10/e p1556)

Q27. Hemorrhage after thyroidectomy is due to:

a. Internal carotid artery
b. External carotid artery
c. Superior thyroid artery
d. Inferior thyroid artery

Ans. c (Bailey 26/e p761)

Q28. All of the following are complications of total thyroidectomy, *except*:

a. Hemorrhage b. Hoarseness
c. Hypercalcemia d. Airway obstruction

Ans. c (Bailey 27/e p815)

Q29. Toxic goiter with low radioiodine uptake may be seen in:

a. Graves' disease
b. Hashimoto's thyroiditis
c. De Quervain's thyroiditis (subacute thyroiditis)
d. Viral thyroiditis

Ans. c

Q30. To reduce the size and vascularity of the thyroid gland before thyroidectomy is done.

a. Iodides b. Propylthiouracil
c. Radioiodine d. Propranolol

Ans. a (Schwartz 10/e p 1533)

Q31. Which of the following is not true about medullary thyroid carcinoma (MTC)?

a. 20–25% are familial
b. Associated diarrhea can be seen in 30% of the patients
c. They secrete calcitonin
d. Medullary carcinoma of the thyroid takes up iodine

Ans. d (Bailey 27/e p820)

SUGGESTED READING

1. Bailey & Love's - Short Practice of Surgery, 27th Edition
2. Schwartz's Principles of Surgery, 18th Edition
3. Textbook of Surgery by David Sabiston, 21st Edition

CHAPTER

29 Parathyroid

"Parathyroid is a New Gland in Man and Fellow Animals, as the "glandulae parathyroidae."

– Monograph on Parathyroid by a Swedish Medical Student, in 1880, Ivar Victor Sandstrom (1852–1889). He discovered the parathyroid gland. Unfortunately, he died by committing suicide at the young age of 37

ANATOMY OF THE PARATHYROID GLAND

In 1925, Mandal in Austria performed the first parathyroidectomy. There are four parathyroid glands, two superior and two inferior, situated over the thyroid gland's back, developed from the third and fourth pharyngeal pouches, weighing around 30 mg and yellow to brown in color. There are more than four parathyroid glands in 5% of individuals. Parathyroid glands are supplied by the inferior thyroid artery (ITA) **(Fig. 1)**.

Superior parathyroid glands are located intrathyroid in 1% of individuals, and 2% have inferior parathyroid glands. In 80% and above, superior parathyroid glands are located at the back of the thyroid gland near the upper pole, around the junction of ITA and recurrent laryngeal nerve (RLN).

Points to remember:
- The superior parathyroid is constant in position, while the inferior is not.
- The superior parathyroid always lies behind the RLN near Zuckerkandl.
- Inferior parathyroid lies anterior to RLA, but is inconsistent.
- The parathyroid gland is approximately 30 g in weight, secretes parathyroid hormone (PTH) (3–5 minutes half-life), which affects bone, kidneys, and gastrointestinal tract (GIT).
- Normal calcium level is 8.5–10.5 mg/dL, and ionized calcium is 4.4–5.5 mg/dL.

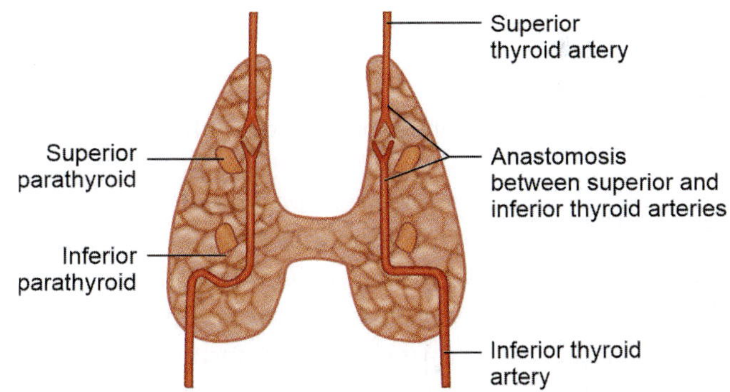

Fig. 1: Anatomy of a parathyroid gland.

PHYSIOLOGY OF THE PARATHYROID GLAND

The parathyroid gland produces a hormone called PTH. It regulates serum calcium levels. It is secreted when the serum calcium level is low and/or the serum magnesium level is high. PTH has half-life of 3–5 minutes if kidney functions are normal. PTH acts on the kidneys, the GIT, and the bones. In kidneys increase in serum calcium levels, and in bone increase in bone turnover leading to higher levels of calcium in the extracellular space. *Calcitonin, which is made by parafollicular C-cells of the thyroid gland, decreases serum calcium levels as it acts against PTH* **(Fig. 2)**.

Goiter

Enlargement of the thyroid gland.

Types

Diffuse/multinodular/retrosternal [nodule may be solitary, palpable with an unpalpable thyroid gland, or solitary palpable node with palpable thyroid gland (dominant nodule)].

PRIMARY HYPERPARATHYROIDISM

Eighty percent and more patients of primary hyperparathyroidism suffer with kidney stones and muscle weakness. It is depicted by a mnemonic. *Bones (Pain in bones/*

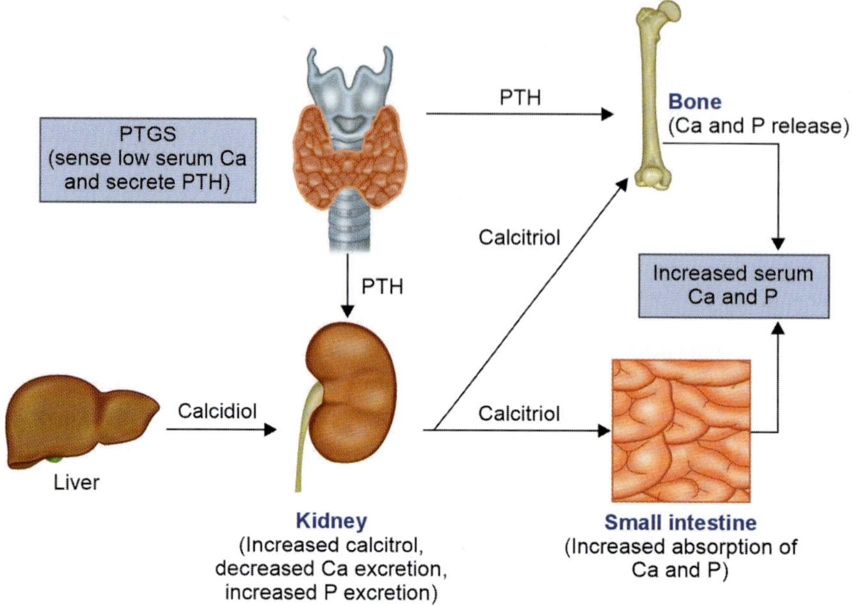

Fig. 2: Physiology of the parathyroid gland. (PTH: parathyroid hormone; PTGS: parathyroid glands)

fractures/subperiosteal bone resorption/salt and pepper), brown tumor of osteitis fibrosa cystica (Von Recklinghausen disease of bone), Stones (renal), Groans (abdominal pain), Maons (lethargy and depression). Primary hyperparathyroidism (PHPT) is reported as <0.5% in the population, usually sporadic, familial, and is a part of MEN type I and IIa; females are three times more affected, and it is seen in late adulthood.

Radiology

- *Tumor:* Adenoma—one gland
- Hyperplasia of all four glands

Risk Factor

The risk factor is radiation exposure.

Investigations

- PTH, serum calcium, and urinary calcium are high.
- USG
- *Scan:* Tc99m sestamibi scan—single photon emission computed tomography (SPECT)
- Localization is done by combining a scan and USG.

Treatment

- *Adenoma:* Removal of the gland with adenoma
- *Hyperplasia:* 3.5 glands removed or all four glands are removed, then half of one gland is autotransplanted in the brachioradialis muscle in the nondominant limb.
- Thymectomy is performed as ectopic parathyroid glands are most commonly found in the thymus gland.

Why is surgery done to remove parathyroid glands in case of a symptomatic hyperparathyroidism?

Due to (Mn = Cocu)

- High serum calcium
- Osteoporosis
- Complications such as renal stones
- *High urinary calcium:* Hypercalciuria (>400 mg/24 hours).

Surgical Treatment for Hyperparathyroidism

The best treatment is surgery, which may be a minimally invasive (focused) parathyroidectomy. Bilateral neck exploration is required when imaging is inconclusive. Kocher's transverse collar incision is used.

Secondary Hyperparathyroidism

It is a derangement in calcium homeostasis that leads to hypersecretion of PTH. It is also called renal hyperparathyroidism as it is a result of chronic renal disease. Secondary hyperparathyroidism is diagnosed by hypocalcemia with increased PTH with high levels of serum phosphate, and low levels of vitamin D. Parathyroid hyperplasia occurs, requires calcimimetics are required to reduce the necessity of surgery (subtotal parathyroidectomy). Calciphylaxis is a syndrome of disseminated calcification in vessels and skin that occurs with secondary hyperparathyroidism. Casanova (Daniel Casanova, Spanish Physician) test is done to detect recurrent disease located in the grafted arm, done by forearm venous sampling for PTH. Renal transplantation is the treatment.

Cause

Hyperplasia.

Investigation

Serum calcium—normal or low/serum phosphorus increases/calcitriol decreases/PTH increases (Calcitriol is the active form of vitamin D3, produced by the kidneys, and it helps in the regulation of calcium levels in body and it also helps in regulation of production of PTH which controls calcium levels in blood).

Treatment

Low phosphate diet with vitamin D3 supplementation—calcimimetic—activates calcium sensing receptors in parathyroid glands. They reduce PTH release and lower serum calcium and phosphate levels.

- Renal transplantation.

Tertiary Hyperparathyroidism

It occurs after kidney transplantation as a persistent autonomous hypercalcemic hyperparathyroidism. It is diagnosed by raised levels of calcium and PTH. Subtotal parathyroidectomy is the treatment.

Not to forget:
- The *Miami criterion* shows a 50% PTH drop from the pre-incision or preexcision estimation of PTH in a blood sample taken 10 minutes after resection of hyperfunctioning of parathyroid glands. If there is no drop of PTH, then multinodular disease or hyperplasia is suspected.
- *Bilateral cervical exploration for parathyroid glands is done in inconsistent images, MEN1 and MEN2, failed Miami criterion, multinodular disease, and lithium-induced hyperparathyroidism.*
- Minimally invasive video-assisted parathyroidectomy (*MIVAP*): It is a new technique through cervical, axillary, postauricular, and transthoracic sites.
- Robotic parathyroidectomy is also in use.
- The first parathyroidectomy was performed by *Mandl in Vienna, Austria in 1925 (Felix Mandl, 1892–1957, Austrian Surgeon).*

HYPERCALCEMIC CRISIS

- It is a life-threatening complication of hypercalcemia.
- It is seen in primary hyperparathyroidism.
- It is also seen in hypercalcemia of malignancy (paraneoplastic syndrome)

Clinical Features

- Calcium level is >14 mg/dL

Mn: CANADA = confusion/abdominal pain/nausea and vomiting/arrhythmia/dehydration/anuria

Most of the patients are asymptomatic, but if the calcium level goes above 3.5 mmol/L will have symptoms. It can be caused by PHPT, renal failure, tumors such as multiple myeloma, lymphoma, and GIT tumors, access of vitamin D and A ingestion, tuberculosis (TB), Paget's disease, and drugs containing lithium. Treatment is based on increasing kidney excretion of calcium and diminishing the release of calcium from bones.

INVESTIGATIONS FOR LOCALIZING PARATHYROID GLANDS

- Sestamibi scanning.
- Sestamibi [2-methoxy-2-methylpropylisonitrile (MIBI)] is the most reliable and accurate way of localizing parathyroid glands.
- Ultrasound
- MRI
- 4D CT
- Parathyroid angiography

Chvostek's (Frantisek Chvostek, 1835–1884, Austrian physician) sign (contraction of fascial muscles of same side on stroking of fascial nerve below the zygomatic bone) and *Trousseau's (Armand Trousseau, 1801–1867, French Physician)* sign (Carpopedal spasm after pressing arm with a blood pressure cuff).

CALCIMIMETICS

Calcimimetics such as cinacalcet increase the sensitivity of the *calcium-sensing receptor (CaR)* to extracellular calcium and decrease PTH synthesis.

PERMANENT HYPOPARATHYROIDISM

It develops postoperatively, is rare but more chances in secondary hyperparathyroidism (4–12%), requires calcium and/or vitamin D supplementation, and there are serum calcium level-related clinical features.

There is mild circumoral or digital numbness, carpopedal spasms with heart arrhythmias, and spasm of laryngeal muscles. Treatment is surgery, but medical treatment is advised for persons who are unfit for surgery or surgery has failed.

You May Be Asked:

- *Postoperative complications* of parathyroidectomy are RLN damage (<1%), permanent hypocalcemia, persistent hyperparathyroidism, and recurrent hyperparathyroidism.
- The most common cause of hyperparathyroidism is solitary adenoma, which is frequently situated in the inferior parathyroid gland.
- *Osteitis fibrosa* is a significant radiological finding of hands (subperiosteal resorption of bones and bone cysts) in advanced PHPT.
- *Hypercalcemic crisis is seen in hyperparathyroidism and malignancy of the parathyroid (paraneoplastic syndrome).* Serum calcium level is >14 mg/dL and leads to confusion, vomiting, abdominal pain, and dehydration with low urine output, even anuria. Treated with aggressive intravenous fluid placement, diuretics, bisphosphates, and dialysis if required.

CALCIPHYLAXIS

It is a rare, painful, and deadly disease in which calcium deposits are formed in blood vessels, blocking blood flow, resulting in the death of the tissue. Usually, patients die within 6 months of diagnosis.

HYPOPARATHYROIDISM

- Most commonly caused by an iatrogenic factor.
- It is a rare disease of decreased function of parathyroid glands with reduced production of PTH. It leads to low levels of serum calcium, causing muscle cramps, twitching of muscles, or tetany.

DIGEORGE SYNDROME

It is a chromosomal disorder causing poor development of many systems of the body. *Mn = HATCH (Hypocalcemia/Atypical facies/Thymic hypoplasia/Cleft lip and palate/Heart anomalies).*

Good to remember:

- Pseudohyperparathyroidism is hypercalcemia of pregnancy, paraneuroplastic syndrome, and even in squamous cell carcinoma (SCC) of the lungs, breast, and prostate.
- *Hungary bone syndrome* is hypocalcemia immediately after excision of parathyroid adenoma due to increased absorption of calcium by bones.

PARATHYROID CARCINOMA

It is a rare malignancy (1%) of PHPT with an unknown cause. It is difficult to diagnose as it resembles PHPT. The only point is the history of neck irradiation. Surgery is the treatment of choice.

IODINE-INDUCED HYPOTHYROIDISM

Clinical Features

Mn = ABCDEFG

Alopecia/bradycardia/constipation/dullness and low energy feel/excess menses (menorrhagia)/freezing and cold intolerance/gaining weight.

THYROIDITIS: INFLAMMATION OF THE THYROID GLAND

- Hashimoto's or lymphocytic thyroiditis
- De Quervain's subacute thyroiditis
- Postpartum thyroiditis
- Riedel's thyroiditis
- Silent or painless thyroiditis
- Drug-induced thyroiditis
- Acute or infectious thyroiditis
- Radiation-induced thyroiditis

HASHIMOTO'S THYROIDITIS

Autoimmune disease, common in females due to autoantibodies against thyroid receptor/thyroglobulin/thyroid peroxidase (TPO) enzymes.

- *Clinical features:* Diffuse goiter
- *Course:* Autoantibodies and lymphocytes—infiltrate thyroid gland tissue—destroy follicles—release hormones—thyrotoxicosis—more destruction of follicles—hypothyroidism.
- *Investigation:*
  - Autoantibody level
  - FNAC
- *Treatment:*
  - Thyroxine
  - Total thyroidectomy

DE QUERVAIN THYROIDITIS

Viral upper respiratory tract infection URTI: Lymphocytic infiltration of the thyroid gland—destruction of follicles—hyperthyroidism, due to follicle destruction. It is a painful neck enlargement associated with human leukocyte antigen (HLA) B35.

RIEDEL'S THYROIDITIS

It is due to fibrosis in the thyroid gland (Woody hard painless enlargement of the thyroid gland) and around it (pressure symptoms due to pressure on the RLN and trachea). Associated with other fibrosis are diseases, such as *Peyronie's disease* and *Dupuytren's contracture*.

- *Differential diagnosis:* Anaplastic carcinoma
- *Investigation:* Core biopsy
- *Treatment:* Steroids and tamoxifen

SOME IMPORTANT QUESTIONS

Q1. Hypoparathyroidism occurs due to:
a. Total thyroidectomy
b. Thyroiditis with secondary atrophy of parathyroids
c. Idiopathic atrophy of parathyroids
d. All of the above

Ans. a

Q2. The most common cause for hyperparathyroidism is:
a. Single adenoma
b. Multiple adenomas
c. Single gland hyperplasia
d. Multiple gland hyperplasia

Ans. a

Q3. A 20-year-old male presents with chronic constipation, headache and habitus, neuroma of the tongue, medullated corneal nerve fibers, and a nodule of 2 × 2 cm in size in the left lobe of the thyroid. The patient is a case of:
a. Sporadic medullary carcinoma of thyroid
b. Familial medullary carcinoma of the thyroid
c. Multiple endocrine neoplasia type 2A (MEN-2A)
d. MEN-2B

Ans. d (Bailey 27/e p856-857)

Q4. In case of parathyroid adenoma, treatment is:
a. Calcitonin and steroid
b. Removal of adenoma
c. Total parathyroidectomy and implantation in the arm
d. Total parathyroidectomy

Ans. b

Q5. The most common organ involved in MEN-1 is:
a. Parathyroid b. Thyroid
c. Adrenal d. Testis

Ans. a (Schwartz 10/e p289)

Q6. Treatment for parathyroid hyperplasia is:
a. Removal of all four glands
b. Calcitonin
c. Removal of 3-1/2 glands
d. Enlarged glands to be removed

Ans. c (Harrison 20/e p2928)

Q7. Intestinal obstruction with jejunal neuromas is found in:
a. MEN-1
b. MEN-2A
c. MEN-2B
d. Familial intestinal polyposis

Ans. c

Q8. Hypocalcemia is a feature of all of the following, *except*:
a. Chronic renal failure
b. Hypoparathyroidism
c. Pseudohypoparathyroidism
d. Total thyroidectomy

Ans. d (Harrison 20/e p2937)

Q9. Common feature of MEN1 and MEN2:
a. Hyperparathyroidism
b. Medullary carcinoma of the thyroid
c. Pheochromocytoma
d. Carcinoids

Ans. a

Q10. An infant is diagnosed with MEN-2B trait. Which of the following will be the best line of management?
a. Prophylactic surgery
b. Clinical observation and follow-up
c. Regular fine needle aspiration cytology (FNAC)
d. All of the above

Ans. a (Schwartz 10/e p1550)

MULTIPLE CHOICE QUESTIONS

Grade I	Simple

Q1. A 20-year-old male presents with chronic constipation, headache and habitus, neuromas of the tongue, medullated corneal nerve fibers, and a nodule of 2 × 2 cm in size in the left lobe of the thyroid. This patient is a case of: (All India 2004)
a. Sporadic medullary carcinoma of thyroid
b. Familial medullary carcinoma of the thyroid
c. MEN2A
d. MEN2B

Q2. True about MEN-1: **(PGI June 2004)**
a. Increased vanillylmandelic acid (VMA) in urine
b. Increased calcitonin
c. Hypergastrinemia
d. Hyperprolactinemia
e. Hypocalcemia

Q3. True about MEN-2A (Sipple syndrome): **(PGI Dec 2006)**
a. Pheochromocytoma
b. Hyperparathyroidism
c. Mucocutaneous neuromas
d. Medullary carcinoma of the thyroid

Q4. In case of parathyroid adenoma, treatment is: **(AIIMS Nov 1995)**
a. Calcitonin and steroid
b. Removal of adenoma
c. Total parathyroidectomy and implantation in the arm
d. Total parathyroidectomy

Grade II | **Difficult**

Q1. The investigation of choice for extra-adrenal pheochromocytoma: **(PGI Dec 2007)**
a. Meta-iodobenzylguanidine (MIBG) scan
b. Magnetic resonance imaging (MRI)
c. Computed tomography (CT)
d. X-ray
e. Ultrasound (USG)

Q2. Primary hyperparathyroidism is caused by: **(PGI 2002)**
a. Parathyroid hyperplasia
b. Adenosis
c. MEN1
d. Thyrotoxicosis
e. Chronic renal failure (CRF)

Q3. All are true about pheochromocytoma, *except*: **(All India 2011)**
a. 90% are malignant
b. 95% occur in the abdomen
c. They secrete catecholamines
d. They arise from sympathetic ganglions

Q4. Parathyroid adenoma most commonly involves which of the following sites: **(AIIMS 2002)**
a. Thyroid substance
b. Superior parathyroid lobe
c. Inferior parathyroid lobe
d. In the mediastinum

Grade III | **Most difficult**

Q1. Features to differentiate parathyroid adenoma from hyperplasia would include which of the following? **(AIIMS 2002)**
a. Presence of excess chief cells
b. High levels of parathormone
c. Infiltration of the capsule
d. Identifying hyperplasia of all four glands at surgery in parathyroid hyperplasia

Q2. The most common cause of hyperthyroidism is: **(All India 1989)**
a. Single adenoma
b. Multiple adenomas
c. Single gland hyperplasia
d. Multiple gland hyperplasia

Q3. Hyperparathyroidism can occur in: **(PGI 2018)**
a. After thyroid surgery
b. DiGeorge syndrome
c. Radical resection of head and neck cancer
d. MEN1

Q4. A 35-year-old woman has had recurrent episodes of headache and sweating. Her mother had renal calculi and died of thyroid cancer. Physical observations revealed a thyroid nodule and ipsilateral enlarged cervical lymph nodes. Before performing thyroid surgery, the woman's physician should order: **(All India 2002)**
a. Thyroid scan
b. Estimation of hydroxyl indole acetic acid in urine
c. Estimation of urinary metanephrines, VMA, and catecholamines
d. Estimation of thyroid-stimulating hormone (TSH) and TRH levels in serum

Q5. A young female with a history of renal calculi complains of bone pain and abdominal cramps. On investigation, multiple fractures were discovered, and serum calcium and parathyroid hormone (PTH) were raised. Which of the following will be the best investigation to arrive at a definitive diagnosis? **(AIIMS 2017)**
a. Contrast-enhanced computed tomography (CECT) scan neck
b. Sestamibi scan
c. Radioiodine scan
d. Ultrasound neck

ANSWERS

Grade I: 1. d (Schwartz 10/e p289); 2. a, c, d (Bailey 27/e p856-857); 3. a, b, d; 4. b

Grade II: 1. b; 2. a; 3. a; 4. c

Grade III: 1. d; 2. a; 3. a, b, c; 4. c; 5. b

MODEL QUESTIONS

Q1. Superior parathyroid glands originate from:

a. Thyroglossal duct
b. Fourth branchial pouch
c. Third branchial pouch
d. Foramen cecum

Ans. b

Q2. Who discovered parathyroid glands in man?

a. Felix Mandl b. Fuller Albright
c. Ivar Sandstorm d. Richard Owen

Ans. c

Q3. Development of parathyroid glands is due to which gene?

a. *RET* b. *GCM2*
c. *CDN1B* d. *pK3*

Ans. b

Q4. Tetany and the parathyroid gland relation were discovered by:

a. Charles Martella b. Eugene Gley
c. Nussbaum d. Irvin

Ans. b

Q5. Parathyroid CA high risk is associated with:

a. Glial cells missing transcription factor 2 (GCM2)
b. Retinoblastoma 1 (RB1)
c. Hyperparathyroidism 2 with jaw tumors (HRPT2)
d. Cyclin-dependent kinase inhibitor 1B (CDKN1B)

Ans. a

Q6. What is the wrong statement?

a. They are less often found in a subcapsular location.
b. They are located anterior and medial to the recurrent laryngeal nerve.
c. The superior thyroid artery is the predominant vascular supply for all parathyroid glands.
d. They are more commonly ectopic and can be found anywhere from the angle of the mandible to the pericardium.

Ans. c

Q7. To raise calcium levels, parathyroid hormone (PTH) stimulates:

a. The activity of osteoblasts
b. The activity of osteoclasts
c. A reduction in calcium absorption from the intestines
d. Calcitonin

Ans. b

Q8. How to locate an ectopic parathyroid gland?

a. Technetium-99m-sestamibi (MIBI) scans
b. Selective arterial catheter sampling for parathormone
c. Magnetic resonance imaging (MRI)
d. Ultrasound (USG)

Ans. a

Q9. Hyperparathyroidism causes all, *except*:

a. Nephrocalcinosis
b. Osteosclerosis
c. Brown tumors
d. Subperiosteal deposition of bone

Ans. b

Q10. How to manage hyperplasia of the parathyroid gland?

a. Removal of two parathyroid glands
b. Removal of three parathyroid glands
c. Cortisol
d. Removal of all parathyroid glands

Ans. b

Q11. Secondary hyperparathyroidism is commonly caused by?

a. Sleeve gastrectomy b. Gastric ballooning
c. Chronic renal failure d. Vitamin D deficiency

Ans. c

Q12. Nephrocalcinosis is caused most commonly due to:

a. Total thyroidectomy
b. Hypoparathyroidism
c. Hyperparathyroidism
d. Hypothyroidism

Ans. c

Q13. Parathyroid glands mainly have a blood supply from:

a. Esophageal arterial branches
b. All four thyroidea ima
c. Inferior thyroid artery
d. Superior thyroid artery

Ans. c

Q14. What is the landmark for the location of the parathyroid glands?

a. Behind the esophagus
b. Tubercle of Zuckerkandl
c. Carotid sheath
d. Recurrent laryngeal nerve

Ans. b

Q15. Most commonly inferior parathyroid glands are located in:

a. Tracheoesophageal groove
b. Behind the esophagus
c. Thymus
d. Superior mediastinum

Ans. c

Q16. False about the parathyroid gland:

a. The number of oxyphil cells in the parathyroid gland decreases with age.
b. The percentage of adipose cells within the parathyroid gland increases with age.
c. The parathyroid glands are usually four in number, situated on the tubercle of Zuckerkandl.
d. Most commonly inferior parathyroid glands are in the thymus gland.

Ans. a

Q17. Tc-99m-sestamibi imaging cell type responsible for identifying parathyroid adenoma?

a. Follicular cell
b. Oxyphil cell
c. Clear cell
d. Parafollicular

Ans. b

Q18. Regulator of PTH is:

a. T3-T4
b. Fibroblast growth factor 23 (FGF 23)
c. Calcium
d. 25-hydroxyvitamin D

Ans. d

Q19. Not a cause of hypercalcemia:

a. Lithium
b. Sarcoidosis
c. DiGeorge's syndrome
d. Hyperthyroidism

Ans. c

Q20. Which of the following is associated with low PTH levels?

a. Vitamin D intoxication
b. Primary hyperparathyroidism (PHPT)
c. Parathyroid hyperplasia
d. Secondary PTH

Ans. a

Q21. Familial hypocalciuric hypercalcemia is associated with:

a. PTH-2R
b. Calcium-sensing receptor (CaSR) of the thyroid gland
c. CaSR of the parathyroid gland
d. Renal CaSR

Ans. d

Q22. Genetic mutation is not related with parathyroid carcinoma:

a. RET
b. RB1
c. GCM2
d. M-22

Ans. a

Q23. The most common bone affected by osteoporosis in hyperparathyroidism is seen at:

a. Scapula
b. Skull
c. Ribs
d. Distal radius

Ans. d

Q24. Which positron emission tomography (PET) tracer is used to detect parathyroid glands?

a. Glucose—fluorodeoxyglucose (FDG)
b. F-18
c. 123I-meta-iodobenzylguanidine (MIBG)
d. 18F-fluorocholine

Ans. d

Q25. In which operation Miami criteria play a role:

a. Parathyroid gland excision
b. Pituitary tumor
c. Total thyroidectomy
d. Excision hemithyroidectomy

Ans. a

SUGGESTED READING

1. Bailey & Love's - Short Practice of Surgery, 27th edition.
2. Schwartz's Principles of Surgery, 18th edition.
3. Textbook of Surgery by David Sabiston, 21st edition.

CHAPTER 30

Adrenal Glands

"Trying to describe a good marriage is like trying to describe your adrenal glands. You know they're in there functioning, but you don't really understand how they work."

– Helen Gurley Brown

INTRODUCTION

There are two adrenal glands weighing about 4 g each, situated near the superior poles of the kidneys in the retroperitoneal area, well encapsulated [Gerota's (Dumitru Gerota, 1867–1939, Romanian Surgeon) capsule]. The right adrenal gland is situated at a lower level than the left adrenal gland, as it lies between the right lobe of the liver and the diaphragm near the inferior vena cava (IVC), and the left gland is situated close to the superior pole of the left kidney near the renal pedicle. *The pancreatic tail and spleen partly cover the left adrenal gland. The adrenal cortex is developed from mesodermal cells, and the medulla from neuroectodermal cells* **(Figs. 1A and B)**.

HISTOLOGY

The adrenal gland is divided into two parts:

- *Cortex*—the external part - it has 3 zones:
  1. *Zona glomerulosa*—having small and compact cells that secrete the hormone aldosterone.
  2. *Zona fasciculata*—having large lipoid-rich cells arranged in radial columns, secretes dehydroepiandrosterone (DHEA), dehydroepiandrosterone sulfate (DHEAS), and cortisol.
  3. *Zona reticularis*—having pigmented and compact cells.
- *Medulla*—large chromaffin cells arranged in a thin layer, they synthesize, keep, and secrete catecholamine.

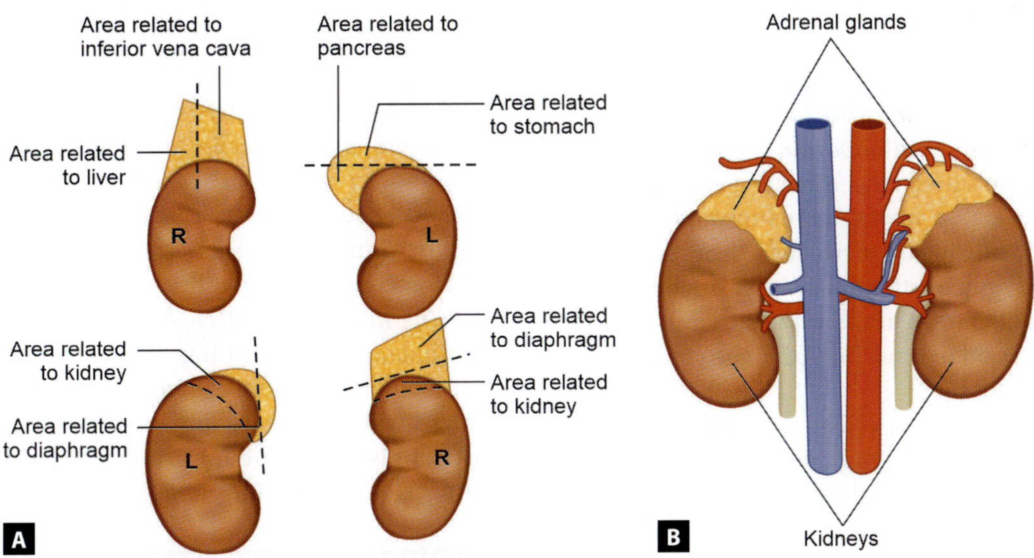

Figs. 1A and B: Location of adrenal glands.

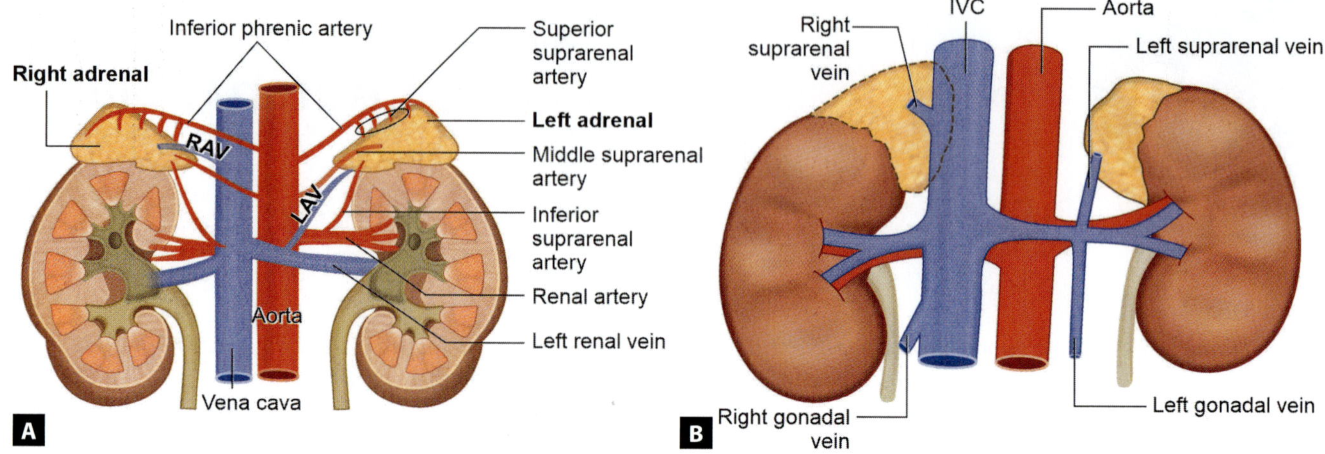

Figs. 2A and B: Arterial blood supply and venous drainage of the adrenal glands. (RAV: right adrenal venous drainage; LAV: left adrenal venous drainage)

BLOOD SUPPLY OF THE ADRENAL GLANDS

The arterial blood supply to the adrenal glands is from the branches of the aorta, the diaphragmatic arteries, and the renal arteries. The arterial supply of the adrenal gland has a lot of variations.

Usually, a single vein drains the adrenal gland, on the right side to the vena cava and on the left side to the renal vein. There are various sites other than renal poles where accessory adrenal tissue is found **(Figs. 2A and B)**.

PHYSIOLOGY OF ADRENAL GLANDS

The "fight or flight" response during stress is having the main role of the adrenal gland secretions. The adrenal cortex secretes corticosteroids, aldosterone, and cortisol, whereas the adrenal medulla synthesizes adrenaline and noradrenaline, which are also known as epinephrine and norepinephrine, and dopamine. These hormones, adrenaline and noradrenaline, directly go to the blood in circulation and act on target organs through receptors, alpha and beta, causing an increase in heart rate and BP. They also cause vasoconstriction in the splanchnic system, but cause vasodilatation in the vessels of muscles. They also cause dilatation of bronchii, stimulate glycogenolysis in the liver and muscles.

The zona glomerulosa cells synthesize aldosterone, which acts on the kidneys, the intestine, salivary glands, and the sweat glands to maintain sodium—potassium equilibrium and homeostasis. It causes the excretion of potassium and the conservation of sodium. The aldosterone secretion is regulated by the concentration of sodium and potassium and the renin-angiotensin organization. Renin is produced in the kidney by juxtaglomerular cells and acts on angiotensinogen, converting it to angiotensin I, which is converted to angiotensin II by angiotensin-converting enzyme (ACE). *Angiotensin I and II stimulate the secretion of aldosterone. If kidney blood supply or flow is reduced, as happens in bleeding, dehydration, low salt, and renal artery stenosis, and low sodium, then secretion of rennin increases, which corrects the low renal blood flow effects (causes sodium retention, potassium excretion, and rise of plasma volume).*

> *Not to forget:*
> *Nelson's (Don H Nelson, 1925–2010, American Physician) syndrome*—due to increased continuous secretion of ACTH, causing hyperpigmentation due to chemical synergies between ACTH and melanocyte-stimulating hormone (MSH).

Dehydroepiandrosterone and sulphate of DHEA, DHEAs are called adrenal androgens, which are made in zona-fasciculata and zona-reticularis with cortisol. Adrenocorticotropic hormone (ACTH), produced by the anterior pituitary, regulates the secretion of cortisol. ACTH is controlled by a hormone called *corticotropin-releasing hormone (CRH).* ACTH is synthesized in the hypothalamus. Cortisol has various functions: Reduces immunological response, increases gluconeogenesis and lipolysis with a decrease in peripheral glucose utilization. Cortisol also causes euphoria (but rarely depression), alertness, wound healing, and bone mineralization.

ADRENAL INCIDENTALOMA

Any lesion of the adrenal gland that is diagnosed incidentally.

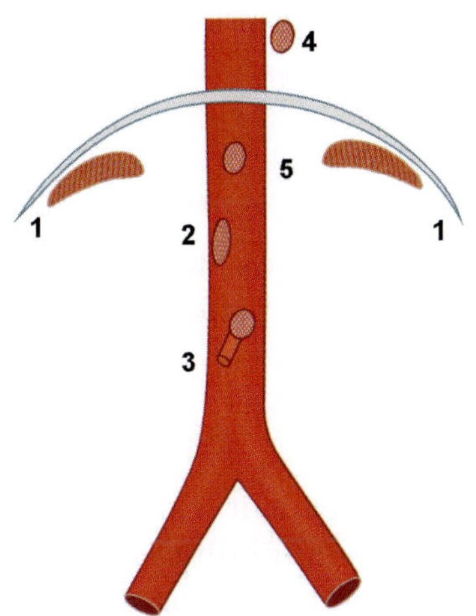

Fig. 3: Accessory adrenal tissue. (1: Below diaphragm, 2: Retroperitoneal along arota, 3: Retroperitoneal along branches of arota, 4: Thorax, 5: Retroperitoneal along pancreas)

Primary hyperaldosteronism (PHA) [Conn's (Jerome William Conn, 1907–1981, American Physician) syndrome].

It is a primary hyperaldosteronism due to increased secretion of aldosterone and causes hypertension. The most common cause of PHA is adrenocortical adenoma, somatic mutations are at KCNJ5. It occurs between 30 and 50 years of age, more commonly in females with muscle weakness, cramps, and headaches. Diagnosis is made by estimating the aldosterone to plasma renin activity ratio with hypokalemia. Computed tomography (CT) and magnetic resonance imaging (MRI) are also required. It is initially treated with spironolactone, then laparoscopic adrenalectomy is done. Accessory adrenal tissue may be found at some sites **(Fig. 3)**.

CUSHING'S SYNDROME

It is the hypersecretion of cortisol due to endogenous synthesis of corticosteroids. Commonly caused by Cushing's disease due to a pituitary adenoma. It may be ACTH dependent (85%) or ACTH independent (15%).

Clinically, the *Cushing (Harvey Williams Cushing, 1869–1939, American Surgeon)* syndrome has diabetes, hypertension, muscle weakness, central obesity, hirsutism, skin striae in the abdomen, menstrual irregularity, depression, osteoporosis, etc. *The diagnosis is made by estimating morning and midnight corticosteroid levels, which are elevated, and dexamethasone fails to reduce 24-hour urinary cortisol excretion.* If there is abnormal cortisol secretion without symptoms, it is called *subclinical Cushing syndrome.* Treatment is adrenalectomy with preoperative preparation with metyrapone or ketoconazole. Postoperatively, cortisol supplement is given as the other adrenal gland is suppressed.

ADRENOCORTICAL CARCINOMA

It is rare, more common in females, and occurs in two peaks (childhood and fourth and fifth decades). It is difficult to differentiate from benign adrenal tumors. Malignant tumors are bigger with necrosis or hemorrhage and capsular or vascular invasion. Most of the patients have Cushing syndrome with abdominal and back pain. CT and MRI are required to diagnose and to exclude pheochromocytoma, chemical investigations are done. The treatment is resection of the tumor, open or laparoscopic adrenalectomy. Postoperative mitotane or with etoposide are given.

Adrenogenital Syndrome (Congenital Adrenal Hyperplasia)

Virilization with adrenal insufficiency is diagnostic. Hypertension and short height are present. Cortisol replacement is sufficient, but may require adrenalectomy.

Points to remember:
- Right side adrenal gland is pyramid shaped and the left side is crescent-shaped.
- ACTH peaks in the early morning.
- Pheochromocytoma adrenal glands scale (PASS) score used to indicate malignancy.
- Extra-adrenal pheochromocytomas secrete only noradrenaline.
- MEN associated pheochromocytoma secretes only adrenaline.
- Malignant pheochromocytoma secretes dopamine and homovanillic acid (HVA).

ACUTE ADRENAL INSUFFICIENCY

It happens as a shock with fever, vomiting, abdominal pain, hypoglycemia, and electrolyte imbalance. *Waterhouse-Friderichsen (Rupert Waterhouse, 1873–1958, British Physician, described this syndrome in 1911. Carl Friderichsen, 1886–1979, Denish Physician mentioned the syndrome in 1918)* syndrome involves both adrenal glands with infraction and meningococcal sepsis. It should be treated as an emergency sickness to avoid death, which is very common.

PHEOCHROMOCYTOMA

It arises from chromaffin cells of the adrenal medulla and sympathetic ganglia. It is a tumor which may be unilateral or bilateral and called "10% tumor" (10% inherited, 10% extra-adrenal, 10% malignant, 10% bilateral, and 10% in children).

Hereditary phaeochromocytomas are seen in: MEN2A, MEN-2B, familial paraganglioma (PG) syndrome (I, III, and IV), *von Hippel-Lindau [Eugen von Hippel, 1867–1939, German Ophthalmologist, Arvid Lindau, 1892–1958, Swedish Pathologist)* (VHL) syndrome and neurofibromatosis (NF I) type I.

Pheochromocytomas are highly vascularized, grayish-pink tumors. They produce certain substances: calcitonin, ACTH, vasoactive intestinal polypeptide (VIP), and parathyroid hormone-related protein (PTHrP).

Clinical Features

- Patients usually feel a headache, palpitations, and sweating intermittently. They are diagnosed by a high level of catecholamine by measuring breakdown products, metanephrine and normetanephrine.
- Weight loss

Investigations

- *Gallium DOTATATE scan:* Metastasis and extra-adrenal pheochromocytoma.
- Screening test 24-hour urinary vanillylmandelic acid (VMA)
- *MRI*: Swiss cheese

Histology

Phaeochromocytoma shows Swiss cheese configuration on histology (Zellballen pattern and salt and pepper nuclei) **(Figs. 4 and 5)**.

Investigation

PET1 (presumably a patient with a primary endocrine tumor) histology/immunohistochemistry positive for synaptophysin and chromogranin, scan is a good technique to show primary tumor, extra-adrenal tumors, and metastasis.

Treatment is adrenalectomy, with a preoperative alpha adrenoreceptor blocker is given to block catecholamine. Postoperatively patient is kept in the intensive care unit (ICU) for 24 hours for hypovolemia and hypoglycemia.

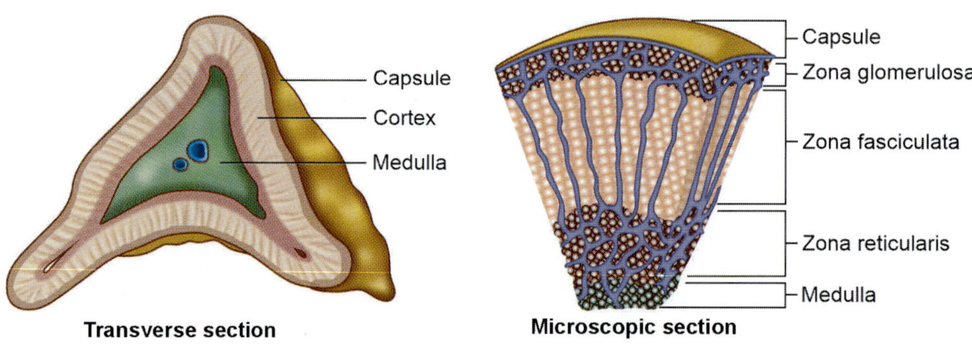

Fig. 4: Histology of the adrenal gland.

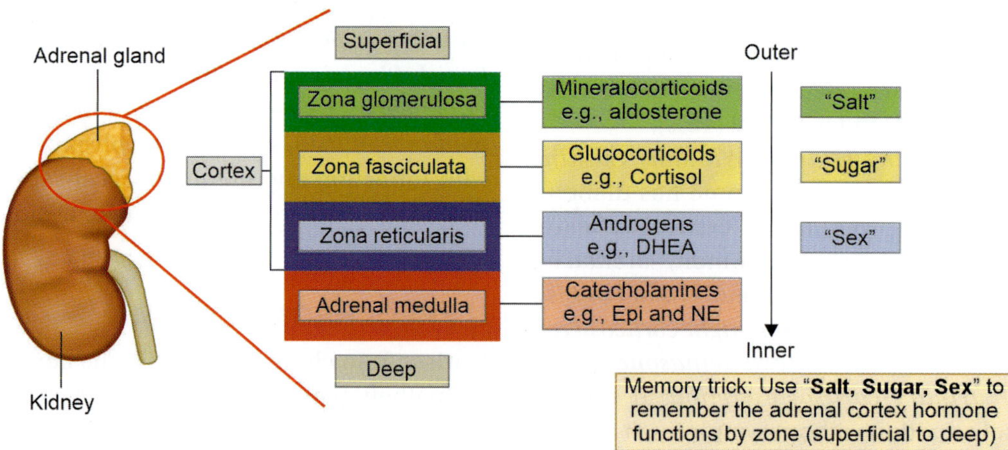

Fig. 5: Functions of the adrenal gland. (Epi: Epinephrine; NE: Norepinephrine)

X-blocker and B-blocker

Malignant pheochromocytoma—X-blocker—adenectomy—chemotherapy.

When the adrenal vein is clamped, there develops sudden hypotension, which is treated with IV fluids and vasopressors.

First and second trimesters in pregnancy—X-blockers are given first, and then surgery.

Third trimester—start X-blocker, then surgery is done after delivery.

Genes associated with a syndrome of familial pheochromocytoma are: RET (MENZA and MEN2B), MF1 (MF Type I), VHL (VHL symptoms), SDHD (Succinate Dehydrogenase Complex Subunit), and Familial paraganglioma.

Malignant Pheochromocytoma

- It occurs in 10% of primary tumors and is treated by alpha blockers. Surgery is the treatment.
- Metastasis is a confirmatory feature.
- Pass score-Ki-67 marker.
    - Vascular invasion
    - Capsular invasion

Adrenal tumors release certain compounds:

- *Pheochromocytoma:* Noradrenaline and adrenaline
- *Paraganglioma:* Noradrenaline
- *Malignant tumor:* Dopamine

> *You may be asked:*
> - *Incidentaloma:* It is an adrenal mass discovered incidentally while imaging. Surgery is the treatment.
> - *Capsular invasion* may be present in benign tumors of the adrenal gland, also, and it is not a solitary feature of malignancy.
> - *Triad of symptoms:* Headache, palpitation, and diaphoresis present in pheochromocytoma.
> - *Hypertension* is the most common feature of pheochromocytoma.

NEUROBLASTOMA

- *It is the most common abdominal malignancy in childhood.* It is a malignant tumor of the adrenal medulla, pale and grey, encapsulated, with areas of calcification, necrosis, and hemorrhage. Metastasis are common. It is diagnosed by biochemical evaluation, 24-hour urinary excretion of VMA and HVA.
- It is of two types:
    1. Sporadic
    2. Familial
- Most common at 5 years of age.
- 60–70% of cases present with metastasis when diagnosed.
- *Metastasis:*
    - It is rare. Bone is the most common metastasis. Other linear skull and lateral nasal processes (LNS).
    - *Atypical metastasis:*
        - Blueberry muffin lesions.
        - Raccoon eye (In 10–20% cases due to retrobulbar metastasis).

Investigation

- MRI (is better)
- CT
- MIBG scan
- *Fine needle aspiration cytology (FNAC)/histopathology:* Small round blue cells (others are Mn BREL = Blastoma, Rhabdomyosarcoma, Ewings tension, Lymphoma—neuro, nephro, retino, hepato, and medulloblastoma).

WILMS TUMOR/NEUROBLASTOMA SYMPTOMS

- Wilms tumor (WT) originates from the kidney, and neuroblastoma (NB) originates from the adrenal gland.
- WT abdominal mass does not cross midline.
- Calcification present in WT and not in NB.

Low-risk patients are treated with surgery, intermediate-risk patients by surgery and chemotherapy, and high-risk patients by chemotherapy.

> *Good to remember:*
> - NB displaces the kidney to the side and down, called the Drooping Lily sign.
> - Pheochromocytoma histology shows salt and pepper nuclei and Zellballen pattern (Nest of chromaffin cells), which is diagnostic of paraganglioma or pheochromocytoma.

GANGLION NEUROMA

It is a benign tumor of the adrenal medulla with mature sympathetic ganglion cells and Schwann cells (Theodore Schwann, 1810–1882, French Anatomist). Appears in all ages and is best diagnosed by CT and MRI. Treatment is adrenalectomy.

Prognosis

- *Good prognosis:*
    - Decrease in 8 months
    - Stage (1, 2A, 2B, and 4S)

- N-MYC—not amplified
- Milk .... Not
  - Better prognosis
  - Poor prognosis

Treatment

Chemotherapy + surgery—etoposide and cisplatin.

CARCINOID TUMORS

Site

- Intestine
- 10% of cases of carcinoid syndrome

Metastasis

Most common in the lungs.

Clinical Features

- C = Cutaneous flushing (most common)
- A = Abdominal pain
- B = Bronchospasm
- L = Weight loss
- E = Valvular lesions
- D = Diarrhea

GASTRINOMA (ZOLLINGER-ELLISON SYNDROME, ZES, ROBERT MILTON ZOLLINGER, 1903–1992, AMERICAN SURGEON, AND EDWIN HOMER ELLISON, 1918–1970, AMERICAN SURGEON)

This condition includes:
- Ulcer diathesis in the stomach, duodenum, etc.
- Recurrent ulceration despite adequate treatment
- Nonbeta islet cell tumors of the pancreas (gastrinoma)

It *occurs in about 20% of PET. The gastrinoma triangle contains the majority of these tumors*. The gastrinoma triangle is made of the head of the pancreas, the superior and descending portions of the duodenum, and the relative lymph nodes.

The progression of gastrinoma is slow, with a 5-year survival rate of 65%. Over 90% of gastrinoma patients have peptic ulcers. Diarrhea, gastroesophageal reflux disease (GERD), and abdominal pain are common symptoms.

Treatment is effectively done by proton pump inhibitors (PPIs) and octreotide. Chemotherapy is used when metastasis is developed. Surgical excision of the tumor is required in patients without diffuse metastases.

SOME IMPORTANT QUESTIONS

Q1. In pheochromocytoma, the urine will contain:
a. Vanillylmandelic acid (VMA)
b. Hydroxyindoleacetic acid (HIAA)
c. Both
d. None

Ans. a

Q2. The most common cause of Cushing syndrome is:
a. Adrenal adenoma b. Carcinoma
c. Hyperplasia d. Atrophy

Ans. c (Harrison 20/e p2724)

Q3. False regarding pheochromocytoma:
a. 10% of nonfamilial adrenal pheochromocytomas are bilateral.
b. Only 10% of hypertensive patients have an underlying pheochromocytoma.
c. 10% of adrenal pheochromocytomas arise in childhood.
d. Fine needle aspiration cytology (FNAC) is a must for diagnosis.

Ans. d

Q4. Indications for surgery in a case of adrenal incidentaloma:
a. Size >5 cm
b. Bilateral adrenal metastasis
c. Functional tumor
d. All of the above

Ans. d (Schwartz 10/e p1589)

Q5. Pheochromocytoma with malignant potential exclusively secretes:
a. Dopamine b. Epinephrine
c. Metanephrine d. Norepinephrine

Ans. a (Bailey 27/e p846)

Q6. Incidental finding in computed tomography (CT) scan, a 3 cm adrenal mass, which of the following is not done?
a. Adrenalectomy
b. Dexamethasone suppression test
c. Measurement of catecholamines
d. Midnight plasma cortisol

Ans. a

Q7. True about pheochromocytoma is:
a. Arises from chromaffin cells of the adrenal medulla

b. Bilateral in 20% of all cases
c. Hypotension rules out pheochromocytoma
d. Almost always a malignant tumor

Ans. a

Q8. A 50-year-old male presents with severe refractory hypertension, weakness, muscle cramps, and hypokalemia; the most likely diagnosis is:

a. Hypoaldosteronism b. Hyperaldosteronism
c. Cushing syndrome d. Pheochromocytoma

Ans. b (Harrison 20/e p2729)

Q9. Which one of the following clinical features is not seen in pheochromocytoma?

a. Hypertension b. Episodic palpitations
c. Weight loss d. Diarrhea

Ans. d (Schwartz 10/e p1586)

Q10. Which one of the following is not a CT feature of an adrenal adenoma?

a. Low attenuation
b. Homogeneous density and well-defined borders
c. Enhances rapidly, contrast stays in it for a relatively longer time, and washes out late.
d. Calcification is rare

Ans. c

MULTIPLE CHOICE QUESTIONS

Grade I	Simple

Q1. Mrs Neena noted an abdominal mass in the left side of her 6-month-old child, while showed calcification near the left kidney. What will be the cause? (AIIMS Nov 2000)

a. Leukemia
b. Neuroblastoma
c. Renal cell carcinoma (RCC)
d. Lymphoma

Q2. Opsoclonus-myoclonus is a phenomenon seen in: (PGI 1997)

a. Wilm's tumor
b. Neuroblastoma
c. Meningioma
d. Cortical tuberculoma

Q3. Investigation of choice in case of a patient with episodic hypertension, headache, and thyroid nodule: (AIIMS Nov 1997)

a. Urinary HIAA
b. Urinary catecholamine and aspiration of the nodule
c. Thyroid function test only
d. Urinary basic amino acid metabolite

Q4. A patient presented with a headache and flushing. He has a family history of his relative having died of a thyroid tumor. The investigation that would be required for this patient would be: (AIIMS June 1999)

a. Chest X-ray
b. Measurement of 5-HIAA
c. Measurement of catecholamine
d. Intravenous pyelography

Q5. During bilateral adrenalectomy, the intraoperative dose of hydrocortisone should be given after: (AIIMS 2004)

a. Opening the abdomen
b. Ligation of the left adrenal vein
c. Ligation of the right adrenal vein
d. Excision of both adrenal glands

Q6. A young female presents with hypertension with vanillylmandelic acid (VMA) >14 mg/day, associated with: (PGI 2002)

a. Medullary carcinoma of the thyroid
b. Von Hippel–Lindsay disease
c. Surge–Weber syndrome
d. Graves' disease
e. Neurofibromatosis

Q7. False statement about pheochromocytoma: (All India 1997)

a. 10% are bilateral.
b. Arises from chromaffin cells.
c. Extra adrenal tumor—increased noradrenaline levels.
d. Increased VMA levels in urine

Q8. A most common cause of Addison's disease in India: (AIIMS 2011)

a. Tuberculosis
b. Postpartum
c. Autoimmune
d. Human immunodeficiency virus (HIV)

Q9. Not seen in neuroblastoma is: (UP 1996)

a. Diarrhea b. Proptosis
c. Splenomegaly d. Bone involvement

Q10. A known patient with renal stone disease developed pathological fractures along with abdominal pain and certain psychiatric symptoms. He should be investigated for: (UPSC 1996)

a. N-myc amplification
b. Rat sarcoma (RAS) oncogene
c. Hyperdiploidy
d. Translocations

Grade II	Difficult

Q1. An accidental finding of an incidentaloma (an Adrenal mass) on ultrasound (USG) is detected. The following is/are to be ruled out. (PGI Dec 2006)

a. Cushing's disease
b. Metastasis
c. Adrenal adenoma
d. Carcinoma
e. Adrenal hyperplasia

Q2. A most common cause of hypercalcemic crisis is: (AIIMS 1987)

a. Parathyroid adenoma
b. Parathyroid hyperplasia
c. Carcinoma breast
d. Paget's disease

Q3. Which one of the following is not a CT feature of an adrenal adenoma? (AIIMS Nov 2010)

a. Low attenuation
b. Homogeneous density and well-defined borders
c. Enhances rapidly, contrast stays in it for a relatively longer time, and washes out late.
d. Calcification is rare.

Q4. Hypocalcemia in the immediate postoperative period following excision of parathyroid adenoma is due to: (AIIMS 1992)

a. Stress
b. Increased uptake by bones
c. Hypercalciuria
d. Increased calcitonin

Q5. Kamli Rani, a 75-year-old woman, presents with postmyocardial infarction after 6 weeks with mild congestive heart failure (CHF). There was a past history of (H/O) neck surgery for parathyroid adenoma 5 years ago, and an electrocardiogram (EKG) shows slow atrial fibrillation. Serum Ca^{+2} is 13.0 mg/L, and urinary Ca^{+2} is 300 mg/24 h. On examination, there is a small mass in the paratracheal position behind the right clavicle. Appropriate management at this time is: (All India 2002)

a. Repeat neck surgery
b. Treatment with technetium-99
c. Observation and repeat serum Ca^{+2} in 2 months
d. USG-guided alcohol injection of the mass

Q6. Hypoparathyroidism can occur in: (PGI May 2018)

a. After thyroid surgery
b. DiGeorge syndrome
c. Radical resection of head and neck cancer
d. Multiple endocrine neoplasia, type 1 (MEN1)

Q7. Episodic hypertension is a feature of: (JIPMER 2010)

a. Carcinoid tumor
b. Insulinoma
c. Pheochromocytoma
d. Zollinger–Ellison syndrome

Q8. The investigation of choice for extra-adrenal pheochromocytoma: (PGI Dec 2007)

a. Metaiodobenzylguanidine (MIBG) scan
b. Magnetic resonance imaging (MRI)
c. CT
d. X-ray
e. USG

Q9. A 20-year-old male presents with chronic constipation, headache, and palpitations. On examination, he had marfanoid habitus, neuromas of the tongue, medullated corneal nerve fibers, and a nodule of 2 × 2 cm in size in its lobe of the thyroid. This patient is a case of: (All India 2004)

a. Sporadic medullary carcinoma of the thyroid
b. Familial medullary carcinoma of the thyroid
c. MEN-IIA
d. MEN-IIB

Q10. MEN-2A includes adverse event: (PGI June 2004)

a. Ganglioneuromas
b. Cutaneous lichenoid amyloids
c. A mutation in the RET in chromosome 10
d. Parathyroid adenoma
e. Adrenal adenoma

Grade III | **Most difficult**

Q1. Investigation useful for detecting extra-adrenal pheochromocytoma: (PGI May 2011)
a. USG
b. CT
c. T2-weighted MRI with gadolinium contrast
d. MIBG

Q2. Neuroblastomas: A good prognostic factor is: (PGI June 2000)
a. N-myc amplification
b. RAS oncogene
c. Hyperdiploidy
d. Translocations

Q3. True about neuroblastoma: (PGI Dec 2006)
a. Seen in adrenal glands
b. Increased VMA/homovanillic acid (HVA)
c. Lymphatic metastasis is more common than blood metastasis
d. Presents with abdominal mass.
e. Old age presentation implied a good prognosis.

Q4. Which of the following statements about neuroblastoma is not true? (All India 2009)
a. The most common extracranial solid tumor in childhood
b. >50% present with metastasis at the time of diagnosis
c. Lung metastasis are common.
d. Often encase the aorta and its branches at the time of diagnosis

Q5. Tumor arising from olfactory nasal mucosa is: (All India 2012)
a. Nasal glioma
b. Adenoid cystic carcinoma
c. Nasopharyngeal carcinoma
d. Esthesioneuroblastoma

Q6. All are true about pheochromocytoma, *except*: (All India 2011)
a. 90% are malignant.
b. 95% occur in the abdomen.
c. They secrete catecholamines.
d. They arise from sympathetic ganglions.

Q7. A 35-year-old woman has had recurrent episodes of headache and swelling. Her mother had renal calculi and died of thyroid cancer. Physical observations revealed a thyroid nodule and ipsilateral enlarged cervical lymph nodes. Before performing thyroid surgery, the woman's physician should order: (All India 2002)
a. Thyroid scan
b. Estimation of hydroxyl indole acetic acid in urine
c. Estimation of urinary metanephrines, VMA, and catecholamines
d. Estimation of thyroid-stimulating hormone (TSH) and thyrotropin-releasing hormone (TRH) levels in serum

Q8. In case of parathyroid adenoma, treatment is: (AIIMS Nov 1995)
a. Calcitonin and steroid
b. Removal of adenoma
c. Total parathyroidectomy and implantation in the arm
d. Total parathyroidectomy

Q9. Which of the following is true about MEN-1? (PGI June 2004)
a. Increased VMA in urine
b. Increased calcitonin
c. Hypergastrinemia
d. Hyperprolactinemia
e. Decreased CA^{2+}

Q10. Palpation of the costovertebral angle produces pain and tenderness in acute adrenal insufficiency. This is: (AIIMS 1989)
a. Rotch's sign
b. Rossolimo's sign
c. Rogoff's sign
d. Osler's sign

ANSWERS

Grade I: 1. b; 2. b (Schwartz 10/e p1638-1640); 3. b; 4. c; 5. d; 6. a, b, c, d; 7. None; 8. a; 9. c (Bailey 27/e p847); 10. c (Bailey 27/e p858)

Grade II: 1. All; 2. c (Harrison 19/e p2470); 3. c; 4. b (Schwartz 10/e p81); 5. d (Harrison 19/e p2470); 6. a, b, c (Sabiston 20/e p925); 7. c; 8. b; 9. d (Schwartz 10/e p289); 10. a

Grade III: 1. c; 2. c (Bailey 27/e p847); 3. a, b, d; 4. c; 5. d; 6. a; 7. c (Schwartz 10/e p289); 8. b (Harrison 19/e p2473-2475); 9. a, c, d; 10. c

SECTION 7 Gastrointestinal Diseases

CHAPTER 31

Hernia

"The most essential part of a student's instruction is obtained, not in the lecture room, but at the bed side."

– Oliver Wendell Holmes (1867)

INTRODUCTION

"Hernia is a protrusion of a viscus or a part of a viscus through an abnormal opening or weakness in the wall of the cavity that contains it." Although a hernia can occur at various sites of the body, these defects most commonly involve the abdominal wall, particularly the inguinal region.

Hernia is a Latin word, which means *"a tear or rupture."* In Greek, it means *"offshoot"* or *"a budding,"* or *"a bulge."* The Egyptian literature has mentioned hernia around 1500 BC. Hernia was mentioned in the Egyptian Papyrus of Ebers in 1552 BC. Hernia surgery has been performed in India since ancient days. Hindus were known to use an abdominal or preperitoneal approach for cases of strangulated hernia. Hippocrates (460–375 BC) described umbilical hernia, causing pain and vomiting. Bassini carried out his operation for the first time in 1884, but did not present until 1887, before the Italian Association of Surgery. In 1890, he published an article in *"Archiv Fur Klinische Chirurgie,"* and it was only then that his method became known outside Italy. Irving L Lichtenstein, in 1984, used the term *"tension-free hernioplasty"* with the use of polypropylene mesh.

Types of hernia:
- *Reducible hernia*
- *Irreducible hernia:* Irreducible, obstructed, strangulated

A complicated hernia is a hernia with complications, such as obstruction and strangulation. Obstructed hernia should be treated as a strangulated hernia unless proved otherwise to avoid serious and even lethal complications.

INGUINAL HERNIA

Inguinal hernia is of two types: Indirect inguinal hernia and direct inguinal hernia.

Inguinal ligament: Inguinal ligament is a line connecting anterior superior iliac spine (ASIS) and pubic tubercle. ASIS lies at the level of the sacral promontory. The inguinal ligament lies beneath the skin fold in the groin and can be felt along its full length.

Anterior superior iliac spine: ASIS is easy to see and feel, but the pubic tubercle is sometimes difficult to feel.

Inguinal canal: It can be marked by two parallel lines, 1 cm apart, 1.25 cm above the medial half of the inguinal ligament.

Deep inguinal ring: It is marked as an oval opening 1.25 cm above the midinguinal point.

Superficial inguinal ring: It is marked as a triangle just above the pubic tubercle, with its center 1 cm above and lateral to the pubic tubercle and its apex facing upward.

Midinguinal point: It is a point at the center between ASIS and pubic symphysis.

Middle point of inguinal ligament: It is a point at the center between ASIS and pubic tubercle. *Inferior epigastric vessels:* It is a line drawn from the midinguinal point to the umbilicus; the lower two-thirds of this line represents the inferior epigastric vessels **(Figs. 1 and 2)**.

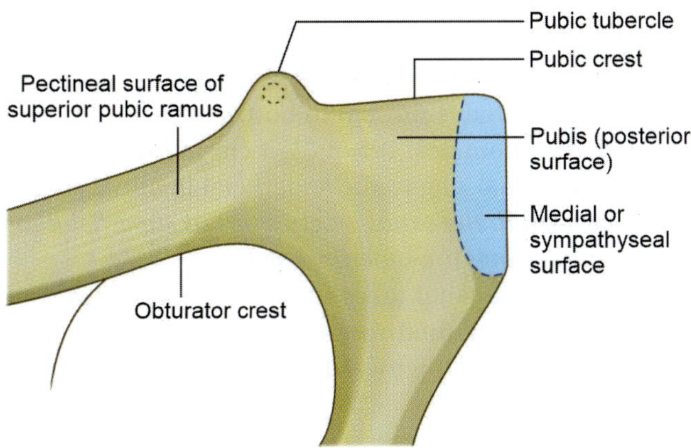

Fig. 1: Bony landmarks in the groin.

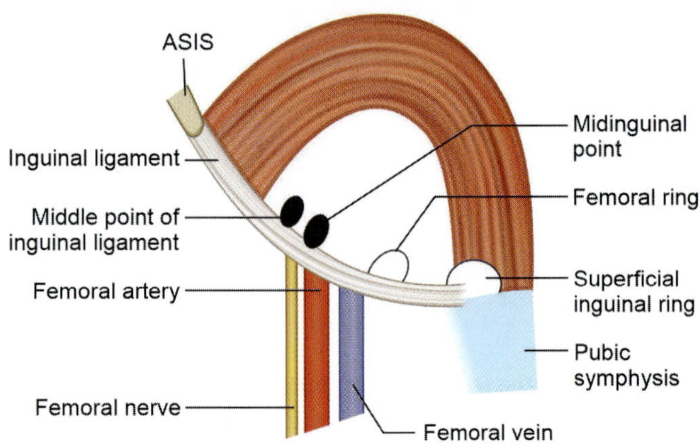

Fig. 2: Surface anatomy of the groin. (ASIS: anterior superior iliac spine)

Pubic Tubercle

It lies beneath the skin crease of the lower abdomen, 2–3 cm away from the midline. To find the pubic tubercle, put your finger on the center of the abdominal crease, push deep until you feel the pubic crest, then move your finger sideways until you reach the tubercle. You can also feel the pubic tubercle by invaginating the scrotum with an examining finger. Pubic tubercle and ASIS are important to the hernia surgeon because various musculoaponeurotic and ligamentous structures are attached to them. Pubic tubercle can be palpated in a female through the lateral margin of the labium majus.

Pubic Crest

It is a ridge of bone on the upper surface of the body of the pubis, medial to the pubic tubercle.

The inguinal canal is a passage in the lower anterior abdominal wall formed due to the migration of the testis out of the abdominal cavity to the scrotum for a favorable environment for spermatogenesis. It weakens this area of the anterior abdominal wall, making it prone to hernia. The inguinal canal is present in both sexes. It is larger in males than in females. It is 3.75–4 cm in an adult from the deep inguinal ring to the superficial inguinal ring. *In a newborn child, the canal is very short as superficial and deep inguinal rings are superimposed.*

The inguinal canal takes its direction as it descends from the deep inguinal ring to the superficial inguinal ring as follows: Downward, forward, and medially **(Figs. 3 to 5)**.

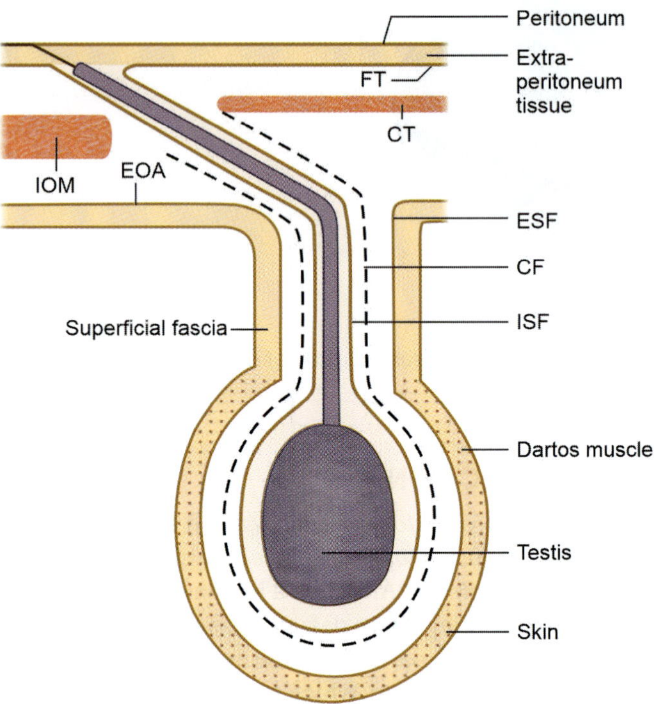

Fig. 3: Coverings of the inguinal canal. (CF: Camper's fascia, CT: conjoint tendon, EOA: external oblique aponeurosis, ESF: external spermatic fascia, FT: fascia transversalis, IOM: internal oblique muscle, ISF: internal spermatic fascia)

Deep or internal inguinal ring: It is a "U"-shaped opening in fascia transversalis, which forms the posterior wall of the inguinal canal. It is situated 1.25 cm above the midinguinal point (a point at the center of line joining ASIS and pubic symphysis). It is lateral to inferior epigastric artery. It is the internal end of the inguinal canal. Internal spermatic fascia arises from the margins of the deep inguinal ring. It has two margins: Superior margin and inferior margin. It is made by following structures: The iliopubic tract, the inferior epigastric vessels, and interfoveolar ligament (Hesselbach's ligament).

Superficial or External Inguinal Ring

Superficial or external inguinal ring is a triangular defect in the external oblique aponeurosis. The base of the triangle is formed by a pubic crest. It is pointing obliquely, medially, and down. It is situated 1.25 cm above the pubic tubercle. The two margins of the superficial inguinal ring are called crura. There are two crura: the Superomedial crus and the inferolateral crus.

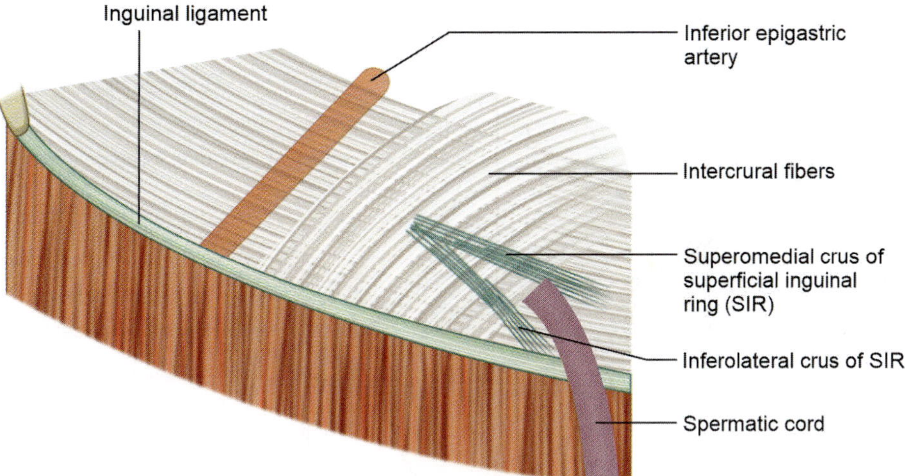

Fig. 4: Inguinal region.

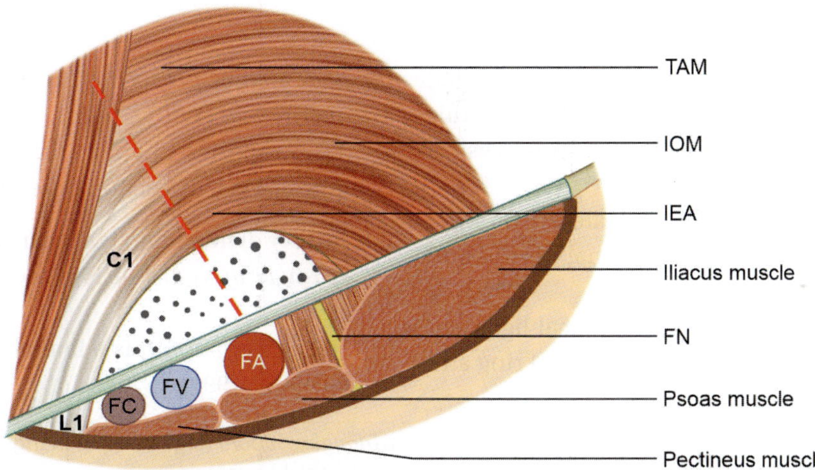

Fig. 5: Important structures of the groin. (FA: femoral artery, FC: femoral canal, FN: femoral nerve, FV: femoral vein, IEA: inferior epigastric artery, IOM: internal oblique muscle, TAM: transversus abdominis muscle.)

LAPAROSCOPIC GROIN ANATOMY

Before the start of practice of laparoscopic hernia surgery, familiarity with the anatomy of the posterior wall of the inguinal canal was not much required, and it was also not much understood. But now it is a must for every surgeon who wishes to practice laparoscopic groin hernia repair. Most of the surgeons are well versed with an anterior view of groin anatomy and not with a posterior view of groin anatomy. During an open hernia repair procedure, some structures are visible, which are not seen during a laparoscopic approach, and vice versa. *It is essential to know the laparoscopic groin anatomy for proper repair and fixation of mesh, and to avoid complications and injuries to organs.* The posterior or inner or abdominal or laparoscopic view of the lower abdominal wall shows five peritoneal folds and six fossae.

The five peritoneal folds are as follows **(Fig. 6)**:

- *Median umbilical ligament or fold:* It is in the midline. It is the remnant of the urachus.
- *Medial umbilical ligaments or folds:* These are two folds, one on either side of the midline. These are formed by peritoneal fold over obliterated umbilical arteries. These folds go up to internal iliac artery.
- *Lateral umbilical ligaments or folds or plica epigastrica:* These are two folds, one on either side. These are formed by peritoneal fold covering inferior epigastric vessels. These folds are lateral to medial umbilical folds.

Six Peritoneal Fossae

The five peritoneal folds divide the lower anterior abdominal wall into six fossae:

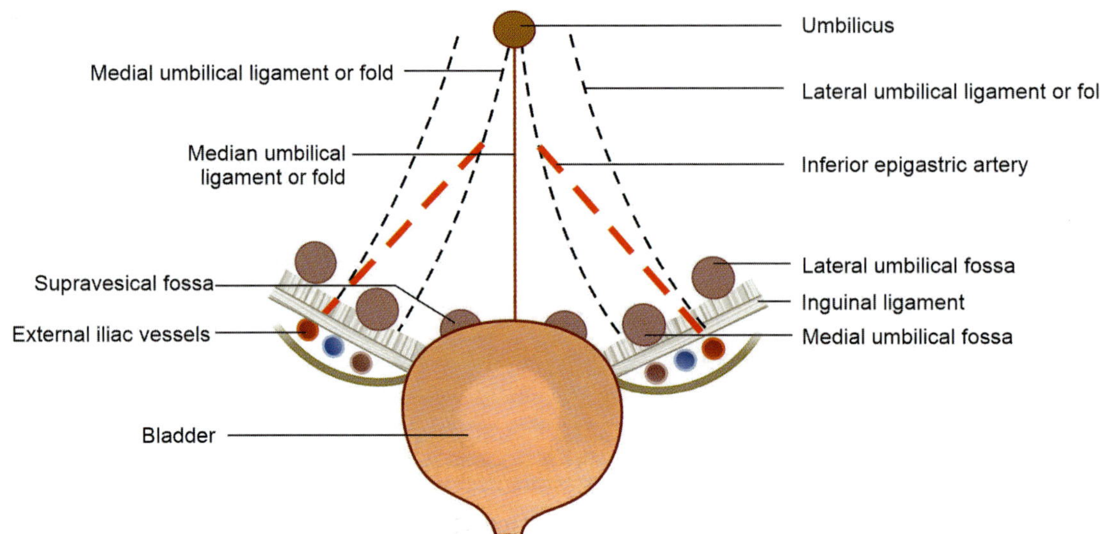

Fig. 6: Peritoneal folds and fossae.

- *Supravesical fossa:* It is in between median and medial umbilical ligament on each side. Hernia is rare in this region due to rectus muscle. It is the site of supravesical hernia.
- *Medial fossa:* It is between medial and lateral umbilical ligaments. It is the site of direct inguinal hernia and femoral hernia.
- *Lateral fossa:* It is lateral to lateral umbilical ligament on both sides. It is the site of internal inguinal ring and indirect inguinal hernia.

> *Points to remember:*
> *Structures pass through the inguinal canal:*
> - Spermatic cord and its coverings in males or the round ligament of the uterus in females
> - *Ilioinguinal nerve:* It enters the inguinal canal midway and comes out through the superficial inguinal ring.
> - *Vestigial remnant of processus vaginalis:* It is the prolongation of the peritoneum, which accompanies the descent of the testis in the scrotum.

Anatomical landmarks are important areas to be identified to avoid complications.

Important anatomical landmarks are described in the following text.

"Trapezoid of Disaster" (Seid) or "Square of Doom" (Annibali and Fitzgibbon)

Injury to vessels residing in the retroperitoneum is the most feared complication, as the associated mortality rate is significant. *These usually occur during initial access to the abdomen or preperitoneal space in the case of a total extraperitoneal (TEP) repair.*

It is a trapezoid-shaped area, which can lead to serious complications if dissection is performed here **(Fig. 7)**.

It is further divided into two triangles:
1. *Triangle of doom:* It is a medially placed triangular area.
2. *Triangle of pain:* It is a laterally placed triangular area (SPAW in 1991).

> *Triangle of doom* **(Fig. 8)***:* It is a triangular area that contains the external iliac vessels.
> - *Importance:* Any dissection in this area can cause injury to the external iliac vessels and may lead to serious bleeding. No dissection should be performed in this area, and no staples should be applied here.
> - *Contents:*
>   - External iliac artery
>   - External iliac vein
>   - Origin of inferior epigastric vessels
> - *Boundaries:* This triangle is formed by:
>   - *Apex:* Meeting point of the vas deferens and testicular vessels at the deep inguinal ring.
>   - *Medial boundary:* Vas deferens.
>   - *Lateral boundary:* Testicular vessels.
> - *Base:* An imaginary line connecting the lower part of the medial border and lateral border or peritoneal reflection.

Triangle of pain—**(Fig. 9)** *(Annibali and Fitzgibbon):* It contains most of the nerves of this area.

- *Importance:* This triangle contains some nerves, which can be damaged by dissection or application of staples here, so no dissection or staples should be applied here.

- *Contents:* The nerves in the triangle of pain are:
  - Femoral nerve
  - Femoral branch of genitofemoral nerve
  - Lateral femoral cutaneous nerve

During laparoscopic repair, lateral femoral cutaneous and genitofemoral nerves are most often affected, usually best treated by repeated exploration with neurectomy. Mesh removal is usually needed as well.

- *Boundaries:*
  - *Apex:* Meeting point of iliopubic tract and testicular vessels at deep inguinal ring
  - *Inferiomedially:* Testicular vessels
  - *Superolaterally:* Iliopubic tract
- *Base:* An imaginary line drawn from lateral part of iliopubic tract to testicular vessels

The trick to avoid injury in triangle of doom and triangle of pain is to not to put any suture or staple below the level of iliopubic tract.

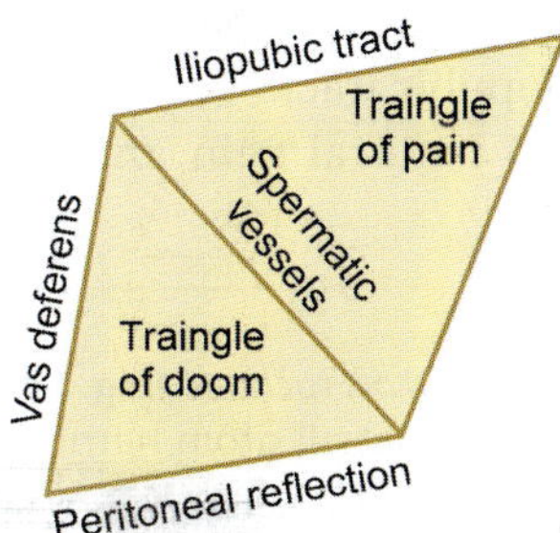

Fig. 7: Trapezoid of disaster.

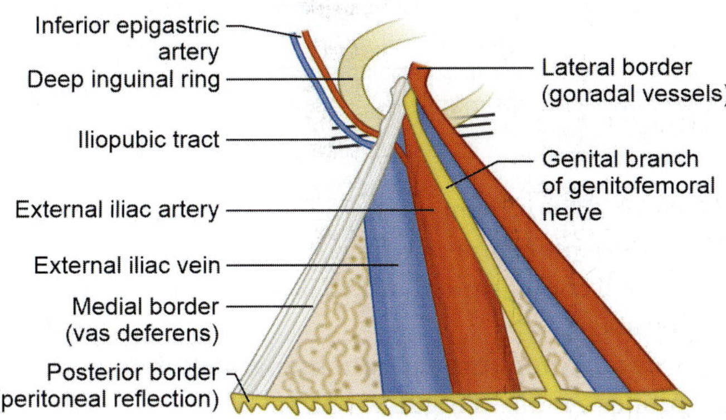

Fig. 8: Triangle of doom.

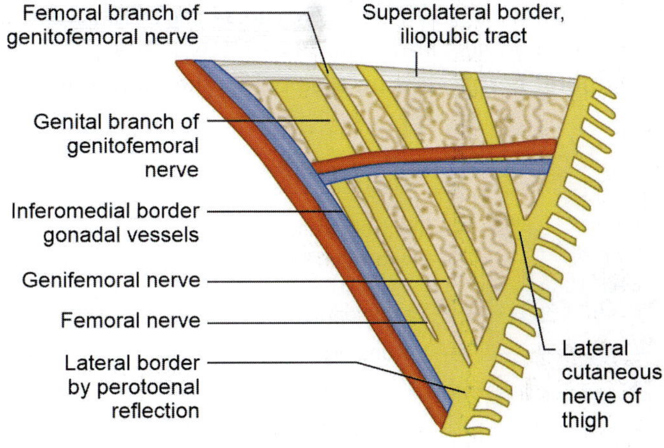

Fig. 9: Triangle of pain.

Corona Mortis or Crown of Death or Circle of Death (Fig. 10)

The pubic branch of the inferior epigastric artery travels down and anastomoses with the obturator artery, a branch of the internal iliac artery. In 20–30% of cases, a pubic branch is enlarged and it replaces the obturator artery, and then it is called the accessory or aberrant obturator artery. The aberrant obturator artery forms an anastomosis between the external and internal iliac arteries. The injury to this artery leads to severe hemorrhage. The aberrant obturator artery is present at the neck of the femoral hernia sac, and it can be damaged with massive bleeding during femoral hernia repair by laparoscopy. Due to this reason, this arterial circle is known as "corona mortis." Injury in this area usually occurs during the fixation of mesh in hernioplasty.

Major hemorrhage from the corona mortis is not common but rare and is dealt with by an experienced hand and requires urgent laparotomy. There is no place for laparoscopic management of major vessel injury. Wantz GE has reported a case of major vessel injury hemorrhage,

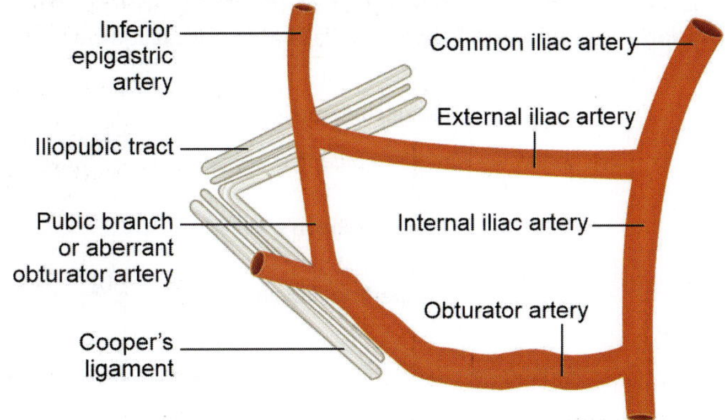

Fig. 10: Corona mortis or crown of death or circle of death.

after 4,114 Shouldice's hernia repair. *Branches of the obturator vein can be damaged while dissecting around Cooper's ligament.* The veins in this area also can be troublesome, especially iliopubic, obturator, and their tributaries as they may be larger than their accompanying arteries.

Inferior Epigastric Vessels

These are the branches of the external iliac vessels.

- *Importance:*
  - Bleeding from their injury is quite brisk and irksome.
  - These are most prominent near its origin from medial side of external oblique artery.
  - They form the lateral border of Hesselbach's triangle **(Fig. 11)**.
  - Direct inguinal hernia is identified as medial to these vessels and indirect inguinal hernia is lateral to these vessels.
- *Branches:* They give the following branches:
  - Cremasteric branch
  - Pubic branch
  - Muscular branches
  - Cutaneous branches

Cremasteric branch: It runs laterally and upward and penetrates the transversalis fascia and goes through internal inguinal ring with spermatic cord.

> *Pubic branch:* The pubic artery goes down vertically on the medial side and crosses the Cooper's ligament and anastomoses with the obturator artery at the obturator foramen. The anterior pubic artery is large in 25–30% of individuals and can replace the obturator artery; then it is called the aberrant obturator artery. This artery passes over the lacunar ligament from inside and thus can be damaged during the femoral hernia operation when the lacunar ligament is divided. The inferior epigastric vessels run upward at the medial aspect of the deep inguinal ring, raising a peritoneal fold called the "lateral umbilical ligament."

Cooper's Ligament (Fig. 12)

- It is a condensation of fascia transversalis and periosteum adherent to pubic ramus.
- It joins iliopubic tract and lacunar ligament.
- It is seen as white curvilinear structure.
- The adipose tissue surrounding Cooper's ligament has to be removed to visualize it properly.

Femoral Canal

- It is the site of a femoral hernia.
- It is behind iliopubic tract.
- It is medial to femoral vein and lateral to lacunar ligament.

> *Not to forget:*
> *Myopectineal orifice (MPO) of Fruchaud* **(Fig. 13)**: Henry Fruchaud, 1956, gave the theory that all groin hernias occur through a weak area in the groin, "MPO", which is now called as "myopectineal orifice of Fruchaud." Fruchaud's contribution to inguinal herniology was to examine the common anatomic etiology of direct, indirect, and femoral hernia. Adequate exposure of the MPO of Fruchaud is required in laparoscopic hernia repair for proper covering and fixation of mesh. MPO is divided by the iliopubic tract into two compartments.
> 1. Superior compartment
> 2. Inferior compartment

Superior compartment is further divided into two compartments by inferior epigastric vessels:

a. Medial compartment, which is prone to direct inguinal hernia
b. Lateral compartment containing deep inguinal ring prone to indirect inguinal hernia

Inferior compartment is also divided into two further compartments:

1. *Medial compartment* or *lacuna vasculorum* having femoral vessels and femoral canal, which is prone to femoral hernia; it is an area below the iliopubic tract

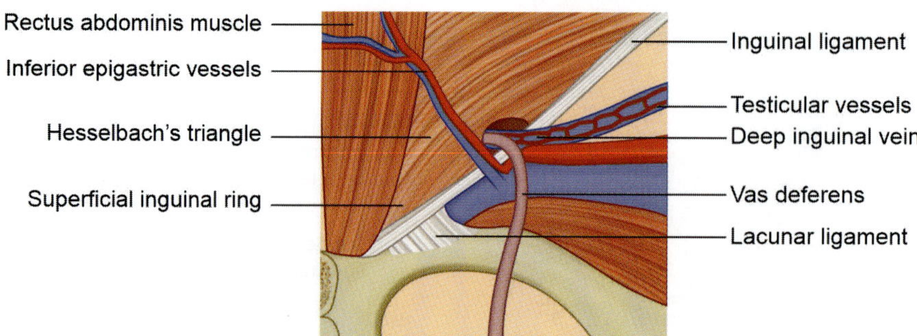

Fig. 11: Hesselbach's triangle, laparoscopic view.

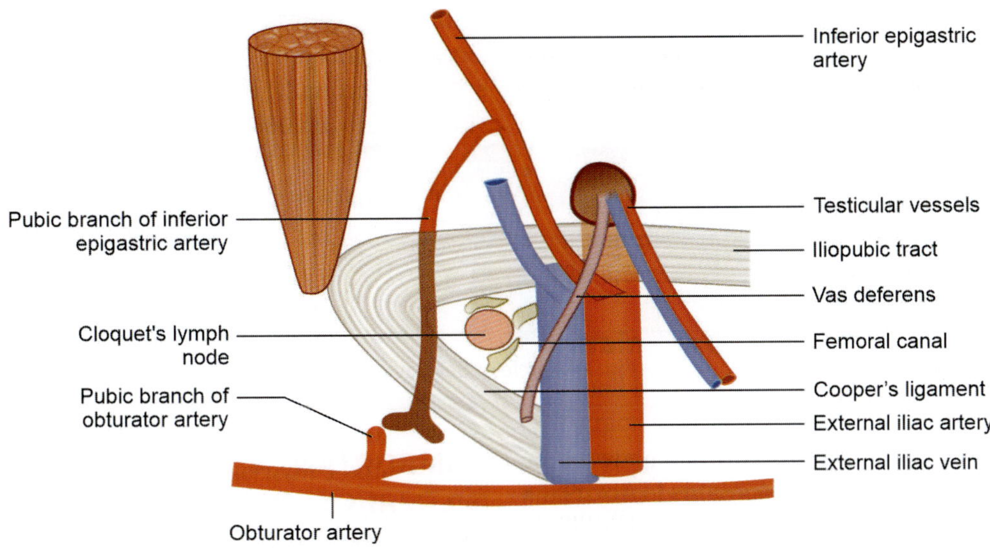

Fig. 12: Cooper's, lacunar, and inguinal ligament, laparoscopic view.

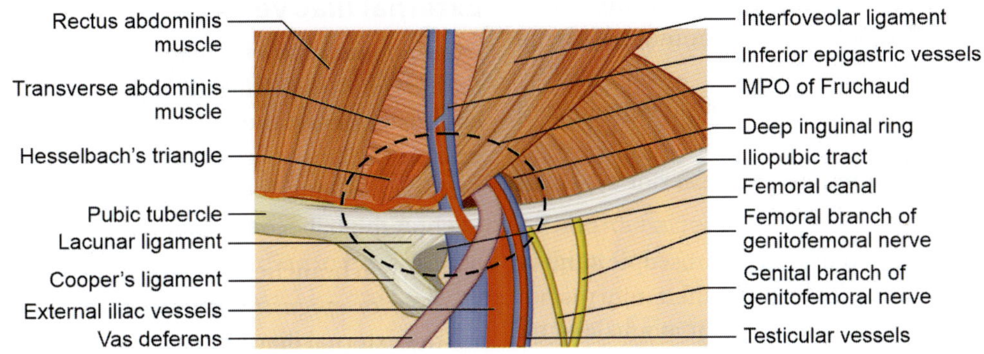

Fig. 13: Myopectineal orifice (MPO) of Fruchaud, laparoscopic view.

through which external iliac vessels cross the pelvis and reach femoral triangle in thigh. It is a neurovascular compartment through which femoral nerve and iliopsoas muscles reach thigh.

2. *Lateral compartment or lacuna musculorum:* It contains the iliopsoas muscle. It is a neuromuscular compartment that also has the femoral nerve. From the posterior side, you can see the posterior surface of the rectus muscle attached to the pubic bone. The pubic bone forms the center, and below it is the urinary bladder. Pubic bone's lateral part is the site of Cooper's ligament, which extends laterally. The iliopubic tract is attached in Cooper's ligament medially and then extends along superior pubic ramus, crossing the external iliac vessels, forming the inferior border of deep inguinal ring, attaching to iliopsoas fascia and then to the ASIS.

Lacunar Ligament

It is seen as a triangular ligament between the iliopubic tract and Cooper's ligament, forming the medial border of the femoral canal.

You may be asked:
Venous circle of Bendavid (R Bendavid) **(Fig. 14)**
- It is a network of veins.
- It is situated in the space of Bogros.
- *It receives tributaries from:*
  - Deep inferior epigastric vein
  - Iliopubic vein
  - Rectusial vein
  - Suprapubic vein
  - Retropubic vein
  - Aberrant obturator vein (in 70% person)

Importance of a circle of Bendavid: The veins in this area can be troublesome. It is important to know about these

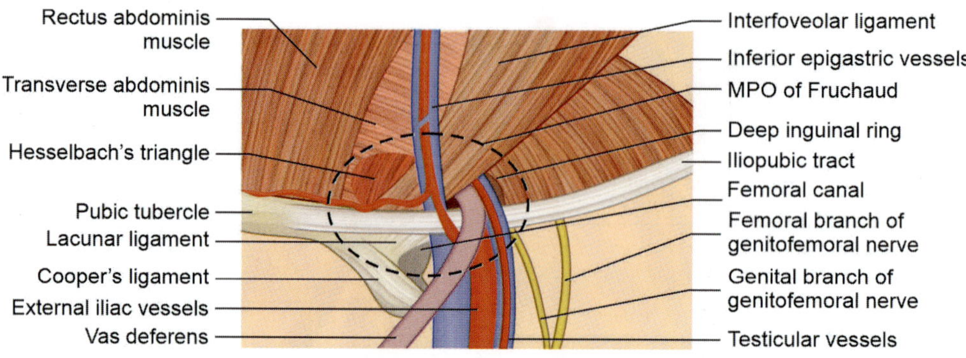

Fig. 14: Circle of Bendavid.

minor-looking veins as their injury during laparoscopic hernia surgery can lead to hemorrhage and hematoma formation. Sometimes it is difficult to stop such bleeding, and panic can cause damage to important structures.

- *Rectusial vein:* It runs along the lateral border of rectus muscle and forms venous anastomosis with the iliopubic vein.
- *Iliopubic vein:* It runs deep to the iliopubic tract and joins inferior epigastric vein.
- *Retropubic vein:* It is found on the posterior aspect of pubic ramus.

These veins are collapsed during laparoscopic surgery due to high carbon dioxide pressure and their injury is not visualized at that time, but they form a hematoma later on when carbon dioxide is removed.

NERVES IN PREPERITONEAL SPACE

The main nerves in inguinofemoral region are situated in a triangular area. This triangular area is called "triangle of pain." It contains following nerves:

- Genitofemoral nerve is on psoas muscle on medial side.
- Genital branch of genitofemoral nerve crosses the lower part of external iliac artery and pierces the iliopubic tract and enters the deep inguinal ring.
- Femoral branch of genitofemoral nerve goes along distal part of psoas muscle.
- Femoral nerve is lateral to genitofemoral nerve. It lies between psoas and iliacus muscles.
- Lateral cutaneous nerve of thigh is medial to ASIS.

IMPORTANT BLOOD VESSELS IN LAPAROSCOPIC HERNIA REPAIR

Important blood vessels in laparoscopic hernia repair are discussed further.

External Iliac Vessels

External iliac artery becomes femoral artery when it crosses the iliopubic tract. It lies on psoas muscle. External iliac vein lies posterior and medial to it. The external iliac artery and vein are the largest vessels in the area. They are seen medial to the psoas muscle and going down under iliopubic tract to enter thigh, becoming femoral vessels.

It gives two branches from its distal part:

1. *Inferior epigastric artery*—from the medial aspect of the external iliac artery
2. *Deep circumflex iliac artery*—from the lateral aspect of the external iliac artery

Both branches of the external iliac artery are given approximately at the same level, just before going deep into the iliopubic tract.

Good to remember:

- *Pampiniform plexus of veins:* Latin: Pampinus—tendril, shaped like a tendril; these veins drain into testicular veins, which in turn drain into:
  - Inferior vena cava on right side
  - Renal vein on the left side
- The pampiniform plexus of veins are classified into four groups:
  1. *Group I:* A tight plexus of veins around a testicular artery.
  2. *Group II:* Plexus of veins in fatty tissue.
  3. *Group III:* Plexus of veins located between groups I and II.
  4. *Group IV:* Arteriovenous anastomosis with testicular artery.

INGUINAL HERNIA

The inguinal region is a weak part in anterior abdominal wall. The weakness is due to presence of the following structures in inguinal canal:

- Inguinal canal
- Deep inguinal ring
- Superficial inguinal ring

COMPOSITION OF HERNIA

Any hernia consists of three parts:

1. Sac of hernia
2. Contents of the sac
3. Coverings of the sac

Contents of Hernia

The contents of the hernia are the viscera or the part of the viscus, which protrude through weak area of abdominal wall and lie within the sac of hernia.

A hernia may contain any of the following structures:

- Omentum
- Intestine
- A hernia containing part of circumference of intestine is called Richter's hernia, after August Gottlieb Richter (1742–1812), a lecturer in surgery. Richter's hernia is the most common in femoral hernia.
- A part of urinary bladder may be present in a hernia.
- Ovary or fallopian tube
- Meckel's diverticulum
- Peritoneal fluid
- Amyand's hernia

Coverings of Indirect Inguinal Hernia

From inside out to the side, the structures are:

- Peritoneum
- Extraperitoneal fat
- Internal spermatic fascia (derived from transversalis fascia at deep inguinal ring)
- Cremasteric fascia and muscles (derived from internal oblique and transversus abdominis muscles)
- External spermatic fascia (derived from external oblique aponeurosis at superficial inguinal ring)
- Superficial fascia including dartos muscle of the scrotum are:
  - Camper's fascia
  - Scarpa's fascia

Coverings of Direct Inguinal Hernia

- Skin
- *Superficial fascia:*
  - Camper's fascia
  - Scarpa's fascia
- External oblique aponeurosis
- Conjoint tendon
- Fascia transversalis
- Peritoneum

Richter's Hernia

"A portion of circumference of the bowel becomes herniated." It was described by August Gottlieb Richter (1742–1812), lecturer in surgery, Göttingen, Germany. Richter's hernia is commonly seen in:

- Femoral hernia
- Obturator hernia

It usually undergoes strangulation, producing obstruction to the lumen of loop of intestine. Intestinal obstruction is not present until half of the circumference of the bowel is involved.

Complete or Inguinoscrotal Hernia

- *Bubonocele:* Hernial sac protrudes only in the inguinal canal and does not descend further down as the inguinal canal is closed at the superficial inguinal ring. Bubon is a Greek word means "groin." It presents as a swelling in the groin. History is usually short. Most of the patients are young adults.
- *Funicular:* Sac comes up to the upper end of the scrotum but is separated from testis as the processus vaginalis is closed just above the epididymis. Hernial sac lies above the testis, and both are separate. Testes can be separately palpated. Funiculus is a Latin word which means a "small cord." It occurs in adults, and a long-standing history is present.
- *Complete or scrotal:* Hernia reaches up to the lower part of scrotum and testis and lies within them; however, you can palpate the testis, but with difficulty. The inguinal canal is patent throughout its length. The hernia sac is continuous with tunica vaginalis of testis. It is not seen at birth but is present in infancy, adolescent, and adulthood. The hernia goes down up to the bottom of scrotum. Hernia sac lies in front and at sides of the testis. Testis can be palpated posteriorly. Indirect hernia is a congenital hernia and occurs in children and yet may not appear until adolescent or adult life.

Congenital Indirect Inguinal Hernia

Congenital indirect inguinal hernia in children or in adults can be of the following variety:

- *Vaginal:* The processus vaginalis does not occlude, so hernia descends up to base of scrotum. The testis lies behind and is difficult to palpate separately.
- *Funicular:* The processus vaginalis is occluded just above the testis, so the hernia comes above the level of the testis, and the testis can be palpated separately.
- *Infantile:* It is similar to the funicular variety, but a process of processus vaginalis is formed in front of hernia, which goes as high as the superficial inguinal ring, so when operating, a peritoneal sac is found in front of the hernia sac. It is due to a diverticulum of the processus vaginalis being stuck at the external inguinal ring during development.
- *Encysted:* A process of the peritoneum is present in front of the sac. It also goes up to the external inguinal ring. It is also due to a diverticulum of the processus vaginalis stuck to the superficial inguinal ring. It is closed at two sites.
- *Interstitial:* A diverticulum develops, which gets caught between the layers of the anterior abdominal wall during development. This is of three types:
    1. *Superficial extraparietal interstitial hernia*—between superficial fascia and external oblique aponeurosis.
    2. *Interparietal or intramuscular*—between the internal and external oblique muscles.
    3. *Preperitoneal or retroperitoneal*—between fascia transversalis and peritoneum.

Direct Inguinal Hernia (Fig. 15)

Direct inguinal hernia occurs due to weakness in anterior abdominal wall with weak muscles and transversalis fascia. Occasionally it occur after sudden physical effort causing transverse fascia split and sudden appearance of hernia. It comes out directly through posterior wall of inguinal canal. Direct inguinal hernia occurs through Hesselbach's triangle. Hesselbach's triangle is divided into lateral and medial part by obliterated umbilical artery (lateral umbilical ligament), so direct hernia is divided into:

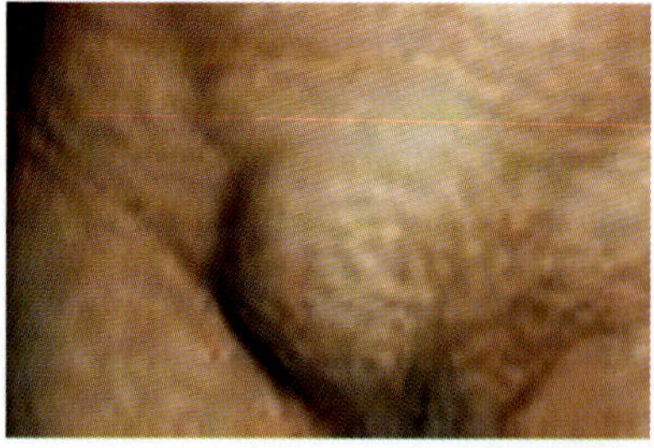

Fig. 15: Right direct inguinal hernia.

- Lateral direct inguinal hernia
- Medial direct inguinal hernia
- Neck of sac in indirect inguinal hernia lies lateral to inferior epigastric vessels.
- Neck of sac in direct inguinal hernia lies medial to inferior epigastric vessels.
- In inguinal hernia, the neck of the sac is above and medial to pubic tubercle.
- In femoral hernia, the neck of sac is below and lateral to pubic tubercle.
- Obliteration of deep inguinal ring with thumb does not allow indirect hernia to pop out, but direct inguinal hernia comes out.
- Occasionally, a direct inguinal hernia occurs suddenly after an awkward sudden physical effort, which causes sudden rise of intra-abdominal pressure. This causes split of fascia transversalis, leading to sudden appearance of direct inguinal hernia and is known as a "rupture."

Pantaloon or Saddlebag or Dual Hernia

It is a combination of both **direct and indirect inguinal hernia**.

- It has two sacs, striding over inferior epigastric vessels.
- It occurs in 5% of all inguinal hernia.
- Sometimes one sac of it is overlooked during the operation and a recurrence occurs, which is a false recurrence due to a missed hernia.

Maydl's Hernia (Hernia-en-W)

Two loops of small bowel form a "w." The outer loops remain in a sac, and the connecting loop remains within the abdomen and often strangulates.

- Tenderness is found above the inguinal ligament.
- Signs of intestinal obstruction are found.
- On operation, the loops of intestine in the sac are found normal, and the strangulated loop lies within the abdomen, so traction brings out the strangulated loop in the sac. The spread of peritonitis is early as the strangulated loop is inside the abdomen.
- Maydl's hernia is also called "retrograde strangulation."
- Strangulated loop of "W" lies within the abdomen, and the normal loop in the hernia sac.

CLINICAL FEATURES OF INGUINAL HERNIA

- General considerations
- History
- Examination

The accuracy of diagnosing a direct hernia is a little better than 50%, while an indirect hernia can be correctly diagnosed in 90% of patients.

History

- *Age:* It can occur at any age, and may even be present at birth.
- *Sex:* Inguinal hernia occurs in both males and females.
- *Occupation:* It is common among workers with strenuous work and heavy weightlifting. It causes strain on abdominal muscles, leading to a hernia.
- *Side:* Indirect inguinal hernia occurs more commonly on the right side due to late descent to the right testis and late closure of the right processus vaginalis.
- *Pain:* There may be no pain, but only discomfort or a lump in the groin is noticed, or there may be a dragging pain, which gets worse as the day passes.
- *Symptoms of intestinal obstruction* (pain, absolute constipation, distension, and vomiting) may be present, then think of: Obstructed hernia, strangulated hernia.
- *Symptoms of causative factors, especially of straining:* Ask history of chronic cough, dysuria, and frequency of micturition for BPH, bladder neck obstruction, urethral stricture, and constipation.

Past history of: Appendicectomy—It is important in direct inguinal hernia, the previous appendicectomy might have damaged subcostal or ilioinguinal nerve, history of previous hernia surgery as this hernia may be recurrent, history of lower segment cesarean section (LSCS), history of surgical removal of lower ureteric stone, and history of lumbar sympathectomy.

METHOD OF EXAMINATION

- Patient is examined in standing and then in supine position.
- Clothes are removed from umbilicus to midthigh.
- A swelling is present in inguinal region, which may be reaching up to scrotum.
- Patient stands and you sit in front of patient. Ask the patient to see on other side (to avoid saliva falling on you) and cough.
- First examine from front.
- Then examine from side—stand at the side of patient on hernia side. Place one hand on patient's back to support and other hand on lump. Now find the following facts: Site, size, shape, position, color, temperature, surface, tenderness, composition (gas/solid/fluid).

SIGNS

There are some characteristic diagnostic signs of a hernia. These are:

- Occurs at a congenital or acquired weak spot
- Reducibility
- Expansile cough impulse
- Reducibility and expansile cough impulse may be absent in irreducible or strangulated hernia, but it does not exclude the diagnosis of hernia.
- *Getting above the swelling:* This test is used to differentiate a scrotal swelling from an inguinal scrotal hernia.

Malgaigne's Bulge

Weakness of abdominal muscles below the umbilicus and in the inguinal region is shown by raising both legs simultaneously. This was described by Joseph-Francois Malgaigne (1806–1865), professor of surgery, Paris, France. See for Malgaigne's bulging, ask the patient to raise head or raise legs straight; bulgings developed in the inguinal area, which indicates weak abdominal musculature. Direct inguinal hernia may be associated with Malgaigne's bulging.

DIAGNOSTIC TESTS FOR INGUINAL HERNIA

The accuracy with which indirect and direct inguinal hernia are clinically distinguished is low.

Zieman's Technique (After Stephen a Ziemann, Surgeon, Providance Hospital, Mobile, Alabama, USA)

This technique is used to differentiate and diagnose indirect, direct inguinal, and femoral hernia **(Fig. 16)**.

Method:

- Ask the patient to lie supine.
- Reduce the hernia.

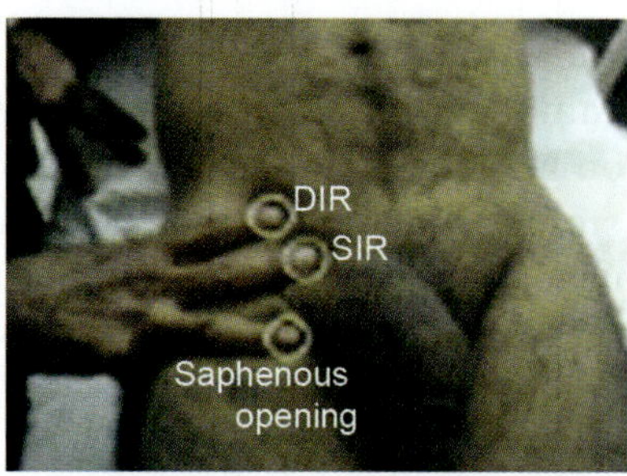

Fig. 16: Zieman's technique. (DIR: deep inguinal ring; SIR: superficial inguinal ring)

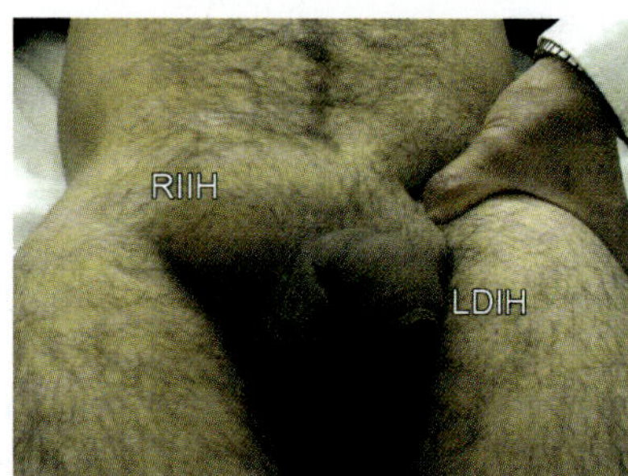

Fig. 17: Deep inguinal ring occlusion test. (LDIH: left direct inguinal hernia; RIIH: right indirect inguinal hernia)

- Then put:
  - Index finger over deep inguinal ring
  - Middle finger over the superficial inguinal ring
  - Ring finger over the saphenous opening
- Then ask the patient to cough and feel the expansible impulse on coughing by finger and diagnose the hernia according to site of impulse.
- Impulse felt by index finger—indirect inguinal hernia
- Impulse felt by the middle finger—direct inguinal hernia
- Impulse felt by ring finger—femoral hernia

Deep Inguinal Ring Occlusion Test (Fig. 17)

Aim: It is done to differentiate between indirect from direct inguinal hernia.

Deep inguinal ring occlusion test is a confirmatory test others while are complementary tests.

Method: Before starting the test, surface marking is required—mark the following landmarks.

- *ASIS:* It is the first bony prominence felt while tracing the inguinal ligament from medial to lateral.
- Deep inguinal ring
- Pubic symphysis
- *Midinguinal point:* Deep inguinal ring is half an inch above the midinguinal point. It is the middle point between ASIS and pubic symphysis.
- Ask the patient to lie supine.
- Reduce the hernia.
- Occlude the deep inguinal ring by the thumb just above the midinguinal point.
- Ask the patient to cough.

Result:

- *Deep inguinal ring blocked and swelling appeared:* Direct inguinal hernia.
- *Deep inguinal ring blocked and swelling did not appear:* Indirect inguinal hernia.

> *Fallacies of occlusion test:*
> - In pantaloon hernia, indirect hernia component will be occluded but direct hernia will pop out.
> - If this test is not done properly, then it will cause confusion.

Finger Invagination Test

Aim: This test is used to differentiate indirect from direct inguinal hernia.

Method:

- *Ask the* patient to lie supine.
- Reduce the hernia.
- Invaginate skin of scrotum with little finger from bottom of scrotum and push up to pubic tubercle. Now rotate the finger and pulp of finger faces toward abdomen of the patient, and now feel the superficial inguinal ring by pulp of your finger further push the finger in inguinal canal. Now ask the patient to cough and feel the impulse on finger.
- If impulse is felt at tip of finger, it is indirect inguinal hernia.
- If impulse is felt at pulp of finger, it is direct inguinal hernia.

Inguinal hernia in females:

- Finger invagination test is difficult as skin over labia is thick.
- Labium majus is found thickened on palpation in an inguinal hernia.

Fallacy: It cannot be done in females as the skin of the labia is thick and not lax.

Ladd method in children is a surgical procedure named after *William Edwards Ladd, American physician (1880–1967).* Roll the spermatic cord forth and back transversely between thumb and index finger. Thickening of the spermatic cord is demonstrated in this way. It is done in infants and children to diagnose inguinal hernia.

TABLE 1: Difference between indirect and direct inguinal hernia.

Difference	*Indirect inguinal hernia*	*Direct inguinal hernia*
Age	Common in young people and children	Common in elderly people
Site	• Usually unilateral • One-third of cases are bilateral • Common on the right side, especially in children due to the later descent of the testis of right side	• Usually unilateral • 50% of cases are bilateral
Site of defect	• Deep inguinal ring • Lateral to inferior epigastric artery	• Hesselbach's triangle • Medial to inferior epigastric artery
Relation to spermatic cord	• Lies within the covering of the spermatic cord • Anterior to cord	• Lies outside covering of cord • Posterior to cord
Shape	Pear-shaped or pyriform when complete and oval shape when incomplete	• Globular or spherical in shape • It is always incomplete
Relation to pubic tubercle	Above and medial to pubic tubercle	Below and lateral to pubic tubercle
Reducibility	Requires manipulation	Spontaneous
Direction of bulge on coughing	• Forward • Downward • Medially	• Forward • Downward
Sex	Males are affected 20 times	Females are not affected usually
Zieman's technique	Impulse is felt at index finger	Impulse is felt at middle finger
Invagination test	Impulse is felt on the tip of a finger	Impulse is felt on the pulp of finger
Ring occlusion test	Hernia will not show a bulge	A bulge will be seen
Cause	Preformed sac	Weakness of the posterior wall of inguinal canal
Malgaigne's bulging	Absent	May be present
Complications	Common due to narrow neck	Uncommon due to a wide neck

General Examination

- Examine the chest
- Do a digital rectal exam (DRE) for the prostate
- *Examine—stricture of the urethra*

The differences between indirect and direct inguinal hernia are described in **Table 1**.

- Plain X-ray of abdomen
- Ultrasonography (USG)
- Computed tomography (CT) scan
- Color Doppler study
- Herniography
- Magnetic resonance imaging (MRI)
- Diagnostic laparoscopy

Ventral hernias are abdominal wall hernias, i.e., epigastric, umbilical, paraumbilical, Spigelian, lumbar, parastomal, incisional, and traumatic.

THS has classified into midline [M–M1 (subxiphoidal), M2 (epigastric), M3 (umbilical), M4 (infraumbilical), and M5 (suprapubic)], and lateral [L–L1 (subcostal), L2 (flank), L3 (Iliac), and L4 (lumbar)].

CLASSIFICATION OF INGUINAL HERNIA

- *European Hernia Society (EHS) classification:* As per location (L—lateral/indirect, M—medial/direct, F—femoral), primary, recurrent, finger breadth (FB) into 0, 1, 2, 3, *x*.
- *Nyhus classification:* Type I (indirect inguinal hernia with normal ring), II (indirect with enlarged ring), III (IIIa—direct hernia with a posterior wall defect, IIIb—indirect hernia with posterior wall defect and enlarged internal ring, IIIc—femoral hernia), IV (recurrent hernia—direct/indirect/femoral/combinations).

Bochdalek hernia: It is the most common hernia of defective development of the pleuroperitoneal canal or membrane, commonly on the left posterolateral side, having the stomach, spleen or/and transverse colon.

Morgagni hernia: It is less common than Bochdalek hernia, with a defective central tendon of the diaphragm on the right anteromedial side, having the transverse colon.

These hernias cause pulmonary hypoplasia and hypertension to be managed by intermittent positive-pressure ventilation (*IPPV*) and extracorporeal membrane oxygenation (*ECMO*) if required.

DIFFERENTIAL DIAGNOSIS OF INGUINOSCROTAL SWELLING

- Infantile hydrocele
- Encysted hydrocele of cord
- Varicocele
- Lymph varix or lymphangiectasis
- Funiculitis
- Diffuse lipoma of cord
- Torsion of testis
- Retractile testis
- Tubercular lymphadenitis
- Malignant extension to cord from tumor of testis

INGUINAL HERNIA IN INFANTS AND CHILDREN

- Indirect inguinal hernia is less common in girls than boys (1:9).
- Repair of the congenital inguinal hernia is the most common operation in children.
- 3–5% of infants are born with an inguinal hernia.
- 80–90% of inguinal hernias occur in boys.
- Inguinal hernias are found on the right side in 60% of cases and on the left side in 30%, and bilaterally in 10 cases.
- Undescended testes or ectopic testes are associated with inguinal hernia in 90% of cases.
- Incidence of incarceration is 12%, most occur within the first 6 months of life.

Management

- 80% cases of incarcerated hernia in infants and children are managed conservatively.
- Inguinal hernia in infants and children needs surgery due to the high risk of incarceration.
- The operation is herniotomy.

Truss: Truss may cure a hernia in a newborn baby, but not in others. The truss is used to avoid protrusion of the hernia from the deep inguinal ring to inguinal canal and out of superficial inguinal ring.

STRANGULATED INGUINAL HERNIA

- *Causes of strangulation:* Narrow neck, rigid rim of neck.
- *Strangulation is common in the following hernia:* Femoral hernia, obturator hernia, and indirect inguinal hernia
- *Constriction factors in strangulated inguinal hernia:* Neck of sac, external inguinal ring in children, adhesions between contents and sac wall
- *Contents of sac in inguinal hernia:* Small intestine—most common, omentum—common, large intestine—less common, ovary and fallopian tube in females—occasionally
- Urgent surgery is required to save life.

TREATMENT OF INGUINAL HERNIA VIA SURGERY

- *Herniotomy*—removal of the sac of the hernia and reduction
- *Herniorrhaphy*—repair of the defect without mesh
- *Hernioplasty*—mesh placement to cover the defect

Surgery can be performed by the open or laparoscopic method (Lichtenstein's tension-free mesh hernioplasty). Laparoscopic surgery can be performed by TEP repair or transabdominal preperitoneal repair (TAPP).

Complications of open surgery: These include hemorrhage, injury to nerve or cord structures, nerve entrapment (ilio-hypogastric nerve), chronic inguinal pain (inguinodynia), seroma formation, infection, and recurrence.

Types of mesh:
- *Synthetic:* Prolene, Vipro (Vicryl + Prolene), polytetrafluoroethylene (PTFE)
- *Biological:* Human dermis or porcine dermis

Mesh is fixed gradually by fibrous growth through holes (larger holes preferred) after anchoring the mesh during surgery. The mesh should cover at least 5 cm on each side of the defect. Plug mesh is also used.

SLIDING HERNIA (HERNIA EN GLISSADE)

"Sliding hernia occurs due to slipping of the posterior parietal peritoneum on the underlying retroperitoneal structures." The posterior wall of the sac is formed by not only the posterior parietal peritoneum but also by retroperitoneal structures. On the right side, caecum forms the posterior wall of the hernia with peritoneum. The appendix may also be there.

On left side, the sigmoid colon and its mesentery form the posterior wall of the hernia with peritoneum.

FEMORAL HERNIA

Femoral hernia is more common in females due to a wider pelvis. It is especially more common in multiparous elderly women due to stretching of pelvic ligaments during pregnancy.

- It represents 2–4% of all groin hernias.
- It is the third most common hernia after inguinal and incisional hernia.
- It accounts for 20% of hernias in females and 5% in adult males.
- Femoral hernia is never congenital.
- Pregnancy is the most important causative factor. Increased abdominal pressure by repeated pregnancy is one of the reasons for femoral hernia.

Femoral ring: It is an oval opening of 1.25 cm in diameter. It is larger in females than in males. It is closed by thickened extraperitoneal tissue from inside, which is called the *femoral septum*. It is pierced by a few lymphatics.

Femoral sheath: Femoral sheath envelopes femoral vessels. The sheath rests upon pectineus and adductor longus muscles medially and psoas major and iliacus muscles laterally. Femoral canal lies in front of pectineus muscle. It has three compartments **(Fig. 18)**:

1. Medial compartment contains femoral canal.
2. Intermediate compartment contains femoral vein.
3. The lateral compartment contains a femoral artery.

Differential Diagnosis of Femoral Hernia

- Inguinal hernia
- Saphena varix
- Enlarged femoral lymph node
- Lipoma in the femoral triangle
- Femoral artery aneurysm
- Psoas abscess
- Rupture of adductor longus muscle
- An enlarged psoas bursa

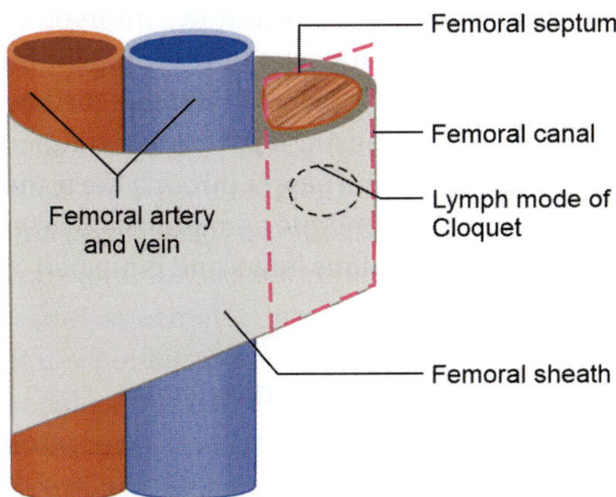

Fig. 18: Femoral sheath.

Operative Treatment

- High operation or McEvedy operation
- Middle approach or inguinal approach, or Lotheissen's operation
- Low operation or Lockwood operation.
- *Laparoscopic repair of femoral hernia:* Iliopubic tract is approximated with Cooper's ligament by polypropylene sutures. A small piece of mesh is introduced in the femoral canal and fixed.

UMBILICAL HERNIA AND PARAUMBILICAL HERNIA

Umbilical hernias develop at umbilical ring as may be present at birth or later. Umbilical hernias are present in approximately 10% of all newborns and are more common in premature infants. A defect <1 cm in size closes in 95% spontaneously. A defect greater than 1.5 cm in diameter seldom closes spontaneously.

Following variety of umbilical hernias are present:

- *Umbilical hernia at birth or exomphalos or omphalocele:* It is present at birth:
  - Exomphalos minor
  - Exomphalos major
- Umbilical hernia of infants and children
- Umbilical hernia of adults

Difference between Gastroschisis and Exomphalos

- *Omphalocele* is a covered defect of the umbilical ring into which abdominal contents herniate.
- *Gastroschisis:* It is a defect of the anterior umbilical wall lateral to the umbilicus with intact umbilical cord **(Table 2)**.

TABLE 2: Difference between gastroschisis and omphalocele.

Omphalocele	*Gastroschisis*
Covered the defect of the umbilical ring	Uncovered defect of the anterior abdominal wall lateral to the umbilicus
Peritoneal sac is present	No peritoneal sac
In 50% of cases, there are associated abnormalities in males	<10–15%
Liver eviscerated	No evisceration of the liver
Mortality is 37%	Mortality is 90%
Surgical closure is the treatment	Surgical closure is the treatment

Treatment

In small hernia (<2 cm), *subumbilical incision and edge-to-edge suturing*; in larger hernia (>2 cm), *Mayo's repair*; and in hernia >4 cm, *prosthetic mesh hernioplasty*.

Paraumbilical Hernia

In umbilical hernia, the bulge occurs under the umbilicus, but in paraumbilical hernia, the bulge occurs either above or below the umbilicus.

Etiological factors:
- Obesity
- Weak and flabby musculature of the anterior abdominal wall due to:
  - Lack of abdominal wall exercise
  - Presence of excessive fat
- Repeated pregnancies

EPIGASTRIC HERNIA

"Epigastric hernia is a protrusion of extraperitoneal fat through the linea alba between the umbilicus and the xiphisternum." Usually, it contains extraperitoneal fat, which is why it is also called "fatty hernia of linea alba." When the hernia starts, it contains only extraperitoneal fat, but as it grows, it pulls a pouch of peritoneum, which is empty or contains a portion of omentum. It does not contain a viscus as the neck of the sac is very narrow. Epigastric hernia was earlier considered a congenital defect, but is now considered an acquired lesion.

Treatment

If the gap is <2 cm, then a simple repair of the linea alba with a nonabsorbable suture is done. If the gap is >2 cm, then vertical Mayo's repair is done. If the gap is >4 cm, then polypropylene mesh hernioplasty is done. Where exploration of the sac is done, if the omentum is found healthy, then it is pushed back into the abdomen. If found strangulated, then it is excised.

INCISIONAL HERNIA

In adults, incisional hernia accounts for 80% or more of ventral hernias. Incisional hernia is also called "postoperative hernia" or "ventral hernia." It usually follows a laparotomy wound as deeper layers of the wound give way during the early postoperative period. Incisional hernia occurs in 14% of abdominal operations.

Treatment

Suture repair or Mayo repair, or tension-free anatomical approximation.

Open mesh repair: In >3 cm size defect—onlay repair, inlay repair, and sublay repair.

Laparoscopic repair: Laparoscopic approach in incisional hernia repair gives better visualization than an open method in multiple fascial defects. Complete visualization of the fascia underlying the previous incision allows for the identification of smaller "Swiss-cheese" defects that could be missed in an open approach.

Ramirez technique: This method includes release and medial advancement of the anterior rectus sheath, rectus muscle, and internal oblique to close the defect. It can cover a defect of 20 cm by advancing structures on both sides of the midline by 10 cm.

SPIGELIAN HERNIA

Adriaan van den Spiegel, 1576–1625, Professor of Anatomy, Padua, Italy. He was born in Brussels and educated in Padua. Spigelian hernia is the protrusion of preperitoneal fat or a peritoneal sac containing or not containing an intraabdominal organ, across a congenital or acquired defect in the Spigelian line. The semilunar line of Spigelian is not clearly seen during surgery. The Spigelian line is a semilunar line visible on the anterior abdominal wall, which marks the transition from muscular to aponeurotic area in the transversus abdominis. It extends from the costal margin to the pubic tubercle. It is convex laterally and concave medially. The lateral border of the rectus is also marked similarly, but the Spigelian line is different from it. The Spigelian aponeurosis is the aponeurosis in between these two lines. The Spigelian aponeurosis is widest between the umbilicus and the interspinal level. >90% of Spigelian hernia occur in this Spigelian hernia belt. *Arcuate line or fold or line of Douglas* is the lower end of the posterior rectus sheath. It is between the umbilicus and pubis. Spigelian hernia passes through the transversus abdominis and internal oblique aponeurosis. The external oblique aponeurosis remains intact and is pushed out with the skin.

Surgery for Spigelian Hernia

The sac is identified, opened, contents reduced, sac ligated, and excised. Repair transversus abdominis, internal and external oblique muscles. Prefix, a mesh plug, can be used to block the opening of a hernia. A polypropylene mesh can be used in big hernial defect.

INTERNAL HERNIA

Operation should be performed at the earliest opportunity to avoid strangulation. Hernia is reduced, and the bowel is assessed for viability after giving 100% oxygen and applying moist packs application. If gangrene is developed, then resection is done.

Defects are closed with nonabsorbable sutures.

LUMBAR HERNIAS

Hernia in the lumbar region of the abdomen is called a lumbar hernia. Lumbar hernia is of the following types: Superior lumbar hernia (SLH) and inferior lumbar hernia (ILH). Both of these are primary hernias. Primary lumbar hernia—rare. Secondary lumbar hernia, or acquired lumbar hernia or incisional lumbar hernia, occurs after open renal surgery. "Secondary lumbar hernia is the protrusion of abdominal contents through the inferior lumbar triangle" and is more common than SLH. Hernias in the inferior lumbar triangle are most often small and occur in young athletic women. *Inferior lumbar triangle or triangle of Petit, defined by Jean Louis Petit 1674-1750, Director of the Academie de Chirurgia, Paris, France,* as its lower border has the iliac crest. Medial border—anterior border of latissimus dorsi muscle; lateral border—posterior border of external oblique muscle. Excision of the sac and herniorrhaphy is the treatment of choice.

RARE HERNIAS

- *Interstitial hernia:* It is defined as a hernia in which the sac emerges between the anterior abdominal muscles. Exploratory laparotomy is done, then Prolene mesh is applied; but if the wound is contaminated, then mesh is not used, and if recurrence occurs, then elective prosthetic repair is done.
- *Ogilvie hernia:* It is a type of direct inguinal hernia. It is also called funicular direct inguinal hernia. There is a congenital defect in the conjoint tendon. Strangulation is the common feature of this hernia. If it contains the urinary bladder, then the history of swelling becomes less prominent after micturition is present.
- *Obturator hernia:* It is a hernia through the obturator foramen; strangulation is common; it is treated by hernioplasty.
- *Gluteal hernia:* It is a rare hernia. It occurs through the greater sciatic foramen. It occurs either from above or below the pyriformis muscle. Sac is excised. Contents are reduced. The defect is repaired by nonabsorbable sutures.
- *Sciatic hernia:* It is the rarest hernia of the abdominal wall. It occurs through the lesser sciatic foramen. Sac is excised. Contents are reduced. A defect is repaired by nonabsorbable sutures.
- *Perineal hernia:* It is a rare hernia. Protrusion occurs through the pelvic floor. Usually, the sac is wide-necked. Obstruction is rare. Repair is usually done by an abdominal approach.
- *Supravesical hernia:* It is a hernia whose sac protrudes through the supravesical fossa.

SOME IMPORTANT QUESTIONS

Q1. In the treatment of femoral hernia, Lockwood's operation refers to:

a. Low operation
b. High operation
c. Inguinal operation
d. Laparoscopic surgery

Ans. a

Q2. A child is complaining of fluid coming out of the umbilicus on straining. What is the diagnosis?

a. Gastroschisis
b. Patent vitellointestinal duct
c. Umbilical hernia
d. Patent urachus

Ans. d

Q3. Femoral hernia is characteristically..... the pubic tubercle.

a. Lateral and below
b. Medical and above
c. Lateral and above
d. Medial and below

Ans. a

Q4. A patient developed loss of sensations in root of penis after a laparoscopic hernia surgery. Which of the following nerves would have been damaged?

a. Ilioinguinal nerve
b. Iliohypogastric nerve
c. Genitofemoral nerve
d. Lateral cutaneous nerve

Ans. a

Q5. As per European Hernia Society Classification, incisional hernia at the level of the umbilicus is given the term:

a. M1 b. M2
c. M3 d. M4

Ans. c

Q6. Regarding the boundaries of laparoscopic anatomy of inguinal hernia, the false statement is:

a. Medial boundary of the triangle of doom is the vas deferens
b. The lateral boundary of the triangle of pain is the iliopubic tract
c. Myopectineal orifice is bounded by the internal oblique and transversus abdominis superiorly
d. Myopectineal orifice bounded by the iliopubic tract inferiorly

Ans. d

Q7. Match the following (nerves injured in surgery):

Nerve injured	*Surgery*
1. External laryngeal nerve	a. Laparoscopic hernia surgery
2. Long thoracic nerve	b. Video-assisted thymectomy
3. Phrenic nerve	c. Modified radical mastectomy
4. Hypoglossal nerve	d. Thyroidectomy
5. Lateral cutaneous nerve	e. Submandibular gland surgery

Ans. 1. d, 2. c, 3. b, 4. e, 5. a

Q8. In the operation theater (OT), a hernia surgery is going on. The sac is found medial to the inferior epigastric artery. What is the hernia, and what is the treatment for it?

a. Direct, Bassini repair
b. Indirect, Bassini repair
c. Direct, Lichtenstein repair
d. Indirect, Lichtenstein repair

Ans. c

Q9. A 50-year-old male presented with swelling on the right groin. While occluding the deep inguinal ring, the swelling reappears. What kind of hernia is it?

a. Indirect b. Direct
c. Femoral d. Pantaloon

Ans. b

Q10. A 30-year-old obese male patient presents with a complete inguinal hernia, and on examination, doughy consistency is felt with a dull note on percussion. This suggests that the contents of the hernia sac contain:

a. Omentum
b. Large intestine
c. Small intestine
d. Encysted ascitic fluid

Ans. a

Q11. A 30-year-old female presented with a mass in the inguinal region, which produced a gurgling sound on reduction, and the mass completely disappears on pressing it through the deep inguinal ring. What is your diagnosis?

a. Indirect inguinal hernia
b. Direct inguinal hernia
c. Femoral hernia
d. Strangulated hernia

Ans. a

Q12. What is the type of hernia shown here?

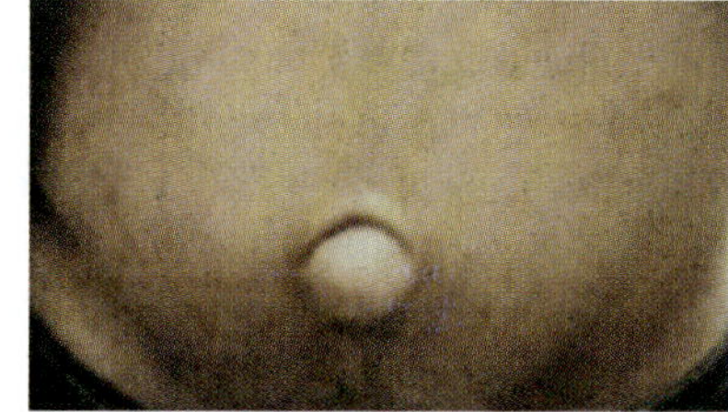

a. Umbilical hernia b. Paraumbilical hernia
c. Incisional hernia d. Epigastric hernia

Ans. b

Q13. A patient has presented with herniation of an intestinal loop, which passes along the spermatic cord and reaches till scrotum/cremaster muscle?

a. Femoral hernia
b. Direct inguinal hernia
c. Indirect inguinal hernia
d. Paraumbilical hernia

Ans. c

Q14. Which one of the following is not performed in Lichtenstein tension-free hernioplasty?

a. High ligation of the indirect hernia sac
b. Mesh sutured to the conjoint tendon and inguinal ligation
c. Conjoint tendon sutured to inguinal ligament
d. The spermatic cord is placed in the two tails of the internal ring

Ans. c

Q15. Femoral hernia in Nyhus classification:
a. IIIA
b. II
c. IIIC
d. IV

Ans. c

Q16. Which one of the following is not performed in Lichtenstein tension-free hernioplasty?
a. High ligation of the indirect hernia sac
b. Mesh sutured to the conjoint tendon and inguinal ligament
c. Conjoint tendon sutured to inguinal ligament
d. Spermatic cord is placed in the two tails of the internal ring

Ans. c

Q17. True statement regarding direct inguinal hernia: (UPPG 2008)
a. The most common inguinal hernia in women is direct
b. Direct hernia is medial to inferior epigastric artery
c. Repair of the transversalis fascia and the internal ring
d. Descends downward and inward toward the scrotum

Ans. b

Q18. The content of epilocele is:
a. Omentum
b. Intestine
c. Colon
d. Urinary bladder

Ans. a

MULTIPLE CHOICE QUESTIONS

Grade I	*Simple*

Q1. A patient operated for direct inguinal hernia developed anesthesia at the root of the penis and adjacent part of the scrotum, the nerve likely to be injured is: (AIIMS Nov 2001)
a. Genital branch of genitofemoral nerve (supplies the dartos muscle)
b. Femoral branch of genitofemoral nerve
c. Iliohypogastric nerve
d. Ilioinguinal nerve

Q2. During repair of indirect inguinal hernia, while releasing the constriction at the deep inguinal ring, the surgeon takes care not to damage one of the following structures: (AIIMS Nov 2009)
a. Falx inguinalis (conjoint tendon)
b. Interfoveolar ligament
c. Inferior epigastric artery
d. Spermatic cord

Q3. Desmoid tumor, treatment is: (AIIMS Nov 2009)
a. Local excision
b. Wide excision
c. Wide excision with radiotherapy
d. Radiotherapy

Q4. Mesh for hernioplasty should be: (AIIMS 2020)
a. Heavy-weight large pore
b. Small-weight small pore
c. Heavy-weight small pore
d. Small-weight large pore

Q5. True about epigastric hernia is: (AIIMS May 2012)
a. Located below the umbilicus and always in the midline
b. Located above the umbilicus and always in the midline
c. Located above the umbilicus and on either side
d. It can be seen anywhere on the abdomen

Q6. What is false regarding gastroschisis and omphalocele? (AIIMS Nov 2000)
a. Intestinal obstruction is common in gastroschisis
b. The liver is the content of the omphalocele
c. Gastroschisis is associated with multiple anomalies
d. The umbilical cord is attached in the normal position in gastroschisis

Q7. A child presented with a swelling in the right groin region. When the swelling was reduced, a gurgling sound was heard. Which of the following is an incorrect statement? (AIIMS Nov 2015)
a. This type of hernia is most common in children
b. The hernia lies above and medial to the pubic tubercle
c. Patent processus vaginalis
d. The sac contains only omentum

Q8. During laparoscopic inguinal hernia repair, a tacker was accidentally placed below and lateral to the iliopubic tract. Postoperatively, the patient complained of pain and soreness in the thigh. This is due to the involvement of: (AIIMS Nov 2015)
a. Lateral cutaneous nerve of thigh
b. Ilioinguinal nerve
c. Genital branch of genitofemoral nerve
d. Obturator nerve

Q9. Howship-Romberg sign is seen in: (JIPMER SS 2006)

a. Sliding hernia
b. Obturator hernia
c. Lumbar hernia
d. Paraduodenal hernia

Q10. Strangulation most commonly occurs in: (MCI Sept 2005)

a. Femoral hernia
b. Direct inguinal hernia
c. Indirect inguinal hernia
d. Lumbar hernia

Q11. Which structures live immediately lateral to the femoral hernia? (AIIMS Nov 2011)

a. Lateral cutaneous nerve of thigh
b. Femoral nerve
c. Femoral artery
d. Femoral vein

Q12. True statement(s) about indirect inguinal hernia: (PGI June 2004)

a. 25% is bilateral
b. In children, if an inguinal (indirect) hernia is present in one side, then processus vaginalis is intact on the other side
c. In bubonocele sac lies in the inguinal canal
d. Equal incidence in males and females

Q13. True about inguinal hernia: (PGI June 2008)

a. It is more common in females.
b. Right sided is more common than left side
c. Direct hernia is less likely to undergo strangulation
d. Femoral hernia is more common in females

Q14. The following are the risk factors for inguinal hernia: (PGI Dec 2007)

a. Family history of inguinal hernia
b. Weightlifter
c. Chronic obstructive pulmonary disease (COPD)
d. Female
e. Obesity

Q15. Spigelian hernia is a type of hernia occurring at: (PGI June 2000)

a. Medial border of rectus abdominis
b. Lateral border of rectus abdominis
c. Lumbar region
d. Femoral canal

Q16. True about hernia: (PGI Dec 2000)

a. Direct hernias are usually acquired
b. The femoral is the most common hernia to strangulate
c. External abdominal hernia are the most common
d. 50% of old people suffer from direct type of hernia with strangulation
e. The treatment of choice for an indirect inguinal hernia is surgery

Q17. About inguinal hernia surgery, all of the following are true, *except*: (AIIMS Nov 2012)

a. Hernia in children is treated with herniotomy
b. Absorbable mesh should not be used for surgery
c. Surgery should not be done unless the patient becomes symptomatic
d. Surgery can be done using laparoscopy

Q18. During laparoscopic inguinal hernia surgery, a tacker was accidentally placed below and lateral to the iliopubic tract. Postoperatively, the patient complained of pain and soreness in the thigh. This is due to the involvement of: (AIIMS Nov 2015)

a. Ilioinguinal nerve
b. Genital branch of the genitofemoral nerve
c. Lateral cutaneous branch of the iliohypogastric nerve
d. Lateral cutaneous nerve of the thigh

Q19. The medial boundary of a femoral ring of formed by: (JIPMER 2011)

a. Inguinal ligament
b. Pectineal ligament
c. Lacunar ligament
d. The septum separating it from a femoral vein

Q20. All are true about Spigelian hernia, *except*: (JIPMER GIS 2011)

a. Usually occurs above the arcuate line
b. Picked up by ultrasound (USG) or computed tomography (CT)
c. Hernia sac will be posterior to the external oblique aponeurosis
d. Usually small and asymptomatic

Q21. Spigelian hernia is a type of hernia occurring at: (PGI June 2000)

a. Medial border of rectus abdominis
b. Lateral border of rectus abdominis

c. Lumbar region
d. Femoral canal

Q22. Spigelian hernia is: (MCI March 2005)
a. Passes through the obturator canal
b. Hernia occurring through the linea alba
c. Hernia through the triangle of Petit
d. Hernia occurring at the level of the arcuate line

Grade II	***Difficult***

Q1. Type IIIA in Nyhus classification of hernia: (MCI Nov 2017)
a. Direct inguinal hernia
b. Indirect inguinal hernia
c. Femoral hernia
d. Umbilical hernia

Q2. The following are the risk factors for inguinal hernia: (PGI Dec 2007)
a. Family history of inguinal hernia
b. Weight lifter
c. COPD
d. Female
e. Obesity

Q3. Most common type of hernia in females is: (JIPMER GIS 2011)
a. Direct inguinal hernia
b. Indirect inguinal hernia
c. Femoral hernia
d. Umbilical hernia

Q4. True about inguinal hernia: (PGI June 2003)
a. It is more common in females.
b. Right sided is more common than left side
c. Direct hernia is less likely to undergo strangulation
d. Femoral hernia is more common in females

Q5. All of the following statements are true about repair of groin hernias, *except*: (AIIMS Nov 2004)
a. Lichtenstein tension-free repair has a low recurrence rate
b. TEP repair is an extraperitoneal approach to laparoscopic repair of groin hernia
c. In Shouldice repair, nonabsorbable mesh is used
d. The surgery can be done under local anesthesia in selected cases

Q6. The treatment of choice for inguinal hernia in infants is: (MCI June 2018)
a. Herniotomy
b. Herniorrhaphy
c. Truss
d. Hernioplasty

Q7. The triangle of doom is bounded by all of the following, *except*: (AIIMS Nov 2008)
a. Cooper's ligament
b. Vas deferens
c. Gonadal vessels
d. Peritoneal reflection

Q8. Which of the following is correct regarding the boundaries of a triangle of doom? (AIIMS May 2018)
a. Medially, vas deferens, laterally gonadal vessels, inferiorly peritoneum
b. Laterally vas deferens, medially gonadal vessels, inferiorly peritoneum
c. Laterally medial umbilical ligament, medially gonadal vessels, inferiorly peritoneum
d. Laterally gonadal vessels, medially lateral umbilical ligament, inferiorly peritoneum

Q9. True regarding indirect inguinal hernia are all, *except*: (MCI March 2008)
a. Most common type of hernia
b. Always unilateral
c. Inguinal herniotomy is the basic operation
d. Transillumination distinguishes it from a hydrocele

Q10. Most common type of hernia in the young age-group: (MCI Sept 2006)
a. Femoral hernia
b. Direct inguinal hernia
c. Indirect inguinal hernia
d. Umbilical hernia

Q11. The least recurrence rate in incisional hernia repair is which of the following? (JIPMER 2010)
a. Onlay mesh repair
b. Intraperitoneal mesh repair
c. Inlay mesh repair
d. Shouldice repair

Q12. Shouldice repair is: (PGI SS June 2007)
a. Multilayered repair of inguinal canal
b. Conjoint tendon is sutured to inguinal ligament
c. Conjoint tenson is sutured to Cooper's ligament
d. Transabdominal repair

Q13. Are true about hernia repair, *except*: **(JIPMER GIS 2011)**
a. Bassini's repair is between the inguinal ligament and the conjoint tendon
b. Shouldice repair is involvement of the posterior wall strengthening
c. McVay's repair is for femoral hernia
d. Lichtenstein is a tension-free mesh repair

Q14. A child presented with a swelling in the right groin region. When the swelling was reduced, a gurgling sound was heard. Which of the following is an incorrect statement? **(AIIMS Nov 2015)**
a. The sac contains omentum only
b. The hernia lies above and medial to the pubic tubercle
c. Patent processus vaginalis
d. This type of hernia is most common in children

Q15. A 3-year-old child comes with a hydrocele of the hernia sac. Management will include: **(AIIMS May 2015)**
a. Herniotomy
b. Herniorrhaphy
c. Observation only
d. Operation after 5 years of age

Q16. Which of these would you like to do for a case of strangulated hernia? **(PGI June 2002)**
a. X-ray
b. USG abdomen
c. Aspiration of the contents of the sac
d. Correction of hypovolemia
e. Prepare OT for urgent surgery

Q17. In a case of strangulated hernia, management is: **(PGI June 2006)**
a. USG abdomen
b. X-ray abdomen
c. Aspirate contents
d. Immediate surgery
e. IV fluids

Q18. Which of the following is not done in case of an obstructed inguinal hernia? **(PGI June 2003)**
a. Aspiration of the sac for diagnosis
b. X-ray abdomen
c. USG abdomen
d. Do early surgery

Grade III	*Most difficult*

Q1. False about paraduodenal hernia: **(PGI Nov 2009)**
a. Congenital
b. Found in fossa of Kolb
c. Found in fossa of Landzert
d. Common on right side

Q2. False about paraduodenal hernia: **(AIIMS GIS 2003)**
a. Left-sided is found in the fossa of Landzert
b. Right sided is found in the fossa of Kolb
c. Congenital
d. More common on the right side

Q3. True about epigastric hernia is: **(AIIMS May 2012)**
a. Located below the umbilicus and always in the midline
b. Located above the umbilicus and always in the midline
c. Located above the umbilicus and on either side
d. It can be seen anywhere on the abdomen

Q4. About hernia, false statements: **(PGI Dec 2003)**
a. In children, indirect inguinal hernia is treated medically.
b. In Richter's hernia, absolute constipation is seen.
c. Indirect inguinal hernia is the MC type.
d. The deep inguinal ring is lateral and above the pubic tubercle.

Q5. True about hernia: **(PGI Dec 2003)**
a. External abdominal hernia is common
b. Direct hernia is usually acquired
c. Strangulation is common in femoral hernia
d. Direct hernia is acquired in old age
e. TOC for indirect inguinal hernia is surgery

Q6. Hernia prone to reoccur after primary repair: **(JIPMER 2013)**
a. Femoral
b. Epigastric
c. Spigelian
d. Incisional

Q7. All of the following structures pass through the inguinal canal in females, *except*: **(All India 2012)**
a. Ilioinguinal nerve
b. Round ligament of the uterus
c. Lymphatics from the uterus
d. Inferior epigastric artery

Q8. The most common presentation of abdominal desmoid tumor is: (AIIMS Nov 2017)

a. Abdominal pain
b. Abdominal mass
c. Fever
d. Rectal prolapse

Q9. A newborn presents with discharge of urine from the umbilicus for 3 days. Diagnosis is: (UPPG 2008)

a. Meckel's diverticulum
b. Mesenteric cysts
c. Urachal fistula
d. Umbilical hernia

Q10. A child complains of fluid coming out of the umbilicus on straining. What is the diagnosis? (AIIMS Nov 2014)

a. Urachal fistula
b. Gastroschisis
c. Patent vitellointestinal duct
d. Congenital umbilical hernia

Q11. A newborn presents with a midanterior abdominal wall defect with characteristic spontaneous disappearance at age 4 years: (UPPG 2008)

a. Patent urachus
b. Omphalocele
c. Ectopia vesicae
d. Umbilical hernia

Q12. A most common cause of umbilicus not separated at the age of 2 years: (UPPG 2008)

a. Raspberry tumor
b. Leukocyte adhesion deficiency
c. Patent urachus
d. Umbilical granuloma

Q13. All of the following are true about hernia surgery, *except*: (AIIMS Nov 2012)

a. Surgery should not be done unless the patient becomes symptomatic
b. Hernia in children is treated with herniotomy
c. Absorbable mesh should not be used for surgery
d. Surgery can be done using laparoscopy

Q14. True statement regarding Spigelian hernia is: (PGI May 2018)

a. Protudes through the linea alba
b. Occurs at the termination of the transverse abdominis muscle
c. Occurs at the lateral edge of the rectus abdominis muscle
d. The content of a hernia mostly includes the small intestine
e. Surgery is the treatment of choice

Q15. Most useful investigation in sliding hernia in females: (UPPG 2008)

a. Fluoroscopy
b. Barium-meal
c. Palpation method
d. Ultrasound

Q16. True about obturator hernia in adults: (PGI Nov 2009)

a. More common in the space of Lorentz
b. Common in females
c. Chronic constipation risk factor
d. Surgical treatment should be done
e. May present with intestinal obstruction

ANSWERS

Grade I: 1. d; 2. c; 3. b; 4. d; 5. b; 6. c; 7. d; 8. a; 9. b; 10. a; 11. d; 12. b, c (Bailey 27/e p124); 13. b, c, d (Bailey 27/e p1031); 14. a, b, c, e (Bailey 27/e p1023); 15. b (Bailey 27/e p1041); 16. a, b, c, e; 17. c; 18. d; 19. c; 20. a; 21. b; 22. d

Grade II: 1. a; 2. a, b, c, e (Schwartz 10/e p1500); 3. b; 4. b, c, d; 5. c (Bailey 27/e p1032); 6. a; 7. a (Sabiston 20/e p1101); 8. a; 9. b; 10. c; 11. b; 12. a; 13. None; 14. a; 15. a; 16. d; 17. d (Bailey 27/e p1034); 18. a, b, c

Grade III: 1. d (Sabiston 20/e p1083); 2. d; 3. c; 4. a, b, d; 5. a, b, c, d, e; 6. d; 7. d; 8. b; 9. c; 10. a; 11. d; 12. b; 13. a; 14. c, d, e; 15. b; 16. b, c, d, e

MODEL QUESTIONS

Q1. In Laugier's hernia opening is in the:

a. Lacunar ligament
b. Conjoint tendon
c. External oblique
d. Peritoneum

Ans. a

Q2. Pascal's law is used in which technique of hernia repair?

a. Lichtenstein mesh repair
b. Stoppa's preperitoneal repair
c. Bassini's repair
d. Darning repair

Ans. b

Q3. After retrocolic gastrojejunostomy, a hernia occurring through a window in the transverse mesocolon is:
- a. Stammer's hernia
- b. Left paraduodenal hernia
- c. Right paraduodenal hernia
- d. Hernia en glissade

Ans. a

Q4. Omphalocele is caused by:
- a. Duplication of intestinal loops
- b. Abnormal rotation of the intestinal loop
- c. Failure of the gut to return to the body cavity from its physiological herniation
- d. Reversed rotation of the intestinal loop

Ans. c

Q5. Umbilical hernia in a child—indications for surgery is/are:
- a. Failure to disappear by 3 years
- b. >2 cm size
- c. Sympathetic
- d. All of the above

Ans. d

Q6. What is false regarding gastroschisis and omphalocele?
- a. Intestinal obstruction is common in gastroschisis
- b. Gastroschisis is associated with multiple anomalies
- c. Umbilical cord is attached in a normal position; there is gastroschisis
- d. The liver is the content of an omphalocele.

Ans. b

Q7. Incidence of exomphalos:
- a. 1 in 1,000
- b. 1 in 3,000
- c. 1 in 5,000
- d. 1 in 10,000

Ans. c

Q8. True regarding gastroschisis is:
- a. An omphalocele
- b. An anterior abdominal wall tumor
- c. A variant of gastric carcinoma
- d. Herniation of abdominal contents through a body wall

Ans. d

Q9. In omphalocele abdominal wall defect is more than:
- a. 0.5 cm
- b. 2.5 cm
- c. 4 cm
- d. 6 cm

Ans. c

Q10. The hernia, which often simulates a peptic ulcer, is:
- a. Umbilical hernia
- b. Fatty hernia of the linea alba
- c. Incisional hernia
- d. Inguinal hernia

Ans. b

Q11. The sac contains the onlay portion of the circumference of the intestine:
- a. Richer's hernia
- b. Littre's hernia
- c. Spigelian hernia
- d. Lumbar hernia

Ans. a

Q12. Strangulation without obstruction is seen in:
- a. Inguinal hernia
- b. Femoral hernia
- c. Richter's hernia
- d. Littre's hernia

Ans. c

Q13. Which of the following is the content of Littre's hernia?
- a. Urinary bladder
- b. Meckel's diverticulum
- c. Circumference of the intestinal wall
- d. Appendix

Ans. b

Q14. Hernia containing Meckel's diverticulum is:
- a. Richter's hernia
- b. Pantaloon hernia
- c. Littre's hernia
- d. Maydl's hernia

Ans. c

Q15. Incisional hernia, not true is:
- a. Faulty operative technique
- b. There is distension of the abdomen
- c. Associated with infection of the wound
- d. Caused by the use of local anesthesia

Ans. d

Q16. Regarding desmoids tumor, which is not correct?
- a. Often seen below the umbilicus
- b. Unencapsulated

c. More common in women
d. Metastasis does not occur
e. Highly radiosensitive

Ans. e

Q17. What is the treatment of choice in desmoids tumors?

a. Irradiation
b. Wide excision
c. Local excision
d. Local excision following radiation

Ans. b

Q18. Regarding desmoid tumor, true is:

a. Mostly females are affected
b. Well-capsulated tumor
c. Common above the level of the umbilicus
d. Radiotherapy is the treatment of choice

Ans. a

Q19. Funicular hernia is type of:

a. Direct inguinal hernia
b. Indirect inguinal hernia
c. Femoral hernia
d. Umbilical hernia

Ans. b

SUGGESTED READING

1. Bailey & Love's - Short Practice of Surgery, 27th edition.
2. Essentials of Abdominal Wall Hernias, 1st edition.
3. Schwartz's Principles of Surgery, 18th edition.
4. Textbook of Surgery by David Sabiston, 21st edition.

CHAPTER 32

Esophagus

"For me no good food is illuminated without acidity."

– Alexander Guaranaschelli

DEVELOPMENT

When organs start appearing in the fetus, the gut develops by folding patterns. During development, the foregut differentiates into the trachea, lungs, and esophagus. At approximately the sixth week of development, the circular and longitudinal muscular layers begin to form, and ganglion cells of the myenteric plexus appear. Moving into week 7, cells of mesoderm originate and proliferate into the submucous layer, forming the eventual blood supply to the esophagus. The muscular layers, which began in week 6, are completed by the Ninth week. Initially, the esophagus is very short, but it elongates rapidly with the growth of the fetus. *The epithelium of the esophagus proliferates and almost obliterates the lumen, but recanalization occurs at a later age. The respiratory system arises as the laryngotracheal diverticulum from the primitive pharynx.* It grows gradually and becomes separated. *Congenital anomalies may arise if there is interference with the normal development of the trachea and esophagus.*

ANATOMY OF ESOPHAGUS

The esophagus is a muscular tube that basically functions as a pathway to transfer food from the pharynx to the stomach. When there is no food in the esophagus, it remains empty and deflated with a 2–3 cm diameter. The esophagus can distend and stretch to some degree (>2–3 cm) to accommodate a bigger bolus of food. The esophagus in an adult is approximately 25 cm long. It starts from the cricoid cartilage (C6 vertebra) and ends at the esophagogastric junction (T11 vertebra) **(Figs. 1A and B)**.

During its course, the esophagus encounters three anatomic constrictions:

1. At the level of the *cricopharyngeus muscle*.
2. As it travels posterior to the aortic arch/left mainstem bronchus
3. At the level of the esophageal hiatus of the diaphragm. These areas of constriction are considered the most frequent sites for a foreign body or food impaction to occur.

PARTS OF ESOPHAGUS

The esophagus has three parts:

1. Cervical esophagus
2. Thoracic esophagus
3. Abdominal esophagus

Cervical Esophagus

It is 5–6 cm long. The cervical esophagus travels between the lower border of the cricoid cartilage and the thoracic inlet. An important feature of the cervical esophagus is that the recurrent laryngeal nerve travels on each side in a space between the esophagus and trachea.

Thoracic Esophagus

It is present in the superior and posterior mediastinum between the trachea and vertebral column, and in the posterior mediastinum, it comes anterior to the aorta. It extends from the thoracic inlet to the diaphragm.

Abdominal Esophagus

It is about 2.5 cm in length and lies on the posterior surface of the left lobe of the liver. It is covered by the peritoneum on its front and left side **(Fig. 2)**.

Relations of the abdominal esophagus: It lies at the level of the 11th and 12th thoracic vertebrae.

Anterior: Posterior surface of left lobe of liver, left vagus nerve, and esophageal plexus.

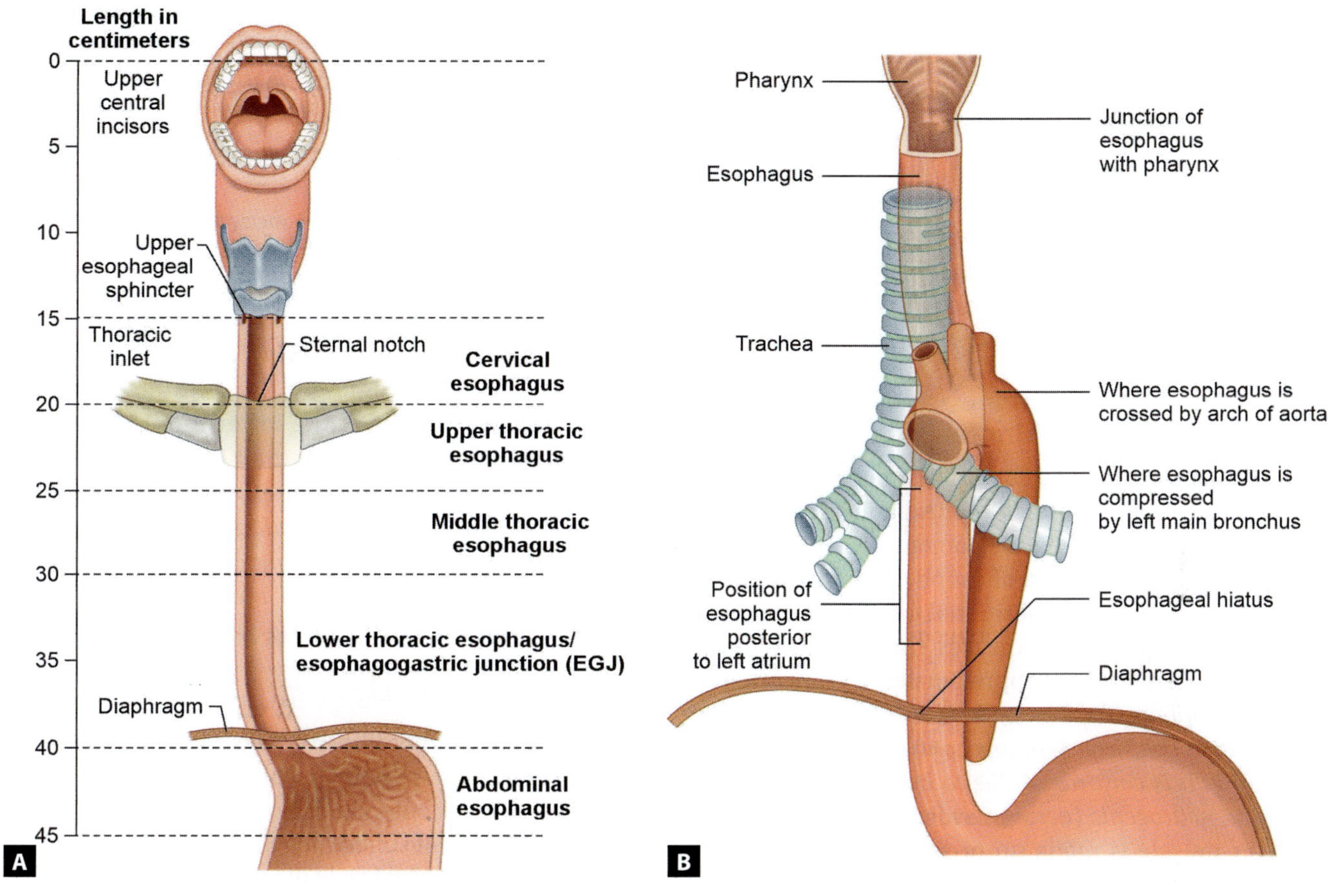

Figs. 1A and B: Esophagus in its course.

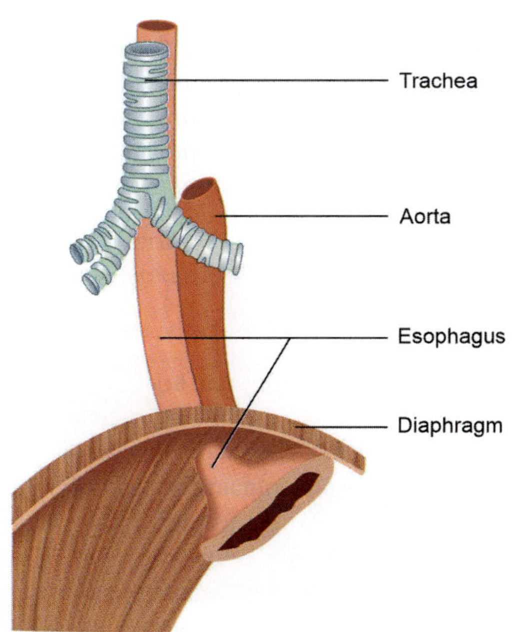

Fig. 2: Thoracic and abdominal parts of the esophagus.

Posterior: Crura of the diaphragm, aorta, and left inferior phrenic artery.

Right: The caudate lobe of the liver.

Left: Gastroesophageal or esophagogastric junction.

The function of the median arcuate ligament is like a barrier. It is a tough band of muscle fibers, 1–3 mm wide. It is the condensation of fibers of the medial crus of the diaphragm.

GASTROESOPHAGEAL JUNCTION

It is the site where the esophagus meets the stomach. It is not a well-marked area. Gastroesophageal junction (GEJ) acts as a sphincter, and it is a complex sphincter. GEJ has two parts:

1. Extrinsic or external part—diaphragmatic part
2. Intrinsic or internal part—lower esophageal sphincter (LES)

So, GEJ has both a diaphragmatic element, skeletal muscle, and LES, the smooth muscle.

Extrinsic or External Junction

It lies in the abdomen below the diaphragm.

Intrinsic or Internal Junction

The histological junction between the esophagus and the stomach is marked by an irregular boundary between the stratified squamous epithelium of the esophagus and the gastric simple columnar epithelium. External and internal junctions do not coincide with each other as the mucosal level changes due to very loose submucosal connective tissue.

Lower Esophageal Sphincter

The LES consists of muscle fibers. It has two components:

1. The extrinsic part is formed by the diaphragmatic crura and the phrenoesophageal ligament.
2. *Intrinsic part:* It is made of esophageal muscle fibers, which are under neurohormonal force. The size of the esophageal sphincter increases gradually after birth, and the LES matures at approximately 2 years of age.

Lower esophageal sphincter is made up of smooth muscles, and then sphincter remains contracted except during swallowing. It is contracted due to both myogenic (muscular) and neurogenic (nerve) factors. The diaphragmatic sphincter muscle is made up of skeletal muscle fibers. The myogenic contraction by gastrointestinal smooth muscle contracts and relaxes.

The LES is innervated by both parasympathetic (vagus) and sympathetic (splanchnic) nerves.

The sphincter at the lower end of the esophagus is helped by several other structures: *The angle (of His) at which the esophagus enters the stomach, the pinchcock action of the diaphragm, a plug of loose esophageal mucosa* (*mucosal rosette*), the phrenoesophageal membrane, and the sling of oblique fibers of the gastric musculature.

Transient Lower Esophageal Sphincter Relaxation

Lower esophageal sphincter relaxation (LESR) is one of the most common processes of causing gastroesophageal reflux disease (GERD), even when the LES pressure is normal. During the swallowing process, LES relaxation occurs for <10 seconds. LESRs are a normal mechanism in healthy persons with normal LES. It is a dominant phenomenon in GERD, as in it, LESR occurs too frequently and for longer periods (>10 seconds). Most GERD attacks occur during LESRs. LESRs are not associated with the swallowing phenomenon.

Intrinsic component of LES: Esophageal smooth muscle fiber.

Extrinsic components of LES:

- Diaphragmatic crura
- Phrenoesophageal ligament

Right Crus of the Diaphragm

The esophageal hiatus of the diaphragm is located in the right crus of the diaphragm. LES is made up of smooth muscles. It is 2–4 cm in size. LES is fixed to the esophageal hiatus of the diaphragm by the phrenoesophageal ligament, which inserts at the lower esophagus. LES is a high-pressure zone. At rest, the LES is in the state of contraction, in the high-pressure zone state. *During the swallowing of food, it relaxes and opens up to allow food to pass into the stomach. The right crus of the diaphragm causes an extrinsic squeeze to the intrinsic LES.* This requires approximately 10 mm Hg pressure to LES **(Fig. 3)**.

Phrenoesophageal Ligament

This so called ligament consists of the following structures:

- Pleura
- Subpleural fascia (endothoracic)
- Phrenoesophageal fascia of Laimer
- Transversalis (endoabdominal subdiaphragmatic) fascia
- Peritoneum

Phrenoesophageal ligament acts as a seal around the esophagus, which is airtight. The seal must be strong enough to resist abdominal pressure that tends to push the stomach into the thorax and flexible enough to give with the pressure changes incidental to breathing and the

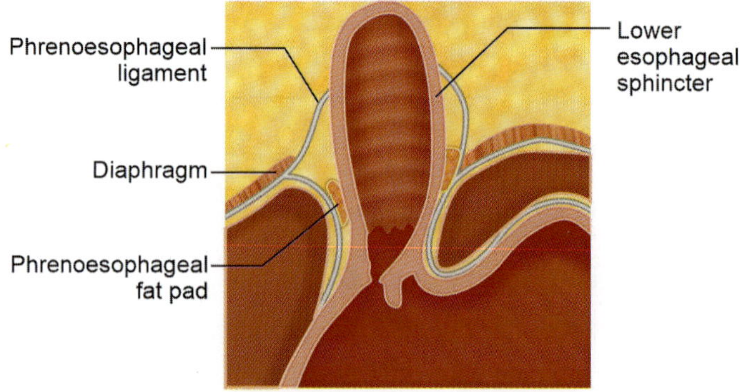

Fig. 3: Gastroesophageal junction and phrenoesophageal ligament.

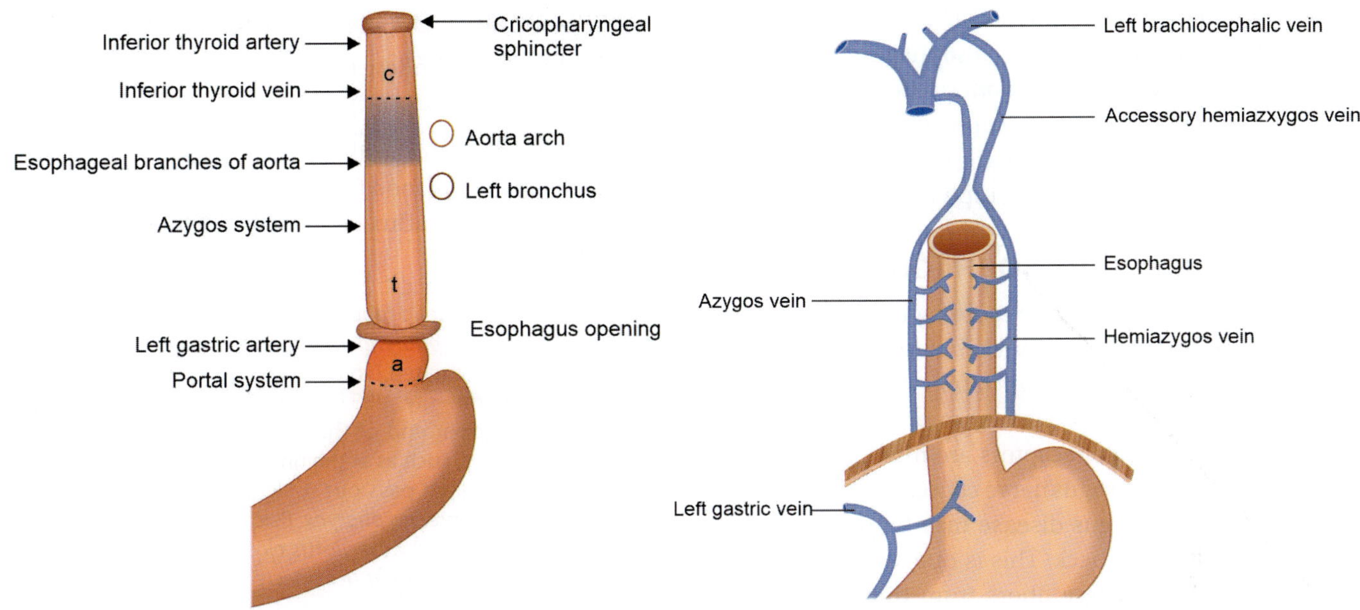

Fig. 4: Blood supply of the esophagus.

Fig. 5: Venous drainage of esophagus.

movement incidental to swallowing. The first and last of these elements provide the requirement for airtightness; the middle three provide flexibility and strength. The ligament exists in infants, is attenuated in adults, and does not exist in adult patients with hiatus hernia.

BLOOD SUPPLY OF ESOPHAGUS

The blood supply of the esophagus is from three directions **(Fig. 4)**:

1. The upper part is supplied by branches of the inferior thyroid artery.
2. The main part of the esophagus is supplied by the esophageal branches of the aorta.
3. The lower part of the esophagus is supplied by the branches of:
   a. Gastric arteries
   b. Inferior phrenic artery

VENOUS DRAINAGE OF ESOPHAGUS

The blood from the esophagus is drained in three directions as follows **(Fig. 5)**:

1. Cervical esophagus veins drain into the inferior thyroid vein, leading to the brachiocephalic veins.
2. *Thoracic esophagus veins drain:*
   i. On the right side into the superior vena cava through the azygos system
   ii. On the left side, veins drain into the brachiocephalic vein through the left hemiazygos system.

- *Veins from the esophagogastric junction drain into:*
  - Coronary veins
  - Splenic veins
  - Retroperitoneal veins
  - Inferior phrenic vein
  - These veins ultimately drain into portal and caval systems.

LYMPHATIC DRAINAGE OF ESOPHAGUS

Lymphatics of the esophagus lie in the submucosa, and here they run up and down. They penetrate the muscle layer of the esophagus and reach the outer surface of esophagus. There are three main drainage systems of the lymphatics of the esophagus:

1. Lymphatics from upper one-third of esophagus drain into deep cervical lymph nodes and then lymph goes to thoracic duct.
2. Lymphatics from middle one-third of esophagus drain into superior and posterior mediastinal lymph nodes.
3. Lymphatics from distal one-third of esophagus drain into the gastric and coeliac lymph nodes.

The lymphatics of these three systems interconnect well. There are three types of lymph nodes according to their sites:

1. *Paraesophageal lymph nodes:* These are present on the wall of the esophagus.

2. *Periesophageal lymph nodes:* These are situated on structures just adjacent to the esophagus.
3. *Lateral esophageal lymph nodes:* These lymph nodes are situated lateral to the esophagus. The lymphatics from paraesophageal and periesophageal nodes drain into the lateral esophageal lymph nodes.

NERVE SUPPLY OF ESOPHAGUS

Both vagus nerves supply the esophagus. The esophagus contains cholinergic receptors, and vagus nerves stimulation leads to the contraction of the esophagus. In LES, both cholinergic and adrenergic receptors are present, but adrenergic receptors are more numerous, so the stimulation of the vagus nerve causes relaxation of LES.

Pain from esophagus disease may be referred to the neck, arm, chest, and back. This is due to the association of afferent visceral nerve fibers from the esophagus to somatic sensory fibers of the intercostal and phrenic nerves.

The angle of His is present at the junction of esophagus and stomach. It is an acute angle between stomach and esophagus. It is between the wall of esophagus and greater curvature of stomach. It helps in preventing the back flow or reflux of gastric contents and acid from entering esophagus. It prevents GERD. It is not well developed in infants; that is why acid regurgitation is common in infants. It is created by:
- Collar sling fibers
- The circular muscles around this GEJ

"Angle of His" was described by a German physician and anatomist, Dr. Wilhelm His Jr. (1864–1934). He also described the atrioventricular "Bundle of His."

Functions of the Angle of His

Functions are as follows:
- It prevents reflux of gastric contents and acid in the esophagus from the stomach and also helps in the prevention of GERD.
- When air distends the fundus of the stomach then this balloon-type distension pushes the GEJ to the right side from the left side and closes the gastroesophageal valve.

The upper esophageal sphincter (UES) is made up of skeletal muscle fibers at the upper end of the esophagus. It has muscle fibers of two muscles:
1. Inferior pharyngeal constrictor muscle
2. Cricopharyngeus muscle

PHYSIOLOGY OF THE ESOPHAGUS

The esophagus is a hollow tube with muscular sphincters at both ends, from the pharynx to the stomach.

The esophagus has primarily two functions:
1. Transportation of food from the mouth to the stomach.
2. Preventions of reflux or retrograde flow of gastric contents.

Esophagus transmits solid food and liquids ingested by mouth to the stomach. The cricopharyngeus and inferior constrictor muscles form UES. UES is a striated (voluntary) muscle structure. UES is a high-pressure zone site. UES is approximately 1 cm in length. UES keeps the upper end of the esophagus closed. It opens only when required, such as at the time of swallowing or letting the gas from stomach pass out (belching). *UES also prevents reflexated material entering pharynx. Belch induces UES relaxation which is also associated with glottis closure. Stress and anxiety increase UES pressure whereas sleep decreases UES pressure.*

Hydrochloric acid (HCl) is produced in our stomach to help digest food and also to kill any virus or bacteria if they may enter with food in the stomach to avoid developing an infection. The acid is mixed with gastric juice and disintegrates the food to prepare it for digestion. The inner lining of the stomach is covered with mucus, which acts as a protective coat to prevent acid from damaging the stomach wall. Mucus helps in the passage of food in the esophagus.

The esophagus is also called the food pipe or gullet. It has the following functions:
- It is a long, muscular pipe that transports the food after ingestion from the pharynx to the stomach.
- The muscle in the wall of the esophagus contracts, which mixes the food well with saliva and moves it downwards.
- The esophagus also contains glands that secrete mucus. Esophageal lining glands only secrete mucus and no other substance. The wall of the esophagus is thin but has the ability to distend and contract to allow food to enter and pass forward. The mucus thus secreted in the esophagus works in two ways:
    1. It makes the passage of food in the esophagus smooth.
    2. It helps avoid the esophageal inner lining being damaged by the reflux of acid from the stomach.

When the food is swallowed, the UES opens and allows food to enter the esophagus. The peristalsis in the esophagus moves the food down, and the LES opens at this time to allow the food to enter the stomach. *The food bolus presses the wall of the esophagus, and the muscles in the wall of the esophagus contract, increasing local pressure, but below the food bolus, there is no pressure on the wall of the esophagus, so having the pressure somewhat low moves the food bolus down.* Food bolus moves from high high-pressure area in the esophagus to low pressure area.

Esophageal Peristalsis

Normally esophagus does not show spontaneous peristalsis. Swallowing of food and liquids and gaseous distension starts peristalsis. Esophageal peristalsis is of two types:

1. *Primary esophageal peristalsis:* This type of peristalsis is started by the swallowing of food. This peristalsis involves the whole esophagus, from up to down.
2. *Secondary esophageal peristalsis:* This type of peristalsis is initiated as a response to regional dilatation of the esophagus by air or fluid. It starts at the dilatation site of the esophagus.

PHYSIOLOGY OF GASTROESOPHAGEAL JUNCTION

Gastroesophageal junction is actually not a simple union of the tubes, but it is a valvular junction that allows the food to go down to the stomach but prevents it from refluxing back to the esophagus. It is actually a valve having two muscular components:

1. Smooth muscle component, i.e., LES.
2. Skeletal muscle component, i.e., diaphragmatic part.

This combination makes the GEJ a competent junction. Any defect or weakness on the part of component (1) or (2) makes this junction incompetent, and gastroesophageal reflux occurs. The common reason is either that the tension of LES is low, or it is quick, recurrent, and momentary relaxations called transient relaxation.

The GEJ is also the site of transition of stratified squamous epithelium to columnar epithelium.

The cause of mucosal injury to the lower esophagus leading to esophagitis is due to:

- Period of contact of the refluxate with the esophageal mucosa
- Acidic potency of refluxate

The higher the period of contact of refluxate with the esophageal mucosa, the higher is the chances of mucosal injury. Similarly higher is the acidic potency of the refluxate, the higher is the chances of injury to the esophageal mucosa.

PHYSIOLOGY OF THE LOWER ESOPHAGEAL SPHINCTER

When food enters the stomach, the churning of food happens in the stomach to make it a paste so that it to move forward smoothly. The LES and pyloric sphincter close tightly for the churning of food. If LES is not tightly closed, then acid with gastric contents leaks to the esophagus.

The lower esophageal sphincter is innervated by parallel sets of parasympathetic excitatory and inhibitory pathways. It remains closed because of its intrinsic myogenic tone, which is modulated by the excitatory and inhibitory nerves. The function of the LES is supplemented by the striated muscle of the diaphragmatic crura, which surrounds the LES and acts as an external LES. Relaxation of LES without esophageal contraction occurs during belching and gastric distention. *Gastric distention evoked transient lower esophageal sphincter relaxation (tLESR) is a vasovagal reflex.* Fatty meals, smoking, and beverages with high xanthine contents (tea, coffee, and cola) also cause a reduction in sphincter pressure. Muscarinic M2 and M3 receptor agonists, alpha-adrenergic agonists, gastrin, substance P, and prostaglandin F2α cause contraction. *Nicotine, β-adrenergic agonists, dopamine, cholecystokinin, secretin, VIP, calcitonin gene-related peptide (CGRP), adenosine, prostaglandin E, and nitric oxide donors, such as nitrates, reduce sphincter pressure.*

Weak Lower Esophageal Sphincter (Fig. 6)

- Overeating
- Smoking
- Alcohol
- Overweight
- Certain medicines, i.e., calcium channel blockers and sleeping pills
- Fatty food
- Chocolate
- Peppermint
- Secretin hormone
- Cholinergic antagonists

Strong Lower Esophageal Sphincter (Fig. 7)

- High protein containing foods, i.e., meat, eggs, and lentils
- Moderate use of nuts, avocado, etc.
- Medicines, i.e., bethanechol
- Strengthening exercises
- Meditation
- Yoga

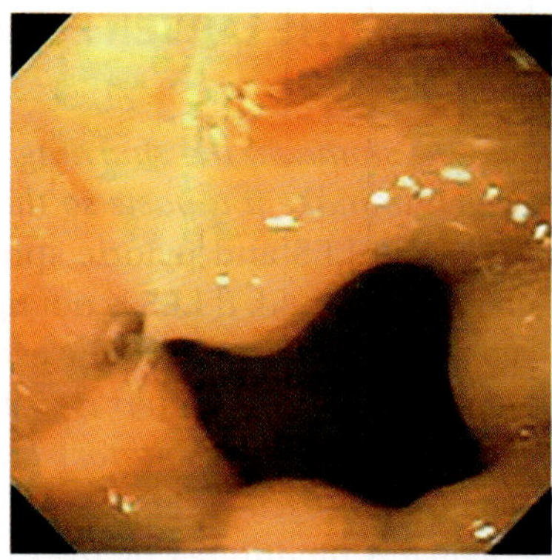

Fig. 6: Weak lower esophageal sphincter (LES).

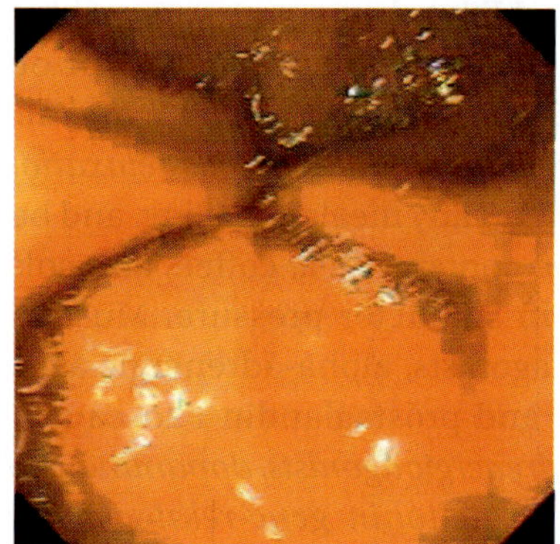

Fig. 7: Strong lower esophageal sphincter (LES).

It has been indicated by researchers that only 10 mm Hg pressure is sufficient at the LES to stop gastroesophageal reflux, but the resting LES pressure is approximately 30 mm Hg, as if God knows that humans will not lead a healthy lifestyle but will choose an unhealthy lifestyle due to their desires. So, HE kept the difference of pressure threshold. The LES is a high-pressure zone part of the lower esophagus, but pressure in the LES does not remain the same all the time. The pressure in a normal resting situation of rest is about 10–13 mm Hg. The pressure of LES increases at night and becomes highest, whereas it is lowest after meals. Recent studies with drugs that work through the cholinergic mechanism have important therapeutic considerations. Anticholinergic agents produce a definite decrease in LES pressure and are to be provided in the treatment of patients with reflux symptoms. On the other hand, cholinergic drugs such as bethanechol have been shown to increase LES pressure in normal subjects and in patients with chronic sphincter incompetence. As the LES does not possess dilator muscles, its opening relies solely on the relaxation of the smooth muscles. At the intracellular level, LES relaxation occurs due to suppression of a resting chloride conductance by nitric oxide (NO) or activation of a potassium conductance, resulting in smooth muscle hyperpolarization. Suppression of calcium influx occurs, leading to the cessation of myosin phosphorylation and muscle relaxation. Excitatory cholinergic nerves release ACh to promote smooth muscle contraction, which enhances the tonic, myogenic property of the LES, and favors contraction. In contrast, the nitrergic pathway releases NO and favors inhibition, opposing the contractile properties of LES. Overall, the combination of these forces favors contraction over relaxation. Thus, the LES remains contracted even when entirely denervated owing to its myogenic property.

ESOPHAGEAL ACID CLEARANCE

Esophageal acid clearance helps in the reduction of esophageal mucosal damage in GERD, and defective esophageal acid clearance increases the changes of esophageal mucosal injury.

The esophageal acid clearance acts in two ways:

1. Volume clearance
2. Chemical clearance

NUTCRACKER ESOPHAGUS

It is also called hypertensive peristalsis. It is a mobility disorder of the esophagus. It is called a "nutcracker" esophagus as there is increased pressure during peristalsis. Using conventional manometry, nutcracker esophagus was defined as a mean distal esophageal peristalsis amplitude (measured 3 and 8 cm above EGJ) >180 mm Hg in the context of normal LES relaxation.

JACKHAMMER ESOPHAGUS

Jackhammer esophagus is an extreme pattern of hypercontractility. The main symptom of Jackhammer esophagus is chest pain, and it gets worse when you eat food. There is no known cure from this disorder. Early semisolid soft foods help.

CORKSCREW ESOPHAGUS

It is a rare disorder of the mobility of the esophagus, characterized by high-amplitude abnormal contractions. They are discoordinated contractions. It is a finding of diffuse esophageal spasm in barium Studies. Abnormal contractions lead to curling of the esophagus like a corkscrew. It is also called as rosary bead esophagus as it gives the appearance of rosary beads. Symptoms are chest pain and dysphagia.

ESOPHAGEAL MUCOSAL RESISTANCES

Esophageal mucosa is stratified squamous epithelium. It serves as a barrier between the luminal contents of the esophagus and the deeper layers of the wall of the esophagus. The esophageal mucosa repairs itself after getting damaged by the acid of the refluxate. Normal individuals also have GERD, but not routinely with symptoms, due to tissue resistance, which is of three types:

1. *Preepithelial:* The mucus covering of the esophageal mucosa is a barrier, but not strong. Pre-epithelial factors comprising tissue resistance include a mucus layer, an unstirred water layer, and bicarbonate ions entrapped within these layers. For the stomach and duodenum, the preepithelial defense is well developed, creating a substantial buffer zone between luminal content and epithelial surface. The esophagus, unlike the stomach and duodenum, has a very limited surface buffer zone, with luminal pH of 2.0 yielding a surface pH of 2.0–3.0. The reasons for this are that the esophagus lacks a mucus layer, and its cells do not secrete bicarbonate ions.
2. *Epithelial:* Mucosa of the esophagus is stratified squamous. The epithelial defense consists of structural and functional components. Structural components include the cell membrane and intercellular junctional complexes of the esophageal mucosa. The esophageal mucosa is a relatively tight epithelium that resists ionic movement at the intercellular, as well as, at the cellular level. The functional components of tissue resistance include the ability of the esophageal epithelium to buffer and extrude hydrogen ions. Intracellular buffering is accomplished by negatively charged phosphates and proteins, as well as bicarbonates.
3. *Postepithelial:* The blood supply of the esophagus also acts as a part of tissue resistance due to its buffering property. Notably, the blood supply and its capacity to deliver HCO_3 is a dynamic and not a static process so that under conditions of increasing luminal activity, esophageal blood flow increases, and some of the known mediators of this increase are through the release within the tissue of histamine, nitric oxide, and calcitonin gene-related peptides.

HISTOLOGY OF ESOPHAGUS

The esophagus is a cylindrical tube and consists of layers, which are mentioned here.

Mucosa

It is stratified squamous epithelium, which is thick and nonkeratinizing, and it continues upward with the mucosa of the oropharynx. It also contains a layer of connective tissue called lamina propria and is external to it. It contains a thin layer of muscle fibers called muscularis mucosa. The mucosa of the esophagus is pink, smooth, and even. Normal GEJ appears as an irregular line, called as z-line or ora serrata. This line separates the esophageal mucosa, which is of lighter color, from the gastric mucosa, which is dark in appearance. The esophageal mucosa is nonkeratinized stratified squamous epithelium. It is a multilayer structure and has three layers, which are functionally different from each other:

1. *Stratum corneum:* It functions as a permeability defender between the lumen of the esophagus with contents on one side and blood in blood vessels on the other side, separating two entities.
2. *Stratum spinosum:* It has cells that are metabolically active and tissue defenders.
3. *Stratum germinativum:* These cells can reproduce.

Submucosa

It is made up of dense connective tissues. It contains blood vessels, veins, lymphatic vessels, nerves, and mucus-secreting glands. Mucosa is surrounded by a layer of loose connective tissue. The submucosa is the thickest and strongest part of the esophagus wall structures. It is highly vascular and contains esophageal glands, which also secrete mucus.

Muscle Layer

The muscles of the esophagus are arranged into two layers:

1. Internal circular layer
2. External longitudinal layer

The upper one-fourth of the esophagus contains a muscle layer, which is made up of striated or voluntary muscle.

In the middle one-fourth, they are a combination of striated (voluntary) and smooth (involuntary) muscles.

In the lower half, only smooth or involuntary muscle fibers are present **(Fig. 8)**.

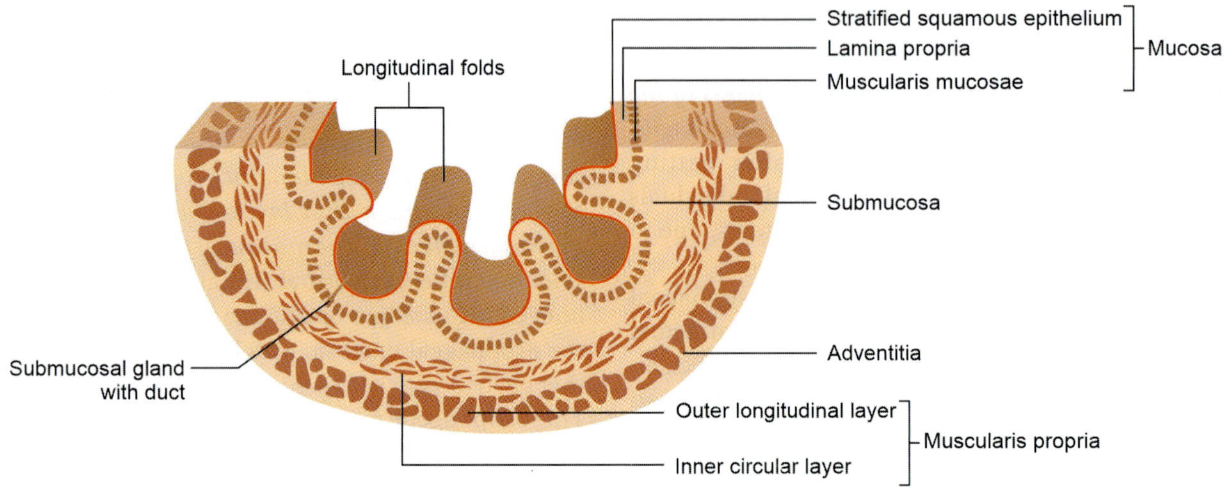

Fig. 8: Structure of esophagus, different layers.

Outermost Layer or Adventia

- It is made up of connective tissue and covers the muscle layer of esophagus.
- Nonerosive reflux disease (NERD) is characterized by the presence of troublesome reflux symptoms, abnormal pH monitoring, absence of endoscopically visible lesions, but with histological changes of squamous epithelium, which is microscopic esophagitis.

The esophagus is having mucosal lining of stratified squamous epithelium, which is nonkeratinizing. The columnar epithelium lines the inside of the stomach wall. The area where the esophagus meets the gastric folds is called GEJ or "Z-line," and normally, GEJ is at a squamocolumnar junction (SCJ). In GERD, SCJ moves up due to metaplasia.

In chronic GERD, the stratified squamous epithelium gets injured due to exposure to acid, and healing happens, which changes the squamous epithelium to columnar epithelium as squamous epithelium is not much resistant to acid attacks, but columnar epithelium is more resistant to acid attacks. This is nature's protective more.

Histology of the lower esophagus is important in GERD, though various researchers feel it is of not much importance. In NERD, the endoscopical picture may be normal, but after endoscopic biopsy, histology may show mucosal injury in a large percentage of cases. Histological changes in GERD mainly include proliferative changes of the squamous epithelium, such as basal cell layer hyperplasia, papillary elongation, and intercellular space dilation, but also intraepithelial inflammatory cell infiltration by eosinophils, neutrophils, and mononuclear cells. Inflammation due to chronic GERD causes metaplastic changes. *This may lead from multilayered epithelium (MLE) to (cardiac mucosa) CM, and ultimately to intestinal metaplasia and Barrett's esophagus.*

SYMPTOMS OF ESOPHAGEAL DISEASES

- Heartburn
- Acid regurgitation
- Chest pain
- Pain in the abdomen
- Belching
- Dysphagia
- Long-standing sore throat
- Nausea and vomiting
- Stomatitis
- Teeth enamel erosion
- Noncardiac chest pain (NCCP)
- Chronic cough
- Asthma
- Posterior laryngitis
- Globus sensation
- Recurrent pneumonitis
- Sleep disorders
- Dental erosion

Heartburn

Heartburn is also called pyrosis. It is a feeling of burning sensation in the upper abdomen and the retrosternal area of the chest. It sometimes behaves as a heart attack. Everybody must have suffered with heartburn sometime in life. The heartburn symptom of GERD has no relation with heart, but sometimes patients may feel that he is having a heart attack, and in such a situation, it is better to consult a clinician.

> *Points to remember:*
> - *Foreign body in esophagus:* It is most common in children and can be best diagnosed by anterior and lateral views of X-ray. It can be removed endoscopically, especially the bottom batteries, as they can cause perforation by corrosion.
> - *Corrosive trauma of the esophagus:* It can be caused by acid or alkali substances. Acid causes the coagulation of protein and penetrates superficially, but alkali causes saponification and causes deeper injuries. Corrosive traumas caused by acid and alkali can lead to stricture formation, which may need dilatation or esophagectomy.
> - *Zargar's classification of esophageal corrosive injuries:* It is divided into grades 0 (normal), 1 (superficial injury), 2a (mucosal superficial inflammation), 2b (deep mucosal inflammation, circumferential), 3a (transmural ulceration and focal necrosis), 3b (transmural ulceration with extensive necrosis), and 4 (perforation).

Most of us may feel heartburn occasionally, which is a normal feature, but GERD patients may feel it more frequently and even daily. Heartburn is the most common symptom of GERD. It occurs due to:

- Reflux of gastric contents with acid into the esophagus due to a relaxed or incompetent LES.
- In overeating, the stomach becomes full and distended and applies pressure on the LES, due to this pressure LES relaxes and opens, so that gastric contents with acid leak into the esophagus.
- In pregnancy, the enlarging uterus with fetus puts pressure on the stomach, which leads to reflux.
- It is also common in smokers as nicotine relaxes the LES by making it weak.
- *Lifestyle:* Heartburn is common in persons leading an unhealthy lifestyle, i.e., obesity, alcohol consumption, smoking, fatty and spicy food, eating too much citrus foods, chocolates, and certain medicines.
- *Obesity:* Obesity also puts pressure on the LES, making it weak. Weight gain frequently results in the development of new symptoms of GERD and the worsening of symptoms in patients with preexisting GERD.
- *Hobby:* Any hobby or a game or exercise, such as lifting of heavy weights or bending forward, which elevates the intra-abdominal pressure, can lead to relaxation of LES pressure and cause reflux, leading to heartburn.
- *Old age:* No age is exempted from heartburn. Although there is a tendency to reduced symptom frequency of the usual complaints of heartburn and acid regurgitation in older patients, the frequency of GERD complications such as erosive esophagitis, esophageal stricture, Barrett's esophagus, and esophageal cancer is significantly higher. An elderly man may have mild heartburn, but on endoscopy may reveal Barrett's esophagus. For example, Collen et al. found an increase of esophagitis and Barrett's esophagus in patients over 60 years of age compared to those younger, 81% versus 47%. The burning feeling of heartburn starts from the upper abdomen or lower chest and moves up in chest and neck. *Occasionally, it involves both arms and radiates to the back. In GERD, the heartburn may be mild or severe, occasionally or daily. Interestingly, the severity of heartburn (e.g., patients with severe heartburn may have a normal-appearing esophagus on endoscopy, and those with severe esophagitis or Barrett's esophagus may at times have mild or even no symptoms). Heartburn is most frequently noted within 1 hour after eating, particularly after the largest meal of the day.* Sugars, chocolate, onions, carminatives, and foods high in fat may aggravate heartburn by decreasing LES, LES pressure.

Acid Regurgitation

Regurgitation of acid into the mouth from the stomach through the esophagus gives a bitter or salty fluid. It is a common symptom of GERD and commonly occurs at night. Night regurgitation of acid causes sleep disturbance. If night regurgitation becomes chronic, then the chances of its complications, i.e., erosive esophagitis, Barrett's esophagus, increase. A person can spit the ingested food and rechew it or spit it out. It is called *"Rumination Syndrome."* It usually occurs within half an hour after taking food. The exact cause of this syndrome is not known, but an increase in abdominal pressure can cause it. It is also considered a psychological problem. *Acid reflux or backwash occurs due to relaxation of the LES and backflow of acid from the stomach to the esophagus.*

The most common or cardinal symptoms of GERD are heartburn and regurgitation. Regurgitation occurs with varying degrees of severity in approximately 80% of GERD patients.

Water Brash

Water brash is also a symptom of GERD, which produces excessive saliva. Saliva mixes with refluxed acid, causing a salty taste. A person with waterbrash may also feel heartburn.

Reflux esophagitis develops in GERD due to acid exposure when the mucosa's resistance becomes low. It may lead to:

- Mild esophagitis with microscopic mucosal changes and leukocytic infiltration. No endoscopic changes
- *Erosive esophagitis:* Inflammation with superficial ulceration and endoscopic changes
- *Peptic stricture:* When ulcers heal, they heal by fibrosis, and this leads to stricture formation, causing dysphagia.

Chest Pain

Gastroesophageal reflux disease is the most common gastrointestinal cause of "noncardiac chest pain." Following exclusion of a cardiac cause of chest pain, an evaluation of the esophagus is, therefore, appropriate. Chest pain of GERD may look like heart attack pain. It is a squeezing or constricting type of pain in the sternal region of the chest. It may involve the whole chest and radiate to the neck, arms, and even the back. The pain can last for minutes to hours. Pain usually gets reduced or disappears with antacids, histamine H2 receptor antagonists (H2Ras), and proton pump inhibitors (PPIs).

Chest pain in GERD is due to probably spasms of the muscles of esophagus. There are chemoreceptors in the esophageal wall which are sensitive to acid. So, the exposure of these chemoreceptors to acid of GERD causes chest pain. The esophagus and heart are located at the same place and have the same nerve supply; therefore, there is a similarity in the pain of GERD and angina pectoris. Chest pain due to GERD is the most common chest pain, only second to angina pectoris. A GERD patient can also have severe chest pain resembling myocardial infarction, but this pain differs from cardiac pain:

- Usual cardiac pain in the left side of the chest. GERD pain occurs in the center of the chest or may occur in the right side of the chest.
- There will be a past history of classical symptoms, such as heartburn in the GERD case.
- GERD pain may change with deep inhalation position and PPIs.
- Most patients with chest pain in GERD will also have heartburn of the same line. Several studies have demonstrated that the prevalence of GERD ranges 21–60% of patients with NCCP compared to patients with cardiac angina. Those with NCCP are usually younger, less likely to have typical symptoms, and more likely to have a normal resting electrocardiogram.

Not to forget:

- *Tracheoesophageal fistula (TEF):* These are of various types: Type A (esophageal atresia, EA), B (proximal TEF with distal EA), C (proximal EA with distal TEF), D (proximal and distal TEF), E (TEF, but not EA), and F (esophageal stenosis).
  It occurs before birth and can be diagnosed by a scan in pregnancy, but if after birth, then drooling of saliva, coiling of the tube inserted, and respiratory distress. It may be associated with anomalies, such as cardiac, anorectal, spinal, renal, and extremity abnormalities.
  Surgery is the treatment of TEF, it depends upon the weight of the baby, complications, and the type of TEF.
  - Type A—anastomosis with the stomach.
  - Type B, C, D, E—Kamron Haight Surgery—anastomosis after cutting the fistula.

Dysphagia

Dysphagia means difficulty in swallowing that may occur in the oral, pharyngeal, or esophageal phases of swallowing. Nonobstructive GERD is the most common identifiable cause of esophageal dysphagia.

Dysphagia is not an uncommon symptom of GERD. It is common in chronic cases of GERD. Cases of dysphagia are:

- GERD-induced severe inflammation in the esophagus.
- *Schatzki's ring:* It is a membranous ring-type of structure which develops in lower esophagus at squamocolumnar junction or at Z-line. It is made up of mucosa and submucosa of the wall of esophagus. A Schatzki's ring does not contain any muscle. Schatzki's ring is also called B ring. GERD of long standing can cause Schatzki's ring and also hiatus hernia can cause it. The treatment of Schatzki's ring is esophageal dilatation.
- Hiatus hernias

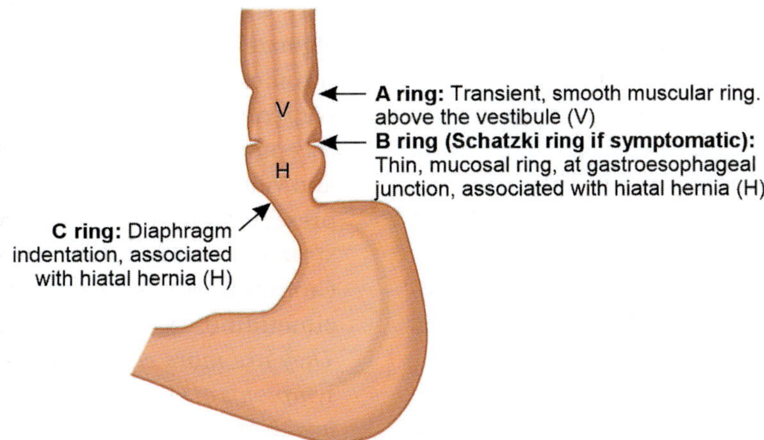

Fig. 9: Rings of dysphagia.

Ring A

It is above the vestibule and is transient.

Ring B

Schatzki's ring

Ring C

Develops in case of hiatus hernia

Vestibule of Esophagus

It is a space in esophagus just above the stomach at the level of diaphragm and goes down in the abdomen. It lies between rings A and B. It is named after the German American physician Rich and Schatzki **(Fig. 9)**.

Painful Swallowing or Odynophagia

It is a problem with the highly inflamed esophagus in GERD. The painful swallowing is both for solids as well as liquids. The diagnosis of odynophagia is confirmed by upper GI endoscopy. Pain can occur in the throat or chest. Odynophagia may be due to viral, bacterial, fungal, or protozoan infection. The inflammation may be mild, moderate, or severe. Pain may vary from a dull ache in the retrosternal area to pain in the neck during swallowing. In severe cases, sometimes a patient cannot even swallow solid foods. Endoscopic biopsy is required in case of odynophagia with dysphagia, as carcinoma of the esophagus is also an odynophagic factor.

INVESTIGATIONS IN ESOPHAGEAL DISEASES

- Radiography—CT and MRI
- Upper gastrointestinal endoscopy (UGIE)
- Endosonography (EUS)
- Esophageal manometry
- 24-hour pH and pH-impedance recording

BAROTRAUMA [BOERHAAVE'S (HERMANN BOERHAAVE, 1668–1738, PROFESSOR OF MEDICINE, LEIDEN, NETHERLANDS) SYNDROME]

It is due to an increase in pressure inside the esophagus when the patient vomits, and the glottis is closed. *It has severe chest pain and the presence of air in the mediastinum on X-ray. It can be managed by surgical repair.* Some other perforations can be managed by nonsurgical methods. Primary repair is not advised in a patient who presents late.

Mallory–Weiss Syndrome

It is a mucosal tear at the cardia of the stomach. *It is a vertical wound caused by recurrent severe vomiting and presents as hematemesis.* Surgery is rarely required, diagnosed by UGIE.

GASTROESOPHAGEAL REFLUX DISEASE

Gastroesophageal reflux disease is due to the reflux of acid from the stomach to the esophagus.

Gastroesophageal reflux disease is *diagnosed by history, physical examination, acid suppression tests, UGIE and biopsy, 24-hour pH monitoring, and manometry.*

Gastroesophageal reflux disease mimics peptic ulcer disease (PUD), nonulcer dyspepsia (NUD), angina pectoris, cholelithiasis, chronic gastritis, hiatus hernia, esophageal diverticulitis, stricture, and carcinoma of esophagus.

If GERD is not treated well, it can lead to esophagitis, Barrett's esophagus, strictures, ulcers, hemorrhage, perforation, and cancer.

Management of Gastroesophageal Reflux Disease

Gastroesophageal reflux disease is a common problem and is gradually increasing all over the globe. The reason for increasing incidence is probably and most commonly is our faulty lifestyle. Smoking, alcohol, fatty food, stress, anger, over worked and spicy food are common risk factors of today's life.

The following are the modalities of treatment of GERD:

- *Lifestyle changes:*
  - Elevate the head end of the bed—about 9."
  - Maintain a healthy weight.
  - Stop smoking.
  - Stop alcohol.
  - Go to bed 3 hours after a meal.
  - Avoid foods that trigger reflux, such as fatty foods, coffee, and spicy foods.
  - Avoid large meals and take small, frequent meals.
- *Antacids: Antacids are normally suggested to neutralize acid in the stomach. Antacids can give relief from symptoms of mild GERD, but cannot heal the esophageal inflammation or erosion. These are only used when a person has occasional heartburn.* For best results, antacids should be taken about an hour after a meal. Antacids can treat you symptomatically but cannot cure. Calcium carbonate (chalk) is a very commonly used antacid. It is quite effective. Eno is also commonly used for heartburn commonly. It is an effervescent antacid and neutralizes stomach acid. Antacids come in two forms, liquid and tablet. Tablets are chewable. Liquid antacids act quickly to relieve heartburn. Liquid antacids act faster than chewable tablet antacids. Alginic acid products are found to be more effective than other antacids. Usually, they contain sodium alginate, sodium bicarbonate, and calcium carbonate. It comes as a liquid as well as a tablet.
- *H2 receptor antagonists (H2RAs):* These histamine-2 receptor antagonists are available over the counter, and you can purchase them without having a doctor's prescription. They decrease acid production in the stomach, especially postprandial acid secretion. Common H2RAs (also called H2 blockers) are cimetidine, ranitidine, famotidine, and nizatidine. *They are more effective than any antacid in treating symptoms of GERD. A course of 8 weeks with H2RA can heal almost half the cases of GERD (50%). Rarely, H2RAs can cause cytopenias, gynecomastia, liver function test disturbances, and antiandrogenic effects.*

  The following are some examples of H2RAs:
  - Cimetidine
  - Ranitidine
  - Famotidine
  - Nizatidine

Mechanism of Action

Acid is secreted by parietal cells of the gastric mucosa; H2 receptors are situated on the surface of parietal cells. These H2RAs do a completion with histamine at H2 receptors and H2 receptors take H2RAs instead of histamine so get blocked by H2Ras, so they function as antagonists. When after a meal, histamine is released from the stomach to combine with H2 receptors on parietal cells of the stomach to release acid, but H2RAs are blocking the H2 receptors, and so histamine stimulation of parietal cell acid secretion does not occur, H2RAs suppress both stimulated and basal gastric acid secretion induced by histamine. *To get a proper effect in GERD, H2RAs should be given in two divided doses for at least 8 weeks, and then, if required, on single-dose maintenance therapy. Healing rates of esophagitis with H2RAs are good but not as good as with PPIs.*

Proton pump inhibitors:
- PPIs are more effective than H2RAs in treating symptoms of GERD.
- PPI after a course of 8 weeks of treatment has better healing in erosive esophagitis than H2RAs.
- Common PPIs are omeprazole, lansoprazole, esomeprazole, pantoprazole, rabeprazole, and dexlansoprazole.

Some researchers have believed that esomeprazole 40 mg is best at treating GERD.

- PPIs block the major pathways of gastric acid production, and they do this better than H2RAs.
- *A single study showed that esomeprazole at doses of 20 and 40 mg is more effective than 20 mg once a day in both healing and symptoms resolutions in GERD patients with reflux esophagitis, with a tolerability profile comparable to that of omeprazole.* A randomized controlled treatment compared esomeprazole 40 mg to lansoprazole 30 mg. Esomeprazole was surprised in healing and symptom control, with superiority highest in more severe degrees of esophagitis. PPIs have suppression of acid secretion significantly and more than irritable digestive reflexes of the abdomen (IDRAs).

Proton pump inhibitors block the gastric H, K-ATPase, inhibiting gastric acid secretion. Because of the H, K-ATPase is the final step of acid secretion, an inhibitor of this enzyme is more effective than receptor antagonists in suppressing gastric acid secretion. PPIs after 8 weeks of treatment have a better rate of healing than H2RAs in esophagitis in GERD. It is better to use PPI twice a day before meals for 8 weeks to seek the best results of PPIs in GERD.

Esomeprazole is found to have better effects than omeprazole and lansoprazole in esophagitis of GERD, but omeprazole is better for nighttime acid suppression. PPIs are very safe medicines and have only minimal side effects, such as headache and diarrhea, which is why they are in maximum use in GERD.

- *Baclofen:* It is used to treat as a muscle relaxant to treat muscle spasms. It is not a pain killer but relieves pain by relaxing the muscles in spasm. It gives some relief in some patients with GERD.
- *Prokinates:* Some prokinates are as follows:
  - Cisapride
  - Metoclopramide
  - Domperidone
  - Mesopride
  - Itopride
  - Renzapride

Surgical Treatment of Gastroesophageal Reflux Disease

Antireflux surgery is widely accepted as a way of treatment when medical treatment fails, or the disease becomes resistant to medical treatment. The most common surgical procedure is Nissen's (Rudolph Nissen, 1896–1981, a Turkey-born Swiss surgeon) fundoplication.

Endoscopic Treatment Procedures for Gastroesophageal Reflux Disease

Now a days, various endoscopic antireflux procedures have been developed to treat GERD. All these methods are not very common at present. These procedures are:

- Radiofrequency ablation (RFA)
- Transoral incisionless fundoplication (TIF)
- Medigus ultrasonic surgical endostapler (MUSE)
- Antireflux mucosectomy (ARMS)

BARRETT'S ESOPHAGUS

Barrett's esophagus is a condition in which an abnormal columnar epithelium that is predisposed to malignancy replaces the stratified squamous epithelium that normally lines the distal esophagus. Barrett's esophagus is diagnosed by a history of GERD, especially chronic, upper GI endoscopy, and endoscopic biopsy of the mucosa at the GEJ site. Histopathology shows the metaplasia of squamous epithelium to columnar epithelium. In general, in the adult population of Western countries, the prevalence of Barrett's esophagus (predominantly short segment) is between 1.6 and 6.8%. The reported rates of Barrett's esophagus (BE) ranged from 2.6% to 23% in Indian patients with GERD symptoms.

When the columnar epithelium replaces the squamous epithelium of the esophagus >3 cm in length at the lower part of the esophagus, it is called "short segment Barrett's esophagus." According to some researches, there may be an increased incidence of the development of malignancy in short-segment Barrett's esophagus.

You may be asked

- *Esophageal infections are of various types:* Candidiasis, cytomegalovirus (CMV), herpes, feline esophagus (GERD/eosinophilic esophagitis). Eosinophilic esophagitis is a chronic immunological disease, diagnosed by biopsy and treated by topical steroids and acid-suppressing drugs.
- *Achalasia cardia:* It is a mortality disorder of the esophagus due to nonrelaxation of the LES, due to the absence of myenteric and Auerbach plexus ganglion cells. It is of two types: Achalasia I—due to ganglion cells absence and Achalasia II—due to *Trypanosoma cruzi* infection [Chaga's (Carlos Justiniano Ribiero Chaga, 1879–1934, Brazilian professor of tropical medicine) disease]. It has common clinical features of regurgitation, dysphagia, and weight loss. Manometry is the best investigation. It is treated by dilatation, botox, and surgery [open, laparoscopic, and peroral endoscopic myotomy (POEM)]. Heller's [Ernst Heller, 1877–1964, German surgeon) Myotomy is the treatment of choice for type I and type II, but POEM is for type III achalasia.

- *Esophageal diverticulum:* Zeneker's (upper esophageal), mid, and lower esophageal. Zeneker's (Friedrich Albert Zeneker, 1825–1898, German pathologist) diverticulum and lower esophageal diverticulum are false diverticulum whereas mid esophageal diverticulum is the true diverticulum. Treatment is by diverticulectomy. Barrium swallow is the best way to diagnose.

High-grade dysplasia (HGD) and early stages of adenocarcinoma may be treated by endoscopic resection or RFA. Columnar-lined esophagus (Barrett's esophagus) was named after Norman Rupert Barrett (1903–1979) in 1950. Even though the condition was originally described by Barrett, it was believed that ulcers were first found by *Philip Rowland Allisorim in 1946.*

According to recent guidelines, those with nondysplastic or low-grade dysplasia (LGD) are managed by annual observation with endoscopy or managed by annual observation with endoscopy, or treatment with RFA. In HGD, the risk of developing cancer might be at 10% per patient year or greater.

Among adult patients who have endoscopic examinations because of GERD symptoms, long-segment Barrett's esophagus is found in 3–5%, whereas 10–20% have short-segment Barrett's esophagus. However, a number of large studies published since 2011 have suggested that the cancer risk for such patients is even lower, in the range of 0.12–0.33%/year.

Factors Responsible for Barrett's Esophagus in Gastroesophageal Reflux Disease

Factors include:

- Low pressure at LES
- Weak esophageal peristalsis
- Impaired esophagogastric junction
- Hyperacid secretion by the gastric mucosa
- Bile reflux
- Diminished secretion of epidermal growth factor (EGF)
- EGF is a salivary protein that helps in the regeneration of cells.

Prague Classification of Barrett's Esophagus

It was given by the *International Working Group for the Classification of Oesophagitis (IWGCO)* in 2004.

This classification uses "C" value for circumferential factor and "M" value for maximum length (tongue-like lesion) **(Figs. 10A and B)**.

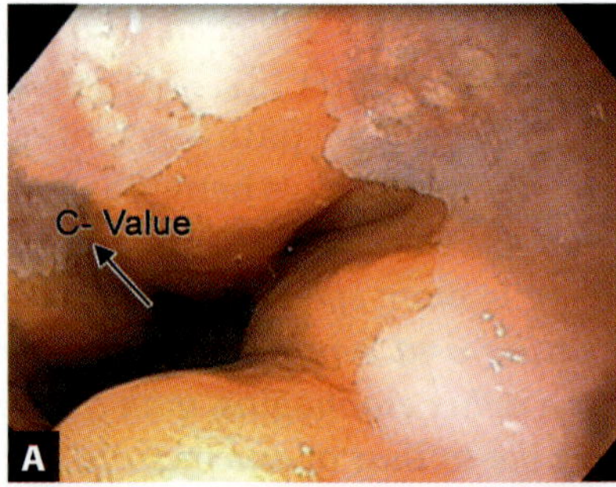

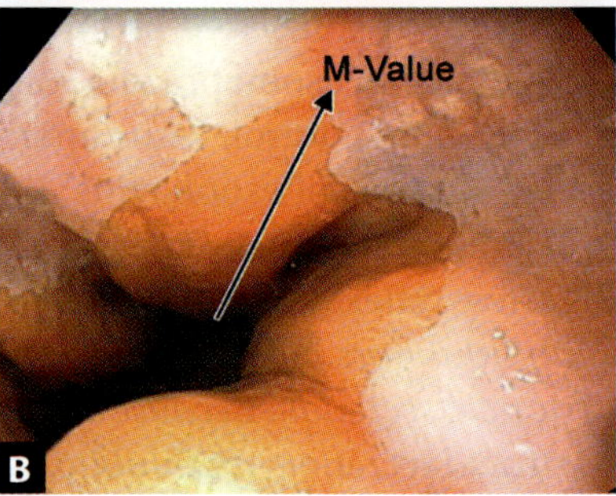

Figs. 10A and B: (A) C value as per the Prague classification of Barrett's esophagus; (B) M value as per the Prague classification of Barrett's esophagus.

Diagnosis

Barrett's esophagus is diagnosed with an upper gastrointestinal endoscopy and mucosal biopsy.

Management of Barrett's Esophagus

- Lifestyle changes
- PPIs
- *Other methods of treatment:*
    - Endoscopic ablative therapy by laser, radiofrequency energy ablation (REA), electrocoagulation, etc.
    - Cryotherapy
    - Photochemical energy
    - Photodynamic therapy (PDT)
    - Endoscopic mucosal resection (EMR)

Lifestyle Changes which are Effective

- Stopping smoking
- Stopping alcohol
- Eating small and frequent meals
- Avoid symptoms triggering foods such as coffee, chocolate, spicing, and fatty foods.

Lifestyle alterations must be tried even when treatment of Barrett's esophagus is on.

Proton Pump Inhibitors

Proton pump inhibitors are the required drugs to treat Barrett's esophagus in the large majority of patients.

Other Methods

Other methods include:

- RFA
- Cryoablation
- EMR
- Esophagectomy
- Endoscopic surveillance for Barrett's esophagus

> Current guidelines for Barrett's esophagus patients recommend endoscopic surveillance intervals of 3–5 years for patients without dysplasia, 6–12 months for those with LGD, and every 3 months for HGD patients.

HIATUS HERNIA

In a hiatus hernia, the upper portions of the stomach are pushed above the diaphragm through an opening or hiatus. Hiatus hernia can cause heartburn, acid regurgitation, chest or abdominal pain, dysphagia, vomiting, etc. **(Figs. 11A to C)**.

Hiatus hernia increases the chances of GERD development through the following factors:

- Hiatus hernia pushes the LES up and so reduces the resting pressure of the LES.
- LES is a high-pressure zone, but due to the upward displacement of LES due to hiatus hernia, the LES gets shortened.
- During straining, LES pressure increases, but hiatus hernia eliminates it.
- Hiatus hernias increase the frequency of LESRs.
- In hiatus hernias, the hernia sac acts as a pocket collecting acid from the stomach (acid pocket), and this develops increased changes of acid reflux.
- The gastric mucosal folds in the acid pocket increase the tendency of reflux.
- LES also opens at a lower pressure in hiatus hernias. The real mechanism of the development of hiatus hernia is not very clear, but raised intra-abdominal pressure, such as heavy weightlifting, may cause hiatus hernia.

An acid pocket in a case of GERD is significantly responsible for acid reflux. In GERD with hiatus hernia, the acid pocket is bigger than in the case of GERD without hiatus hernia, and due to this reason, in the case of GERD with hiatus hernia, acid reflux is much more common and frequent.

Hiatus hernia is a known risk factor for GERD. Hiatus hernias adversely affect the main acid reflux barrier, which is the LES. Hiatus hernia influences LES and reduces its pressure, leading to relaxation of the LES of opening of the LES. Hiatus hernia leads to back leakage of acid into the esophagus from the stomach by the following mechanisms:

- Relaxation of LES by reducing its contraction or pressure
- TLESR, transient LES esophageal relaxation occurs quickly and recurrently by Hiatus hernia.
- Esophageal clearance is delayed.
- Probably the gastric contents in the hiatus hernia sac leak back into the esophagus when the LES relaxes during the swallowing of food.

Types of Hiatus Hernias

There are four types of hiatus hernias:

1. *Type I—sliding type:* >90% of hiatus hernias are of this type. It is usually associated with acid regurgitation or GERD.
2. *Type II—paraesophageal hernia*. Here, a part of the esophagus escapes into the chest parallel to esophagus.
3. *Type III:* It is a combination of sliding and paraesophageal hernia.

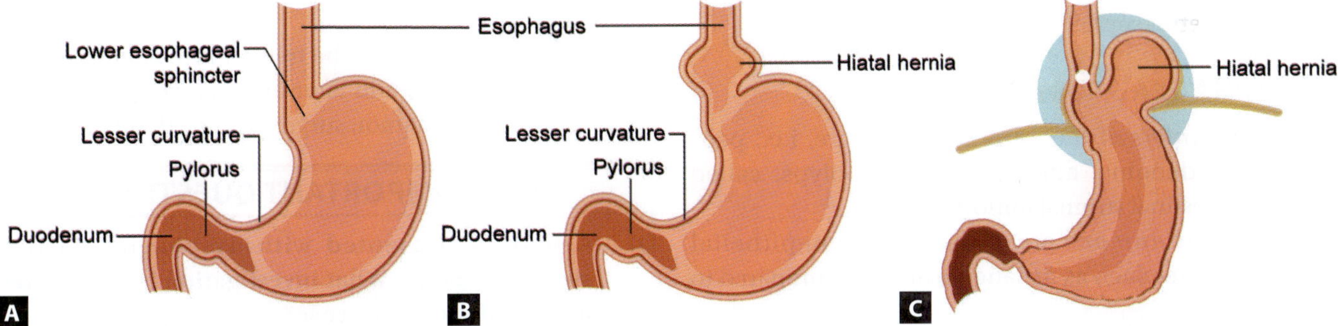

Figs. 11A to C: Hiatal hernia: (A) Normal stomach; (B) Sliding hiatus hernia; and (C) Paraesophageal hiatal hernia.

4. *Type IV:* When, along with the stomach, some other abdominal organ also herniates, such as the small intestine, colon, and spleen.

Type I and Type III are commonly associated with GERD.

Patients with hiatus hernia may not have GERD, and some patients without many significant signs of hiatus hernia have advanced GERD. Hiatus hernias that are in range [>3 (m)] and nonreducible (in which the gastric rugal folds remain above the diaphragm between swallows) are especially prone to reflux.

> *Good to remember!*
> *Esophagectomies:* The surgical removal of the esophagus is location dependent: Transhiatal for the lower one-third of the esophagus, it is called Orringer (Mark Burton Orringer, American surgeon) esophagectomy. Esophagectomy for the middle one-third of the esophagus is through an abdominal incision or right-sided thoracic incision called Ivor Lewis esophagectomy. The esophagectomy for the middle one-third with LN clearance is through the abdomen, right side of the thorax, or even neck (left side), called McKeown's (Kenneth Charles McKeown, 1912–1995, British surgeon) or three-field esophagectomy.

The hiatus hernia is the herniation of part of stomach through esophageal hiatus of the diaphragm. This happens when the esophageal hiatus is weak and lax. When the upper part of the stomach escapes to the chest, the reflux of gastric contents with acid easily flows back to the esophagus, leading to GERD. While small hiatal hernias often require surgery. The most important symptom is heartburn, followed by regurgitation. Regurgitation does not mean GERD, as not every patient with regurgitation in hiatus hernias has GERD. The history of symptoms is important to diagnose hiatal hernia and with GERD. Physical examination in case of hiatal hernia and GERD is of not much importance. Upper gastrointestinal endoscopy is the most important investigation tool to diagnose hiatus hernia with or without GERD. It is also important as it excludes serious esophageal diseases also, such as Barrett's esophagus and saver of esophagus.

ESOPHAGEAL TUMORS

- *Benign tumors* of the esophagus are rare, i.e., papilloma, adenoma, and hyperplastic polyps, called gastrointestinal stromal tumors (GISTs).
- *Malignant tumors* are common. Nonepithelial malignancies such as melanoma are rare compared to carcinoma.

CARCINOMA OF THE ESOPHAGUS

- Squamous cell carcinoma (SCC)
- Adenocarcinoma

The risk factors of carcinoma of esophagus are: Smoking, alcohol, betel nut chewing, very hot drinks, n-nitroso-containing foods (pickles), deficiency of vitamin E and selenium, history of corrosive stricture, history of radiation, persistent vegetative state (PVS), achalasia, GERD, Barrett's esophagus, scleroderma, Zenker's diverticulum, etc. SCC mainly affects the middle one-third of the esophagus, whereas adenocarcinoma affects the lower one-third. GERD and Barrett's esophagus are high-risk factors for adenocarcinoma, whereas smoking and alcohol are high-risk factors for SCC. Dysphagia is the earliest and most common symptom with weight loss. *UGIE with biopsy is the best investigative procedure. Rat tail appearance is a significant feature on barium swallow. EUS shows various bands which are hypo- and hyperechogenic, arranged alternatively.*

TUMOR, NODE, AND METASTASIS CLASSIFICATION

Tis T_1, T_2, T_3, T_4a, T_{4b}, N_0, N_1, N_2, N_3, M_0, and M_1

> - The minimum number of LN to be removed with esophagectomy should not be >15 involved.
> - Esophagus replacement can be done with the stomach, colon, or jejunum, but the best is the stomach.
> - Chemoradiation has better sensitivity and effect on cancer tumors than chemotherapy and radiation alone.
> - Self-expanding metallic stents (SEMS) can be used for malignant TEF, which depends upon the depth of the tumor and stage.

Treatment

- Tia—EMR
- Tib, N_0/T_2N_0—esophagectomy (tumor-free margin should be 5 cm distally and 10 cm proximally to prevent recurrence)
- $T_2N_1/T_3/T_4$—initially to be treated with chemotherapy and radiotherapy, and later on, after contraction and limitation of the tumor, surgery can be done.

SOME IMPORTANT QUESTIONS

Q1. A patient presented with dysphagia. Barium swallow is done. What investigation is not needed and not done in this case?

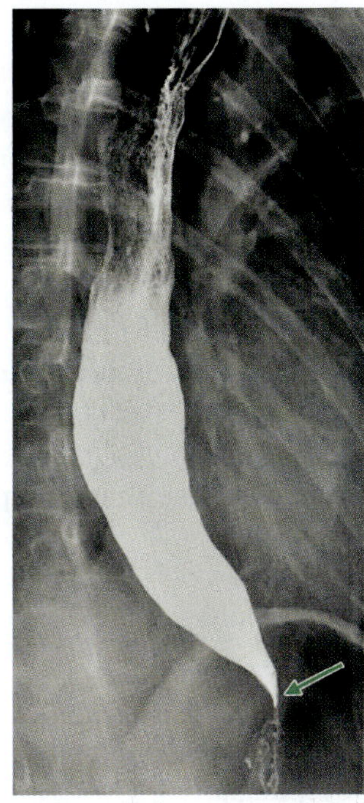

a. Manometry
b. 24-hour pH
c. Endoscopy
d. Contrast-enhanced computed tomography (CECT) chest

Ans. b

Q2. The most common organ that herniates in Morgagni's hernia:

a. Spleen
b. Liver
c. Stomach
d. Transverse colon

Ans. d

Q3. A baby playing unsupervised complained of dysphagia for the past few hours. What is the diagnosis as per the X-ray shown?

a. Tracheal foreign body
b. Esophagus having a coin
c. Soft tissue calcification neck
d. Artifact

Ans. b

Q4. The most common complication seen in hiatus hernia is:

a. Esophagitis
b. Aspiration pneumonitis
c. Volvo's
d. Esophageal stricter

Ans. a

Q5. A patient aged 30 years presents with dysphagia. High-resolution manometry done for that patient showed the following findings. There was panesophageal pressurization with distal contractile integrity as >450 mm Hg cm. What is the diagnosis?

a. Type 1 achalasia
b. Type 2 achalasia
c. Type 3 achalasia
d. Diffuse esophageal spasm

Ans. c

Q6. Water-soluble contrast is made up of:

a. Barium
b. Calcium
c. Iodine
d. Bromine

Ans. c

Q7. The most useful investigation in sliding hernia in females:

a. Fluoroscopy
b. Barium meal
c. Palpation method
d. Ultrasound

Ans. b

Q8. Fundoplication is used in the treatment of:

a. Hiatus hernia
b. Achalasia cardia
c. Chopstick-Handled Perforation Sleeve (CHPS)
d. CA esophagus

Ans. a

Q9. In Nissen's fundoplication, wrapping is done:

a. 1/3
b. 1/4
c. 3/4
d. 1/2

Ans. None

Q10. On endoscopy there is serpentine ulcers in distal esophagus with otherwise normal mucosa seen. Diagnosis is:

a. Herpes simplex
b. Pill induced
c. Cytomegalovirus (CMV)
d. Candidiasis

Ans. c

Q11. A punched-out ulcer in the esophagus on endoscopy in an immunocompromised patient is seen in:

a. Herpes zoster virus
b. Herpes simplex
c. CMV
d. Candidiasis

Ans. b

Q12. A 35-year-old lady presented with dysphagia, nocturnal asthma, and weight loss for 6 years. The most probable diagnosis is:

a. Achalasia cardia
b. Lye stricter of the esophagus
c. Gastroesophageal reflux disease
d. Cancer esophagus

Ans. c

MULTIPLE CHOICE QUESTIONS

Grade I	*Simple*

Q1. Which of the following is the most important determinant of prognosis in neonatal congenital diaphragmatic hernia (CHD)? (All India 2011)

a. Pulmonary hypertension
b. Delay in surgery
c. Size of defect
d. Gestational age at diagnosis

Q2. Which of the following is the least important prognostic factor in congenital diaphragmatic hernia? (All India 2011)

a. Pulmonary hypertension
b. Delay in emergency surgery
c. Size of defect
d. Gestational age at diagnosis

Q3. All are true about Bochdalek hernia, *except*: (GB Pant 2011)

a. Posterolateral
b. Left side
c. Present in the second decade
d. Congenital

Q4. Most common site of Morgagni's hernia: (AIIMS 2006)

a. Right anterior
b. Right posterior
c. Left anterior
d. Left posterior

Q5. The gold standard for diagnosis of gastroesophageal reflux disease (GERD) is: (JIPMER 2014)

a. Barium swallow
b. Endoscopy
c. 24-hour pH monitoring
d. Esophageal manometry

Q6. Which of the following is the earliest indicator of pathological gastroesophageal reflux disease in infants (GERD)? (All India 2011)

a. Respiratory symptoms
b. Postprandial regurgitation
c. Upper GI bleed
d. Stricter esophagus

Q7. The best test to diagnose gastroesophageal reflux disease and quantify acid output is: (AIIMS 2011)

a. Esophagogram
b. Endoscopy
c. Manometry
d. 24-hour pH monitoring

Q8. The most important pathophysiological cause of GERD is: (AIIMS 2012)

a. Hiatus hernia
b. Transient lower esophageal sphincter (LES) relaxation
c. LESS hypotension
d. Inadequate esophagus clearance

Q9. True about Schatzki's ring: (PGI 2010)

a. Has skeletal muscle
b. Located at the lower esophagus
c. Causes dysphagia
d. Contains all layers of the esophagus

Q10. Diaphragm develops from all of the following structures *except*: (All India 2011)

a. Septum transverse
b. Pleuroperitoneal membrane
c. Cervical myotomes
d. Dorsal mesocardium

Q11. Which of the following incisions is taken for diaphragmatic surgery? (AIIMS 2014)

a. Transverse
b. Circumferential
c. Vertical
d. Radial

Q12. Nonprogressive contractions of the esophagus are: (AIIMS 2011)

a. Primary
b. Secondary
c. Tertiary
d. Quaternary

Q13. Which of the following is a contraindication for bag and mask ventilation? (AIIMS June 2000)

a. Septicemia
b. Tracheoesophageal fistula
c. Meconium aspiration
d. Diaphragmatic hernia

Q14. The diagnostic feature of congenital diaphragmatic hernia on prenatal ultrasonography is: (AIIMS June 2001)

a. A cyst behind the left atrium
b. Mediastinal shift with normal heart axis
c. Peristalsis in the thoracic cavity
d. Absence of a gas bubble under the diaphragm

Q15. A neonate with a scaphoid abdomen and respiratory distress has: (All India 1994)

a. Congenital pyloric stenosis
b. Diaphragmatic hernia
c. Volvulus
d. Wilm's tumor

Grade II	Difficult

Q1. Most common complication after Nissen's fundoplication: (AIIMS 2011)

a. Esophageal injury b. Stomach injury
c. Liver injury d. Pneumothorax

Q2. All are true about antireflux surgeries, *except*: (JIPMER 2011)

a. Nissen's is a 360° complete wrap
b. Watson is 90° posterior
c. Toupet is a 270° posterior
d. Dor is a partial fundoplication

Q3. A most common cause of esophagitis is: (AIIMS 2009)

a. Alcohol b. Smoking
c. Spicy and hot food d. Esophageal reflux

Q4. All are true about achalasia, *except*: (JIPMER 2011)

a. It predisposes to malignancy.
b. Body peristalsis is normal.
c. LESS pressure is increased.
d. Dilatation of proximal segment

Q5. Most common motility disorder leading to dysphagia: (JIPMER 2010)

a. Nutcracker esophagus
b. Esophageal web
c. Diffuse esophageal spasm
d. Achalasia cardia

Q6. Which of the following is a true diverticulum of the esophagus? (AIIMS 2016)

a. Zenker's diverticulum
b. Meckel's diverticulum
c. Epiphrenic diverticulum
d. Parabronchial diverticulum

Q7. Not a component of POEMS syndrome: (JIPMER 2010)

a. Polyneuropathy b. Esophageal atresia
c. Endocrinopathy d. Multiple myeloma

Q8. The acronym POEMS stands for: (PGI 2011)

a. Esophageal dismally b. Polyneuropathy
c. Endocrinopathy d. M-protein
e. Scleroderma

Q9. True about Barrett's esophagus: (PGI 2007)

a. Long esophageal segment involved
b. Metaplasia
c. Peptic ulcer
d. Paraesophageal hernia
e. Leads to adenocarcinoma

Q10. Barrett's esophagus is diagnosed by: (AIIMS 2012)

a. Squamous metaplasia b. Intestinal metaplasia
c. Squamous dysplasia d. Intestinal dysplasia

Q11. Premalignant lesions of carcinoma of the esophagus include: (PGI 2011)

a. Tylosis
b. Plummer–Vinson syndrome
c. Barrett's esophagus
d. Achalasia cardia
e. Scleroderma

Q12. Not a predisposing factor for carcinoma esophagus: (AIIMS 2009)

a. Diverticulum
b. Human papilloma virus
c. Mediastinal fibrosis
d. Caustic ingestion

Q13. Which of the following mechanisms cannot prevent gastroesophageal reflux? (AIIMS Nov 1998)

a. Looping fibers of the right crus of the diaphragm
b. Mucosal folds at the gastroesophageal junction
c. Circular muscle fibers of the GE sphincter
d. The angle made by the esophagus with the stomach

Q14. A female patient has dysphagia, intermittent epigastric pain. On endoscopy, the esophagus was dilated above and narrowed at the bottom. Treatment is: (AIIMS May 2012)

a. PPI
b. Esophagectomy
c. Dilatation
d. Heller's cardiomyotomy

Q15. A young patient presents with a history of dysphagia, more to liquids than solids. The first investigation you will do is: (AIIMS June 2000)

a. Barium swallow
b. Esophagoscopy
c. Ultrasound of the chest
d. Computed tomography (CT) scan of the chest

Grade III	Most difficult

Q1. Which of the following is the best indicator of survival in CA esophagus? (AIIMS 2008)

a. TNM stage
b. Resection margin
c. Histology and location
d. Size of tumor

Q2. Best prognosis in CA esophagus: (AIIMS 2010)

a. Polypoidal
b. Fungating
c. Ulcerative
d. Infiltrative

Q3. Characteristic features of LN involvement on endoscopic ultrasonography (EUS) in CA esophagus are all, *except*: (AIIMS 2008)

a. Round contour
b. Sharp border
c. Hyperechogenic
d. Size >1 cm

Q4. The most commonly used chemotherapy regimen in CA esophagus is: (AIIMS 2008)

a. 5FU + cisplatin
b. Cisplatin + vinblastine
c. Cisplatin + paclitaxel
d. Cisplatin + epirubicin

Q5. T-staging of the esophagus is best done by: (AIIMS 2011)

a. EUS
b. CT
c. Magnetic resonance imaging (MRI)
d. Positron emission tomography (PET)

Q6. Treatment of choice for CA esophagus: (PGI 2009)

a. Esophagectomy
b. External radiotherapy
c. Internal radiotherapy
d. Chemotherapy

Q7. A most common complication of placing a stent in the CA esophagus: (AIIMS 2011)

a. Migration
b. Chest pain
c. Perforation
d. Bleeding

Q8. Lymph node metastasis in CA esophagus is best detected by: (JIPMER 2016)

a. PET
b. EUS
c. CT
d. Thoracoscopy + laparoscopy

Q9. In esophagus cancer, prognosis is best determined by: (AIIMS 2015)

a. Cellular differentiation
b. Age of patient
c. T-stage
d. Length of involvement

Q10. The first successful esophagectomy was done by: (AIIMS 2011)

a. Miculikz
b. Kaplan
c. Torek
d. Orringer

Q11. The most common benign tumor of the esophagus: (JIPMER 2014)

a. Leiomyoma
b. Papilloma
c. Adenoma
d. Hemangioma

Q12. Endoscopic treatment of leiomyoma of the esophagus is contraindicated due to: (JIPMER 2011)

a. Infection
b. Chances of dissemination
c. Perforation
d. Perforation and dissemination

Q13. Mackler's triad includes: (PGI 2009)

a. Vomiting
b. Subcutaneous emphysema
c. Lower thoracic pain
d. Peripheral cyanosis
e. Pleural effusion

Q14. Treatment for achalasia is associated with a high rate of recurrence: (All India 2002)

a. Pneumatic dilatation
b. Laparoscopic myotomy
c. Open surgical myotomy
d. Botulinum toxin

Q15. All of the following statements about Zenker's diverticulum are true *except*: (All India 2009)

a. Acquired diverticulum
b. Lateral X-rays on barium swallow are often diagnostic
c. False diverticulum
d. Out pouching of the anterior pharyngeal wall just above the cricopharyngeus muscle.

ANSWERS

Grade I: 1. a (Sabiston 20/e p1863-1864); 2. b; 3. c; 4. a; 5. c (Bailey 27/e p1077); 6. a; 7. d; 8. b (Harrison 19/e p1906); 9. b, c; 10. d; 11. b (Sabiston and Spencer's Surgery of Chest 8/e p chapter 7); 12. c; 13. d; 14. c; 15. d

Grade II: 1. d; 2. b; 3. d; 4. b (Schwartz 10/e p990-992); 5. d; 6. d; 7. b (Harrison 19/e p718); 8. b, c, d; 9. a, b, c, e (Sabiston 20/e p1050); 10. b; 11. a; 12. c; 13. None; 14. d; 15. a

Grade III: 1. a (Sabiston 20/e p1027-1032); 2. a (Sabiston 20/e p1038); 3. c; 4. a; 5. a; 6. a; 7. b (Bailey 27/e p1094); 8. b (Schwartz 10/e p1003-1014); 9. c; 10. c; 11. a (Sabiston 20/e p1032); 12. c; 13. a, b, c; 14. d; 15. d

MODEL QUESTIONS

Q1. In gastroesophageal reflux disease (GERD), what demonstrates the best anatomical picture?

a. Barium swallow
b. 24-hour pH monitoring
c. Endoscopy
d. Manometry

Ans. a

Q2. A young girl presented with reflux and retrosternal discomfort. Best investigation for this:

a. 24-hour ambulatory pH monitoring
b. Upper gastrointestinal (GI) endoscopy
c. Contrast-enhanced computed tomography (CECT)
d. Magnetic resonance imaging (MRI)

Ans. a

Q3. Achalasia cardia is characterized by all, *except*:

a. Most common in women
b. Dysphagia is the most common symptom.
c. Premalignant condition
d. Parrot's beak's appearance

Ans. a

Q4. What is the location of Killian's dehiscence?

a. Below superior constrictor
b. Below the inferior constrictor
c. Below the cricopharyngeal muscle
d. Below upper one-third of the smooth muscle of the esophagus

Ans. b

Q5. Which of the following is not done in carcinoma esophagus?

a. Biopsy
b. pHmetry
c. CT chest
d. PET scan

Ans. b

Q6. All are predisposing factors for carcinoma esophagus, *except*:

a. Achalasia
b. Patterson Brown Kelly syndrome
c. Zenker's diverticulum
d. Ectodermal dysplasia

Ans. d

Q7. A 28-year-old alcoholic patient walks to the hospital with the complaints of binge vomiting, chest pain, fever, and pneumomediastinum. The most probable condition:

a. Boerhaave syndrome
b. Tension pneumothorax
c. Perforated peptic ulcer (PUD) perforation
d. Mallory Weiss tear

Ans. a

Q8. Risk factors for esophagus carcinoma are all, *except*:

a. GERD
b. Betel chewing
c. Nitrate food
d. Antioxidant deficiency

Ans. b

Q9. Which of the following is not a natural constriction of the esophagus?

a. Thyroid position
b. Pharyngoesophageal junction
c. Aortic region
d. Diaphragmatic region

Ans. b

Q10. The stricter esophagus is dilated with.....French dilator?

a. 30
b. 40
c. 50
d. 60

Ans. c

Q11. What is Dohlman's procedure for Zenker's diverticulum?

a. Endoscopic stapling of the septum
b. Endoscopic suturing of the pouch
c. Resection of the pouch
d. Laser excision

Ans. a

SUGGESTED READING

1. Bailey & Love's - Short Practice of Surgery, 27th edition.
2. Schwartz's Principles of Surgery, 18th edition.
3. Textbook of Surgery by David Sabiston, 21st edition.

CHAPTER 33

Stomach and Duodenum

"Every heartburn must be reported to doctor and let him decide whether you need only over the counter drugs or some investigations also."

– Vinod Kumar Nigam

ANATOMY AND PHYSIOLOGY OF THE STOMACH

INTRODUCTION

Stomach is the dilated part of the upper gastrointestinal tract. It is "J-shaped" and is situated in the upper part of the abdomen. It is a muscular, hollow organ connected with the esophagus at the upper end and with the duodenum at the lower end.

DEVELOPMENT OF STOMACH (FIGS. 1A TO E)

In the fourth week of the embryo's life, the foregut develops a fusiform dilatation which grows and forms future stomach. The right wall of the future stomach grows faster than the left wall and this development leads to formation of future greater and lesser curvatures of stomach. *Simultaneously, the stomach rotates on its long axis clockwise up to 90°; so, the ventral border of stomach becomes right border, and dorsal border becomes left border, and the left side becomes ventral surface and right side becomes dorsal surface.*

The vitelline arteries from the celiac artery, the superior mesenteric artery (SMA), and the inferior mesenteric artery supply the areas of the gastrointestinal tract are defined as the foregut, midgut, and hindgut.

STRUCTURE OF STOMACH

The word stomach is derived from the Greek "stomachos," ultimately from stoma, meaning mouth.

Gastro- and gastric (meaning related to the stomach) are both derived from the Greek "gaster," meaning belly.

The stomach lies in the upper left quadrant of the abdomen. It has two curvatures: (1) Lesser curvature and (2) greater curvature (right and left border). A large, fat-laden, double-layered peritoneal fold called the greater omentum hangs from the greater curvature of the stomach, covering almost whole of the abdominal cavity in front. It is also called "abdominal policeman."

The stomach has the following relations with other organs in the abdominal cavity **(Fig. 2)**:

- *Anteriorly:* Anterior abdominal wall, left lobe of liver, and left costal margins.
- *Posteriorly:* Tail of the pancreas, left kidney, spleen, left adrenal gland, and abdominal aorta, transverse colon and its mesocolon, left crus of diaphragm. The posterior relation of the stomach is also called "stomach bed."
- *To the right:* Liver and duodenum.
- *To the left:* Diaphragm and spleen.
- *Superiorly:* Diaphragm, left lobe of liver, and esophagus.
- *Inferiorly:* Transverse, colon, and small intestine.

PARTS OF THE STOMACH

Stomach is a hollow and dilated sac. The stomach can be divided into the following parts **(Fig. 3)**:

- Fundus
- Body
- Pylorus
- Pyloric antrum
- Sulcus intermedius separates the pylorus from the pyloric antrum

The stomach has two surfaces:

1. Anterior surface
2. Posterior surface

The stomach has two borders:

1. Lesser curvature
2. Greater curvature

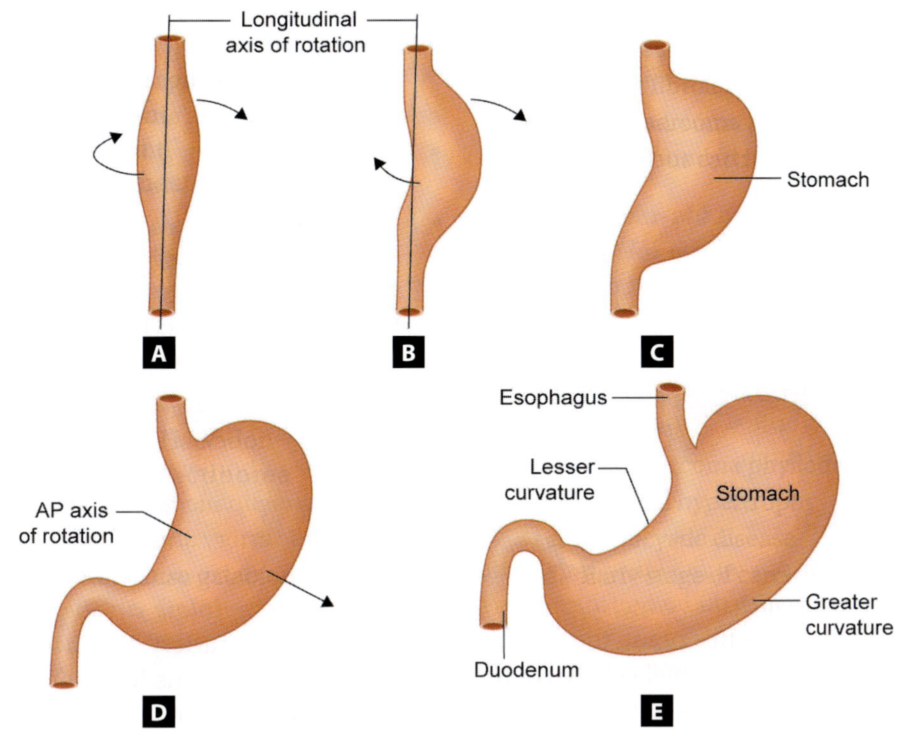

Figs. 1A to E: Development and rotation of the stomach along its longitudinal or vertical axis.

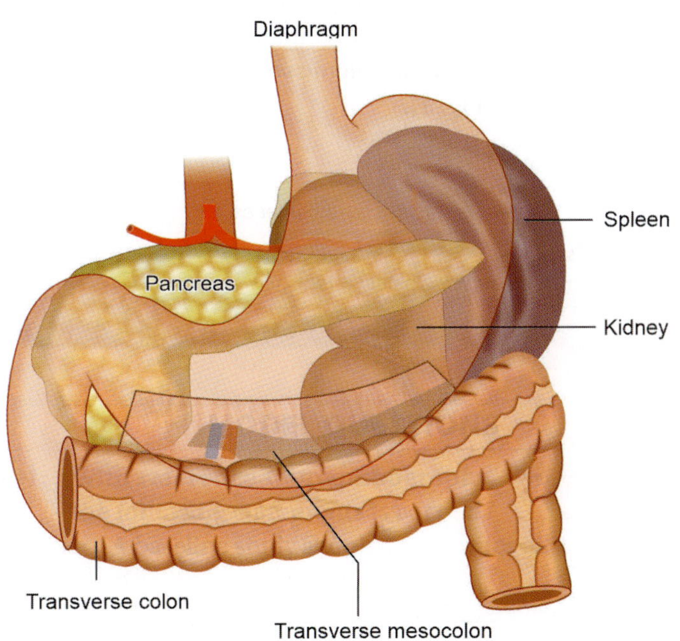

Fig. 2: Stomach and its relations.

The stomach has two ends:

1. One meets the esophagus
2. Other meets the duodenum

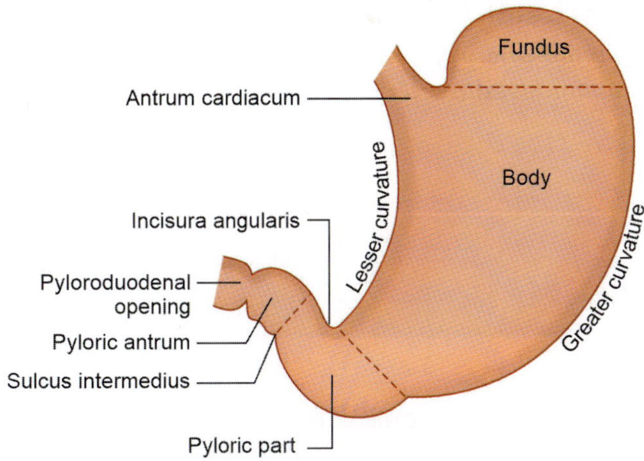

Fig. 3: Parts of the stomach.

The stomach has two sphincters:

1. *Upper:* Gastrojejunal area—lower esophageal sphincter (LES)
2. *Lower:* Pyloric sphincter.

The cardia is where the contents of the esophagus empty into the stomach. The cardia is defined as the region following the "Z-line" of the gastroesophageal junction, the point at which the epithelium changes from stratified squamous to columnar. Near the cardia is the LES. Research has shown that the cardia is not an anatomically distinct region of the stomach but a region of the esophagus.

Pylorus (from Greek "gatekeeper") is the lowest part of the stomach that empties the contents into the duodenum. Pylorus has two parts:

1. Pyloric antrum
2. Pyloric canal

Pyloric antrum: Here, the body of the stomach joins the pylorus.

Pyloric canal: This canal opens in the duodenum, and this opening is called the "pyloric orifice." It marks the junction of the stomach and the duodenum.

INCISURA ANGULARIS

This is an angulation, as a notch on the lower part of the lesser curvature. It is a point at which the body of the stomach separates from the pylorus. Above this point, the mucosa of the stomach contains parietal and chief cells secreting acid, intrinsic factor, and pepsinogen, whereas below this point, the mucosa of the pyloric antrum contains mucin-producing cells and endocrine cells.

ARTERIAL SUPPLY OF THE STOMACH

The celiac artery gives three major arteries, which are the common hepatic artery, the splenic artery, and the left gastric artery. All these branches of the celiac arteries jointly supply the stomach, spleen, liver, etc.

All branches of the arteries supplying the stomach originate from a celiac artery **(Fig. 4)**.

- *Right gastric artery:* It is a branch of the hepatic artery, and it supplies the lower right part of the stomach.
- *Left gastric artery:* It arises directly from the celiac artery. It supplies the lower part of the esophagus along with the upper right part of the stomach.
- *Short gastric arteries:* These arteries originate from the splenic artery and supply the fundus of the stomach. The splenic artery is contained within the splenorenal ligament and runs posterior to the stomach and along the superior border of the pancreas.
- *Left gastroepiploic artery:* This artery originates from the splenic artery and supplies the area of the stomach along with the greater curvature.
- *Right gastroepiploic artery:* It originates from the gastroduodenal artery, which is a branch of the hepatic artery. It supplies the lower portion of the stomach at the greater curvature.

Veins draining the stomach ultimately drain into the portal vein. The veins are the right gastric vein, left gastric vein, short gastric veins, left gastroepiploic vein, and right gastroepiploic vein. These veins drain into a superior mesenteric vein and the splenic vein, which unite to form the portal vein **(Fig. 5)**.

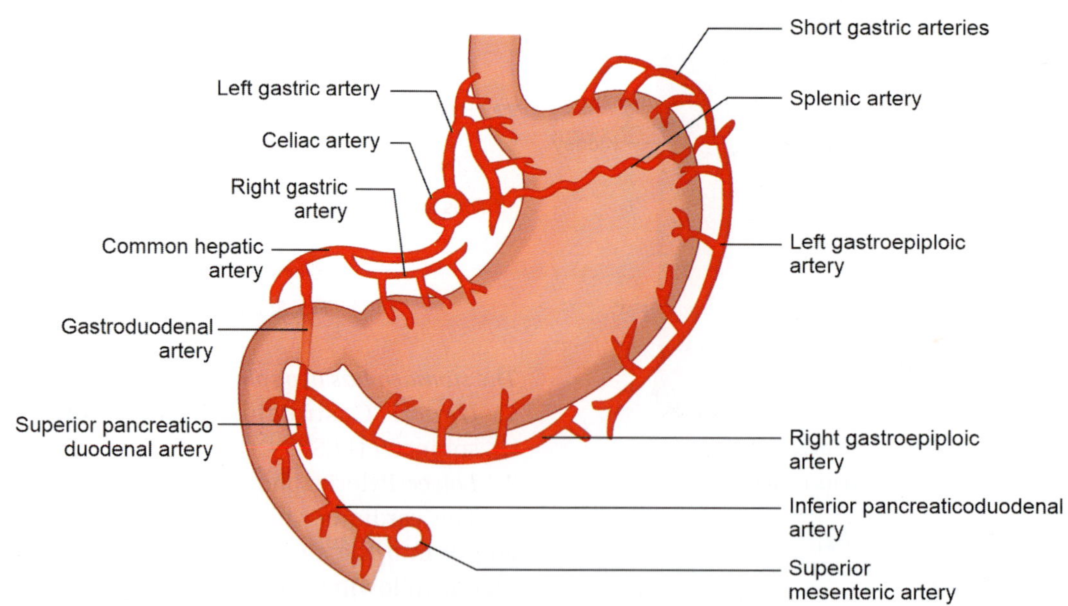

Fig. 4: Arterial supply of the stomach.

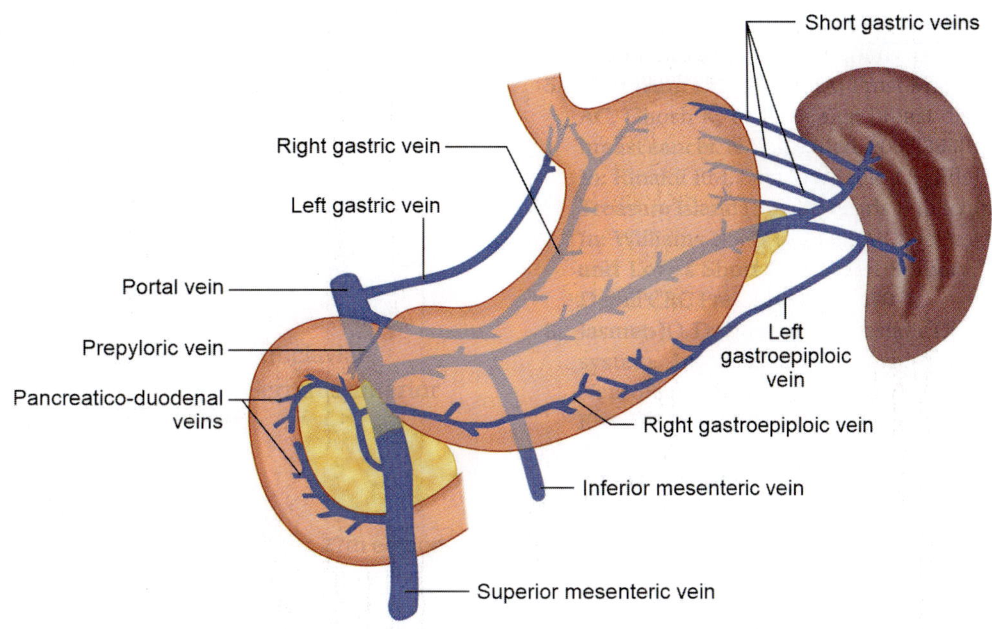

Fig. 5: Venous drainage of stomach.

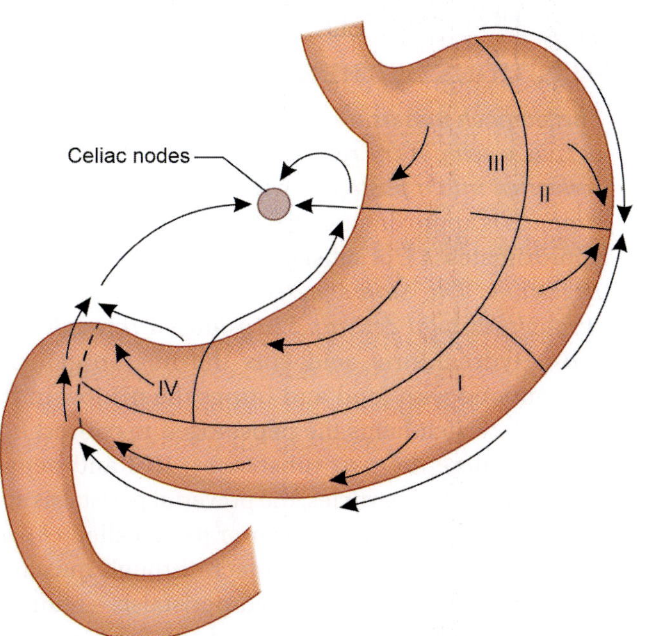

Fig. 6: Lymphatic drainage of the stomach.

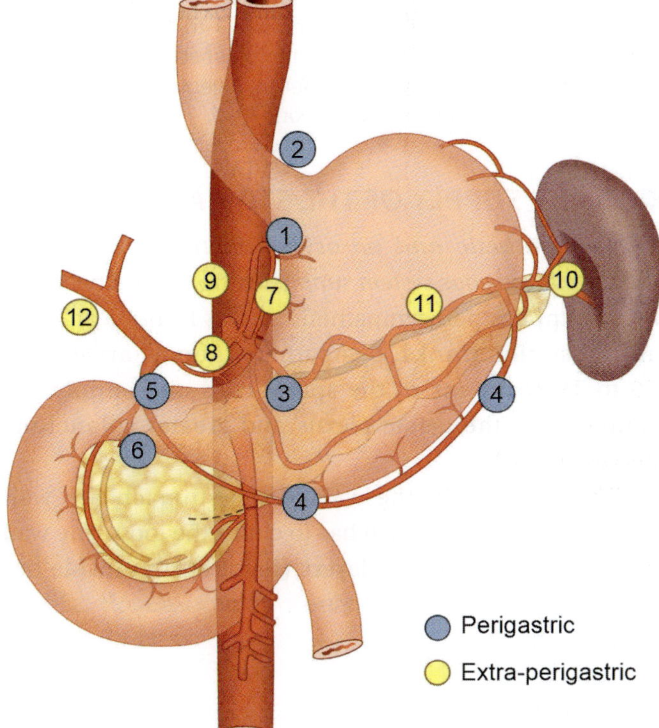

Fig. 7: Lymph node stations of stomach.

Lymphatic Drainage of Stomach (Figs. 6 and 7)

- *Zone I (inferior gastric):* Drains to subpyloric nodes.
- *Zone II (splenic):* Pancreaticosplenic nodes.
- *Zone III (superior gastric):* Superior gastric nodes.
- *Zone IV (hepatic):* Suprapyloric nodes.

The lymphatic system of the stomach is a complex and involves lymph nodes (LNs) and lymphatics. The knowledge of the lymphatic system is known to us from a very long time, several centuries ago, and its detailed description was made by Rouviere in 1932. Most of the lymphatics, after going to other nodes, reach the celiac nodes.

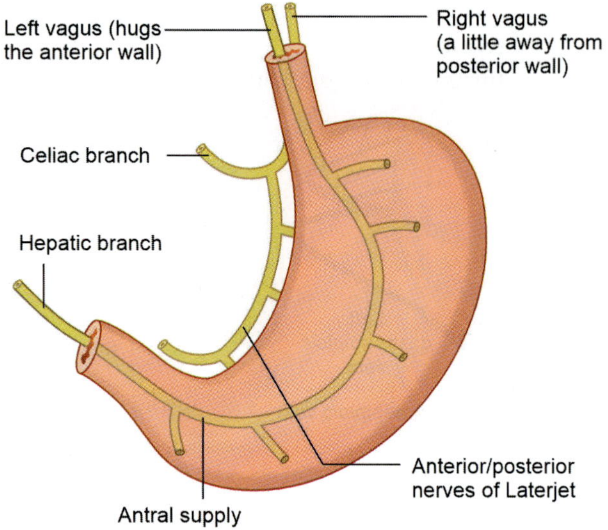

Fig. 8: Nerves supply of stomach.

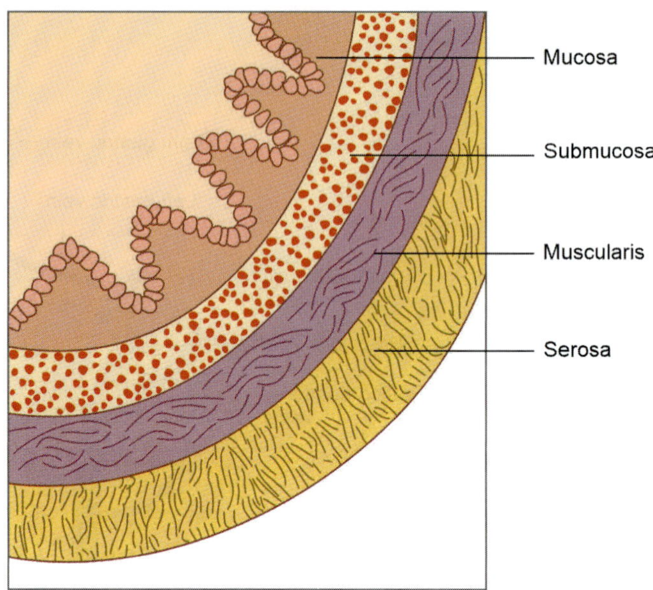

Fig. 9: Layers of stomach wall.

> *Lymph node station:* According to the Japanese Gastric Cancer Association (JGCA), it classifies the gastric LN stations into 16 stations according to their location. The LNs of the stomach are defined and given station numbers from 1 to 16 according to their location, to help in the decision of what type of surgery is required in gastric cancer as per involvement of these LN stations, such as total gastrectomy or partial.

NERVE SUPPLY OF THE STOMACH

The sympathetic and parasympathetic nerves of the autonomic nervous system supply the stomach. The vagus nerve supplies parasympathetic nerves from its anterior and posterior trunks. Sympathetic nerves arise from T6 to T9 segments of the spinal cord and supply the stomach via the celiac plexus and greater splanchnic nerves **(Fig. 8)**.

The muscles in the wall of the stomach are well developed as the stomach has to churn the food. The wall of the stomach has four layers **(Fig. 9)**, from inside out they are:

1. Mucosa
2. Submucosa
3. Muscularis externa
4. Serosa

> *Note:* Auerbach plexus or myenteric plexus lies between the outer longitudinal and middle circular layer. It innervates both muscle layers and is responsible for peristalsis and mixing. *It is named after Leopold Auerbach, a German neuropathologist. George Meissner, 1829–1905, German physiologist.*

PHYSIOLOGY OF STOMACH

FUNCTIONS OF THE STOMACH

- *The stomach acts as a reservoir for food. The stomach acts as a temporary reservoir for food till the food is converted into a paste-like chyme.* The capacity of the stomach is approximately 1 L, but it can accommodate approximately 4 L of substance.
- *Digestion: The Stomach secretes hydrochloric acid through parietal cells and pepsinogen through chief cells.* Hydrochloric acid kills the microorganisms that entered with food and brings the pH low in the stomach, which helps the pepsinogen to convert into pepsin. There are two substances: HCl and pepsin disintegrate food particles, the powerful peristalsis also converts the food into a form of paste called *chyme.* Food is churned by the stomach through muscular contractions of the wall called peristalsis—reducing the bolus before looping around the fundus, which passes ahead through the pyloric canal. Each time, 3 mL of chyme passes to the duodenum. Amylase breaks down carbohydrates in food, pepsin breaks down protein, and lipase breaks down triglycerides (fat).
- *Absorption:* Most of the substances in food are absorbed in the small intestine, but some substances are also absorbed in the stomach, such as:
  - Water
  - *Alcohol:* 10–20% of ingested ethanol

- Amino acids
- Aspirin
- Caffeine
- Intrinsic factor, produced by parietal cells of the stomach, helps in the absorption of vitamin B_{12} in the last part of the small intestine.

- *Waste elimination*
- *Production of HCl, hormones, and enzymes.*
- *Peristalsis*

Glands of stomach: Gastric glands are of three types:
1. Fundic glands or main gastric glands or oxyntic glands—situated in the body and fundus of the stomach
2. Pyloric glands—present in the pyloric part of the stomach
3. Cardiac glands—located in the cardiac region of the stomach

Cells in the glands of the stomach and their secretions **(Fig. 10)**:

- *Fundic glands:*
  - Chief cells:
    - Pepsinogen
    - Renin
    - Lipase
    - Gelatinase
    - Urase
  - *Parietal cells or oxyntic cells:*
    - Hydrochloric acid
    - Intrinsic factor of Castle
  - *Mucus neck cells:*
    - Mucin
    - Enteroendocrine cells
    - Enterochromaffin (EC) cells or Kulchitsky cells: Serotonin
    - Enterochromaffin-like (ECL) cells: Histamine
    - Stem cells
  - *Pyloric glands:*
    - G-cells
    - Mucus cells
    - EC cells
    - ECL cells
  - *Cardiac glands:*
    - EC cells
    - ECL cells
    - Chief cells
    - *G cells:* Gastrin
    - *D cells:* Somatostatin
    - *A cells:* Glucagon
    - *Ghrelin-producing cells:* Ghrelin
    - *Unnamed cells:* Vasoactive intestinal peptide (VIP)

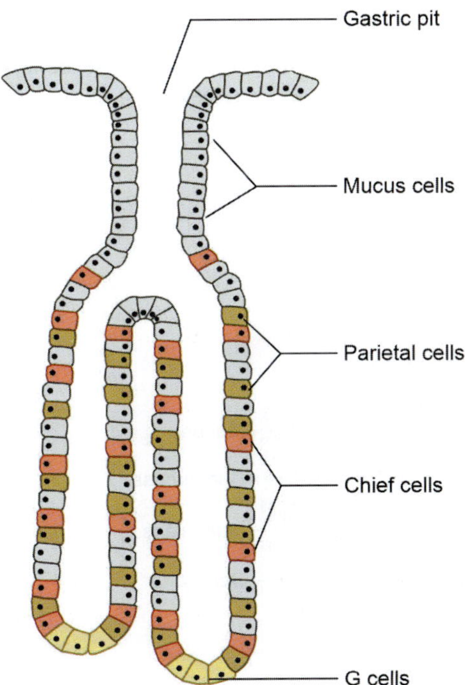

Fig. 10: Cells of the stomach.

GASTRIC JUICE

- Daily 1,200–1,500 mL secreted
- Specific gravity 1.004
- It contains 99.5% water and 5% solid organic and inorganic substances.

Functions of Gastric Juice

- Digestive function
- *Hematopoietic function:* The intrinsic factor secreted by the stomach helps in the absorption of vitamin B_{12} when it is required for the production of red blood cells (RBCs).
- It is protected by mucus when the injury is caused by HCl and pepsin.

Secretion of Hydrochloric Acid

It happens in the canaliculi of the parietal cells. HCl is produced by hydrogen ions from carbonic acid and chloride ions from sodium chloride of blood, and both combine to form HCl **(Fig. 11)**.

Acid secretion in different periods:
- *Cephalic phase:* The thinking, vision, and even smell of food and drinks can stimulate acid secretion. It is mediated by vagal activity, secondary to sensory arousal as first demonstrated by Pavlov (Ivan Petrovich Pavlov, 1849–1936, Russian Physiologist)
- *Gastric phase:* When food enters the stomach, the distention and its pressure on the wall of the stomach stimulate acid secretion by gastrin release.
- *Intestinal phase:* When food, after becoming chyme, enters the duodenum, it stimulates hormone secretions to lead to acid secretion.

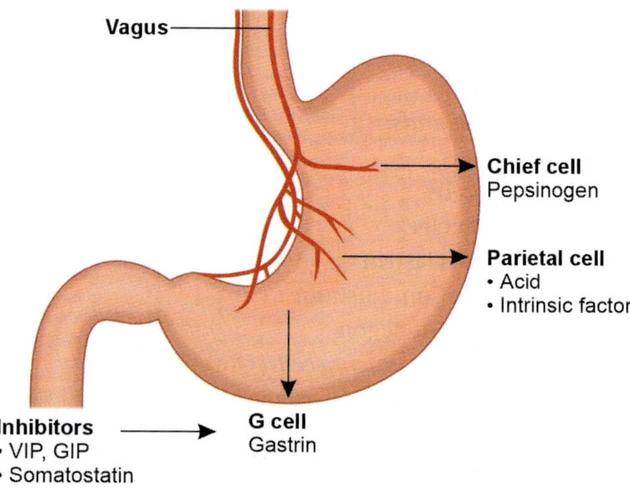

Fig. 11: Gastric juice secretion. (GIP: gastric inhibitory peptide; VIP: vasoactive intestinal peptide)

HISTOLOGY OF STOMACH

INTRODUCTION

The stomach is a dilated portion of the foregut. It is the site for breaking down the food and forming a pulp or paste called "chime." This breakdown of the food is done mechanically (churning) as well as chemically by hydrochloric acid and pepsin.

From inside out, the stomach has the following layers **(Figs. 12 to 15)**:
- Mucosa
- Submucosa
- Muscle coat
- Serosa

MUCOSA

Mucosa is the innermost lining of the stomach. It is made up of simple columnar cells with tubular glands. The mucosa of the stomach is arranged in longitudinal folds called "rugae." These rugae are gathered along the lesser curvature of the stomach and irregularly arranged in other parts of the stomach. When the stomach is distended with food or air, the rugae disappear as the mucosa stretches flat. Various small depressions are found in the mucosa of the stomach called "gastric pits." The gastric glands open in these gastric pits and pour their secretions here. The mucosa and rugae on the lesser curvature make a canal-type of

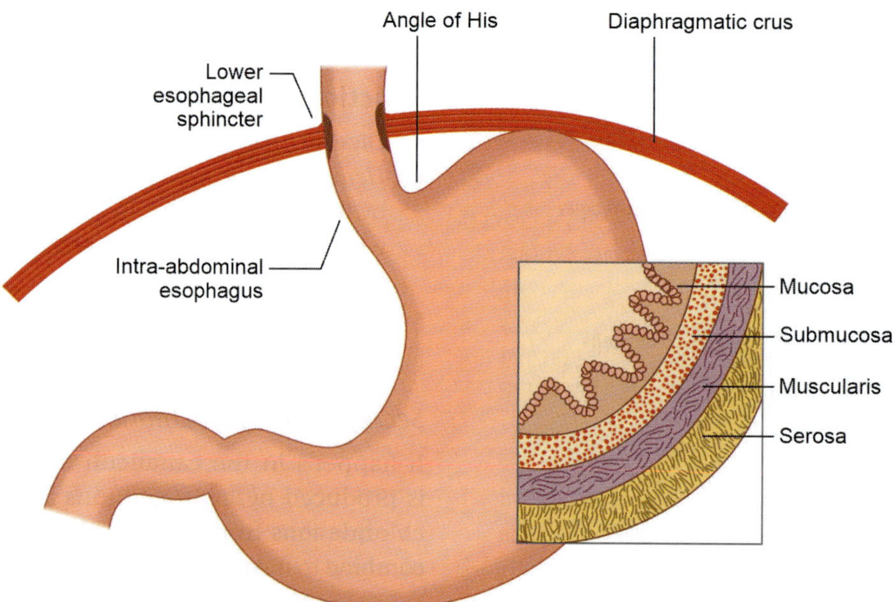

Fig. 12: Layers of stomach wall.

narrow tube called "magenstrasse" (street of the stomach) or gastric canal, which conveys foods and liquids from the esophagus to the pyloric region. The lesser curvature is more prone to ulcers than the greater curvature as it faces the insult from the ingested liquids more than any other part of the stomach. It has gastric glands, pits, and a smooth muscle layer called "*muscularis mucosa*." This muscle layer squeezes out the contents of the gastric glands by contracting. Muscularis mucosa is made up of smooth muscle fibers. Muscularis mucosa consists of two layers of smooth muscle:

1. Outer longitudinal layer
2. Inner circular layer.

Gastric glands, which are situated in the lamina propria, open in the gastric pits **(Fig. 13)**. The lining cells produce mucus, which forms a protective layer over the mucosa, protecting it from the injurious effects of hydrochloric acid and pepsin. These mucus-secreting cells are very important for stomach lining protection, and they are replaced in every 4–6 days of period.

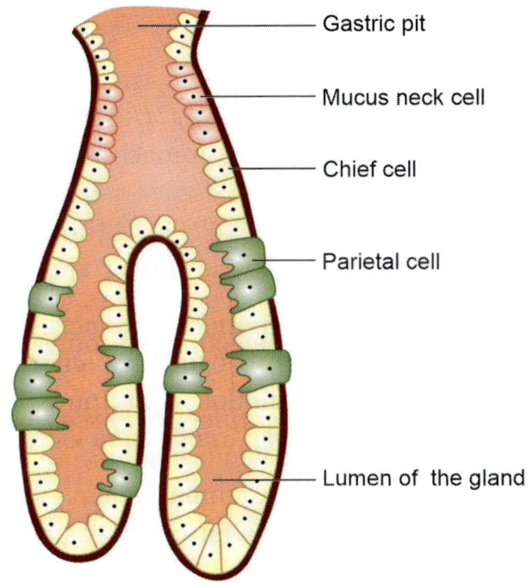

Fig. 13: Gastric glands and pits.

SUBMUCOSA

The submucosa is made up of loose connective tissues. Nerves and blood vessels supplying the stomach lie in the submucosa. It also has Meissner's plexus. This layer contains blood vessels, lymphatics, and nerve plexus (Meissner's plexus). Its function is to support the mucosa and to attach it with the muscularis externa.

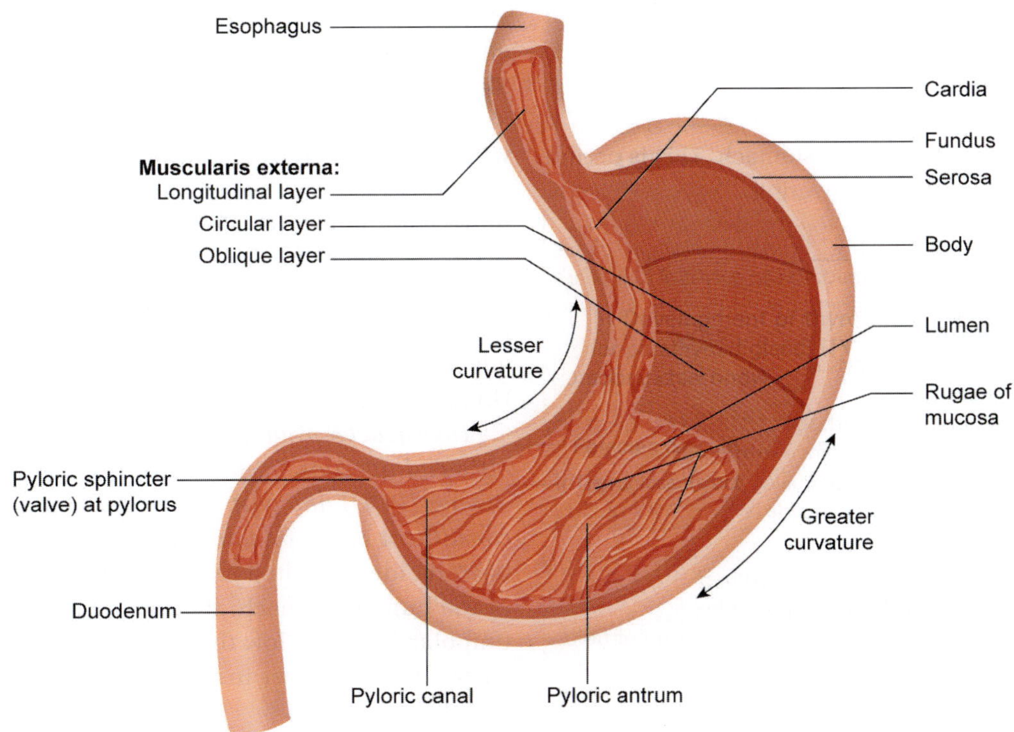

Fig. 14: Muscle layers of the stomach.

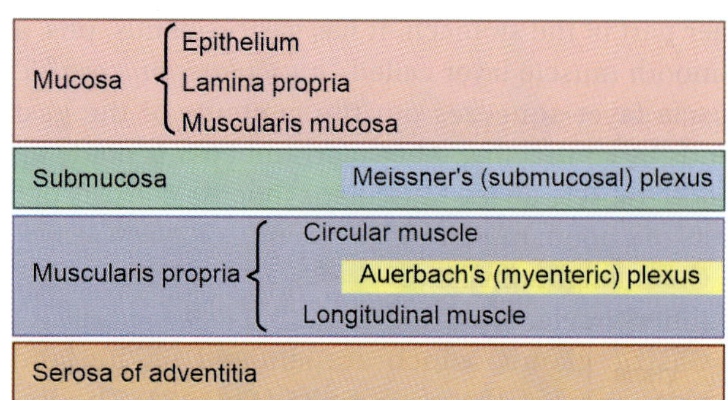

Fig. 15: Layers of stomach wall with nerve plexuses.

MUSCLE COAT

There are three muscle layers in the wall of the stomach **(Fig. 14)**:

1. *Longitudinal muscle fibers:* These fibers make up the outermost layer of muscle fibers.
2. *Circular muscle fibers:* They form the intermediate muscle layer. These fibers form the pyloric sphincter at the pylorus.
3. *Oblique muscle fiber:* They form the innermost layer of muscle fibers. These fibers loop around the cardia. These fibers are thickened and well developed at the lesser curative area, forming the gastric canal during contraction. The gastric canal facilitates the passage of ingested fluids.

SEROSA

It is the outermost coat of wall of stomach. This is peritoneal covering. It is a protective covering.

> *Meissner's (George Meissner, 1829–1897, German physiologist) plexus or submucosal plexus lies in the submucosa.* The nerves of Meissner's plexus are derived from parasympathetic nerves, the plexus around the SMA. Meissner's plexus has mainly two functions:
> 1. To control the secretion of glands
> 2. To control blood flow
>
> Auerbach's plexus (Leopold Auerbach, 1828–1897, German neuropathologist, who described myenteric plexus in 1862) plexus mainly controls mobility by controlling the muscle layers of stomach as it innervating the various muscle layers of the stomach.

> *Why gastric ulcers are common on lesser curvature?*
> The following anatomical factors are responsible:
> - Mucosa for this site faces repeated insults from irritant fluids as this is the site of gastric canal.
> - Epithelium is thin here.
> - Mucosa is not much mobile here over muscle layer.
> - Blood supply is low here.

DUODENUM

It is lined by mucus-secreting columnar epithelium. *Brunner's (Johann Conrad Brunner, 1653-1729, German anatomist) glands* lie beneath the mucosa. Brunner's glands secrete an alkaline fluid which protects from the acid of the stomach.

INVESTIGATIONS

- *Upper gastrointestinal endoscopy (UGIE):* It is the gold standard investigation for the stomach and duodenum.
- *Imaging:* CT scan
- *Endoscopic ultrasound (EUS):* More sensitive investigation for early gastric cancer and duodenal tumors.
- *Laparoscopy:* Good for detecting peritoneal and liver metastasis.
- *Positron emission tomography (PET) scan:* Good for anatomical and functional information.
- *Gastric emptying studies:* Gamma camera.
- *Gastric angiography:* Good for upper gastrointestinal (UGI) bleeding.

HELICOBACTER PYLORI INFECTION

Helicobacter pylori (Hp) infection is the most common chronic bacterial infection in humans globally. Simulations indicate that *H. pylori* spread from East Africa around 58,000 years ago, later evolving into many strains with varying degrees of pathogenicity. Most individuals acquire infection during childhood, and infection is more common in developing countries. In the United States, *H. pylori* infection is more common in Hispanic and black populations, although this may be related to socioeconomic factors, including low income, less education, household crowding, and immigration into the United States.

Helicobacter pylori infection, the most common chronic bacterial infection in the world, is linked to peptic ulcer disease (PUD) and gastric adenocarcinoma and is a key constituent of the human microbiome. They are unique bacteria ideally suited to live in the acidic environment of the human stomach: their spiral shape and multiple unipolar flagella allow them to move freely through the gastric mucosa layer in a microenvironment protected from low gastric pH.

Dr Warren (John Robin Warren, Australian, discovery of *H. pylori*) discovered the spiral bacteria *H. pylori* in 1982. *H. pylori* was known as *Campylobacter pylori*. It is a gram-negative, microaerophilic, and spiral (helical) bacterium. Within a few years, multiple research groups had verified the association of *H. pylori* with gastritis and, to a lesser extent, ulcer to demonstrate that *H. pylori* caused—gastritis and was not merely a bystander, Marshall drank a beaker of *H. pylori* culture. He became ill with nausea and vomiting several days later. An endoscopy 10 days after inoculation revealed signs of gastritis and the presence of *H. pylori*. These results suggested *H. pylori* was the causative agent. *Marshall (Barry James Marshall, Australian, discovery of Helicobacter pylori) and Warren went on to demonstrate that antibiotics are effective in the treatment of many cases of gastritis. In 1994, the National Institute of Health stated that most recurrent duodenal and gastric ulcers were caused by H. pylori and recommended that antibiotics should be included in the treatment regimen.* While initially met with some skepticism, the link between *H. pylori* and peptic ulcer disease served as a pioneering discovery that changed the treatment of PUD and earned Marshall and Warren the Nobel Prize in Medicine in 2005. Medical therapy has proven to be largely successful in combating *H. pylori*, with eradication rates of 70–95% across several trials. The treatment of peptic ulcer has now changed from surgical to medical.

Helicobacter pylori infection can cause gastritis, peptic ulcerations, and even gastric cancer. A persistent infection with H. pylori causes inflammation of the gastric mucosa and gradually causes atrophy of the gastric glands and low production of gastric acid. Later, if not treated well can lead to gastric carcinoma. The World Health Organization (WHO) is of the opinion that the eradication of *H. pylori* is necessary to prevent gastric cancer. The relationship between *H. pylori* infection and gastroesophageal reflux disease (GERD) is a subject of debate. Rapid urease test (RUT) is now a routine test to diagnose *H. pylori* infection.

Many epidemiological studies have shown a protective role of *H. pylori* infection towards GERD. A lower prevalence of *H. pylori* infection in patients affected by GERD in the magnified of 5–10%, when compared with a control population, has been reported by most authors.

The strongest argument for H. pylori as a protective factor in GERD comes from clinical trials. A higher incidence of erosive GERD following successful eradication in patients with duodenal ulcer disease had been reported, but was recently rebutted by the analysis of large clinical trials conducted in patients with duodenal ulcer and gastric ulcer, in whom no increase of GERD following eradication has been documented.

Not to forget:

- The most common site of a duodenal ulcer is the first part of the duodenum.
- Endoscopic treatment of a bleeding UGI ulcer is done either by cautery coagulation or injection of adrenaline.
- Graham's patch repair by omental piece is done for duodenal ulcer perforation.
- Posterior duodenal ulcer is rare and causes a renal vein sign of gas under the right kidney.
- Kocherization (mobilization of the duodenum) is required to see the posterior duodenal ulcer.
- The gastroduodenal artery is involved in duodenal ulcer bleeding, and the left gastric artery in gastric ulcer bleeding.

In 2015, it was estimated that over 50% of the World's population had *H. pylori* in their upper gastrointestinal tracts with this infection (or colonization) being more common in developing countries. In recent decades, however, the prevalence of *H. pylori* colonization of the gastrointestinal tracts has declined in many countries.

It is found by various studies that if the H. pylori infection predominantly affects the antral area of stomach, then it can increase gastric acid production and can result in duodenitis and even duodenal ulcers. If H. pylori infection affects mainly the body of the stomach, excluding the fundus and antral parts of the stomach, it can lead to low production of acid and may increase the risk of gastric carcinoma. While pan gastric infection leads to gastric atrophy and increases the chances of gastric carcinoma. Antral involvement by *H. pylori* causes hyperacidity and acid reflux, but after *H. pylori* eradication therapy, it improves. Atrophic changes markedly increase the risk of gastric ulceration and noncardiac gastric adenocarcinomas, but the lower acid production protects against acid-induced complications of gastroesophageal reflux.

Gastritis

Gastritis caused by *H. pylori,* as chronic gastritis, is one of the most common types of gastritis.

Autoimmune Gastritis

It has atrophy of gastric parietal cells leading to hypochlorhydria, achlorhydria, and pernicious anemia. Hypergastrinemia is caused by G cells involvement.

Stress Gastritis

It is a form of acute gastritis that happens after serious injury, severe burn, or serious illness can lead to ulceration and bleeding.

MENETRIER'S DISEASE

It is a premalignant condition that is refractory to treatment, having hypertrophy of gastric mucosal folds leading to hyperchlorhydria, hypoproteinemia, and anemia. It is probably caused by transforming growth factor-α (TGF-α) and epidermal growth factor (EGF) overexpression.

> *You may be asked:*
> - Vagotomy is at present not usually done as it is replaced by proton pump inhibitors (PPIs).
> - The nerve of Latarjet supplies the pyloric muscle, so gastric emptying is affected if this nerve is cut by chance.
> - Craws foot nerve supplies the antrum.
> - The criminal nerve of Grassi is the cause of postvagotomy ulcer recurrence.
> - Early dumping syndrome hashes 10–15 minutes after a meal, causes nausea, vomiting, and bloating, and deteriorates with food, whereas late dumping happens 30–40 minutes after food, has headache, tachycardia, and sweating, and rebound hypoglycemia, which improves with food.
> - An antidumping diet (avoid sugar, reduce fat, and protein, and have small meals several times a day) helps in continuous dumping.

Peptic Ulcer

It is commonly seen in the lesser curvature of the stomach and the first part of the duodenum, occurring at the junction of the epithelium, where it is minimally resistant to the acid effect. Most commonly caused by nonsteroidal anti-inflammatory drugs (NSAIDs) and *H. pylori*. Duodenal ulcers are more common than stomach ulcers, but gastric ulcers may become cancerous. The main treatment is *H. pylori* treatment. A peptic ulcer can perforate and bleed. It can be treated conservatively or surgically. Peptic ulcer can cause pain with periodicity, nausea and vomiting, weight reduction, bleeding, and anemia. Investigation of peptic ulcer and UGIE is the mainstay.

Black introduced the beta blockers and H2 receptor antagonists. (Sir James Black, 1924–2002, British pharmacologist, was awarded the Nobel Prize for Physiology or Medicine in 1988). In many centers, Polya [Eugene (Jeno) Alexander Polya, 1876–1944, Hungarian Surgeon) gastrectomy is also done. Roux-en-Y (Gsar Roux, 1857, 1934, Swiss Surgeon and Gynecologist, described in 1908) reconstruction is performed as it functions better postoperatively.

Surgery for peptic ulcer is of various types, such as Billroth (Christian Albert Theodore Billroth, 1829–1894, Austrian surgeon, performed the first gastrectomy in 1881) II gastrectomy, gastrojejunostomy, truncal vagotomy and drainage, highly selective vagotomy, and truncal vagotomy and antrectomy. Surgery for a gastric ulcer is Billroth I gastrectomy.

Complications of peptic ulcer surgery can develop in any patient who undergoes surgery, including recurrence, small stomach syndrome, dumping syndrome (early and late), bile vomiting, diarrhea, cancer transformation, nutritional effects (iron-deficiency anemia and B_{12} deficiency).

Peptic ulcer can develop complications such as perforation, bleeding, and stenosis. Perforation is the most common and is treated by emergency surgery, by closing the perforation and pyloroplasty; an omental patch is good for such cases. Postoperatively, *H. pylori* eradication is a must.

> *Good to remember:*
> *Gastric ulcer:* Pain is the main symptom, and it increases with food, and perforation is common. UGIE is the investigation of choice for diagnosis. Biopsy is essential as it may become malignant.
>
> *Johnson's classification divides into five types:*
> - *Type I:* Along the lesser curvature near incisura angularis
> - *Type II:* Preparing and duodenal
> - *Type III:* Pyloric
> - *Type IV:* High up in the body of the stomach, it commonly bleeds
> - *Type V:* Diffuse ulcers by NSAIDs
>
> Treatment is by gastrectomy with PPIs and vagotomy.

Dieulatory's Disease

It is a gastric vascular malformation, very difficult to treat; its bleeding can be healed by itself, sometimes local excision is required.

GASTRIC OUTLET OBSTRUCTION

It is common with PUD and stomach cancer. UGIE with biopsy is mandatory. *H. pylori* eradication therapy is a must. Resection and drainage procedure may be required.

Zollinger–Ellison Syndrome (Robert Milton Zollinger, 1903–1992, American Surgeon, and Edwin Homar Ellison, 1912–1919, American Surgeon, Described in 1955)

It is a gastrin-producing tumor, commonly found in the duodenal loop and pancreas. It may be either sporadic or Multiple endocrine neoplasia (MEN) type I. The most common site is the "gastrinoma triangle" [Passaro (Edward Passaro, 1974–1997, American surgeon)].

Duodenal Adenocarcinoma

It is uncommon in the stomach, but common in the small intestine. *Whipple's (Allen Oldfather Whipple, 1881–1963, American surgeon)* procedure (pancreaticoduodenectomy) is normally required.

Stomach Cancer

It is a major cause of death globally. It does not metastasize at a distance before involving LNs, giving a good period for appropriate treatment. In Japan, the incidence of gastric cancer is maximum in the world. Causes of gastric cancer are many, but *H. pylori* is very important. If diagnosed early, it has a good cure rate. It is of two types: (1) Intestinal and (2) diffuse. Diffuse has a worse prognosis. It is treated by radical surgery. It is also chemosensitive also, so chemotherapy can also be tried. The proximal part of the stomach is the most common area for gastric cancer. Most of the UGI cancers occur at the esophagogastric (EG) junction. In advanced cancer of the stomach, thrombophlebitis, Trousseau's sign (Armand Trousseau, 1801–1867, French physician) is commonly seen.

Gastric cancer is a common tumor of the stomach. It is associated with the following risk factors:

- Smoking
- Alcohol
- *H. pylori* infection
- Smoked/barbecued food
- Gastritis
- Gastric polyps
- Blood group A
- Hypertrophic mucosal folds of the stomach (Menetrier's disease)
- Nitroso preserved foods.

Tumor, Node, and Metastasis Classification

Primary tumors (T) are of Tis, T1a, T1b, T2, T3, and T4 types.

Tis = carcinoma in situ, T1a = invades lamina propria or muscularis mucosa, T1b = invades submucosa, T2 = invades muscularis properties, T3 = invades connective tissue, T4 = invades series and related structures.

Borrmann's Classification of Advanced Gastric Cancer

It divides advanced gastric cancer into four types **(Fig. 16)**.

Treatment is through surgery, chemotherapy, and radiotherapy. Distal gastrectomy or subtotal gastrectomy or total gastrectomy are done according to the site of the tumor. Total gastrectomy is associated with esophagojejunostomy.

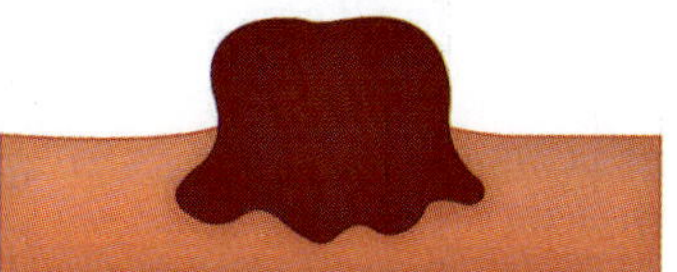

Borrmann 1 type Polypoid tumor

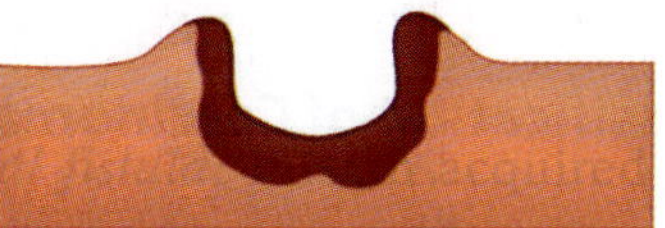

Borrmann 2 type Ulcerated tumor

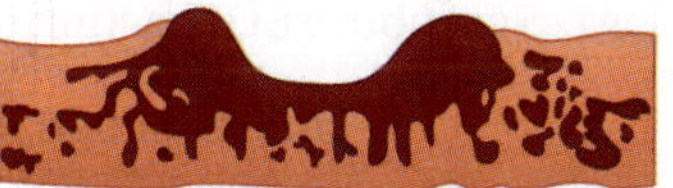

Borrmann 3 type Fungating tumor

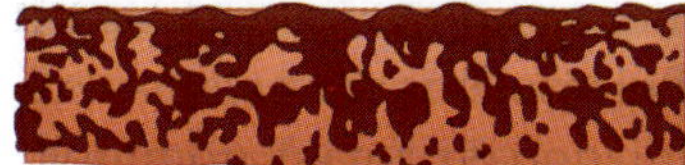

Borrmann 4 type Infiltrating, linitis plastica

Fig. 16: Borrmann's classification.

> *Points to remember:*
> - All gastric ulcers must be biopsied due to the risk of cancer.
> - The most common gastric polyp is the metaplastic polyp caused by *H. pylori.*
> - Advanced gastric cancer, fungating or polypoidal type as type I or with elevated borders with ulcer or fungating growth as type II, ulcer with wall invasion is type III, Linitis plastica is type IV.
> - Gastric carcinoma most commonly presents with a mass in the abdomen, gastric outlet obstruction, abdominal distention, anemia, nausea and vomiting, and loss of appetite.

Lymph node clearance as per Japanese stations: These are 13 stations: 1—right paracardial, 2—left paracardial, 3—lesser curvature, 4—greater curvature, 5—suprapyloric, 6—infrapyloric, 7—left gastric, 8—common hepatic, 9—celiac, 10—splenic phylum, 11—splenic artery, 12—hepatoduodenal ligament, and 13—retropancreatic. 1-6 stations are removed in D1 type of LN clearance, and from 1 to 11 in D2 type of LN clearance.

Chemotherapy: Cisplatin and 5-fluorouracil are commonly used in T3/T4, LN involvement, and muscle involvement.

Radiotherapy is given to the gastric bed.

Minimum LNs removed in GI cancerous tumors:

- *Gastric:* 16 LNs
- *Esophagus:* 15 LNs
- *Small intestine:* 8 LNs
- *Colon:* 12 LNs
- *Breast:* 10 LNs

Siewert Classification of Carcinoma of the Gastroesophageal Junction and Lower Esophagus

- *Type I:* Tumor 1–5 cm above EG junction in esophagus—transhiatal esophagectomy required.
- *Type II:* At 1–2 cm toward the stomach from the EG junction—transhiatal esophagectomy required.
- *Type III:* 2–5 cm below EG junction—total gastrectomy.

Wilkie's Disease

It is also known as SMA syndrome, as SMA pressurizes the third part of the duodenum, leading to gastric outlet obstruction, in young females who are on extreme dieting and are thin. The angle between SMA and aorta (aortomesenteric angle) if becomes <22°, normal is 35–65°. It is treated by releasing pressure on the duodenum by severing Treitz's ligament (a strong procedure).

Watermelon Stomach

The stomach looks like watermelon, happens in elderly females, also called gastric antral vascular ectasia, treated by laser coagulation.

Trichobezoar

It is a collection of hairs (hair ball) in the stomach due to trichophagy. Psychiatric factor is suspected. Usually, it causes a gastric outlet problem with abdominal pain and vomiting. Removal of hairballs by open or endoscopically methods is recommended.

Gastrointestinal Stromal Tumor

Most commonly occurs in the stomach from intestinal pacemaker cells of Cajal. It may be sporadic with Carney's triad or familial with Carney-Stratakis syndrome. It usually presents with pain in the abdomen and a lump, with hemorrhage and perforation commonly seen. *It metastasizes by local invasion, blood, and lymphatics. It is diagnosed by endoscopy, CT, and PET scan. The most common tumor marker is IHC-CD127/c-Kit. Gastrointestinal stomach tumor (GIST) may be borderline (benign) or metastatic (malignant). It is treated by wedge resection and imatinib (tyrosine-kinase inhibitor).*

Carney's triad: Multifocal gastric, pulmonary, and endocrine (paraganglioma and adrenal adenoma) tumors.

Carney-Stratakis syndrome: Inherited disorder marked by gastrointestinal tract tumors with tumors of embryonic nervous tissue in the head, neck, and torso.

Mucosa-associated Lymphoid Tissue Tumor

It is commonly found in the stomach with *H. pylori* infection as of low grade and high grade. These are treated with *H. pyloric* eradication and as you treat lymphoma.

Borchardt's Triad

It occurs in volvulus of the stomach of both organoaxial (vertical) and mesenteroaxial (vertical) types. It has retching, pain, and inability to pass Ryle's tube. Contrast imaging is diagnostic. Surgery is the treatment, i.e., gastropexy, and diaphragmatic repair of a defect after detonation of the stomach.

- *Sister Mary Joseph's [Sister Mary Joseph (Julia Dempsey), 1856–1946, Nursing superintendent, American, noted the presence of an umbilical nodule in many patients of advanced gastric cancer and pointed this out to William Mayo while working at the Mayo Clinic) nodule:* Periumbilical metastasis seen in cancer of the stomach.
- *Krukenberg's tumor:* Stomach cancer can cause bilateral ovarian metastases.
- The most important point in prognosis of gastric cancer is depth of invasion and LNs involvement.

CONGENITAL HYPERTROPHIC PYLORIC STENOSIS

It is a hypertrophy of the pyloric muscle, causing gastric outlet obstruction in the firstborn male child. It presents as projectile nonbilious vomiting, visible peristalsis, and a solid-shaped lump. Contrast imaging shows string, double tract, and mushroom signs. Recurrence of vomiting leads to metabolic alkalosis with hypokalemia, hypothermia, and hypochloremia. Treatment consists of correction on electrolyte abnormalities and Ramstedt's pyloromyotomy. Duodenal atresia has bilious vomiting and the double bubble sign on X-ray.

UPPER GASTROINTESTINAL HEMORRHAGE

Bleeding from the upper gastrointestinal tract is a common problem. It is either caused by esophageal varices or from other causes of esophageal and stomach lesions. Nonvariceal causes of upper gastrointestinal tract buster are as follows:

- *Peptic ulcer disease:* It is the most common cause.
- *Gastritis:* Gastritis can be caused by various reasons:
  - *Type A:* It is caused by an autoimmune factor and mainly involves the body of stomach.
  - *Type B:* It is a bacterial gastritis caused by *H. pylori* with a risk of cancer. It is either antral type or pangastritis.
  - *Stress gastritis:* It is caused by stress on bunch as in head injury (Cushing's ulcer in the parietal cell area where acid is produced in the stomach), and severe burn injuries (Curling ulcer is seen in the first part of the duodenum most commonly).

    AIDS and NSAIDs also cause ulcers in the stomach.
- Mallory–Weiss (George Kenneth Mallory, 1926, American pathologist; Soma Weiss, 1899–1942, American physician) syndrome
- Gastric antral vascular ectasia (GAVE)
- Dieulafoy's (Georges Dieulafoy, 1839–1911, French physician) syndrome
- Menetrier's (Pierre Menetrier, 1859–1935, French physician) disease
- GIST and other tumors of the stomach.

Treatment

The most important part of the treatment is to maintain the BP with a sufficient amount of IV fluids. Variceal bleeding is sometimes very serious and difficult to control. It is treated as:

- *Drugs:* Terlipressin, octreotide, and PPIs.
- Banding of varices
- Sclerotherapy

Sclerosis drugs such as sodium tetradecyl sulfate and ethanolamine pleated are commonly used.

Sclerosing agent stops the bleeding in most of cases, but if not, then the following tubes are used to compress the bleeding spots by pressing.

Sengstaken–Blakemore (Robert William Sengstaken, 1923–1978, American surgeon; Arthur Hendley Blakemore, 1897–1970, American surgeon) tube is most commonly used. The tube must be deflated intermittently at a period of 12 hours to avoid necrosis and perforation of the esophagus. Minnesota balloon and Linton tube are also used.

Shunts are used; the most commonly used is the transjugular intrahepatic portosystemic shunt (TIPS).

It reduces portal pressure.

Transjugular intrahepatic portosystemic shunt is a selective shunt, shunts gut, and splenic blood. Selective shunts such as Inokuchi and Warren shunts are only splenic vein blood.

Esophageal devascularization is rarely done nowadays. It is called the Sugiura method.

SOME IMPORTANT QUESTIONS

Q1. *Helicobacter pylori* has been implicated in all, *except*:

a. Gastric ulcer b. Gastric carcinoma
c. Gastric lymphoma d. Gastric

Ans. d

Q2. *Helicobacter pylori* infection is associated with the development of which malignancy?

a. MALTomas
b. Atherosclerosis
c. Sarcoma
d. Gastrointestinal stomach tumor (GIST)

Ans. a

Q3. Which of the symptoms given below are seen in the child with the following X-ray?

a. Bilious vomiting
b. Palpable mass
c. Hypochloremia and hypokalemia
d. Metabolic alkalosis

Ans. b, c, and d

Q4. Cushing ulcer is seen in:

a. Stress ulcer in head injury
b. Stress ulcer in burn
c. Ulcer in hiatus hernia
d. Ulcer in Crohn's disease

Ans. a

Q5. Posterior perforation of a peptic ulcer drains into:

a. Omental bursa b. Greater sac
c. Foramen of Winslow d. Paracolic gutter

Ans. a

Q6. The stump of the stomach and duodenum is present in:

a. Billroth I operation b. Billroth II operation
c. Whipple's operation d. Truncal vaguely

Ans. a

Q7. Pyloroplasty of choice when the DU (Duodenum) is fibrosed and contracted:
a. Finney's pyloroplasty
b. Billroth type I surgery
c. Billroth type II surgery
d. Ramstedt's operation

Ans. a

Q8. All of the following drugs are used in the management of peptic ulcer, *except*:
a. Alginic acid
b. Sucralfate
c. Misoprostol
d. Ipratropium

Ans. d

Q9. Lesser curvature anterior seromyotomy is indicated in:
a. Gastric ulcer
b. Gastric cancer
c. Duodenal blowout
d. Duodenal ulcer

Ans. d

Q10. In a highly selective vagotomy, the vagaries supply is severed too:
a. Proximal two-thirds of the stomach
b. Antrum
c. Pylorus
d. The whole of the stomach

Ans. a

Q11. A 5-year-old male child presents with acute fulminant liver failure. Which one of the following criteria is not included in the King's College criteria for liver transplant?
a. Age <10 years
b. Prothrombin time is >50 seconds.
c. Bilirubin >300 μmol/L
d. Jaundice <7 days before the development of encephalopathy

Ans. d

Q12. Treatment of symptomatic polycystic liver disease is:
a. Deroofing of cyst
b. Injection of sclerosis
c. Hepatic resection
d. Liver transplant

Ans. a

Q13. Okuda staging contains all, *except*:
a. Bilirubin
b. Tumor size
c. Ascites
d. Alpha-fetoprotein (AFP)

Ans. d

Q14. Ramstedt's operation is performed for:
a. Hirschsprung's disease
b. Congenital hypertrophic pyloric stenosis (CHPS)
c. Duodenal atresia
d. Anorectal malformation

Ans. b

Q15. True about trichobezoar is all, *except*:
a. It is caused by *Trichuris*
b. It is a psychiatric manifestation
c. Ball of hair in the stomach
d. Pulling the hair and sucking the hair is usually seen

Ans. a

Q16. Borchardt's triad is characterized by the following, *except*:
a. Inability to pass a nasogastric tube
b. Vomiting
c. Shock
d. Diarrhea

Ans. b

Q17. With Couinaud's nomenclature, which one of the following segments of the liver has an independent vascularization?
a. Segment I
b. Segment II
c. Segment IV
d. Segment VIII

Ans. a

Q18. The boundary of Morrison's pouch is formed by:
a. Kidney
b. Falciform ligament of liver
c. Spleen
d. Pancreas

Ans. a

Q19. Conjugated hyperbilirubinemia is seen in:
a. Dubin–Johnson syndrome
b. Crigler–Najjar syndrome
c. Crigler–Najjar syndrome II
d. Gilbert syndrome

Ans. a

Q20. The most common surgical cause of obstructive jaundice is:
a. Periampullary carcinoma
b. Gallbladder (GB) carcinoma
c. Carcinoma of the head of the pancreas
d. Common bile duct (CBD) stones

Ans. d

Q21. Primary sinusoidal dilatation of the liver is also known as:
a. Hepar lobatum
b. Peliosis hepatis
c. Von Meyenburg complex
d. Caroli's disease

Ans. b

Q22. Obstruction of inferior vena cava (IVC) leads to:
a. Dilatation of thoracoepigastric veins
b. Caput medusae
c. Hemorrhoids
d. Esophageal varices

Ans. a

MULTIPLE CHOICE QUESTIONS

Grade I	Simple

Q1. Which of the following factors contributes to the development of duodenal ulcers? (PGI 2001)
a. Lysolecithin
b. Gastric acid
c. Alcohol abuse
d. Prostaglandins
e. Smoking

Q2. The most common site of benign peptic gastric ulcer is: (AIIMS 2004)
a. Upper third of lesser curvature
b. Greater curvature
c. Pyloric antrum
d. Lesser curvature near incisura angularis

Q3. Increased gastric acid secretion occurs in: (AIIMS 2011)
a. Type I gastric ulcer
b. Type III gastric ulcer
c. Type IV gastric ulcer
d. All of the above

Q4. Which of the following vessels is the most commonly involved in the hemorrhage of a duodenal ulcer? (All India 2012)
a. IVC
b. Gastroduodenal artery
c. Superior mesenteric artery (SMA)
d. Inferior pancreatic duodenal artery

Q5. Proton pump inhibitors for peptic ulcer disease should be taken: (JIPMER 2011)
a. Before breakfast
b. After breakfast
c. After lunch
d. After dinner

Q6. Which of the following acid reducing surgery does not require drainage procedure? (PGI 2007)
a. Highly selective vaguely
b. Billroth I operation
c. Antrectomy
d. Gastric resection
e. Truncal vaguely

Q7. *Helicobacter pylori* is associated with.....% of gastric ulcers: (JIPMER 2011)
a. 5
b. 20
c. 40–60
d. 80

Q8. Barium meal characteristic feature of a malignant gastric ulcer is: (JIPMER 2017)
a. Hampton line
b. Carman's meniscus sign
c. Ulcer cap
d. Ulcer crater

Q9. Treatment of high-lying ulcer near the gastro-esophageal junction is: (PGI 2009)
a. Pauchet procedure
b. Kelling–Marlene operation
c. Csendes procedure
d. Total gastrectomy
e. Vagotomy and pyloroplasty

Q10. Incorrect about gastric ulcer is: (PGI 2009)
a. Most common on the lesser curvature
b. 70% *H. pylori*-related
c. Type IV ulcer most common type
d. Treatment is primarily medical.
e. 30% of genitourinary (GU) are associated with malignancy.

Q11. Treatment of choice in type III gastric ulcer is: (UPPG 2008)
a. Vagotomy only
b. Vagotomy and antrectomy
c. Vagotomy and pyloroplasty
d. Highly selective vagotomy

Q12. Herpes simplex virus (HSV) is done in: (AIIMS 2006)
a. Menetrier's disease
b. Giant gastric ulcer
c. Gastric mucosal erosions
d. Megaesophagus treatment by esophageal mucosal resection

Q13. A most common metabolic complication of gastrectomy is: (AIIMS 2011)

a. Iron-deficiency anemia
b. Megaloblastic anemia
c. Hypocalcemia
d. Osteoporosis

Q14. All of the following are true regarding focal nodular hyperplasia (FNH), *except*: (AIIMS 2010)

a. Not frequently associated with oral contraceptive pills (OCPs)
b. Surgical resection is required due to the risk of malignancy
c. Stellate scar is diagnostic
d. Typical hepatic vascularity is not seen with the spoke wheel pattern.

Q15. True statement regarding FNH is: (PGI 2011)

a. More common in young women
b. Associated with OCP use
c. May present with abdominal pain
d. Excision biopsy may aid in diagnosis.
e. Progress to cirrhosis

Q16. Similarities between FNH and hepatic adenoma are all, *except*: (AIIMS 2003)

a. Hemoperitoneum is common.
b. Biliary abnormalities are seen.
c. More common in females
d. Associated with OCPs

Q17. Most common benign tumor of liver is: (JIPMER 2011)

a. Hemangioma
b. Hepatic adenoma
c. Hepatoma
d. Hamartoma

Q18. Solitary hypoechoic lesion of liver without septa or debris is most likely to be: (AIIMS 2005)

a. Hydatid cyst
b. Caroli's disease
c. Liver abscess
d. Simple cyst

Q19. Simple hepatic cyst, all are true, *except*: (AIIMS 2006)

a. Asymptomatic
b. Lined by columnar epithelium
c. Intracystic bleeding is common, and reroofing is mandatory
d. Congenital

Q20. Treatment of choice for simple cyst of liver: (JIPMER 2017)

a. Percutaneous drainage
b. Cystoenterostomy
c. Deroofing
d. Aspiration

Q21. In a high-risk population, hepatocellular carcinoma (HCC) is best detected by: (AIIMS 2003)

a. USG
b. CT
c. Magnetic resonance imaging (MRI)
d. Positron emission tomography (PET) scan

Q22. Alpha-fetoprotein (AFP) is elevated in: (PGI 2011)

a. HCC
b. Hepatoblastoma
c. Infant hemangioendothelioma
d. Amebic liver abscess
e. Embryonic sarcoma

Grade II	***Difficult***

Q1. Most common abnormality after gastric resection and Billroth I is: (AIIMS 209)

a. Vitamin B_{12} deficiency
b. Steatorrhea
c. Calcium deficiency
d. Vitamin D deficiency

Q2. A patient of partial gastrectomy presents with neurological symptoms. Most probable diagnosis is: (JIPMER 2011)

a. Folic acid deficiency
b. Thiamine deficiency
c. Vitamin B_{12} deficiency
d. Iron deficiency

Q3. Gastric atony occurs in all, *except*: (AIIMS 2006)

a. Billroth I
b. Billroth II
c. HSV
d. Posterior selective vagotomy with anterior seromyotomy

Q4. Long-term effects of gastrectomy includes: (PGI 2009)

a. Renal calculi
b. Vitamin C deficiency
c. Hypothyroidism
d. Osteomalacia

Q5. All are true about retained antrum syndrome, *except*: (JIPMER 2018)
a. Technetium 99m scan is used for diagnosis.
b. Seen after Billroth l surgery
c. Positive secretin stimulation test
d. Calcium provocation test is negative.

Q6. BLEED risk criteria include all risks, *except*: (AIIMS 2009)
a. Ongoing bleeding b. Low urine output
c. BP < 100 mm Hg d. Altered mental status

Q7. In case of UGI bleeding, all are true about endoscopy, *except*: (AIIMS 2009)
a. Decreases the transfusion requirement
b. Leads to early discharge of the patient
c. Can detect the cause in all cases
d. Best tool for the localization of bleeding

Q8. Bleeding from a Mallory–Weiss tear usually occurs from: (AIIMS 2015)
a. Phrenic vein b. Left gastric artery
c. Short gastric arteries d. Coronary vein

Q9. Gastric lymph node station number 5: (AIIMS 2009)
a. Suprapyloric b. Splenic holling
c. Lesser curvature d. Greater curvature

Q10. Level 9 LN includes: (AIIMS 2010)
a. Celiac nodes
b. Splenic hilum
c. Splenic artery
d. Hepatoduodenal ligament

Q11. The most common site of carcinoma of the stomach is: (JIPMER 2010)
a. Proximal stomach b. Gastric antrum
c. Lesser curvature d. Greater curvature

Q12. Which of the following statements about gastric carcinoma is true? (All India 2011)
a. Squamous cell carcinoma is the most common histological subtype.
b. Often associated with hypochondria/achlorhydria
c. Occult blood in stool is not seen.
d. Highly radiosensitive tumor

Q13. Sister Mary Joseph's nodule is most commonly seen with: (AIIMS 2009)
a. Ovarian cancer b. Stomach cancer
c. Colon cancer d. Pancreatic cancer

Q14. The most common paraneoplastic syndrome of HCC is: (AIIMS 2003)
a. Hypoglycemia b. Hypertension
c. Hypercalcemia d. Erythrocytosis

Q15. Tumor markers for primary blood HCC are all, *except*: (AIIMS 2007)
a. AFP
b. Alpha-2 macroglobulin
c. PIVKA-II
d. Neurotensin

Q16. Hypercalcemia is seen in: (AIIMS 2011)
a. Pancreatic cancer b. HCC
c. Stomach cancer d. GB carcinoma

Q17. All are true about fibrolamellar HCC, *except*: (AIIMS 2009)
a. AFP is not raised.
b. Recurrence is common.
c. Raised neurotensin levels
d. Well demarcated and encapsulated

Q18. Which of the following liver metastases appears hypoechoic on ultrasound? (All India 2012)
a. Breast cancer
b. Colon cancer
c. Renal cell carcinoma (RCC)
d. Mucinous adenocarcinoma

Q19. The most common indication of liver transplantation in children is: (JIPMER 2011)
a. Biliary atresia
b. Indian childhood cirrhosis
c. HCC
d. Hepatitis C infection

Q20. Which is not true regarding the basis of functional division of the liver? (AIIMS 2015)
a. Based on the portal vein and hepatic vein
b. Divided into eight segments
c. There are three major and three minor fissures
d. Four sectors

Q21. All are true about the caudate lobe, *except*: (JIPMER 2011)
a. Blood supply from both right and left hepatic arteries
b. Ductal drainage from both right and left ducts
c. Venous drainage is mainly from the left and middle hepatic veins.
d. Supply of both branches of the portal vein

Grade III	*Most difficult*

Q1. Dieulafoy's lesions: (PGI 2005)
a. Within 6 cm of the GE junction
b. In the esophagus
c. In the ileum
d. In rectum

Q2. All are true about GAVE, *except*: (JIPMER 2011)
a. Dilated submucosal venous plexus
b. Bleeding is the most common presentation.
c. Pain is the most common clinical symptom.
d. Argon laser treatment is established one.

Q3. Thickened gastric folds are found in: (PGI 2003)
a. Lymphoma
b. Menetrier's disease
c. Carcinoma
d. Eosinophilic gastritis
e. Giardiasis

Q4. Which of the following is the most significant risk factor for the development of gastric carcinoma? (All India 2006)
a. Paneth cell metaplasia
b. Pyloric metaplasia
c. Intestinal metaplasia
d. Ciliated metaplasia

Q5. According to Borrmann's classification, Linitis plastica is: (AIIMS 2011)
a. Type I
b. Type II
c. Type III
d. Type IV

Q6. True about GIST all, *except*: (AIIMS 2010)
a. Most common in duodenum
b. Necrosis and ulceration present
c. PET is used to assess the response to therapy
d. Cell circumscribed

Q7. Carney's triad consists of: (PGI 2011)
a. Gastric carcinoma
b. Paraganglioma
c. Pulmonary chordoma
d. Bronchus carcinoma
e. Chondromatosis

Q8. The most common type of gastric sarcoma is: (MCI 2018)
a. Lipoma
b. Glomus tumor
c. Leiomyosarcoma
d. Fibrosarcoma

Q9. All are true about stomach lymphoma, *except*: (GB Pant 2011)
a. The most common type is non-Hodgkin lymphoma (NHL).
b. Large B cell type
c. Chemosensitive
d. The most common site is fungus.

Q10. Indications of surgery in gastric lymphoma are all, *except*: (PGI 2011)
a. Bleeding
b. Perforation
c. Residual disease after chemotherapy
d. Intractable pain

Q11. False about gastric lymphoma is: (AIIMS 2008)
a. The stomach is the most common site.
b. Associated with *H. pylori* infection
c. Total gastrectomy with adjuvant chemotherapy is the treatment of choice.
d. 5-year survival rate after treatment is 60%.

Q12. Which of the following is not a feature of ultrasound in CHPS? (AIIMS 2011)
a. 95% sensitivity by ultrasound
b. Thickness of pylorus >4 mm
c. Channel length >16 mm
d. High gastric residue

Q13. All of the following are seen in chronic pyloric obstruction, *except*: (MCI 2010)
a. Alkaline urine
b. Acidic urine
c. Hypochloremia
d. Hypokalemia

Q14. Which of the following is true about acute dilatation of the stomach? (PGI 2005)
a. Dilatation of the stomach is seen on X-ray.
b. Presents with vomiting
c. Aspiration
d. Immediately open the abdomen
e. Atony of the stomach

Q15. Surgical lobes of the liver are divided on the basis of: (PGI 2002)
a. Hepatic artery
b. Hepatic vein
c. Bile ducts
d. Portal vein
e. Central veins

Q16. In Couinaud's classification, segment IV of the liver is: (AIIMS 2007)

a. Caudate lobe b. Quadrate lobe
c. Right lobe d. Left lobe

Q17. The Couinaud's segmental nomenclature is based on the position of the: (All India 2003)

a. Hepatic veins and portal vein
b. Hepatic veins and biliary ducts
c. Portal vein and biliary ducts
d. The portal vein and hepatic artery

Q18. Liver is divided into two halves by: (AIIMS 2004)

a. Right hepatic vein
b. Portal vein
c. Hepatic artery
d. CBD

Q19. Focal lesions of the liver are best detected by: (AIIMS 2003)

a. MRI b. CT
c. USG d. PET scan

ANSWERS

Grade I: 1. b, c, e; 2. d (Sabiston 20/e p1207); 3. b; 4. b (Schwartz 10/e p1053-1073); 5. a (Bailey 27/e p1119); 6. a; 7. d; 8. b; 9. a, b, c (Sabiston 20/e p1208); 10. c; 11. b; 12. d; 13. a; 14. b; 15. a; 16. a; 17. a; 18. d; 19. c; 20. c; 21. a; 22. a, b

Grade II: 1. a; 2. c; 3. c; 4. d; 5. c; 6. b (Schwartz 10/e p 1060); 7. c; 8. b (Harrison 20/e p2199); 9. a (Bailey 27/e p1165); 10. a; 11. b; 12. b; 13. b; 14. a; 15. b; 16. b; 17. d; 18. a; 19. a; 20. b; 21. c

Grade III: 1. a; 2. c (Schwartz 10/e p1088); 3. a, b, c, d (Harrison 19/e p1931); 4. c; 5. d; 6. a; 7. a, b, c; 8. c; 9. d (Sabiston 20/e p1227); 10. d; 11. c; 12. d; 13. a; 14. a, b, c, e; 15. b, d; 16. b; 17. a; 18. a; 19. a

MODEL QUESTIONS

Q1. A 35-year-old man with gastric outlet obstruction presents to the emergency department with multiple episodes of vomiting. Which of the following fluids is preferred for this patient?

a. Normal saline
b. 20% dextrose with water
c. Ringer's lactate
d. 5% dextrose

Ans. a

Q2. Which is not true about dumping syndrome:

a. Post vagotomy
b. Small, frequent meals are beneficial
c. Starch is beneficial.
d. Clinical features include diarrhea and bloating

Ans. c

Q3. The first gastrectomy was performed in 1881 by:

a. Mikulicz b. Wolfer
c. Billroth d. Moynihan

Ans. c

Q4. Investigation of choice for UGI bleed is:

a. Endoscopy b. Angiography
c. CT d. Barium studies

Ans. a

Q5. A patient who underwent gastrectomy after eating within 20 minutes develops dehydration and giddiness. What could be the cause?

a. Hyperglycemia
b. Early dumping syndrome
c. Late dumping syndrome
d. Hypoglycemia

Ans. b

Q6. Among the following, the least common cause of acute upper GI bleeding is:

a. Vascular extenuating b. Mallory-Weiss tear
c. Ulcer d. Varices

Ans. a

Q7. Mallory-Weiss syndrome is a partial thickness rupture that occurs at:

a. Gastric cardia
b. Esophagus mucosa
c. Gastroesophageal junction
d. Gastroduodenal junction

Ans. a

Q8. A patient underwent total gastrectomy. Which of the following deficiencies would be seen in this patient?

a. Vitamin B_{12} b. Vitamin A
c. Vitamin B_1 d. Vitamin C

Ans. a

Q9. Troisier's sign is:

a. Metastatic left supraclavicular lymphadenopathy
b. Carpopedal spasm in hypocalcemia
c. Migratory thrombophlebitis
d. Any of the above

Ans. a

Q10. The Irish node is most commonly seen in:

a. Stomach cancer
b. Lung cancer
c. Larynx cancer
d. Endometrium cancer

Ans. a

Q11. Calcified liver metastases are seen in:

a. Adenocarcinoma of colon
b. Carcinoid tumors
c. Renal cell carcinoma (RCC)
d. Lymphoma

Ans. a

Q12. The place of the first liver transplant is:

a. Pittsburgh b. Boston
c. Colorado d. Cambridge

Ans. c

Q13. The Pringle maneuver may be required for the treatment of:

a. Injury to the tail of the pancreas
b. Mesenteric ischemia
c. Bleeding esophageal varices
d. Liver lacerations

Ans. d

Q14. Bear claw appearance on the contrast-enhanced computed tomography (CECT) of the abdomen is seen in:

a. Hepatic lacerations
b. Pancreatic lacerations
c. HCC
d. RCC

Ans. a

Q15. The function of hepatic Kupffer cells is:

a. Function of sinusoids
b. Vitamin A storage
c. Increase blood perfusion
d. Phagocytosis

Ans. d

Q16. Dieulafoy's lesion is:

a. Prolapse gastropathy
b. Gastric antral vascular ectasia
c. Gastric hemorrhagic telangiectasia
d. An aberrant vessel in the mucosa that bleeds from a mucosal defect.

Ans. d

Q17. Watermelon stomach is:

a. Prolapse gastropathy
b. Gastric antral vascular ectasia
c. Gastric hemorrhagic telangiectasia
d. An aberrant vessel in the mucosa that bleeds from a mucosal defect.

Ans. b

Q18. The most common gastric polyp is:

a. Hyperplastic polyp
b. Inflammatory polyp
c. Adenomatous polyp
d. Part of familial polyposis

Ans. a

Q19. E-Catherine is more often mutated in:

a. Diffuse type of gastric cancer
b. Intestinal type of gastric cancer
c. Malignant ulcer of the stomach
d. Erosive gastritis

Ans. a

Q20. False about GIST is:

a. The stomach is the most important site.
b. Can present with bleeding
c. Commonly metastasizes to lymph nodes
d. Can present with peritoneal metastasis

Ans. c

Q21. Sunitinib is used in:

a. GIST
b. Rectal cancer
c. Colonic carcinoma
d. Pancreatic carcinoma

Ans. a

Q22. Which is the treatment of choice for duodenal atresia?

a. Duodenoduodenostomy
b. Duodenojejunostomy
c. Bishop-Koop procedure
d. Gastroduodenostomy

Ans. a

SUGGESTED READING

1. A Handbook of Gastroesophageal Reflux Disease, 1st edition.
2. Bailey & Love's - Short Practice of Surgery, 27th edition.
3. Schwartz's Principles of Surgery, 18th edition.
4. Textbook of Surgery by David Sabiston, 21st edition.

CHAPTER 34 Bariatric and Metabolic Surgery

"The true measure of a Bariatric surgery success is not in pounds lost, but in a better quality of life."

- Anonymous

INTRODUCTION

- *Gastric banding:* Adjustable banding is not common nowadays and is replaced by the Pars flaccida technique, band is applied below the gastroesophageal junction (GEJ) through the opening of the lesser omentum. It reduces appetite and hunger considerably and thus causes weight loss **(Fig. 1)**.
- Sleeve gastrectomy **(Fig. 2)**
- Roux-en-Y gastric bypass **(Fig. 3)**
- Banded roux-en-Y gastric bypass
- *Biliopancreatic diversion (BPD):* Sleeve gastrectomy followed by duodenoileostomy and ileoileostomy, good but more nutritionally poor
    - Mini gastric bypass (one anastomosis bypass)
    - *SADI-S*—single anastomosis duodenoileal bypass with sleeve gastrectomy
    - *Sleeve gastrectomy and ileal transposition*

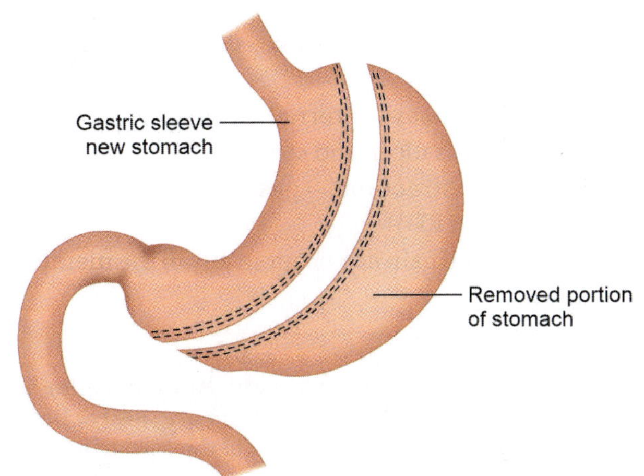

Fig. 2: Sleeve gastrectomy.

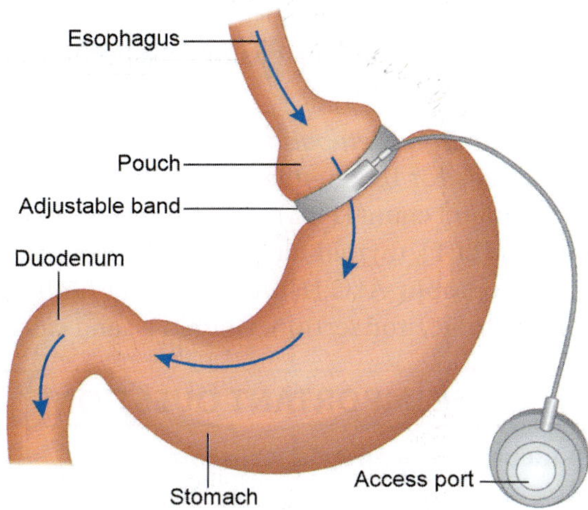

Fig. 1: Gastric banding.

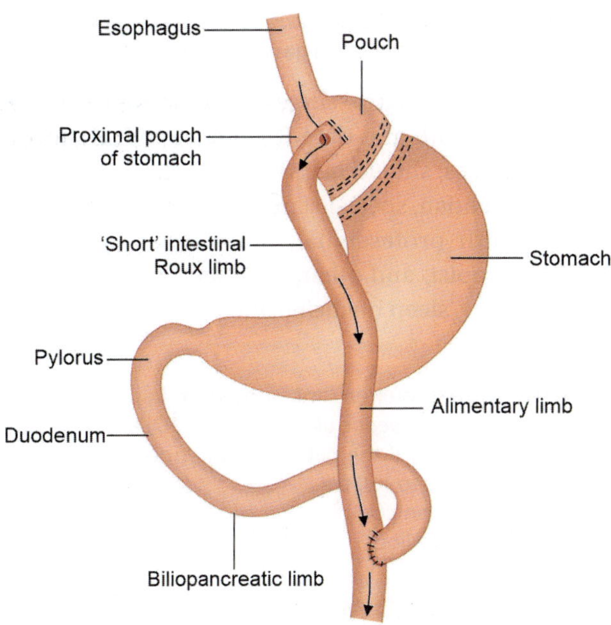

Fig. 3: Roux-en-Y gastric bypass.

Points to remember:
OS-MRS—Obesity Surgery Mortality Risk Score: Risk factors are given one point each, as arterial hypertension, age >45 years, male, body mass index (BMI) >50, and risk factors for pulmonary thromboembolism.

COMPLICATIONS OF BARIATRIC SURGERY

- *Early:*
  - Gastric banding—infection and deep vein thrombosis (DVT)
  - Gastric bypass—anastomosis leak, bleeding, obstruction, DVT
  - Sleeve gastrectomy—leak and DVT
- *Late:*
  - Gastric band—intolerance, slippage, and erosion in the stomach
  - Gastric bypass—internal hernia, malnutrition, anastomosis ulcer, and stricture
  - Sleeve gastrectomy—gastroesophageal reflux disease (GERD)

Weight loss and gain can occur in any of the mentioned procedures.

Not to forget:
Mechanism of weight loss by bariatric surgery is not well understood, but the suspected factors are: Restriction of volume, malabsorption, and reduction of the level of hormone ghrelin.

All bariatric surgery procedures are not reversible, BPD and duodenal switch (DS) are irreversible procedures.

Maximum weight loss in bariatric surgery is with BPD and DS then in sleeve gastrectomy and gastric bypass and bending.

The team of bariatric surgery, according to National Institute for Health and Care Excellence (NICE) accreditation guidelines, should have bariatric surgeon, bariatric physician, dietitian, specialist nurse, appropriately trained mental health professional, anesthetist, radiologist, exercise therapist, and other secondary care specialists, e.g., respiratory/sleep medicine and cardiology.

You may be asked:
The length of the Roux-en limb should be kept as 50 cm in the surgery done for *peptic ulcer disease (PUD)* and 100 cm in bariatric surgery, but if the patient is super obese, the length should be increased to 150 cm.

The most common complication of sleeve gasterectomy is bleeding from staple line.

BARIATRIC AND METABOLIC SURGERY

Obesity is fast increasing and so is its consequences. India will become the world capital of obesity. Obesity reduces life expectancy considerably by 5–20 years, depending on its class:

- *Normal weight:* BMI 18.5—24.9
- *Overweight 0:* BMI 25—029.9
- *Class 1 obesity:* BMI 30—34.9
- *Class 2 obesity:* BMI 35—39.9
- *Class 3 obesity:* BMI 40 and above

Severe obesity increases the risk of the following diseases:

- Hypertension
- Diabetes, specifically type 2
- Dyslipidemia
- Osteoarthritis
- GERD
- Depression
- Cognitive dysfunction
- Others—apnea, fatty liver, etc.

Bariatric surgery is done for weight loss by bypass surgery of the upper gastrointestinal series (UGI) manipulation.

Good to remember:
Nutritional deficiencies are common with bariatric surgery, such as malnutrition, iron deficiency anemia, which is most common, and mineral deficiency. Supplementation should be done postsurgery with multivitamins, minerals, and trace elements.

Why Bariatric Surgery?

It changes the way the body's basal metabolic rate acts with dieting, thus reducing weight loss by about 20% for long-term, as much as two decades, improves life expectancy, and improves quality of life.

METABOLIC SURGERY

The term bariatric is now replaced by the term metabolic surgery as it improves metabolism and helps in metabolic syndrome (diabetes, hypertension, dyslipidemia, and obesity).

British Obesity and Metabolic Surgery Society (BOMSS) gave guidelines for biochemistry after bariatric surgery such as full blood count (FBC), urea and electrolytes, liver function test (LFT), thyroid function test (TFT), ethereum (ETH), hemoglobin A1C (HbA1c), fasting blood sugar (FBS), lipid profile, iron ferritin, vitamin D, and calcium.

SOME IMPORTANT QUESTIONS

Q1. Which gas is used in laparoscopy?

a. CO_2 b. N_2O
c. O_2 d. N_2

Ans. a

Q2. Shoulder pain postlaparoscopy is due to:
a. Subphrenic abscess
b. CO_2 retention
c. Positioning of the patient
d. Compression of the lung

Ans. b

Q3. Minimal invasive surgery includes all, *except*:
a. Functional endoscopic sinus surgery (FESS)
b. Lap cholecystectomy
c. Endoscopic sclerotherapy
d. Percutaneous nephrolithotomy (PCNL)

Ans. d

Q4. During laparoscopy, the intra-abdominal pressure is:
a. 5–10 mm Hg b. 12–15 mm Hg
c. 15–20 mm Hg d. 20–25 mm Hg

Ans. b

Q5. Instrument used to create artificial pneumoperitoneum in laparoscopy:
a. Maryland forceps b. Veress needle
c. Trocar d. All of the above

Ans. b

Q6. Complications of laparoscopy:
a. Diaphragmatic rupture
b. Vascular injury
c. Pneumothorax
d. All of the above

Ans. d

Q7. Complication(s) of obesity is/are:
a. Venous ulcer
b. Pulmonary embolism
c. Increased mortality
d. Prostate cancer
e. Pulmonary hypertension

Ans. a, b, c, d, and e

MULTIPLE CHOICE QUESTIONS

Grade I | **Simple**

Q1. Gases for pneumoperitoneum: (PGI June 2007)
a. CO_2 b. N_2
c. Room air d. N_2O

Q2. Layers that are penetrated with a trocar and a cannula in the production of pneumoperitoneum are: (PGI June 2005)
a. Skin and superficial fascia
b. Deep fascia
c. Rectus abdominis
d. Transversus abdominis
e. Rectus sheath

Q3. Hypothermia is used in all, *except*: (PGI 1998)
a. Cardiac surgery b. Neonatal ischemia
c. Heat stroke d. Cardiac arrhythmia

Grade II | **Difficult**

Q1. Cancers associated with excess fat intake are/is: (PGI December 2000)
a. Breast b. Colon
c. Prostate d. Lung
e. Thyroid

Q2. Physiological changes seen in laparoscopy include all, *except*: (AIIMS May 2015)
a. Increased intracranial pressure (ICP)
b. Decreased functional residual capacity (FRC)
c. Increased central venous pressure (CVP)
d. Increased pH

Q3. Bariatric surgical procedures include all, *except*: (WBPG 2015)
a. Gastric bleeding
b. Gastric bypass
c. Biliopancreatic diversion
d. Ileal transposition

Grade III | **Most difficult**

Q1. The most commonly performed and acceptable method of bariatric surgery is: (AIIMS May 2015)
a. Biliopancreatic diversion
b. Biliopancreatic diversion with ileostomy
c. Laparoscopic gastric banding
d. Roux-en-Y gastric bypass

Q2. All of the following are primarily restrictive operations for morbid obesity, *except*: (All India 2010)
a. Vertical band gastropathy
b. Duodenal switch operation
c. Roux-en-Y operation
d. Laparoscopic adjustable gastric banding

Q3. The intra-abdominal pressure during laparoscopy should be set between: (AIIMS Nov 2003)
a. 5–8 mm Hg b. 10–15 mm Hg
c. 20–25 mm Hg d. 30–35 mm Hg

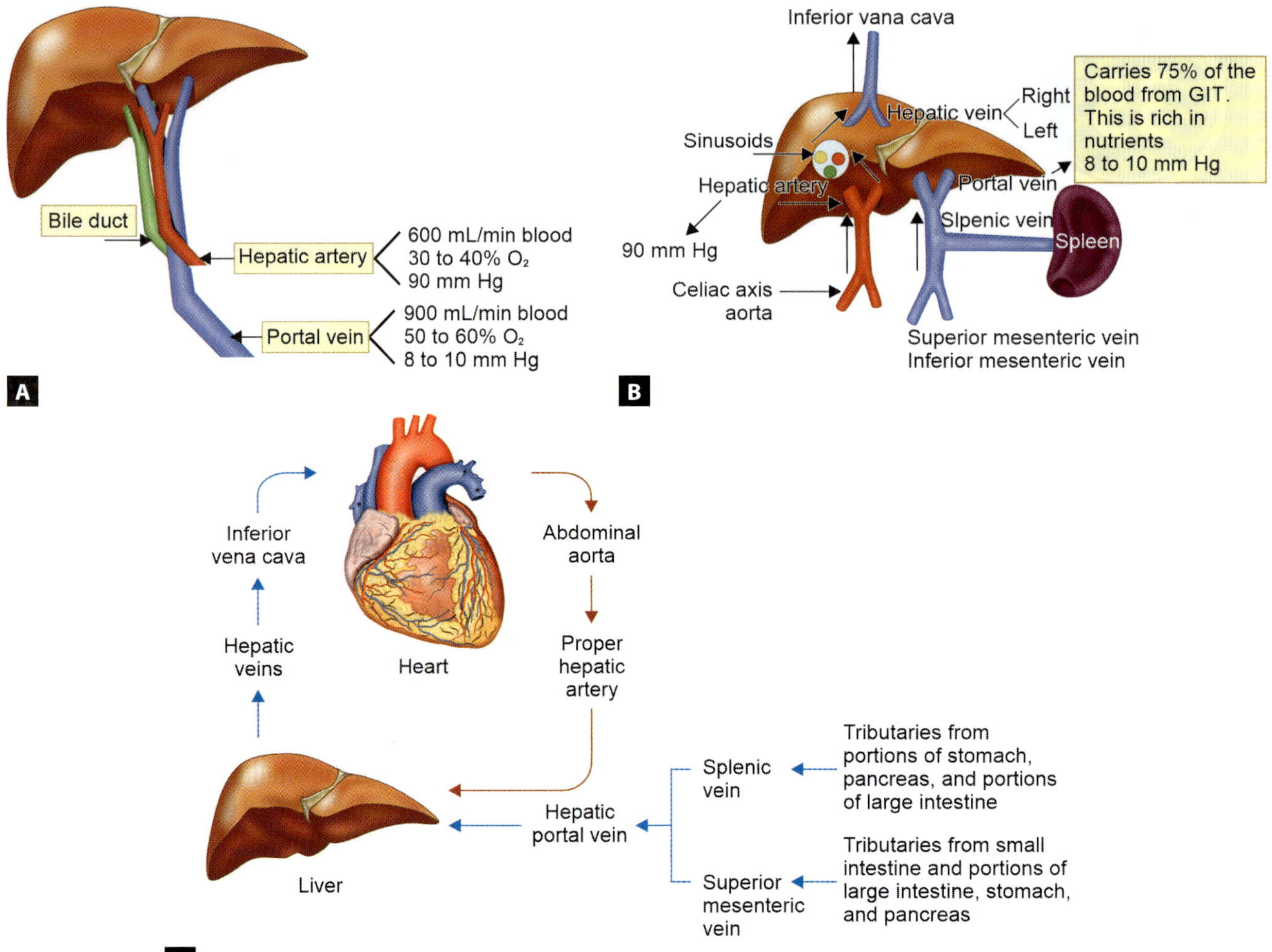

Bile duct
Hepatic artery
600 mL/min blood
30 to 40% O2
90 mm Hg
Portal vein
900 mL/min blood
50 to 60% O2
8 to 10 mm Hg
A
Inferior vana cava
Hepatic vein
Right
Left
Carries 75% of the blood from GIT. This is rich in nutrients 8 to 10 mm Hg
Sinusoids
Hepatic artery
Portal vein
90 mm Hg
Slpenic vein
Spleen
Celiac axis aorta
Superior mesenteric vein
Inferior mesenteric vein
B
Inferior vena cava
Heart
Abdominal aorta
Hepatic veins
Proper hepatic artery
Liver
Hepatic portal vein
Splenic vein
Tributaries from portions of stomach, pancreas, and portions of large intestine
Superior mesenteric vein
Tributaries from small intestine and portions of large intestine, stomach, and pancreas
C

Scheme of principal blood vessels of hepatic portal circulation and arterial supply and venous drainage of liver

Figs. 1A to C: Blood supply of the liver.

Groove for IVC
Cantlie's line
Falciform ligament
Left portal vein
Bare area of the liver m/c involved in amebic liver abscess
Right portal vein
Right hepatic vein
Left hepatic vein
Middle hepatic vein
Fossa segments 4B and 5
• Can be involved in gallbladder cancer→ Resected in radical cholecystectomy
8
4A
7
2
1
3
4B
5
6

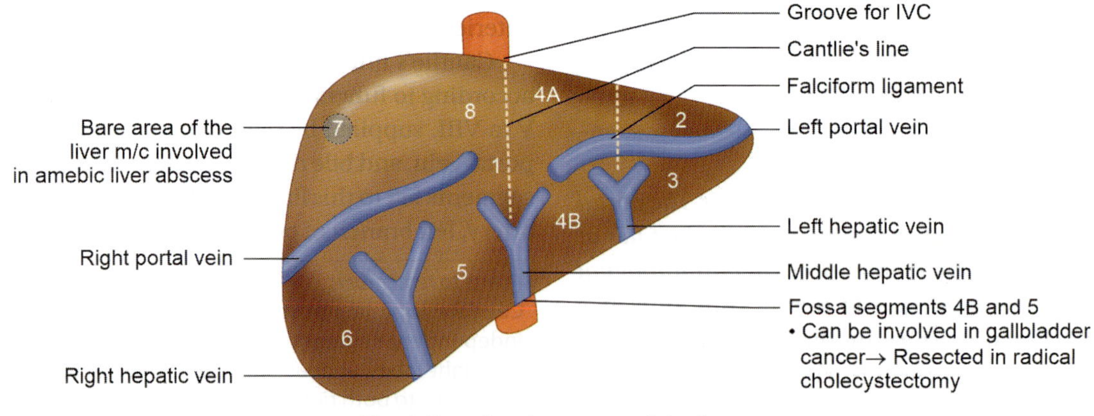

Fig. 2: Functional anatomy of the liver.

LOBULES OF LIVER

The functional unit of the liver is a lobule. A lobule of liver is having three zones: Zone 1—periportal zone, zone 2—intermediate zone, and zone 3—perivenular zone, which is prone to hypoxia and causes central necrosis **(Fig. 3)**.

The quadrate lobe of the liver is situated on the inferior surface of the right lobe **(Figs. 4A and B)**.

FUNCTIONS OF THE LIVER

- Glucose metabolism, gluconeogenesis, and glycolysis
- Bilirubin formation
- Core body temperature maintenance
- pH balance and correction of lactic acidosis
- Clotting factors formation
- Urea synthesis from proteins
- Excretion of drugs and toxins

> *Not to forget:*
> *Brisbane classification of hepatic resection:* Left (4a, 4b, 2, and 3) hepatectomy, right (5, 6, 7, and 8) hepatectomy, left (4a, 4b, 2, 3+5, and 8) trisectorectomy and right (5, 6, 7, 8 + 4a, and 4b) trisectorectomy. GHARBI classification of hydatid cyst is old and has now been replaced by the World Health Organization (WHO) classification.

LIVER FUNCTION TESTS

- Serum bilirubin
- Serum glutamic oxaloacetic transaminase (SGOT)
- Serum glutamic pyruvic transaminase (SGPT)
- Alkaline phosphate (ALP)
- Gamma-glutamyl transpeptidase (GGT)
- Albumin
- Prothrombin time (PT)

INVESTIGATIONS IN LIVER DISEASES

- Liver function test (LFT)
- Ultrasound (USG)
- Computed tomography (CT)

> *How to check liver malfunction?*
> *The functioning of liver is done by scoring systems: Child–Pugh score, model for end-stage liver disease (MELD), and pediatric end-stage liver disease (PELD).* Child–Pugh score system is based on EAST. E: Encephalopathy, A: Ascites, S: Serum albumin and bilirubin, T: PT or INR. Points given are: 1, 2, and 3. MELD is based on SIC, serum bilirubin, INR, and creatinine. PELD is based on A TIGA—albumin, total bilirubin, INR, growth failure, and age <1 year.

LIVER ABSCESS

It is caused by bacteria, most commonly by *Escherichia coli*, and also by *Staphylococcus aureus* and *Klebsiella*. Amoebic liver abscess is caused by *Entamoeba histolytica*. Bacterial pyogenic abscess develops as the infection travels from ascending cholangitis to the liver, causing solitary or multiple abscesses. Amoebic liver abscess develops as the infection ascends up from the intestinal amoebic ulcer through the portal vein. The amoebic ulcers are flask-shaped. The most common site of amoebic liver abscess is the bare area of the liver in segment 7. In amoebic abscess, the pus is like anchovy sauce without any neutrophils, but the pus of pyogenic liver abscess is full of neutrophils. The amoebic abscess patient shows positive serology for *Entamoeba*. *Contrast-enhanced computed tomography (CECT)* is the most important investigation to diagnose liver abscess. The treatment of amoebic liver abscess is by metronidazole, which acts as a tissue amebicide, followed by delocalize, which is a luminal amebicide for

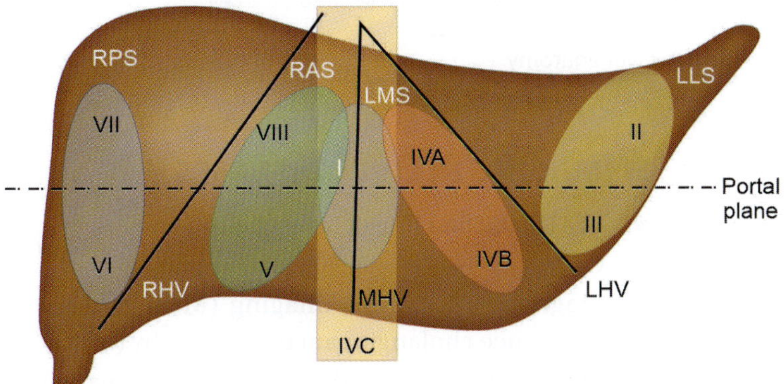

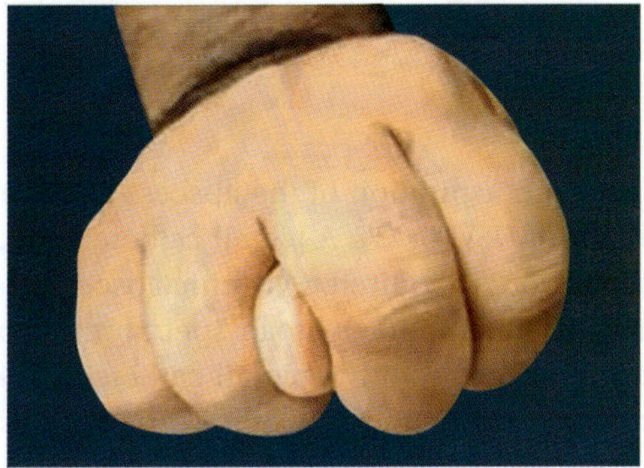

Fig. 3: Liver lobules. (LHV: left hepatic vein; LLS: left lateral segment; LMS: liver measurement for stiffness; MHV: middle hepatic vein; RAS: renin-angiotensin-system; RHV: right hepatic vein; RPS: right posterior segment)

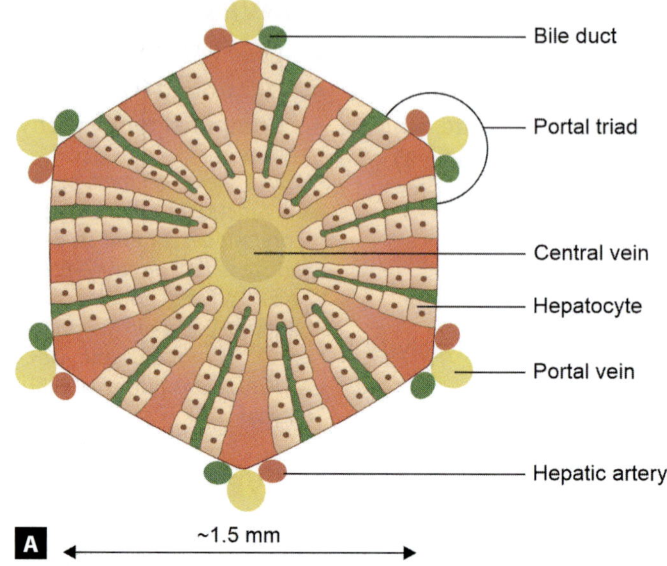

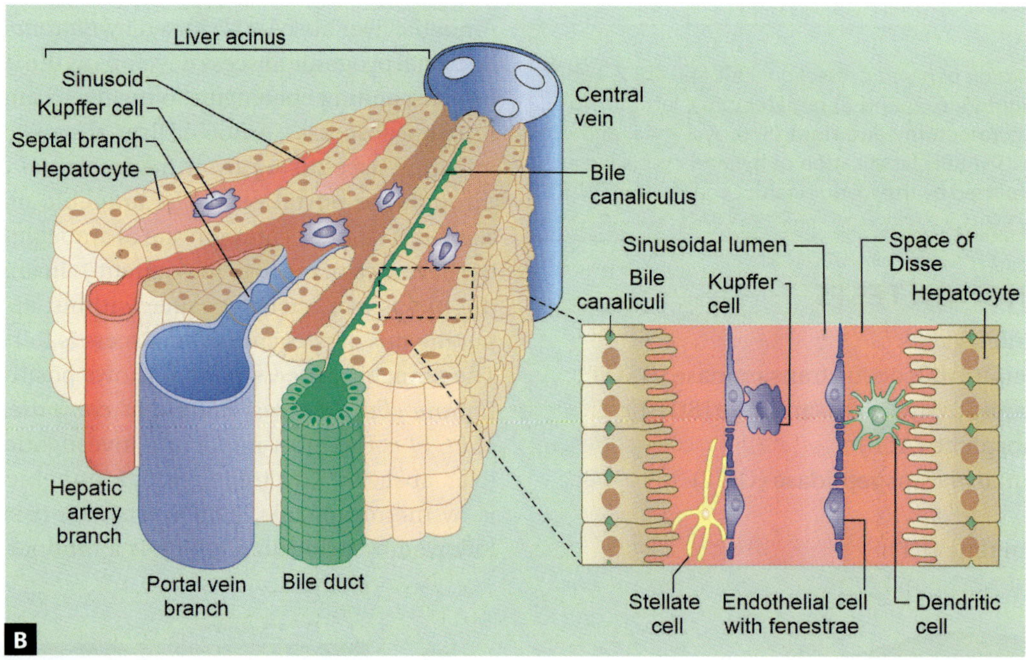

Figs. 4A and B: Liver anatomy.

10 days, and aspiration of the abscess is done under the guidance of USG or CT. A pigtail catheter **(Fig. 5)** is used for aspiration if required. Pyogenic abscess of the liver is treated with intravenous broad-spectrum antibiotics, and aspiration is done with a pigtail catheter if the response of antibiotics is not good. Complications of liver abscess are rupture of the abscess into the peritoneal, pleural, and pericardial cavity, and amoebic abscess getting bacterial secondary infection.

IMAGING IN LIVER DISEASES

- USG is the first line of investigation
- CT
- Magnetic resonance imaging (MRI) and magnetic resonance cholangiopancreaticography (MRCP)
- Endoscopic retrograde cholangiopancreaticography (ERCP)
- Percutaneous transhepatic cholangiography (PTC)

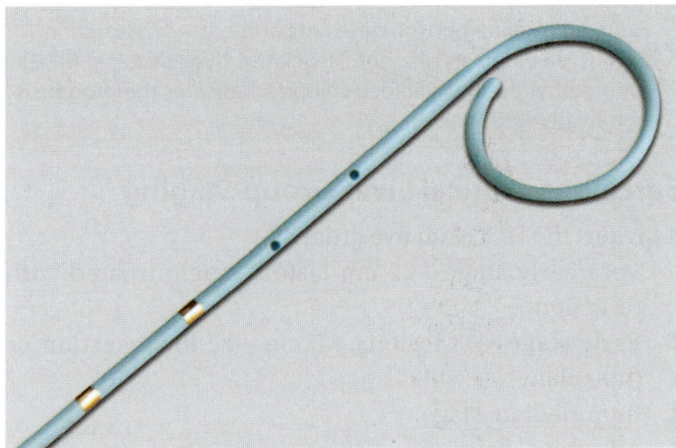

Fig. 5: Pigtail catheter.

- Positron emission tomography (PET) scan
- Hepatic angiography
- Laparoscopy

CHRONIC LIVER DISEASE

Chronic disease of the liver may lead to deterioration of liver function. Common features of chronic liver disease (CLD) are: Lethargy, weakness, jaundice, loss of appetite and weight, coagulopathy, hepatic encephalopathy, ascites, esophageal varices, splenomegaly, etc.

HYDATID DISEASE OF LIVER

It is caused by *Echinococcus granulosus,* but sometimes by *Echinococcus multilocularis,* which is also called malignant hydatid.

You may be asked
- Liver Imaging Reporting and Data System (LI-RADS) scoring system for tumors of the liver.
- It is based on a CT scan.
- *It has five types of reviews:* LR-1 is 100% benign, LR-2 is probably benign, LR-3 is intermediate and probably hepatocellular carcinoma (HCC), LR-4 is probably HCC, and LR-5 is 100% HCC.
- The most common primary malignant tumor in the liver in children is hepatoblastoma, and in adults is HCC, but the most common tumor of the liver is metastasis.

The hosts for this are the dog as the definitive host, and sheep as the intermediate host, and human beings are accidental intermediate hosts. Liver is the most common organ affected by hydatid disease, and lungs at the second most common organ affected. Other organs, such as the kidneys and spleen, are also affected by it sometimes. Most of the cases are without any symptoms, whereas others have pain and tenderness in the right hypochondrium and an enlarged palpable liver. CECT is the investigation of choice.

Which is the basis of the classification of hydatid cysts?
World Health Organization classification
Hydatid cysts of the liver are classified into five types:
- Type 1 or CE-1—Unilocular cyst
- Type 2 or CE-2—Multiseptated (honeycomb or rosette-like)
- Type 3 or CE-3—Floating membrane (water lily sign)
- Type 4 or CE-4—Heterogeneous cyst with calcification
- Type 5 or CE-5—Calcified wall
- Types 1, 2, and 3 are active, and types 4 and 5 are inactive and dead.

Investigations

- CECT is the most important investigation.
- ELISA and Casoni's intradermal test

The most common clinical feature is hepatomegaly without pain. Jaundice and passage of cyst membrane like grapes with stools.

Complications

- Rupture
- Infection

Treatment

Treatment includes albendazole tablets and then percutaneous aspiration infusion of scolicidal agents and reaspiration (PAIR). PAIR is not done if the cyst is superficial in the liver to avoid its rupture, CE2, biliary cyst communication, CE4 and 5, and dead cyst.

BUDD–CHIARI SYNDROME

It is an entity that occurs due to obstruction of venous drainage of the liver by hepatic venous thrombosis or obstruction from a venous web, leading to portal hypertension and cirrhosis. CT scan is the investigation of choice, but the deficiency of protein C and S, along with antithrombin 3, is to be investigated. Treatment depends upon the stage at which the patient has arrived. TIPS and liver transplant are considered.

TUMORS OF LIVER

Benign Tumors

Hemangioma

The most common tumors of the liver. It may be single or multiple, is more common in women, and is usually an incidental diagnosis. USG and delayed contrast enhancement CT (triple-phase CT) are diagnostic. MRI shows "Light bulb sign." It is a plexus of blood vessels. Consumption coagulopathy occurs in very large or giant hemangiomas with bleeding and pain, which is called *Kasabach-Merritt syndrome.* Angioembolization is the treatment if symptomatic.

Hepatic Adenoma

It is common in female adults, solitary, probably due to the use of oral contraceptives. Most of these tumors are found incidentally. USG and CT diagnose them. There is a risk of malignancy in 10% of cases. It may rupture in the peritoneal cavity, leading to hemoperitoneum, which is the second most common cause of hemoperitoneum after trauma. Surgical excision is the treatment.

Focal Nodular Hyperplasia

It is due to the overgrowth of liver supporting tissue of unknown cause. It contains both Kupffer cells and hepatocytes. USG, CT, and MRI are diagnostic. It is the second most common benign liver tumor after hemangioma, common in adult females, and may rupture and bleed. Sulfur colloid liver scan shows a "hot spot" as only Kupffer cells take up colloid. No treatment is required.

HEPATOCELLULAR CARCINOMA

It is a common cancer of the liver, more common in Asia and Africa than in Western countries, due to risk factors associated with the place.

Risk Factors

- Chronic hepatitis B virus (HBV) infection is responsible for more than half of the cases globally. Hepatitis C virus (HCV) infection increases the risk several times.
- Alcohol
- Obesity
- Contrast agent thorotrast increases the risk.
- Diabetes
- Nonalcoholic fatty liver disease (NAFLD)

Good to remember:
- *Liver parenchyma has two types of cells:* Hepatocytes for synthesis and excretion, and Kupffer cells for reticuloendothelial function.
- Hepatobiliary iminodiacetic acid (HIDA) scan is based on the function of hepatocytes, and sulfur colloid scan on the function of Kupffer cells.
- Elevated alkaline phosphatase indicates biliary obstruction.
- GGT is elevated in alcohol associated liver disease. MEGX (Monoethylglycine xylidide), chloride, indicates the prognosis of transplanted liver.

Barcelona Clinical Liver Group Staging

It divides the HCC into five groups:

1. Very early stage—<2 cm lesion, single treated with resection
2. Early stage—<3 lesions, <3 cm size for resection or transplant
3. Intermediate stage
4. Advanced stage
5. Terminal stage

Clinical features are male predominance, hard and nodular enlarged liver, and jaundice.

Paraneoplastic Syndromes with Hepatocellular Carcinoma

- Cushing's syndrome
- Hypoglycemia is most common
- Hypercholesterolemia
- Gynecomastia

Investigations in Hepatocellular Carcinoma

- *CT triple phase:* No contrast, hyperdense (arterial), and early washout (venous)
- Core biopsy
- *Tumor markers:* AFP, protein-induced vitamin K antagonist (PIVKA), and neurotensin B

The treatment is by surgical resection and liver transplant.

Associating liver partition with portal vein ligation for staged hepatectomy (ALPPS).

FUNCTIONAL LIVER RESERVE

- *Ablative therapies:* Percutaneous injection of ethanol and acetic acid or thermal ablation. A tumor if very near to blood vessel will dissolve the thermal effect, called "heat sink effect."
- *Transarterial chemoembolization (TACE) and radioembolization (TARE)* can be used to get local effects on the tumor.

FIBROLAMELLAR TUMOR

It is common in young males. Neurotensin is a tumor marker, good prognosis, and the tumor is resectable.

SOME IMPORTANT QUESTIONS

Q1. Which of the following is not a sign of pulmonary hydatidosis?

a. Water lily sign b. Rising sun sign
c. Meniscus sign d. Drooping lily sign

Ans. d

Q2. Capitonnage is used in the treatment of:

a. Choledochal cyst b. Dermoid cyst
c. Hydatid cyst d. Renal cyst

Ans. c

Q3. A patient with right hypochondriac pain, water lily sign is seen on ultrasound, what is the diagnosis?

a. *Entamoeba* b. Schistosoma
c. Ascariasis d. Hydatid cyst

Ans. d

Q4. Which of the following liver tumors always merits surgery?

a. Hemangioma
b. Hepatic adenoma
c. Focal nodular hyperplasia
d. Peliosis hepatic

Ans. b

Q5. Which of the following is false about a chronic liver disease patient?

a. Model for End-Stage Liver Disease (MELD) used for liver transplant
b. MELD has prothrombin time (PT), albumin, and creatinine
c. The Child–Pugh (CTP) score has international normalized ratio (INR), albumin, and bilirubin
d. CTP has grades A, B, and C

Ans. b

Q6. A chronic alcoholic female patient with chronic liver disease presents with hematemesis. What is the most common cause?

a. Mallory–Weiss tear b. Boerhaave syndrome
c. Bleeding varices d. Perforated ulcer

Ans. c

Q7. A 5-year-old male child presents with acute fulminant liver failure. Which one of the following criteria is not included in the KING's College criteria for liver transplant?

a. Age <10 years
b. Prothrombin time is >50 seconds
c. Bilirubin >300 μmol/L
d. Jaundice <7 days before the development of encephalopathy

Ans. d

Q8. Treatment of symptomatic polycystic liver disease is:

a. Deroofing of cyst b. Injection of sclerosis
c. Hepatic resection d. Liver transplant

Ans. a

Q9. Okuda staging contains all, *except*:

a. Bilirubin
b. Tumor size
c. Ascites
d. Alpha-fetoprotein (AFP)

Ans. d

Q10. Calcified liver metastases are seen in:

a. Adenocarcinoma of colon
b. Carcinoid tumors
c. Renal cell carcinoma
d. Lymphoma

Ans. a

Q11. Place of first liver transplant:

a. Pittsburgh b. Boston
c. Colorado d. Cambridge

Ans. c

Q12. The Pringle maneuver may be required for the treatment of:

a. Injury to tail of pancreas
b. Mesenteric ischemia
c. Bleeding esophageal varices
d. Liver lacerations

Ans. d

Q13. Beer claw appearance on the contrast-enhanced computed tomography (CECT) abdomen is seen in:

a. Hepatic lacerations
b. Pancreatic lacerations
c. Hepatocellular carcinoma (HCC)
d. Renal cell carcinoma (RCC)

Ans. a

Q14. Function of hepatic Kupffer cells:

a. Function of sinusoids
b. Vitamin A storage
c. Increase blood perfusion
d. Phagocytosis

Ans. d

Q15. With Couinaud's nomenclature, which one of the following segments of liver has an independent vascularization?

a. Segment I
b. Segment II
c. Segment IV
d. Segment VIII

Ans. a

Q16. The boundary of Morrison's pouch is formed by:

a. Kidney
b. Falciform ligament of liver
c. Spleen
d. Pancreas

Ans. a

Q17. Conjugated hyperbilirubinemia is seen in:

a. Dubin–Johnson syndrome
b. Crigler–Najjar syndrome
c. Crigler–Najjar syndrome II
d. Gilbert syndrome

Ans. a

Q18. The most common surgical cause of obstructive jaundice is:

a. Periampullary carcinoma
b. Carcinoma of the gall bladder (GB)
c. Carcinoma of the head pancreas
d. Common bile duct (CBD) stones

Ans. d

Q19. Primary sinusoidal dilatation of the liver is also known as:

a. Hepar lobatum
b. Peliosis hepatis
c. Von-Meyenburg complex
d. Caroli's disease

Ans. b

Q20. Obstruction of the inferior vena cava (IVC) leads to:

a. Dilatation of thoracoepigastric veins
b. Caput Medusa's
c. Hemorrhoids
d. Esophageal varices

Ans. a

MULTIPLE CHOICE QUESTIONS

Grade I	*Simple*

Q1. Most common cause of liver abscess: **(AIIMS 2011)**

a. *Escherichia coli*
b. *Proteus*
c. *Klebsiella*
d. *Staphylococcus*

Q2. All are true about pyogenic liver abscess, *except*: **(JIPMER 2011)**

a. The most common route of infection is the biliary tree.
b. The most common site is the right lobe.
c. *Klebsiella* is most common in gas-forming abscess.
d. Percutaneous drainage is the least cured.

Q3. All are true about amoebic liver abscess, *except*: **(PGI 2010)**

a. Metronidazole is the mainstay of treatment.
b. Multifocal abscess cannot be treated by aspiration.
c. More common on the left side
d. More common in female

Q4. Liver abscess ruptures in most commonly in: **(AIIMS 2003)**

a. Pleural cavity
b. Peritoneal cavity
c. Pericardial cavity
d. Bronchus

Q5. True statements regarding pyogenic liver abscess is/are: **(PGI 2018)**

a. Most common on the left side of the liver
b. Surgical drainage is the treatment of choice.
c. The most common organism responsible is *E. coli.*
d. X-rays are diagnostic.
e. Diagnosis is confirmed by aspiration and culture.

Q6. Indications for needle aspiration in liver abscess are: **(PGI 2006)**

a. Recurrent
b. Left lobe
c. Refractory to treatment after 48–72 hours
d. >10 ams in size
e. Multiple

Q7. Not an indication for PAIR (puncture, aspiration, injection, and reaspiration) treatment in hydration cyst: **(PGI 2010)**

a. Size >5 cm
b. Multiloculated
c. Cyst in lung
d. Recurrence after surgery
e. Perforated cyst

Q8. Investigation of choice for hydatid disease is: **(MCI 2009)**

a. Computed tomography (CT) scan
b. Enzyme-linked immunosorbent assay (ELISA)

c. Biopsy
d. Ultrasound (USG)

Q9. All are true about liver adenoma, *except*: (AIIMS 2011)

a. Normal liver architecture
b. Increased fat
c. Increased glycogen
d. Cell arranged in cords

Q10. Most common cause of nontraumatic hemoperitoneum: (AIIMS 2003)

a. Hepatic adenoma
b. Focal nodular hyperplasia (FNH)
c. Hepatocellular carcinoma (HCC)
d. Hemangioma

Q11. What is not included in the model for end-stage liver disease (MELD) score? (AIIMS 2020)

a. Creatinine b. Bilirubin
c. Prothrombin time d. Albumin

Q12. All of the following are true regarding FNH, *except*: (AIIMS 2010)

a. Not frequently associated with oral contraceptive pills (OCPs)
b. Surgical resection is required due to the risk of malignancy.
c. Stellate scar is diagnostic.
d. Typical hepatic vascularity is not seen with the spoke wheel pattern.

Q13. A surgeon excises a portion of liver to the left of the attachment of the falciform ligament. The segments that have been resected are: (All India Nov 2008)

a. Segment 1 to 4 b. Segment 1 and 4b
c. Segment 2 and 3 d. Segment 2 to 4

Q14. All are true about the functional division of the liver, *except*: (AIIMS May 2015)

a. Divided into four sectors
b. Based on the portal vein and hepatic vein
c. Divided into eight segments
d. 3 major and three minor fissures

Q15. All of the following are true about the caudate lobe, *except*: (AIIMS Dec 2010)

a. Blood supply from both the right and left hepatic arteries.
b. Ductal drainage from both right and left ducts.
c. Venous drainage is mainly by the left and middle hepatic veins.
d. Supply by both branches of the portal vein.

Q16. Right hepatic duct drains all, *except*: (AIIMS May 2009)

a. Segment I b. Segment III
c. Segment V d. Segment VI

Q17. False about hepatic duct: (AIIMS May 2009)

a. Left hepatic duct formed in the umbilical fissure.
b. Caudate lobe drains only the left hepatic duct.
c. The right hepatic duct is formed by the V and VIII segments.
d. Left hepatic duct crosses the IV segment.

Q18. Which of the following is not a liver capsular plate? (AIIMS Nov 2011)

a. Portal plate b. Hilar plate
c. Umbilical plate d. Cystic plate

Q19. What percentage of the blood flow to the liver is supplied by the hepatic artery? (JIPMER 1988)

a. 90% b. 20%
c. 40% d. 60%

Q20. True about pyogenic liver abscess: (PGI June 2001)

a. Single and large abscess
b. X-ray features are diagnostic
c. Serology is a confirmatory investigation
d. Systemic complaints, fever, and jaundice are common
e. Liver enzyme abnormalities are common and severe

Grade II ***Difficult***

Q1. True statement regarding FNH: (PGI 2011)

a. More common in young women
b. Associated with OCP use
c. May present with abdominal pain
d. Excision biopsy may aid in diagnosis
e. Progress to cirrhosis

Q2. Similarities between FNH and hepatic adenoma are all, *except*: (AIIMS 2003)

a. Hemoperitoneum is common.
b. Biliary abnormalities are seen.
c. More common in females
d. Associated with OCPs

Q3. Most common benign tumor of liver: (JIPMER 2011)

a. Hemangioma b. Hepatic adenoma
c. Hepatoma d. Harriman

Q4. Solitary hypoechoic lesion of liver without septa or debris is most likely to be: (AIIMS 2005)

a. Hydatid cyst b. Caroli's disease
c. Liver abscess d. Simple cyst

Q5. Simple hepatic cyst, all are true *except*: (AIIMS 2006)

a. Asymptomatic
b. Lined by columnar epithelium
c. Intracystic bleeding is common, and reroofing is mandatory.
d. Congenital

Q6. Treatment of choice for simple cyst of liver: (JIPMER 2017)

a. Percutaneous drainage
b. Cystoenterostomy
c. Deroofing
d. Aspiration

Q7. All are risk factors for HCC *except*: (AIIMS 2006)

a. Tumor markers of HCC
b. Alpha-fetoprotein (AFP)
c. Alpha decorates
d. DCGP (Diabetes Care in General Practicc)
e. Carbohydrate antigen

Q8. In a high-risk population, HCC is best detected by: (AIIMS 2003)

a. USG
b. CT
c. Magnetic resonance imaging (MRI)
d. Positron emission tomography (PET) scan

Q9. AFP is elevated in: (PGI 2011)

a. HCC
b. Hepatoblastoma
c. Infant hemangioendothelioma
d. Amoebic liver abscess
e. Embryonic sarcoma

Q10. Most common paraneoplastic syndrome of HCC: (AIIMS 2003)

a. Hypoglycemia b. Hypertension
c. Hypercalcemia d. Erythrocytosis

Q11. Tumor markers for primary blood HCC are all, *except*: (AIIMS 2007)

a. AFP
b. Alpha-2 macroglobulin
c. Protein induced by vitamin K absence-II (PIVKA-2)
d. Neurotensin

Q12. Hypercalcemia is seen in: (AIIMS 2011)

a. Pancreatic cancer b. HCC
c. CA stomach d. CA GB

Q13. All are true about fibrolamellar HCC, *except*: (AIIMS 2009)

a. AFP is not raised.
b. Recurrence is common.
c. Raised neurotensin levels
d. Well demarcated and encapsulated

Q14. All are true about pyogenic liver abscess, *except*: (JIPMER 2011)

a. The most common route of infection is the biliary tree.
b. The most common site is the right lobe.
c. *Klebsiella* is most common in gas-forming abscess
d. Percutaneous drainage is the least cured

Q15. All are true about liver hemangioma, *except*: (AIIMS Dec 2006)

a. CHF is very common
b. Incidental detection
c. Consumptive coagulopathy can occur
d. Spontaneous regression is seen

Q16. CECT with nodular enhancement is suggestive of: (AIIMS Dec 2006)

a. Hepatic adenoma b. FNH
c. Hemangioma d. HCC

Q17. All are true about hepatic adenoma, *except*: (JIPMER 2011)

a. Usually multiple
b. Oral contraceptive pill (OCP) is a predisposing factor
c. Has cords of benign hepatocytes
d. 50–75% are symptomatic

Q18. Which of the following most significantly increases the risk of HCC? (AIIMS May 2012)

a. Hepatitis B virus (HBV)
b. HAV

c. Cytomegalovirus (CMV)
d. Epstein-Barr virus (EBV)

Q19. True regarding HCC: (JIPMER 2010)
a. Nonalcoholic steatohepatitis is a risk factor:
b. OCPs are a cause
c. Focal nodular hyperplasia may turn malignant
d. Chromosomal abnormalities are common

Q20. Which of the following liver tumors has a propensity to invade the portal or hepatic vein? (AIIMS June 2004)
a. Cavernous hemangioma
b. Hepatocellular carcinoma
c. Focal nodular hyperplasia
d. Hepatic adenoma

Grade III	Most difficult

Q1. Which of the following liver metastases appears hypoechoic on USG? (All India 2012)
a. Breast cancer
b. Colon cancer
c. RCC
d. Mucinous adenocarcinoma

Q2. Most common indication of liver transplantation in children: (JIPMER 2011)
a. Biliary atresia
b. Indian childhood cirrhosis
c. HCC
d. Hepatitis C infection

Q3. Which is not true regarding the basis of the functional division of the liver? (AIIMS 2015)
a. Based on the portal vein and the hepatic vein
b. Divided into 8 segments
c. There are three major and three minor fissures
d. Four sectors

Q4. All are true about the caudate lobe, *except*: (JIPMER 2011)
a. Blood supply from both right and left hepatic arteries
b. Ductal drainage from both right and left ducts
c. Venous drainage is mainly from the left and middle hepatic veins
d. Supply of both branches of the portal vein

Q5. Surgical lobes of the liver are divided on the basis of: (PGI 2002)
a. Hepatic artery
b. Hepatic vein
c. Bile ducts
d. Portal vein
e. Central veins

Q6. In Couinaud's classification, segment IV of the liver is: (AIIMS 2007)
a. Caudate lobe
b. Quadrate lobe
c. Right lobe
d. Left lobe

Q7. The Couinaud's segmental nomenclature is based on the position of the: (All India 2003)
a. Hepatic veins and portal vein
b. Hepatic veins and biliary ducts
c. Portal vein and biliary ducts
d. Portal vein and hepatic artery

Q8. Focal lesions of the liver are best detected by: (AIIMS 2003)
a. MRI
b. CT
c. USG
d. PET scan

Q9. The following are true about hepatocellular carcinoma, *except*: (AIIMS Nov 2003)
a. It has a high incidence in East Africa and South-East Asia.
b. Its worldwide incidence parallels the prevalence of hepatitis B
c. Over 80% of tumors are surgically resectable
d. Liver transplantation offers the only chance of cure in those with irresectable disease.

Q10. All of the following are true about fibrolamellar carcinoma of the liver, *except*: (All India 2001)
a. More common in females
b. Better prognosis than HCC
c. AFP levels are always >1,000
d. Occur in younger individuals

Q11. True about hepatocellular carcinoma: (PGI Dec 2002)
a. Most common tumor of liver
b. Resectable only in 1% of cases
c. >70% of cases show increased AFP
d. USG-guided aspiration biopsy is used for diagnosis

Q12. MELD score does not include: (AIIMS Dec 2011)
a. INR
b. Serum bilirubin
c. Serum creatinine
d. Blood urea

Q13. Auxiliary orthotopic liver transplant is indicated for: (AIIMS May 2008)
a. Metabolic liver disease

b. As a standby procedure until finding a suitable donor
c. Drug-induced hepatic failure
d. Acute fulminant liver failure for any cause

Q14. A 50-year-old male presented with a history of hematemesis—500 mL of blood, and on examination, shows blood pressure (BP)—90/60, pulse rate (PR)—110 beats/min, and splenomegaly 5 cm below the lower costal margin. Most probable diagnosis is: (AIIMS Nov 2006)
a. Mallory-Weiss tear
b. Duodenal ulcer
c. Gastritis
d. Portal hypertension

Q15. A patient with compensated liver cirrhosis presented with a history of variceal bleed. The treatment of choice is this patient is: (AIIMS June 2002)
a. Propranolol
b. Liver transplantation
c. Transjugular intrahepatic portal shunt (TIPS)
d. Endoscopic sclerotherapy

Q16. Which of the following management procedures of acute upper gastrointestinal bleed should possibly be avoided? (AIMMS Nov 2003)
a. Intravenous vasopressin
b. Intravenous β-blockers
c. Endoscopic sclerotherapy
d. Balloon tamponade

Q17. True about TIPS: (PGI June 1998)
a. It is a type of portocaval shunt
b. It is an intrahepatic shunt
c. Performed by passing endoscopes
d. Most suitable for a patient going for a liver transplant

Q18. For treatment of ascites, the LeVeen shunt is placed between the peritoneum and: (AIIMS Nov 2014)
a. Gallbladder
b. Inferior vena cava
c. Cisterna chyli
d. Superior vena cava

Q19. Left-sided portal hypertension is best treated by: (AIIMS June 2001)
a. Splenectomy
b. Portocaval shunt
c. Lienorenal shunt
d. Splenorenal shunt

Q20. In a child's criteria for partial encephalopathy, bilirubin 2.5 mg/dL, albumin 3 g/dL, and controlled ascites indicate: (PGI 1996)
a. Grade A
b. Grade B
c. Grade C
d. More information needed

ANSWERS

Grade I: 1. a; 2. d; 3. c, d (Sabiston 20/e p1449-1452); 4. b; 5. c, e (Bailey 27/e p1168); 6. b; 7. b, c, d, e; 8. b; 9. a; 10. a; 11. a, b, c, d; 12. b; 13. c (Schwartz 10/e p1265); 14. c; 15. c (Sabiston 20/e p1422); 16. b (Sabiston 20/e p1422); 17. b; 18. a (Sabiston 20/e p1423); 19. b (Bailey 20/e p1153); 20. a, d

Grade II: 1. a; 2. a; 3. a; 4. d; 5. c; 6. c; 7. a; 8. a; 9. ab; 10. a; 11. b; 12. b; 13. d; 14. d; 15. a (Schwartz 10/e p1289-1290); 16. c (Schwartz 10/e p1290); 17. a; 18. a (Bailey 27/e p1173); 19. a; 20. b (Bailey 27/e p1174)

Grade III: 1. a; 2. a; 3. b; 4. c; 5. b, d (Schwartz 10/e p1265); 6. b; 7. a; 8. a; 9. c (Bailey 27/e p1175); 10. c (Bailey 27/e p1172); 11. c, d (Schwartz 10/e p1289); 12. d (Schwartz 10/e p1280); 13. d (Sabiston 19/e p1229, 659); 14. d; 15. d; 16. a (Schwartz 10/e p1088); 17. a, b, d (Bailey 27/e p1164); 18. d; 19. a; 20. b (Schwartz 10/e p1280)

MODEL QUESTIONS

Q1. True about amebic liver abscess:
a. Male:female >10:1
b. Not predisposed by alcohol
c. More common in diabetics
d. *E. histolytica* is isolated in >50% from blood cultures

Ans. a

Q2. Not an indication for percutaneous aspiration in amebic liver abscess:
a. Radiographically unresolved lesion after 6 months
b. Suspected diagnosis
c. Left lobe liver abscess
d. Compression or outflow obstruction of the hepatic or portal vein

Ans. a (Sabiston 20/e p1452)

Q3. The most common cause of pyogenic liver abscess is:

a. Aspiration
b. Hematogenous spread from a distant site
c. Direct contact
d. Lymphatic spread

Ans. b

Q4. Anchovy sauce pus is a feature of:

a. Amebic liver abscess b. Lung abscess
c. Splenic abscess d. Pancreatic abscess

Ans. a

Q5. In pyogenic liver abscess most common route of spread is:

a. Hematogenous through the portal vein
b. Ascending infection through the biliary tract
c. Hepatic artery
d. Local spread

Ans. b

Q6. All are used in the treatment of amoebic liver abscess, *except*:

a. Diloxanide furoate b. Chloroquine
c. Metronidazole d. Emetine

Ans. a

Q7. Not true about amebic liver abscess is:

a. Adult forms are seen
b. Conservative treatment is generally seen
c. Larvae are seen
d. Ultrasound (USG) can diagnose it

Ans. c (Bailey 27/e p1169)

Q8. The water lily appearance in a chest radiograph suggests:

a. Metastasis
b. Cavitating metastasis
c. Aspergilloma
d. Ruptured hydatid cyst

Ans. d (Bailey 27/e p1169)

Q9. True treatment regarding hepatic amoebiasis:

a. More common in females
b. Multiple lesions
c. Mostly treated conservatively
d. Jaundice is common

Ans. c

Q10. Capitonnage is used in the treatment of:

a. Choledochal cyst b. Dermoid cyst
c. Hydatid cyst d. Renal cyst

Ans. c

Q11. In the treatment of hydatid cyst, PAIR is contraindicated in:

a. Lung cyst
b. Size >5 cm
c. Not amenable to treatment with albendazole
d. Multiple
e. Inaccessible location

Ans. a and e (Sabiston 20/e p1454)

Q12. A 40-year-old male presents with a painless cystic liver enlargement of 4 years duration without fever or jaundice. The most likely diagnosis is:

a. Amoebic liver abscess b. Hepatoma
c. Hydatid cyst of liver d. Choledochal cyst

Ans. c

Q13. All are complications of hydatid cyst in the liver, *except*:

a. Jaundice b. Suppuration
c. Cirrhosis d. Rupture

Ans. c

Q14. During surgical exploration for hydatid cyst of the liver, any of the following agents can be used as a scolicidal agent *except*:

a. Hypertonic sodium chloride
b. Formalin
c. Cetrimide
d. Povidone iodine

Ans. b

Q15. Ring-like calcification on contrast-enhanced computed tomography (CECT) is seen in:

a. HC b. FNH
c. Liver metastasis d. Hydatid cyst

Ans. d (Sabiston 20/e p1452)

Q16. Which of the following is true about the hydatid cyst of the liver?

a. Surgical management is always done
b. Conservative treatment is effective
c. Aspiration is safe
d. *Echinococcus multilocularis* is the most common cause

Ans. c (Bailey 27/e p1169)

Q17. Treatment of hydatid cyst:

a. Excision of cyst
b. Percutaneous drainage
c. Conservative management
d. None

Ans. b

Q18. Consider the following features: Asian Male, alcoholic cirrhosis, hypervascular lesion during the arterial phase of CT, and portal vein thrombosis. The above features are mostly suggestive of:

a. Cholangiocarcinoma
b. Hepatocellular carcinoma
c. Metastatic colorectal carcinoma
d. Neuroendocrine tumors

Ans. b

Q19. The screening for HCC in chronic liver disease is:

a. Serial USG + alpha-fetoprotein (AFP)
b. Serial liver function test (LFT) + AFP
c. Serial LFT + CT scan
d. Serial USG + serial LFT

Ans. a

Q20. All are true about hepatoblastoma, *except*:

a. Present in childhood
b. Common in cirrhosis of the liver due to hepatitis B virus (HBV)
c. Chemosensitive
d. Surgical resection is the treatment of choice

Ans. b

Q21. AFP is raised in:

a. 100% of hepatoblastoma
b. 90% of hepatoblastoma
c. 100% of HCC
d. 90% of HCC

Ans. b

Q22. All are true about hemangioendothelioma, *except*:

a. Adult variant is benign
b. More common in females
c. Multiple and involve bilateral lobes
d. An indication of a liver transplant

Ans. a

Q23. Contraindications to major hepatic resection for metastatic disease include all of the following, *except*:

a. Total hepatic involvement
b. Advanced cirrhosis
c. Extrahepatic tumor involvement
d. Jaundice from extrinsic ductal obstruction

Ans. d (Sabiston 20/e p1470)

Q24. The minimum amount of normal perfused liver parenchyma to be left intact when a hepatic resection is planned is:

a. 10%
b. 20%
c. 50%
d. 75%

Ans. b

Q25. The left medial sector contains the segment:

a. III, IV
b. II, III
c. I, II
d. I, IV

Ans. a

SUGGESTED READING

1. Blumgart's Surgery of the Liver, Biliary Tract and Pancreas, 6th edition.
2. Schwartz's Principles of Surgery, 18th edition.
3. Textbook of Surgery by David Sabiston, 21st edition.

CHAPTER 36

Spleen

"Spleen is the most common organ ruptured in blunt abdominal trauma."

– Vinod Kumar Nigam

DEVELOPMENT OF SPLEEN

It develops from the condensation of mesoderm in the dorsal mesogastrium. Tissue between the fetal spleen and the fetal stomach forms the gastrosplenic ligament, and tissue between the fetal spleen and the left fetal kidney forms the lienorenal ligament.

ANATOMY OF SPLEEN (FIG. 1)

Spleen is situated in the right upper quadrant of the abdomen, weighing about 75–250 g, along the 10th rib, between the kidney and the stomach. There is a notch on its inferolateral border, called the anterior notch, which is palpable on physical examination. The splenic artery is a

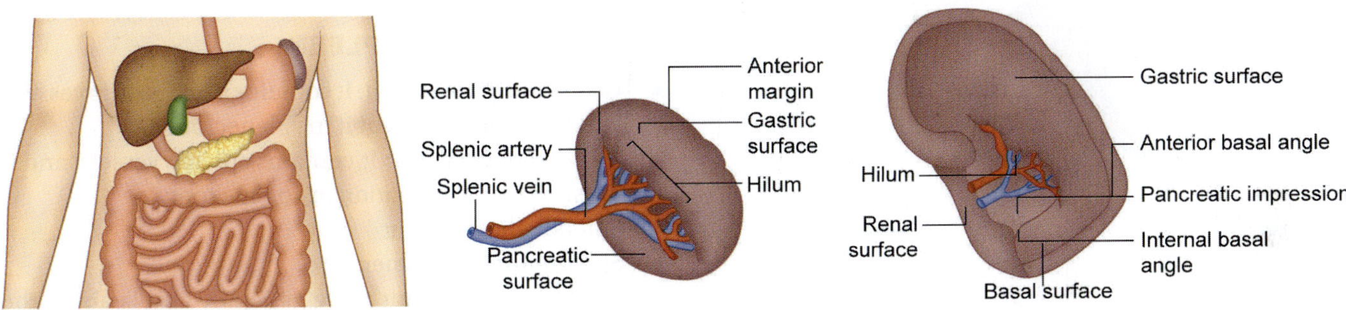

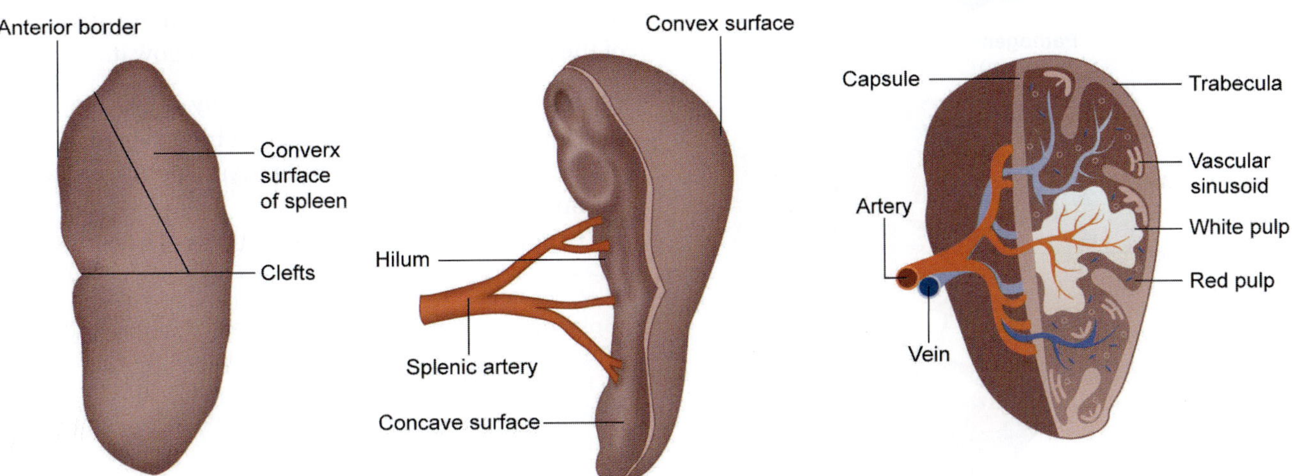

Fig. 1: Anatomy of the spleen.

branch of the celiac axis, which divides into superior and inferior branches. *The splenic vein is made at the hilum of the spleen by several tributaries and joins with the superior mesenteric vein to form the portal vein. The splenic pulp has red and white pulp. Sympathetic nerves come from the celiac plexus.*

FUNCTIONS OF SPLEEN (FIG. 2)

The rate of blood flow through the spleen is 300 mL/min.

- The spleen functions as a reservoir for red blood cells (RBCs), white blood cells (WBCs), and platelets, which is why the removal of the spleen is associated with a rise in these cells in the blood.
- Immunological functions are the production of various antibodies, immunoglobulin M (IgM), and pushing into circulation when required; that is why, after splenectomy, the chances of infection increase.
- *It filters the nonfunctional blood cells; that is why it is called the graveyard of blood cells. It is also called culling.*
- Hematopoiesis, physiological in idiopathic ulcerative laryngitis (IUL), and pathological in myeloproliferative diseases.
- *Pitting:* It removes inclusions in RBC.

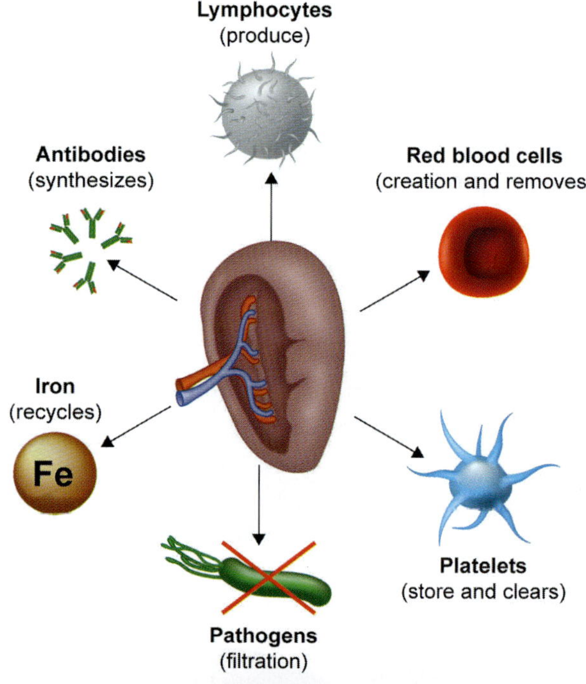

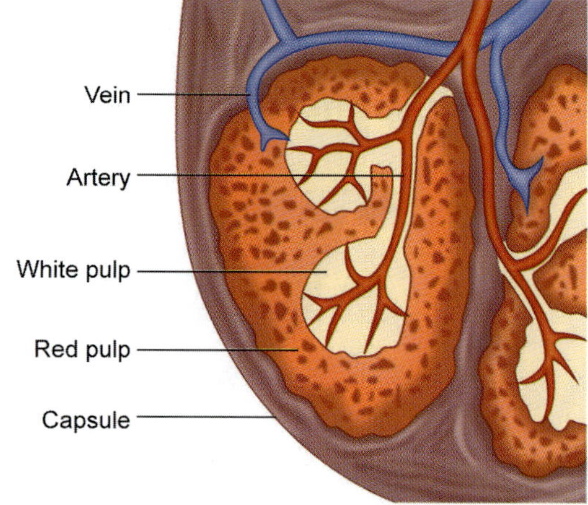

Fig. 2: Functions of the spleen.

> *Points to remember:*
> *How to prevent postsplenectomy infections?*
> Vaccination prevents opportunistic postsplenectomy infections (OPSIs). Pneumococcal vaccine, meningococcal vaccine, and *Haemophilus influenzae* vaccine are given 10 weeks before splenectomy; in case of trauma, where the splenectomy is done as an emergency procedure, the vaccines are given 2 weeks after splenectomy.

LIGAMENTS OF SPLEEN

- *Gastrosplenic ligament:* It contains short gastric vessels, and it is required to cut it in splenectomy.
- *Lienorenal ligament:* It contains splenic vessels, and it must be cut after ligation in splenectomy.
- Splenocolic ligament
- Splenophrenic ligament

Spleen weighs about 150 g generally and is about the size of a fist, 12 × 7 × 3 cm. The splenic artery is the largest branch of the celiac trunk, and it runs on the upper border of the pancreas with the splenic vein below it.

Blood changes occur after splenectomy as:

- Howell–Jolly bodies are seen in blood smear.
- Heinz bodies are denatured hemoglobin and are seen on a smear.
- Pappenheimer bodies are particles of iron in RBCs.

> *Not to forget:*
> Splenectomy causes some permanent changes in the blood structure:
> - Howell Jolly bodies
> - Reticulocytes
> - Basophilic stippling
> - Hypersegmented WBCs
> - Transient leukocytosis can be mistaken for infection.
> - Transient platelet count reduction increases the risk of thrombosis, so it to be treated with aspirin.

SPLENICULI

These are accessory splenic tissues. They are most commonly found in the hilum of the spleen.

SPLENDID

It is normal splenic tissue that gets attached to the omentum and intestines after trauma to the spleen and appears like a tumor.

SPLENIC CYST

It may be a false or true cyst. A false cyst is not lined by epithelium and results from trauma, and treatment is not recommended as it resolves by itself. True cysts are hydatid, epidermoid, and dermoid cysts.

> *You may be asked!*
> Tumors are not very common, but the most common benign tumor of spleen is hemangioma, and most common malignant tumor of spleen is lymphoma. Metastasis in the malignant tumors of spleen is very rare, but if occurs, it occurs in lung and breast. Colorectal and ovarian cancers cause metastasis in spleen. Malignant melanoma is a common malignant tumor of spleen.

SPLENIC ABSCESS

It is most commonly seen in patients with immunodeficiencies, commonly caused by Staphylococcus, and contrast-enhanced computed tomography (CECT) is diagnostic. It is drained with a pigtail catheter if single, but splenectomy is required if multiple.

SPLENIC ARTERY ANEURYSM

It is the most common aneurysm in an artery of an organ. It is usually asymptomatic but may rupture. It is diagnosed by CT angiography. Treatment is embolization and splenectomy if required.

SPLENIC INFARCTION

It is commonly seen in portal hypertension, usually asymptomatic, but may have pain in the left hypochondrium. CECT is the investigation of choice. Treatment is conservative, but splenectomy may be required.

> *Good to remember:*
> Splenectomy is done for trauma and diseases of spleen, but it is also the part of en bloc resection in the cancer of stomach and pancreas. Splenectomy can also be done as therapeutic in hemangioma and lymphoma of spleen.

SOME IMPORTANT QUESTIONS

Q1. What is the treatment of choice for idiopathic thrombocytopenic purpura (ITP)?

a. Blood transfusion
b. Steroids
c. Intravenous (IV) immunoglobin
d. Splenectomy

Ans. b

Q2. Best time to give platelets in immune thrombocytopenic purpura (ITP), 48,000/μL:

a. After ligation of the splenic artery
b. Preoperatively
c. Postoperatively
d. After ligation of the splenic vein

Ans. a

Q3. Splenectomy can be curative in all of the following, *except*:

a. Thalassemia
b. Sickle cell disease
c. Hereditary spherocytosis
d. ITP

Ans. b

Q4. Splenectomy is indicated in:

a. Spherocytosis
b. Pyropoikilocytosis
c. Elliptocytosis
d. All

Ans. d

Q5. Splenectomy is done to tide over the acute crises of uncontrollable.

a. ITP
b. Thrombotic thrombocytopenic purpura (TTP)
c. Hemolytic uremic syndrome (HUS)
d. All of the above

Ans. a

Q6. Autosplenectomy is seen in one of the following hemolytic anemias:

a. Hereditary spherocytosis
b. Sickle cell anemia
c. Thalassemia
d. Immunohemolytic anemia

Ans. b

Q7. Vaccine for postsplenectomy infection is given against all, *except*:

a. *Streptococcus pneumoniae*
b. *Haemophilus influenzae*
c. *Neisseria meningitidis*
d. *Escherichia coli*

Ans. d

MULTIPLE CHOICE QUESTIONS

Grade I	*Simple*

Q1. M/C (Most common) immediate complication of splenectomy: (FMGE 2019)
a. Hemorrhage
b. Fistula
c. Bleeding from the gastric mucosa
d. Pancreatitis

Q2. All are true about immune thrombocytopenic purpura (ITP), *except*: (JIPMER GIS 2011)
a. Low platelet count, normal bone marrow seen
b. In adults, most common in young women
c. Chronicity, if it occurs in children, is common in girls
d. Remission occurs in 70% of cases of adult ITP

Q3. An evidence that splenectomy might benefit a patient with idiopathic thrombocytopenic purpura includes which of the following: (UPSC 2007)
a. A significant enlargement of the spleen
b. A high reticulocyte count
c. Patient's age <5 years
d. An increase in platelet count on corticosteroid therapy

Q4. During splenectomy in ITP, platelet infusion is given: (DPG 2008)
a. Immediately after lighting the splenic artery
b. Immediately after the removal of the spleen
c. After incision
d. The next day of surgery

Q5. Which of the following does not fit into the definition of hypersplenism? (JIPMER GIS 2011)
a. Bone marrow hypoplasia
b. Splenomegaly
c. Pancytopenia
d. Antiplatelet antibodies

Q6. Most common complication of splenectomy: (AIIMS GIS Dec 2011)
a. Overwhelming postsplenectomy infection (OPSI)
b. Avascular necrosis of the greater curvature of the stomach
c. Pancreatitis
d. Atelectasis

Q7. In the contemporary world, the most common indication for splenectomy is: (JIPMER GIS 2011)
a. Trauma
b. Hemolytic anemia
c. ITP
d. Infections

Q8. Which of the following is not an absolute indication of splenectomy? (All India 2000)
a. Splenic abscess
b. Hereditary spherocytosis
c. Fibrosarcoma
d. Autoimmune hemolytic anemia

Q9. Splenectomy is not done in: (AIIMS June 2001)
a. Myelofibrosis
b. Sickle cell anemia
c. Hereditary spherocytosis
d. Splenic abscess

Q10. A female patient who had steroid-resistant ITP underwent splenectomy. On day 3 postlaparoscopic surgery patient developed a fever. Which of the following conditions is most likely to cause the fever? (AIIMS May 2015)
a. Port site infection
b. Left lower lobe consolidation
c. Urinary infection
d. Intra-abdominal collection

Q11. The most common complication after splenectomy is: (AIIMS June 1994)
a. Chest infection
b. Hematemesis
c. Subphrenic collection
d. Acute dilation of the stomach

Q12. In which case pneumococcal vaccine is most effective? (AIIMS Nov 1997)
a. When given preoperatively
b. When given postoperatively
c. Against all strains of bacteria
d. Against gram-negative bacteria

Grade II	*Difficult*

Q1. Which of the following is not an absolute indication of splenectomy? (All India 2000)
a. Splenic abscess
b. Hereditary spherocytosis
c. Fibrosarcoma
d. Autoimmune hemolytic anemia

Q2. Splenectomy is most useful in: (All India 1996)
a. Sickle cell anemia
b. Thalassemia
c. Hereditary spherocytosis
d. Acquired autoimmune hemolytic anemia

Q3. The most common complication of splenectomy is: (AIIMS Nov 1993)
a. Hematemesis
b. Left lower lobe atelectasis
c. Peritoneal effusion
d. Acute dilatation of the stomach

Q4. Postsplenectomy sepsis is common in: (PGI June 2000)
a. ITP
b. Thalassemia
c. Hereditary spherocytosis
d. Trauma

Q5. The most common complication of splenectomy is: (AIIMS 1992)
a. Pancreatic leak
b. Pulmonary complications
c. Pneumococcal peritonitis
d. Hemorrhage

Q6. Management of grade 3 splenic trauma in a stable child. (PGI November 2010)
a. Embolization
b. Partial splenectomy
c. Total splenectomy
d. Conservative

Q7. Postsplenectomy sepsis is common in: (PGI June 2000)
a. ITP
b. Thalassemia
c. Hereditary spherocytosis
d. Trauma

Q8. Which is the commonest postsplenectomy infection? (All India 2000)
a. *Streptococcus pyogenes*
b. *Staphylococcus aureus*
c. *Streptococcus pneumoniae*
d. *Pseudomonas aeruginosa*

Q9. All of the following are true about overwhelming postsplenectomy infection (OPSI), *except*: (PGI June 2009)
a. Maximum risk is within 1 year of splenectomy
b. Begins with mild appearing prodrome
c. May present with septic shock
d. Usually does not respond to antibiotic treatment
e. Develops 1–5 years after splenectomy

Q10. Vaccine for postsplenectomy infection is given against all, *except*: (MCI Sept 2009)
a. *Streptococcus pneumoniae*
b. *Haemophilus influenzae*
c. *Neisseria meningitidis*
d. *E. coli*

Q11. Most common tumor of spleen is: (All India 2000)
a. Lymphoma
b. Sarcoma
c. Hemangioma
d. Metastasis

Q12. The most common malignancy affecting the spleen is: (PGI June 1997)
a. Angiosarcoma
b. Hamartoma
c. Secondaries
d. Lymphoma

Grade III | Most difficult

Q1. All of the following are true regarding splenic rupture *except*: (MCI Sept 2009)
a. Elevation of the left dome of the diaphragm
b. Obliterated psoas shadow
c. Obliterated colonic gas shadow
d. Obliterated splenic outline

Q2. The most common cause of isolated splenic metastasis is: (All India 2012)
a. Carcinoma pancreas
b. Carcinoma stomach
c. Carcinoma ovary
d. Carcinoma cervix

Q3. True regarding hemangioma of the spleen: (MCI March 2005)
a. Least common benign tumor of the spleen
b. May transforms into a hemangiosarcoma
c. Malignant transformation may be managed conservatively
d. None of the above

Q4. The most common cysts of the spleen are: (All India 2010)
a. Hydated cyst
b. Dermatoid cyst
c. Pseudocyst
d. Lymphangioma

Q5. Spleniculi are seen in: (PGI June 1995)
a. Colon
b. Hilum
c. Liver
d. Lungs

Q6. Accessory spleen is found at all sites, *except*: (AIIMS 1994)

a. Hilum
b. Presacral area
c. Tail of the pancreas
d. Greater omentum, small bowel mesentery

Q7. True statement about splenosis: (PGI Nov 2017)

a. Occurs after traumatic rupture of the spleen
b. Functions as normal spleen
c. Multiple small implants of splenic tissue on the peritoneal surfaces
d. Peritoneal nodules of metastatic carcinoma
e. Benign tumor so the spleen

Q8. Right-sided isomerism is associated with: (All India 2011)

a. Asplenia
b. One spleen
c. Two spleens
d. Polysplenia

Q9. Most common splanchnic aneurysm: (AIIMS GIS 2003)

a. Splenic artery
b. Hepatic artery
c. Gastroduodenal artery
d. Superior mesenteric artery

Q10. Downward displacement of an enlarged spleen is prevented by: (All India 1998)

a. Lienorenal ligament
b. Phrenicolic ligament
c. Upper pole of the right kidney
d. Sigmoid colon

Q11. Kehr's sign, seen in splenic rupture, is: (AIIMS Nov 1993)

a. Pain over left shoulder
b. Pain over right scapula
c. Periumbilical pain
d. Pain over the renal angle

Q12. In splenic injury, conservative management is done in: (AIIMS June 1999)

a. Hemodynamically unstable
b. Young patient
c. Shattered spleen
d. Extreme pallor and hypotension

ANSWERS

Grade I: 1. a; 2. d; 3. d; 4. a; 5. a; 6. d; 7. a; 8. d (Bailey 27/e p1180); 9. None (Schwartz 10/e p1432); 10. b (Schwartz 10/e p1443); 11. a (Schwartz 9/e p1260); 12. a (Schwartz 10/e p1438)

Grade II: 1. d; 2. c; 3. b; 4. a, b, c; 5. b; 6. d; 7. a, b, c (Schwartz 10/e p1444); 8. c (Schwartz 10/e p1438); 9. a (Schwartz 10/e p1440); 10. d (Sabiston 19/e p1558); 11. c; 12. d

Grade III: 1. c; 2. c; 3. d; 4. c (Sabiston 20/e p1563-1564); 5. b; 6. b; 7. a, b, c; 8. a; 9. a; 10. b; 11. a; 12. b (Schwartz 10/e, p457)

MODEL QUESTIONS

Q1. The most common infection after splenectomy is:

a. Anaerobic
b. Staphylococcal
c. Streptococcal
d. Pneumococcal

Ans. d

Q2. The innovative method for the treatment of moderate splenic injury:

a. Conservative management
b. Mesh repair
c. Splenorrhaphy
d. Splenectomy

Ans. a

Q3. Kehr's sign is seen in:

a. Splenic injury
b. Liver injury
c. Renal injury
d. Mesenteric hematoma

Ans. a

Q4. The most important radiological sign of splenic rupture is:

a. Obliteration of psoas shadow
b. Obliteration of splenic shadow
c. Indentation of the left side air bubble
d. Fracture of one or more lower ribs on the left side

Ans. b

Q5. The most common site of accessory spleen is:

a. Lienorenal ligament
b. Hilum of spleen
c. Gastrosplenic ligament
d. Around the tail of the pancreas

Ans. b

Q6. Splenic vein thrombosis is most commonly caused by:

a. Chronic pancreatitis
b. Carcinoma pancreas
c. Spleen trauma
d. Perforation of the duodenum

Ans. a

Q7. Tropical splenomegaly is caused by:

a. Malaria
b. Kala-azar
c. Schistosoma
d. All of the above

Ans. d

SUGGESTED READING

1. S Das Textbook of Surgery, 3rd edition.
2. Schwartz's Principles of Surgery, 18th edition.
3. Textbook of Surgery by David Sabiston, 21st edition.

CHAPTER 37

Gallbladder and Bile Ducts

"Gallstone is tomb stone erected in the memory of organisms which lie dead within them."

– Lord Moynihan

INTRODUCTION

The gallbladder (GB) is pyriform-shaped with a capacity of approximately 50 mL but can accommodate even up to 300 mL of bile. It is 7.5–12 cm in length. It is divided into fundus, body, neck, and Hartmann's pouch, which terminates infundibulum, which ends as the cystic duct. The cystic duct is approximately 3 cm in length and 1–3 mm in diameter. Cystic duct joins the supraduodenal part of the common bile duct (CBD) in 80% of cases. The cystic duct wall has spiral mucosal folds called valves of *Heister (Lorenz Heister, 1683–1758, German Professor of Surgery),* which have no valvular function and also have a sphincter called the sphincter of Lutkens (Ulrich Lutkens, German Surgeon, discovered in 1926). Right and left hepatic ducts join to form the common hepatic duct (CHD), which is 2.5 cm in length. The cystic duct and CHD join to form the CBD, which is about 7.5 cm in length and 4 mm in diameter. The left hepatic duct is larger than the right hepatic duct. The mucous membrane dips in muscle quote, called crypts of Luschka (Hubert Luschka, 1820–1875, German Professor of Anatomy) **(Figs. 1 to 3)**.

The common bile duct has four parts ***(Fig. 4)****:*

1. Supraduodenal—2.5 cm
2. Retroduodenal
3. Infraduodenal
4. Intraduodenal

It passes through the second part of the duodenum, surrounded by the *sphincter of Oddi (Ruggero Oddi, 1845–1906, Physiologist, Italy)* and opens in the ampulla of *Vater (Abraham Vater, German Professor of Anatomy, 1684–1751).*

The cystic artery is the branch of the right hepatic artery, which arises behind CHD, in 15% of cases in front of CHD. Calot's triangle or hepatobiliary triangle is named after *Jean Francois Calot (Jean Francois Calot, 1861–1944, French Surgeon).*

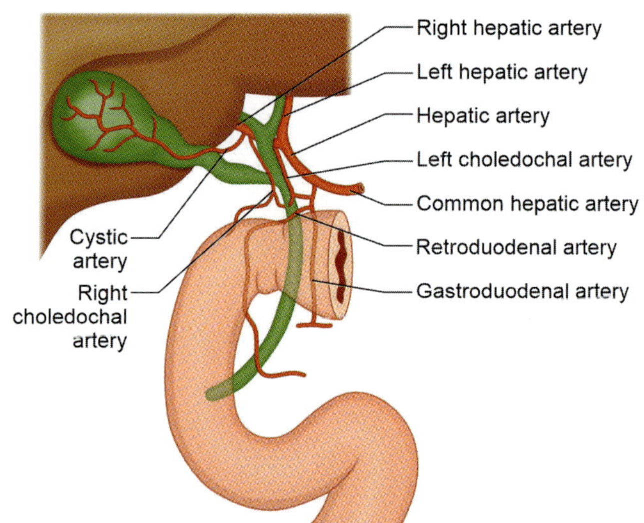

Fig. 1: Biliary tract.

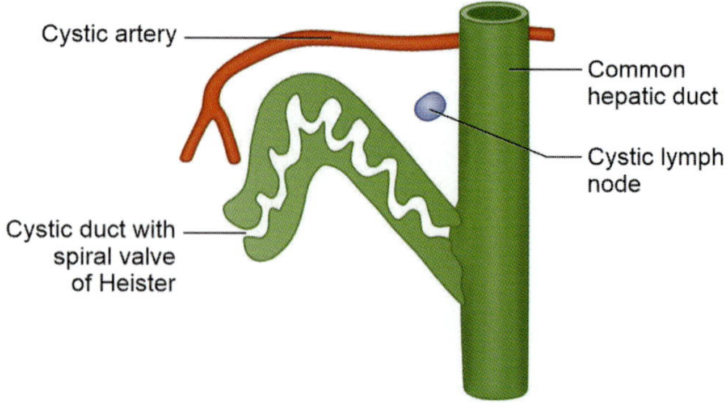

Fig. 2: The spiral valve of Heister.

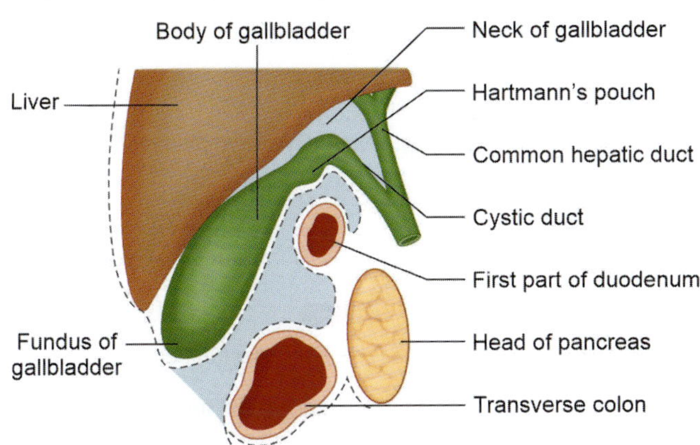

Fig. 3: Position of bile ducts.

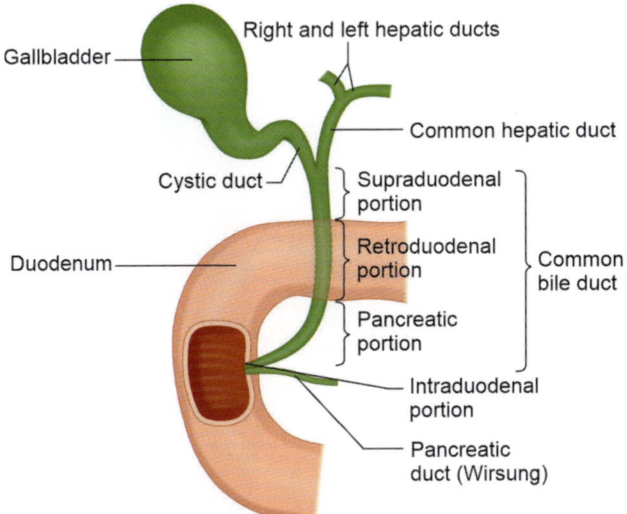

Fig. 4: Parts of the common bile duct (CBD).

BORDERS OF CALOT'S TRIANGLE (FIG. 5)

- Above—inferior border of the liver
- Medial—CHD
- Lateral—cystic duct

The cystic artery passes through Calot's triangle. It has most dangerous anomaly called Moynihan's [Berkeley George Andrew Moynihan (Lord Moynihan), 1865–1936, Professor of Clinical Surgery, Leads, UK] hump/caterpillar turn—common hepatic artery or right hepatic artery takes a tortuous turn in front of cystic duct **(Fig. 6)**.

HEPATOCYSTIC TRIANGLE

It is formed by cystic duct and GB below, CHD medially, and liver above.

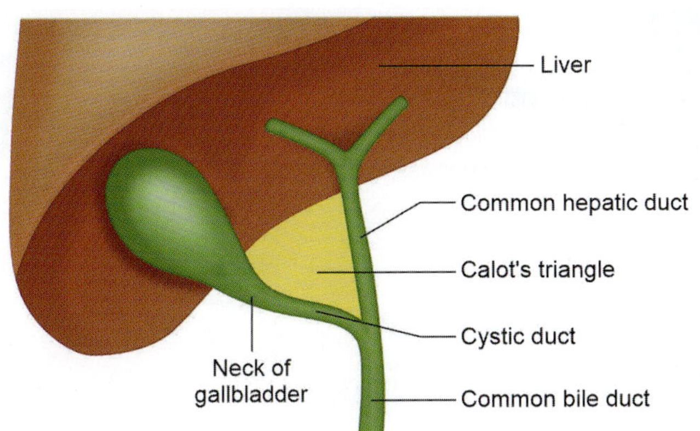

Fig. 5: Calot's triangle.

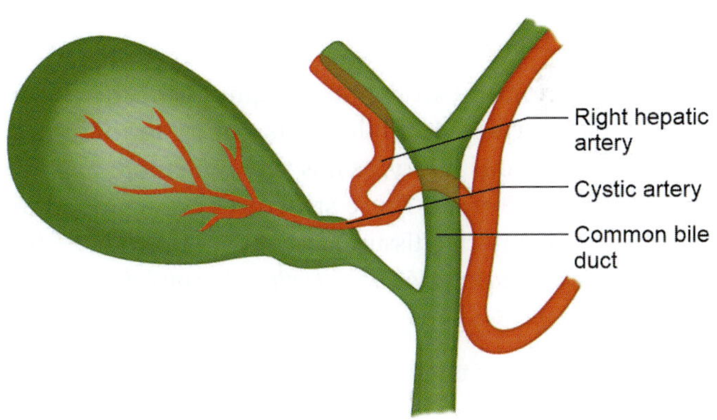

Fig. 6: Moynihan hump.

CYSTIC PLATE

It lies in GB fossa in the liver, continues with the capsule of liver. It is exposed during cholecystectomy, critical view of safety.

R4U LINE

It is an imaginary line from the roof of the Rouviere's sulcus to the base of segment 4 of the liver. This line is a safety line during dissection for cholecystectomy. It separates the safe and danger zones during dissection. The safe zone lies above this line, and the danger zone lies below this line. Rouviere's sulcus—segment 4 of liver—umbilical fissure **(Fig. 7)**.

ROUVIERE'S SULCUS

It is a cleft from the right side of the liver hilum to segment 1 of the liver. It is normally 2–3 cm long and contains the portal triad. It indicates the plane of CBD.

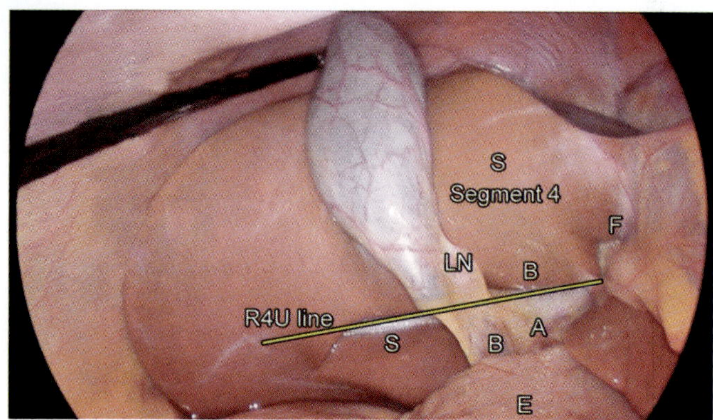

Fig. 7: R4U line. B: Bile duct, base segment 4; S: Sulcus Rouviere, segment 4; A: Artery hepatic; F: Fissure umbilical; E: Enteric structure (duodenum/stomach).

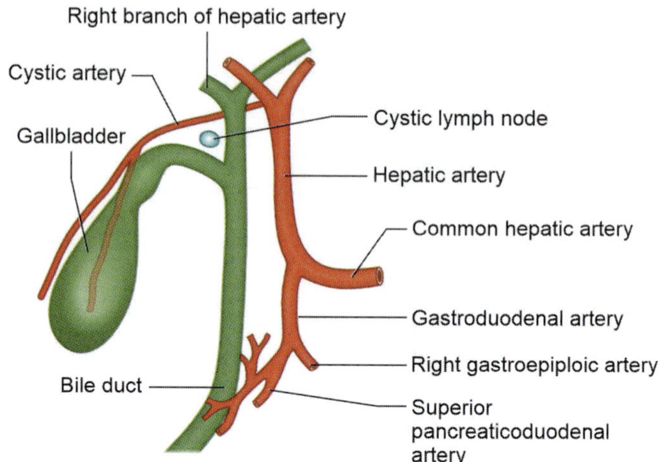

Fig. 8: Arterial supply of biliary tree.

PORTAL TRIAD

It is a collection of extrahepatic segments of the portal vein, hepatic artery, and bile ducts. Injury to the portal triad is a dangerous injury, as it is very difficult to manage such traumatic events. These structures are wrapped up in a sleeve of connected tissue. *Mnemonic—DAVE—D = bile ducts, A = hepatic artery, V = portal veins, E = epiploic foramen.*

Charcot's triad

It is a combination of three clinical features in cholangitis:
1. Intermittent pain
2. Intermittent jaundice
3. Intermittent fever

ARTERIAL SUPPLY OF BILIARY APPARATUS (FIG. 8)

- The cystic artery is the main source of blood supply.
- Branches from the posterior superior pancreaticoduodenal artery.
- Right hepatic artery.
- Accessory cystic artery, a branch of the common hepatic artery.

VENOUS DRAINAGE OF BILIARY APPARATUS

- Tributaries of the hepatic veins
- Cystic veins
- Portal vein

NERVE SUPPLY

Cystic Plexus of Nerves

Parasympathetic nerves supply the muscles of the GB and ducts. It is inhibitory to the sphincters. Sympathetic nerves, from T7 to T9, are vasomotor and motor to the sphincters.

Pain travels from GB through vagus to the stomach, through sympathetic nerves to the inferior angle of the right scapula and through phrenic nerve to right shoulder.

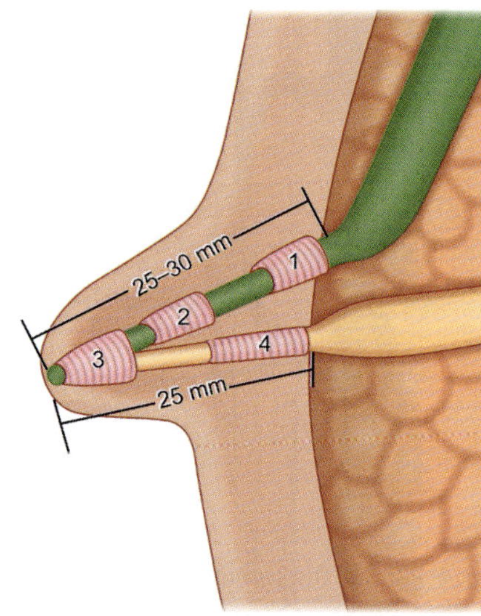

Fig. 9: Sphincter of Oddi: (1) Upper sphincter choledochus, (2) lower sphincter choledochus, (3) sphincter ampullae, and (4) pancreatic sphincter.

SPHINCTER OF ODDI

It has three sphincters **(Fig. 9)**:
1. At the end of the bile duct (sphincter choledochus), divided into the upper and lower sphincter choledochus.
2. At the end of the pancreatic duct (pancreatic sphincter).
3. Around the ampulla (sphincter ampullae).

LYMPHATIC DRAINAGE OF THE GALLBLADDER

Subserosal and submucosal lymphatics drain into the lymph node of Lund (Fred Bates Lund, American Surgeon, 1865–1950) or the lymph node of Mascagni (Paolo Mascagni, Italian physician and anatomist, 1755–1815), at the fork made by the CHD and cystic duct. From the lymph node of Lund, lymph goes to the liver and the celiac lymph nodes. Subserosal lymphatics join subcapsular lymphatics of the liver, and carcinoma of the GB spreads to the liver through this route **(Fig. 10)**.

FUNCTIONS OF THE GALLBLADDER

Bile is formed in the liver and stored in the GB **(Fig. 11)**.

- Stores bile
- Concentration of bile (5–10 times)
- Secretion of mucus (20 mL/day)

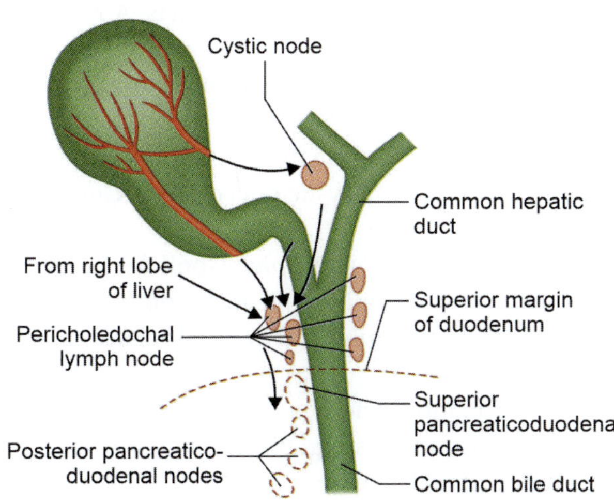

Fig. 10: Lymphatic drainage of the gallbladder.

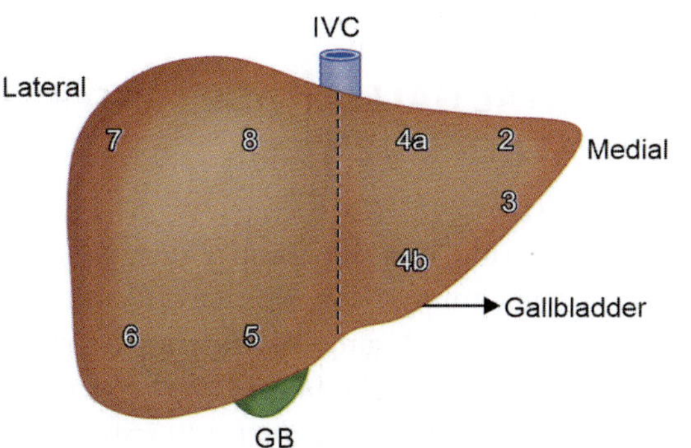

Fig. 11: Gallbladder and liver lobes 4b and 5 (Couinaud segments: Functional division).

COUINAUD SEGMENTS

The Couinaud classification divides the liver into eight separate segments each having own branch of bile duct, hepatic artery, and portal vein (Claude Couinaud, 1922–2008, French Surgeon and anatomist, first to describe segmental anatomy of liver).

CHOLEDOCHOLITHIASIS

Stones in the bile ducts are 90% gallstones, and 10% stones form in the CBD.

Clinical Features

Common bile duct stones may remain asymptomatic or present with symptoms of pain, jaundice, and fever *(Charcot's triad) and Reynold's pentad.* CBD stones can cause complete obstruction of the CBD, leading to obstructive jaundice.

Investigation

- Magnetic resonance cholangiopancreatography (MRCP)
- Endoscopic ultrasound (EUS)

Treatment

- Stone detected before laparoscopic cholecystectomy—laparoscopic cholecystectomy after endoscopic retrograde cholangiopancreatography (ERCP).
- Stone detected during laparoscopic cholecystectomy—laparoscopic exploration and removal of CBD stone + T-tube insertion **(Figs. 12 and 13)**—If residual

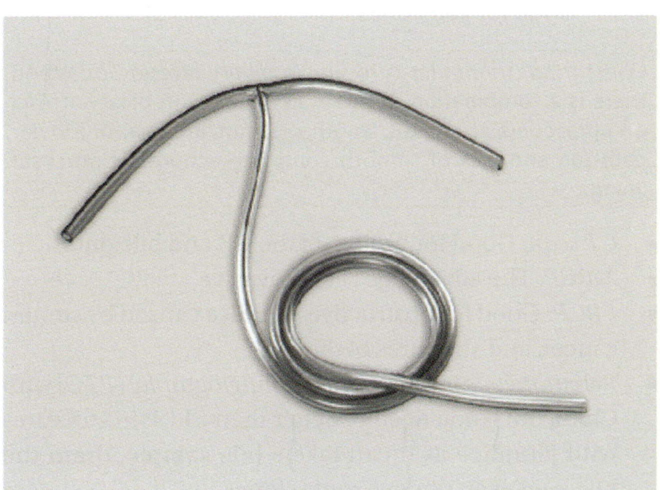

Fig. 12: T-tube.

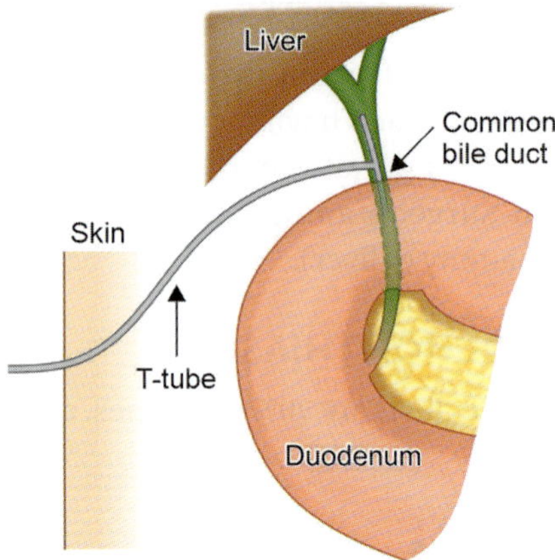

Fig. 13: Placement of T-tube.

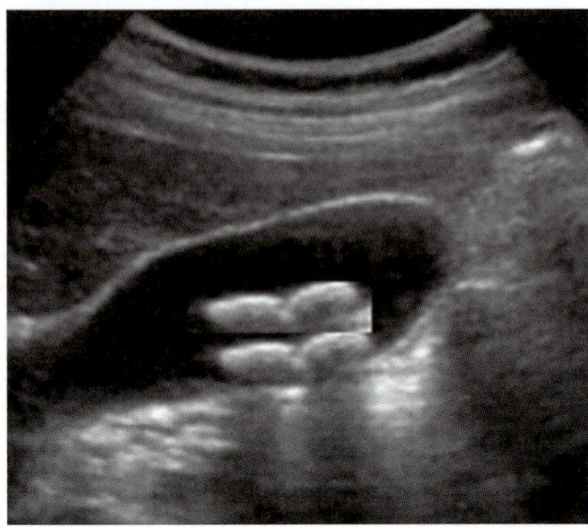

Fig. 14: Ultrasound of abdomen for gallstones.

stones—Burhenne technique (removal of stones by choledochoscope)

- Stones detected after laparoscopic cholecystectomy—ERCP + sphincterotomy

INVESTIGATIONS IN GALLBLADDER DISEASE

- *Plain X-ray*:
  - 10% radiopaque
  - 90% radiolucent
  - Gas in the center of the stones shows a Mercedes-Benz or seagull sign
  - Porcelain GB—calcified GB—5% develop carcinoma—cholecystectomy is the treatment
- *Ultrasonography* ***(Fig. 14)***:
  - Transabdominal
  - EUS
  - Good for gallstones

> *Ghost triad (triangular cord sign in biliary atresia GB)*: When there is a combination of three GB features on biliary atresia on ultrasound, atretic GB, length <19 mm, irregular or lobular contour, and lack of smooth/complete echogenic mucosal lining.

- *CT scan:* Good for tumors of the GB and bile ducts.
- *MRCP:* The advantage is noninvasive.
- *ERCP:* Good for obstructive jaundice caused by stones, cancer, and strictures of the CBD.
- *Percutaneous transhepatic cholangiography (PTC)* with Chiba or Okuda needle. Better than ERCP in strictures with jaundice as it can take a bile sample, drain the bile, and even remove some stones.
  - Intraoperative cholangiogram is the gold standard for diagnosis of acute cholecystitis [hepatobiliary iminodiacetic acid (HIDA) also known as cholescintigraphy or hepatobiliary scintigraphy. It is for the liver, GB, and bile ducts. A radioactive tracer is injected.
- *Preoperative cholangiography* through the cystic duct contract is injected.
- *Choledochoscopy*: During the operation an endoscope is passed through the cystic duct or CBD. Good for the removal of stones.
- *Laparoscopic ultrasonography*: Good for biliary and pancreatic tumors for identification and staging.
- *Oral cholecystography (OCG)*: It is also called as Graham-Cole test.
  - Dye—iopanoic acid
  - Dye in IV cholecystography is biligraffin
  - OCG is of no value in:
    - Intestinal malabsorption
    - Obstruction jaundice
    - Hepatic failure
    - Vomiting

CONGENITAL GALLBLADDER AND BILE DUCTS ABNORMALITIES

- *Agenesis of GB*
- *Phrygian cap* (like hats of people of Phrygia, an ancient country in Asia minor)—in 5% cases **(Figs. 15 and 16)**.
- *Floating GB*—the GB hangs on the mesentery
- *Low insertion of cystic duct* + on CBD
- *Accessory cholecystohepatic duct*—directly from the GB to the liver, must be identified and closed in surgery.

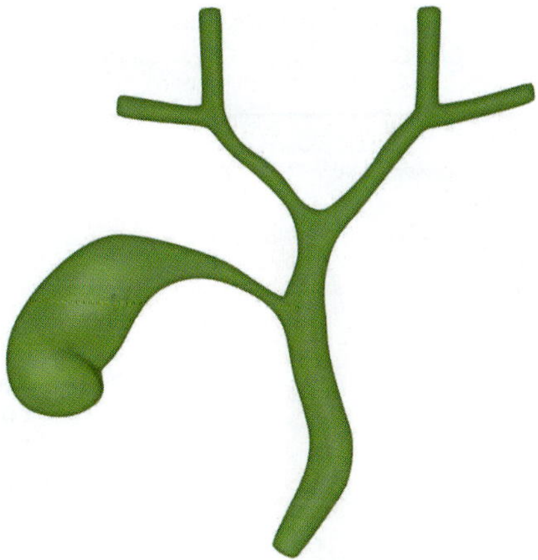

Fig. 15: Phrygian cap gallbladder.

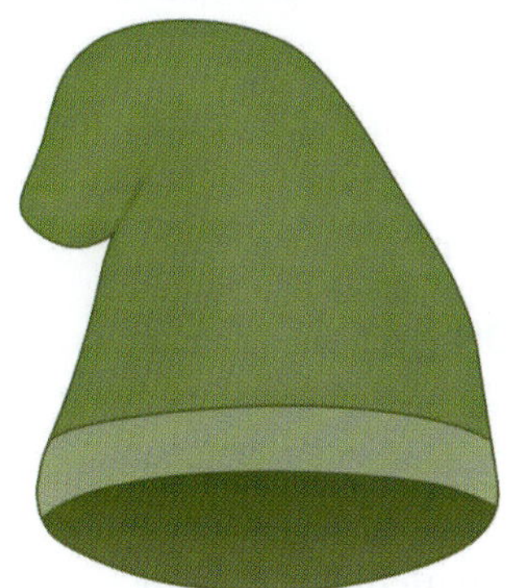

Fig. 16: Phrygian cap.

- *Caroli's disease* (Jacques Caroli, a French Gastroenterologist) congenital dilatation of intrahepatic ducts.
  - Limited disease—resection of the liver
  - Diffuse disease—liver transplant
- *Choledochal cyst*:
  - Diagnosed by US/magnetic resonance imaging (MRI)/MRCP/CT
  - Increased risk of cholangiocarcinoma

Choledochal Cyst

It is a dilatation of part of the biliary tree, which leads to infection and poor drainage of bile, causing jaundice. There is a 10% risk of cholangiocarcinoma.

Types of Choledochal Cysts (Todani Classification) (Fig. 17)

- *Type I* fusiform—most common
- *Type II* diverticulum of CBD, within the duodenum
- *Type III* dilatation

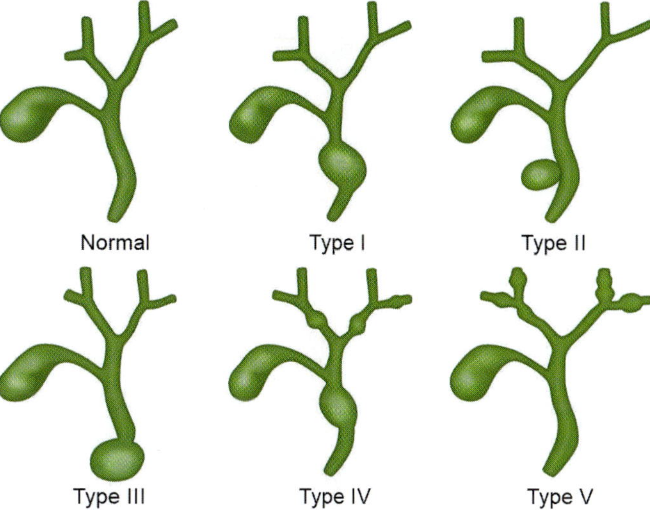

Fig. 17: Types of choledochal cysts.

- *Type IV*:
  - Multiple dilatation both intra- and extrahepatic
  - Multiple dilatations only extrahepatic
- *Type V*—only intrahepatic multiple dilatation called Caroli's disease

Clinical Presentation

- Fever
- Jaundice
- Pain
- Right hypochondrial mass

  Treatment is the excision of cyst.

> *Risk factors of cholangiocarcinoma:*
> - Choledocal cyst
> - Obesity
> - Diabetes
> - Hepatitis B virus (HBV)/hepatitis C virus (HCV)
> - Thorotrast—a radioactive material used as contrast.
> - Abnormal pancreaticobiliary duct junction (APBDJ)
> - Sclerosing cholangitis

Cholangiocarcinoma

It is a carcinoma of the bile ducts.

Clinical Features

- Obstructive jaundice and CBD tumor.
- Klatskin tumor—hilar cholangiocarcinoma.

Investigation

- MRCP

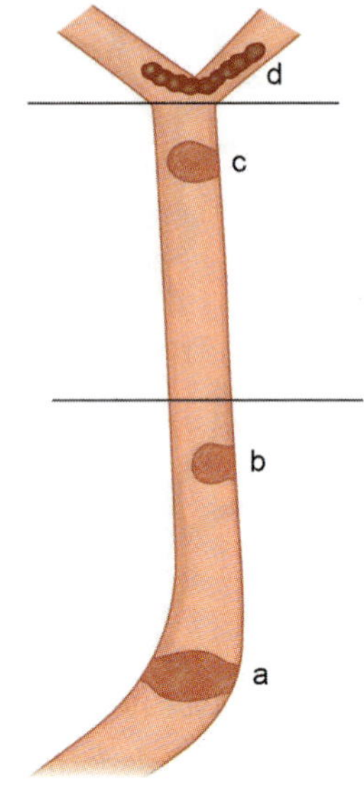

Fig. 18: Resectable treatment.

TABLE 1: Difference between hemobilia and bilhemia.

	Hemobilia (biliary tree bleeding)	***Bilhemia (bile leaks into blood vessels)***
Cause	Post-ERCP and trauma	Post-ERCP and trauma
Symptoms	Pain, jaundice, melena	Jaundice
Investigation	CT angiography	ERCP
Treatment	Self-limiting	ERCP + stenting
	Can lead to death if it reaches lungs	Can lead to liver abscess and cholangiocarcinoma

Treatment

- Resectable—distal CBD (Whipple's operation), supraduodenal CBD (choledochojejunostomy), CHD (hepaticojejunostomy), and Klatskin tumor (portoenterostomy) **(Fig. 18)**
- Nonresectable palliative treatment—ERCP + stenting **(Table 1)**

EXTRAHEPATIC BILIARY ATRESIA

- 1 in 12,000 births
- If untreated, death before 3 years of age due to liver failure
- Type I is restricted to CBD
- Type II atresia of CHD
- Type III atresia of CHD right and left hepatic ducts

Clinical Features

- Jaundice at birth

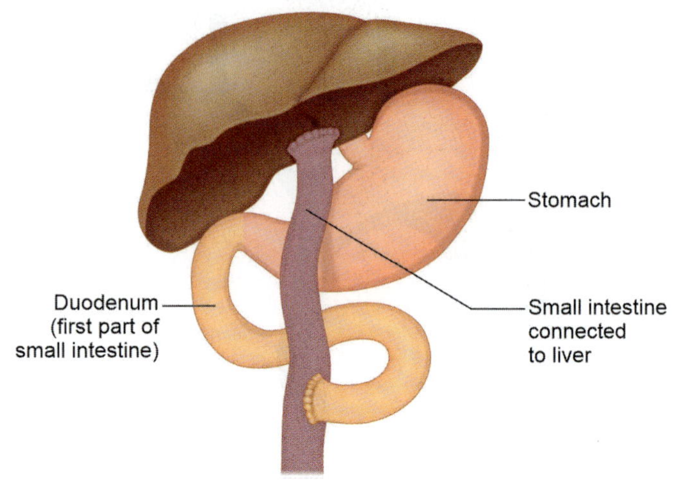

Fig. 19: Kasai operation.

- Liver function test (LFT) derailed as in obstructive jaundice
- Pruritus

Differential Diagnosis

Neonatal hepatitis.

Treatment

- Roux-en-Y hepaticojejunostomy
- Kasai operation (Roux-en-Y of jejunum to exposed area of liver after excision of all bile ducts up to capsule of liver **(Fig. 19)**

SPHINCTER OF ODDI DYSFUNCTION

It is of two types:

1. Biliary
2. Pancreatic

   Both are of three types, types I, II, and III.

Milwaukee classification of sphincter of Oddi dysfunction (SOD) is presented in **Table 2**.

GALLSTONES

Types of Gallstones (Fig. 20)

Cholesterol		***Pigment***	
Pure	***Mixed***	***Black***	***Brown***
10%	70%	15–20%	15–20%
(Mixed stones are actually 80–90%)			
• Single		• Multiple	
• Large			
• Yellow	• Yellow	• Green	• Black

TABLE 2: Milwaukee classification.

	Biliary type SOD	*Pancreatic type SOD*
Type I	• Biliary type pain • Dilated CBD (>12 mm in diameter) • Enzymes two times • Prolonged biliary drainage time (>45 minutes)	• Pancreatic-type pain • Dilated pancreatic duct (increased to 6 mm) • Amylase two times • Prolonged pancreatic drainage time (>9 minutes)
Type II	Biliary type pain +1 or 2 above features	Pancreatic-type pain One or two above features
Type III	Biliary type pain only	Pancreatic-type pain only

(CBD: common bile duct; SOD: sphincter of Oddi dysfunction)

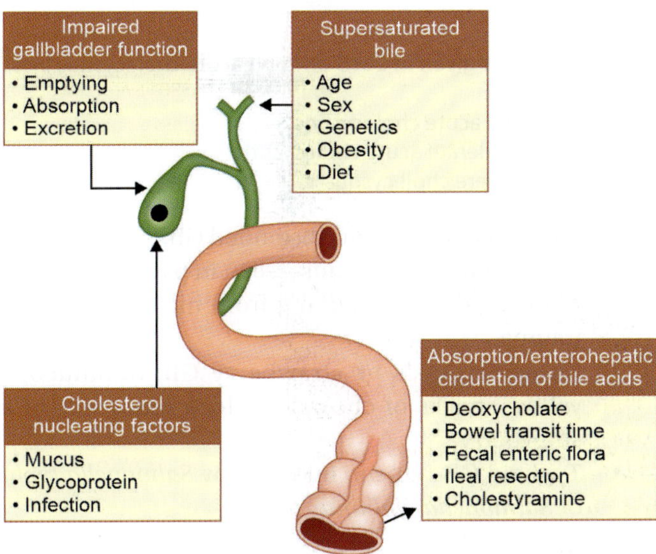

Fig. 20: Formation of gallbladder stones.

- Lithogenic bile
- Stasis
- Nucleation

Bile acids and phospholipid—lecithin micelles with cholesterol

Factors Necessary for Stone Formation

Any mechanism which increases the cholesterol in bile, or decreases bile acids (salts) or lecithin makes the bile supersaturated or lithogenic.

Factors Increasing Biliary Cholesterol

- Obesity
- High calorie and cholesterol rich diet
- Clofibrate therapy

Factors Decreasing Bile Acids

- Primary biliary cirrhosis.
- Oral contraceptives
- Genetic factors—*CYPTAI* gene

Cholesterol stones are made of crystalline cholesterol monohydrate **(Figs. 21A to C)**.

Black stones are made up of:

- Insoluble bilirubin pigment polymer
- Calcium phosphate
- Calcium bicarbonate

Brown stones are made up of:

- Calcium bilirubinate
- Calcium palmitate
- Calcium stearate
- Cholesterol

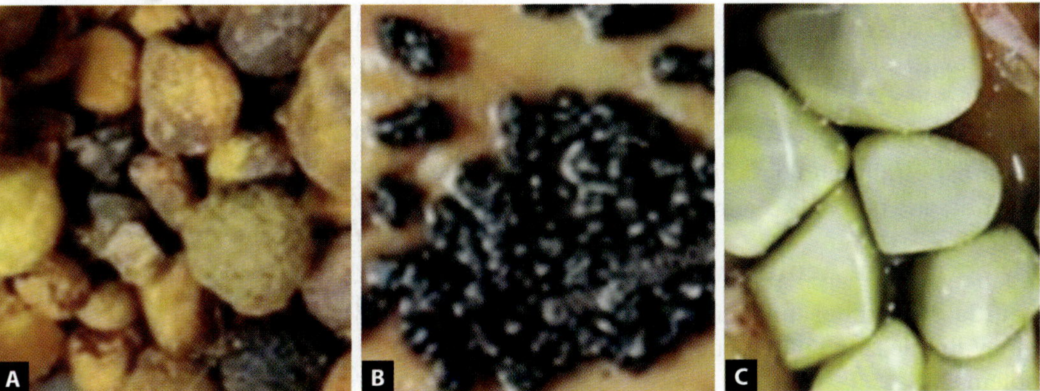

Figs. 21A to C: Brown, pigment, and mixed gallbladder stones.

Gallstones affect 10–15% of the European population. It is about 4.3% in India.

Cholesterol is insoluble in water and is formed by the liver. The liver excretes bile approximately 40 mL/h. Micelles formed by phospholipids hold cholesterol when the bile is supersaturated with cholesterol or bile acid concentration is low, cholesterol crystals are formed, and stones may form.

Clinical Presentation

- Asymptomatic
- *Symptomatic*:
  - Pain in right hypogastrium and epigastrium
  - Dyspepsia
  - Flatulence
  - Nausea and vomiting
  - Biliary colic
  - Jaundice
  - Ileus

Complications of Gallbladder Stones

- Pain—biliary colic
- Acute cholecystitis
- Chronic cholecystitis
- Empyema mucocele
- Perforation
- Biliary obstruction
- Acute cholangitis
- Acute pancreatitis
- Gallstone ileus

A painless palpably enlarged gallbladder accompanied with mild jaundice is unlikely to be caused by gall stones.

—Courvoisier's Law, 1890

(Ludwig Courvoisier, 1843–1918, Professor of Surgery, Basle, Switzerland)

Complications of Gallstones

Gallstones usually cause severe pain as biliary colic, but can also cause some other problems, which may prove serious. GB surgery is done specially to remove the chances of complications, especially cholecystitis, obstructive jaundice, pancreatitis, and probably carcinoma of the GB.

Differential Diagnosis of Acute Cholecystitis

Acute cholecystitis sometimes becomes difficult to diagnose as it may mimic some of the common painful abdominal problems.

- *Common abdominal painful problems*:
  - Acute pancreatitis
  - Perforated duodenal or gastric peptic ulcer
  - Acute appendicitis
- *Uncommon problems*:
  - Pneumonia—right lower lobe
  - Myocardial infraction
  - Acute pyelonephritis

Diagnosis

- History
- *Physical examination*:
  - Tenderness in right upper quadrant (RUQ) of abdomen
  - Murphy's sign
  - Mass
  - Palpable and nontender GB

Tokyo consensus guidelines for severity grading of acute cholecystitis was given in 2018 dividing acute cholecystitis into three categories:
1. *Grade I*—mild acute cholecystitis
2. *Grade II*—moderate acute cholecystitis
3. *Grade III*—severe cholecystitis

- Empyema of GB—pus distended GB.
- A calculous cholecystitis—seen in patients who are critically ill or recovering from major surgery or trauma.
- Cholesterolosis or strawberry GB. Submucous yellow specks of cholesterol look like seeds of a strawberry.
- Typhoid GB—due to infection by *Salmonella typhi* or *Salmonella typhimurium*.

Treatment

- *Cholecystectomy*:
  - Open
  - Laparoscopic

Critical View of Safety

The most important part of dissection in laparoscopic cholecystectomy is proper dissection at Calot's triangle and clearly dissecting out the structures here and their identification. According to the critical view of safety cystic artery and cystic duct are clipped separately, and then the GB is removed **(Fig. 22)**.

Types of Cholecystectomy as Per Time

- Early cholecystectomy within 2–3 days.
- Delayed or interval cholecystectomy 6–8 weeks after.

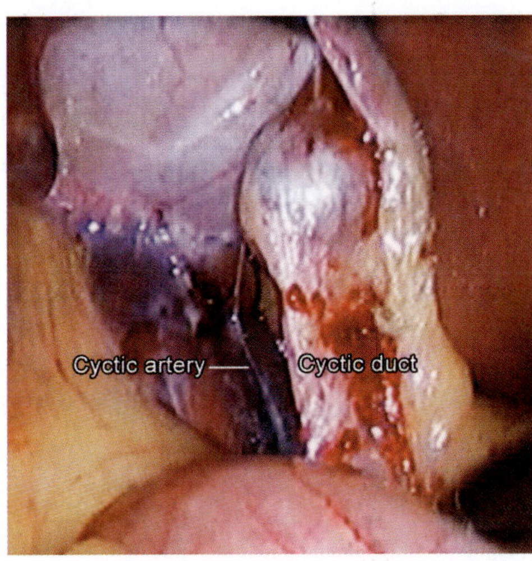

Fig. 22: Critical view of safety.

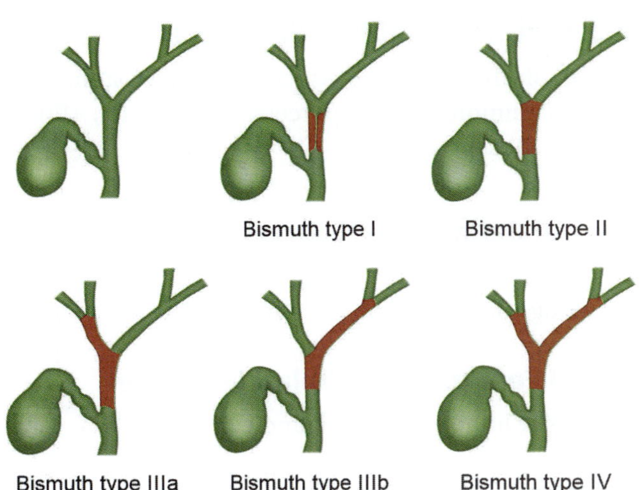

Fig. 23: Bismuth classification of stricture of the bile duct.

- Emergency for empyema, emphysema, and perforation of the GB.

> Partial and subtotal cholecystectomy when Calot's triangle structures are having adhesions and cannot be identified.

Indications for Choledochotomy

- History of jaundice
- History of cholangitis
- Palpable CBD stones
- CBD dilated—above 6 mm
- Raised alkaline phosphatase

Complications of Cholecystectomy

- *Infection*:
  - In 10–15% of cases.
  - Operative mortality is <1%.
- Bleeding
- Bile leak
- Biliary duct injury (0.5%)
- Cholangitis
- Late choledocholithiasis

> *What to do if Calot's triangle is found frozen?*
> It is difficult to proceed in such situations, so either abort the cholecystectomy or convert to open and do cholecystectomy or subtotal cholecystectomy as a bailout procedure. Nigam's Classification of Subtotal Cholecystectomy According to the Level of Resection (NCSC-LR) classifies the subtotal cholecystectomies in three categories, level 1: Resection through lower part of the body of gallbladder, level 2: Resection through the infundibulum, and level 3: Resection through the neck. NCSC-LR is important in late development of post-operative complications.

Choledochotomy

A longitudinal cut is made in the CBD, and a "T" tube is inserted.

STRUCTURE OF BILE DUCT

Biliary strictures produce obstruction or impedance in the flow of bile in the biliary tree and may also lead to complete obstruction. The most common cause of biliary stricture is injury of the bile ducts during the operation of removal of the GB **(Fig. 23)**.

PRIMARY SCLEROSING CHOLANGITIS

Idiopathic fibrosing inflammatory conditions of intra- and extrabiliary ducts.

TUMORS OF BILE DUCTS

- Benign tumors
- Malignant tumor

Treatment

- 10–15%—suitable for resection
- 85–90%—liver transplant (without distant metastasis)
- After resection, 35% survived for 5 years

GALLBLADDER CANCER

- 9–10% of all biliary diseases, more in north India than south India
- More in females
- Risk factors include chronic cholecystitis, gallstones, and calcification of the GB (porcelain GB)

Risk Factors of Gallbladder Cancer

- 90% of GB cancers are associated with GB stones.
- It is commonly seen in porcelain gallbladder, APBDJ, and GB polyps.

Types of Gallbladder Cancer

Adenocarcinoma—infiltrating, nodular, and papillary. Infiltrating adenocarcinoma is most dangerous.

Clinical Features of Gallbladder Cancer

Gallbladder lump, pain, and jaundice.

Spread of Gallbladder Cancer

- Direct—liver
- Lymphatic—subserosal lymphatics—liver
- Hematogenous—liver and lung

Investigation in Gallbladder Cancer

- Contrast-enhanced computed tomography (CECT)
- Fine-needle aspiration cytology (FNAC)
- Biopsy

Staging of Gallbladder Cancer

Staging of GB cancer is presented in **Table 3**.

TABLE 3: 8th AJCC (2017) TNM classification of carcinoma gallbladder.

T1a	Lamina propria invasion
T1b	Muscular invasion
T2	Invade the perimuscular connective tissue: • *T2a*: Invade the perimuscular connective tissue on the peritoneal side with no extension to serosa • *T2b*: Invade the perimuscular connective tissue on the hepatic side with no extension into the liver
T3	Serosal perforation and/or direct invasion of the liver (regardless of extent) and/or invasion of any other single extrahepatic organ
T4	Tumor invades the main portal vein, hepatic artery, or two or more extrahepatic organs
N1	Metastasis to one to three regional nodes
N2	Metastasis to four or more regional nodes
M1	Distant metastasis

(AJCC: American Joint Committee on Cancer; TNM: tumor, node, and metastasis)

Treatment

- Hepatectomy
- Advanced disease—metastasis—palliative treatment

Structures removed in radical en bloc resection of GB:

- Segmental or extended liver resection
- GB
- Bile ducts
- Regional lymph nodes

Predisposing Factors for Cholesterol Gallstone Formation

- Loss of weight
- Obesity
- By birth (genetic)
- Stasis
- Therapy—clofibrate
- Estrogen
- Reduced bile acid secretion
- Reduced phospholipid secretion
- Increasing age

Predisposing Factors for Pigment Stones

- Genetic
- Hemolysis
- Cirrhosis
- Pernicious anemia
- Chronic infection of the biliary tract
- Increasing age
- Ileal resection
- Cystic fibrosis

Important Signs of Acute Cholecystitis

- *Murphy's sign or Naunyn's sign*—inspiratory arrest with deep palpation in the RUQ.
- *Boas sign*—Hyperesthesia below the scapula.

Historical Milestones in Gallbladder Disease

- In 1985, the first laparoscopic cholecystectomy was done by German Surgeon Erich Müle.
- Carl Johann August Langenbuch, a German physician, performed the first cholecystectomy in 1882.
- Gallstones were found in the mummy of Princess Amentum of Thebes, dating back 1500 BCE.

Rigler's Triad—a Radiological Sign

- Small bowel obstruction (SBO)

- Pneumobilia (presence of gas in the biliary system)
- Atypical mineral shadow

Rx—laparotomy and enterotomy without ruling out stone.

Bouveret's Syndrome

Duodenal obstruction by gallstones
Rx—duodenostomy

Important indications of cholecystectomy in asymptomatic gall stones:
- Solitary large stone, >3 cm due to risk of cancer
- Multiple stones chances of CBD obstruction
- Signs of adenomyomatosis of GB (overgrowth of mucosa) on ultrasound
- Comet tail artifacts
- No chance of malignancy

Adenomatous Polyps of the Gallbladder

- These are the most common benign tumors of the GB.
- If bigger than 2 cm, almost always cancerous.

Emphysematous Gallbladder

It is caused by *Clostridium welchii.*

Mirizzi Syndrome (Fig. 24)

- Biliary obstruction due to an impacted stone in Hartmann's pouch or the cystic duct.
- Type I—compression at CHD
- Type II—stone erodes into CHD
- Causing cholecystocholedochal fistulas

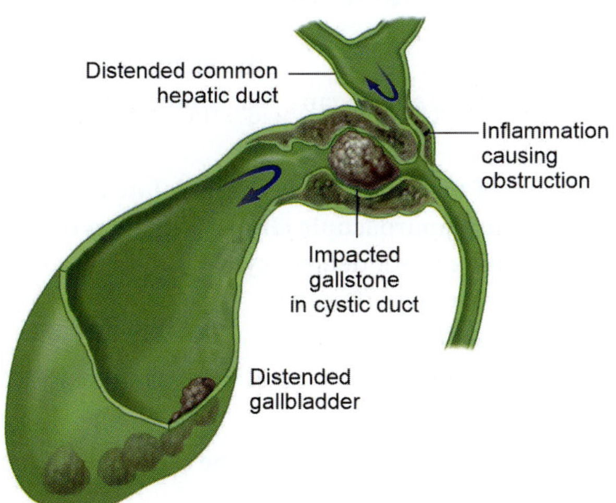

Fig. 24: Mirizzi syndrome.

Management of Gallbladder Cancer

- TIa stage—simple cholecystectomy
- Stage Ib, II, early stage III—extended cholecystectomy
- Stage IV—palliative therapy

Common Risk Factor for Carcinoma Gallbladder (90% of Carcinomas have GB Stones)

- Adenomatous polyp
- Choledochal cyst
- Porcelain GB

5-Year Survival Rate after Resection in Gallbladder Carcinoma

- *T1*—85-100%
- *T2*—80-98%
- *T3*—15-63%
- *T4*—2-25%

Treatment of Choice for Common Bile Duct Stone

Endoscopic retrograde cholangiopancreatography + sphincterotomy + stone removal.

CHOLANGITIS

- Ascending bacterial infection of bile ducts causes:
  - Gallstones
  - Strictures
  - Instrumentation
  - Parasites
  - Organism
  - *Escherichia coli*
- Cholangitis may progress to *Reynold's pentad (Charcot's triad + shock + mental status alteration).*
- ERCP is the gold standard to diagnose CBD stones.

Pregnancy and Cholelithiasis

During pregnancy, GB stones are formed due to increased cholesterol secretion and delayed GB emptying due to low bile acid secretion.

- *First trimester*—conservative treatment
- *Second trimester*—laparoscopic cholecystectomy
- *Third trimester*—conservative treatment

BILE DUCT INJURY

Laparoscopic cholecystectomy is the gold standard procedure for gallstones, acute and chronic cholecystitis in today's time, but this procedure has increased the incidence of bile duct injuries. Bile duct injuries should be managed properly and cautiously so as not to get in serious complications of this event.

Strasberg Classification of Bile Duct Injuries (Fig. 25)

- *Type A*—cystic duct leak
- *Type B*—injury to the sectoral duct with no bile leak
- *Type C*—injury to the sectoral duct with bile leak
- *Type D*—lateral injury to major bile ducts
- *Type E*—circumferential injury to major bile ducts
- *Type E is divided into:*
    - *Type E1*—low CHD stricture
    - *Type E2*—proximal CHD stricture
    - *Type E3*—hilar stricture, no CHD, and confluence of hepatic duct present
    - *Type E4*—hilar stricture, no CHD, confluence of hepatic duct not present
    - *Type E5*—stricture of CHD with involvement of the aberrant right sectoral hepatic duct

Treatment of Bile Duct Injuries

Repair of CBD/CHD/other bile duct injury
Duct < 3 cm—repair
>3 cm—repair/T-tube
Other—Roux-en-Y hepaticojejunostomy, Roux-en-Y choledochojejunostomy

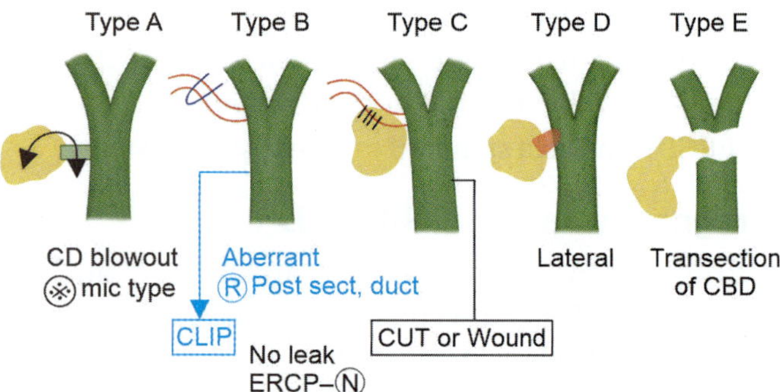

Fig. 25: Strasberg classification of bile duct injuries. (CBD: common bile duct; CD: cystic duct; ERCP: endoscopic retrograde cholangiopancreatography)

Postcholecystectomy Cystic Duct Bile Leak

- Conservative with the drain
- ERCP with stenting

SOME IMPORTANT QUESTIONS

Q1. All of the following are essential for the formation of gallstones, *except*:

a. Bile stasis
b. Nucleation
c. Crystallization
d. Lithogenic bile

Ans. c

Q2. The true color of cholesterol stone is:

a. Black
b. Brown
c. Dark yellow
d. Pale yellow

Ans. d

Q3. Best investigative modality for the gallbladder (GB):

a. Oral cholangiography (OCG)
b. Percutaneous transhepatic cholangiogram (PTC)
c. Ultrasound (USG)
d. Intravenous cholangiogram

Ans. c

Q4. About gallstones, false is:

a. Intervention should be done if gallstones are present in the bile duct, irrespective of the duct diameter
b. Operation should be done in most cases
c. Can be caused due to parasitic infestation
d. Can lead to cholecystitis

Ans. b

Q5. Indications of prophylactic cholecystectomy are all, *except*:

a. Diabetes
b. Hemoglobinopathy
c. Gallstone size >3 cm
d. Porcelain GB

Ans. a

Q6. Which of the following is the absolute contraindication for laparoscopic cholecystectomy?

a. Clotting factor deficiency
b. Perforation peritonitis
c. Empyema of the GB
d. Adhesions

Ans. a

Q7. Acalculous cholecystitis can be seen in all, *except*:

a. Dengue hemorrhagic fever
b. Malaria

c. Leptospirosis
d. Enteric fever

Ans. b

Q8. Indications of cholecystectomy in GB polyp removal are all, *except*:
a. Size >1 cm b. With stone
c. >3 in number d. Locally invasive

Ans. c

Q9. True about CA, GB, and gallstones:
a. 3% association b. 30% association
c. 50% association d. 90% association

Ans. d

Q10. All are risk factors for CA GB, *except*:
a. Adenomyosis
b. Anomalous pancreaticobiliary ductal junction (ABPDJ)
c. Gallstones
d. Adenomatous polyps

Ans. a

Q11. True about CA GB:
a. T1a can be treated and cured by laparoscopic cholecystectomy
b. T1b needs radical operation in all cases
c. Port site metastasis is a localized disease
d. Preoperative diagnosis of CA GB has different survival rates according to stage

Ans. a

Q12. What is the most common GB malignancy?
a. Adenocarcinoma
b. Squamous cell carcinoma
c. Mucinous cystadenocarcinoma
d. Serous cystadenocarcinoma

Ans. a

Q13. Bleeding adjacent to the "triangle of Calot" should be controlled by:
a. Pressing the artery manually
b. Blind clipping
c. Kocher's artery forceps
d. Stitching

Ans. a

Q14. Pain at the tip of the shoulder is due to all, *except*:
a. Peptic ulcer b. Pancreatitis
c. Cholecystitis d. Appendicitis

Ans. d

Q15. Abdominal pain, fever, and jaundice. This triad is known as:
a. Charcot's triad b. Saint's triad
c. Virchow triad d. Reynold's triad

Ans. a

Q16. 3 days after cholecystectomy, the patient developed severe abdominal pain with fever. Her liver function test (LFT) was normal, serum amylase was also normal. What is the most likely cause of her condition?
a. Bile leak b. CBD stone
c. Acute pancreatitis d. Liver abscess

Ans. a

Q17. A lady was incidentally diagnosed with a 0.5 cm solid mass in her GB on USG, which was nonmobile, diagnosed as a GB polyp. She is asymptomatic. What is the next step in the management?
a. Reassure the patient and follow-up
b. Laparoscopic cholecystectomy
c. Open cholecystectomy
d. Contrast-enhanced computed tomography (CECT) abdomen

Ans. a

Q18. What do you expect from a lady after GB removal, most commonly?
a. Weight loss b. Steatorrhea
c. High cholesterol d. Hypoglycemia

Ans. b

Q19. A patient has a USG finding of a gallstone abutting the cystic duct with dilatation of the common hepatic duct. What is the most likely diagnosis?
a. Acute cholecystitis b. Porcelain GB
c. GB polyp d. Mirizzi syndrome

Ans. d

Q20. Cholesterol gallstones are made up of:
a. Crystalline cholesterol monohydrate
b. Crystalline cholesterol dehydrate
c. Amorphous cholesterol monohydrate
d. Amorphous cholesterol dehydrate

Ans. a

Q21. Gallstones do not contain:
a. Oxalate b. Cholesterol
c. Phosphate d. Carbonate

Ans. a

Q22. The predominant constituent of the pale yellow gallstones in the GB is:

a. Mucin glycoprotein
b. Calcium carbonate
c. Cholesterol
d. Calcium phosphate

Ans. c

Q23. Which is true about gallstones?

a. Pigment stones are the most common
b. Bacterial nidus of infection may be seen
c. Even if an asymptomatic GB should be removed
d. They are mostly solitary

Ans. b

Q24. Mercedes–Benz sign or Seagull sign is seen in:

a. Gallstones
b. Renal stones
c. CBD stones
d. Hydatid cyst

Ans. a

Q25. Which of the following is a contraindication for medical management of gallstones?

a. Radiopaque stones
b. Radioluscent stones
c. Normal functioning GB
d. Small stones

Ans. a

Q26. Which of the following is not an indication for cholecystectomy?

a. GB polyp with stone
b. Asymptomatic polyp >1 cm
c. Multiple GB polyps
d. Symptomatic GB polyps

Ans. c

Q27. Contraindications of laparoscopic cholecystectomy are:

a. Coagulopathy
b. Obstructive pulmonary disease
c. End-stage liver disease
d. All of the above

Ans. d

Q28. Laparoscopic cholecystectomy is largely preferred for all of the following reasons to conventional laparotomy, *except*:

a. Decrease pain
b. Decreased incidence of bile duct injuries
c. Smaller scar
d. Decreased stay in hospital

Ans. b

Q29. Cholesterolosis is:

a. Disease of defective metabolism of choline
b. Concerned with epithelial tumors of the brain
c. Diffuse deposition of cholesterol in the mucosa of the GB
d. Disease concerned with obstructive jaundice

Ans. c

Q30. After laparoscopic cholecystectomy, if biopsy reveals in situ cancer of the GB (Stage I), then the appropriate management is:

a. Follow-up
b. Extended cholecystectomy
c. Excision of all port sites
d. Radiotherapy

Ans. a

MULTIPLE CHOICE QUESTIONS

Grade I	*Simple*

Q1. False about brown pigmented stones: **(AIIMS GIS May 2008)**

a. Associated with disorders of biliary motility and associated bacterial infection
b. More common in Caucasians
c. Soft and earthy in texture
d. High content of cholesterol and calcium palmitate

Q2. Gallbladder stone formation is influenced by all, *except*: **(All India 1998)**

a. Clofibrate therapy
b. Hyper alimentation
c. Primary biliary cirrhosis
d. Hypercholesterolemia

Q3. Which among the following does not lead to pigment gallstones? **(PGI June 1999)**

a. Total parenteral nutrition (TPN)
b. Clonorchis sinensis
c. Hemolytic anemia
d. Alcoholic cirrhosis

Q4. A gallstone gets impacted most commonly in which part of the common bile duct? **(JIPMER 1987)**

a. Supraduodenal
b. Retroduodenal
c. Ampulla of Vater
d. Common hepatic duct

Q5. Calculous cholecystitis is associated with all of the following, *except*: (MCI March 2005)

a. Oral contraceptives
b. Estrogen
c. Obesity
d. Diabetes

Q6. Investigation of choice in acute cholecystitis: (PGI Dec 2005)

a. Oral cholecystography (OCG)
b. Hepatobiliary iminodiacetic acid (HIDA) scan
c. Ultrasound (USG)
d. Computed tomography (CT)

Q7. Investigation for assessing proper functioning of the biliary system: (MCI March 2007)

a. USG
b. CT scan
c. HIDA scan
d. All of the above

Q8. Ursodeoxycholic acid is a: (PGI June 95)

a. Urinary stone dissolving drug
b. Thrombolytic drug
c. Gallstone dissolving drug
d. Antifibrinolytic

Q9. All are true about gallstone ileus, *except*: (AIIMS GIS 2003)

a. May be diagnosed with an abdominal X-ray
b. Most common fistula is to duodenum
c. Tumbling obstruction
d. Cholecystectomy should be done in the same episode

Q10. Rigler's triad consists of: (PGI May 2011)

a. Intestinal obstruction
b. Gas in the bile duct
c. Cholangitis
d. Ectopic gallstone
e. Biliary stenosis

Q11. The indications of cholecystectomy are: (PGI Dec 2007)

a. Strawberry gallbladder
b. Mucocele of the gallbladder
c. Gallbladder polyp
d. Asymptomatic gallstone disease
e. Symptomatic cholelithiasis

Q12. Prophylactic cholecystectomy is done in: (AIIMS GIS 2003)

a. Calcified GB
b. Diabetes
c. Asymptomatic gallstones
d. Family history of gallstones

Q13. A 69-year-old male patient having coronary artery disease was found to have gallbladder stones while undergoing a routine USG of the abdomen. There was no history of biliary colic or jaundice at any time. What is the best treatment advice for such a patient for his gallbladder stones? (AIIMS Nov 2003)

a. Open cholecystectomy
b. Laparoscopic cholecystectomy
c. No surgery for gallbladder stones
d. Endoscopic retrograde cholangiopancreatography (ERCP) and removal of gallbladder stones

Q14. The treatment of choice for silent gallbladder stones is: (All India 1997)

a. Observation
b. Chenodeoxycholic acid
c. Cholecystectomy
d. Lithotripsy

Q15. The most common malignancy after cholecystectomy is of: (PGI SS Dec 2005)

a. Colon
b. Stomach
c. Pancreas
d. Ileum

Q16. In cholecystectomy, fresh plasma should be given: (UPPG 2008)

a. Just before the operation
b. At the time of operation
c. 6 hours before operation
d. 12 hours after the operation

Q17. Acalculous cholecystitis are caused by: (PGI Dec 2006)

a. Diabetes mellitus (DM)
b. Total parenteral nutrition (TPN)
c. Leptospirosis
d. Estrogen therapy

Q18. Acute emphysematous cholecystitis is caused by: (JIPMER 2012)

a. *Pseudomonas aeruginosa*
b. *Staphylococcus*
c. *Clostridium perfringens*
d. *Streptococcus pyogenes*

Q19. Precancerous lesions of GB are all, *except*: (AIIMS GIS Dec 2010)

a. Porcelain GB
b. Typhoid carrier
c. ABPDJ
d. Biliary ascariasis

Q20. In a male, after laparoscopic cholecystectomy, a specimen is sent for histopathology, which shows carcinoma gallbladder stage T1a. Appropriate management is: (AIIMS May 2011)

a. Conservative and follow-up
b. Extended cholecystectomy
c. Excision of all port sites
d. Radiotherapy

Q21. Best prognosis in CA GB is seen in: (PGI SS Dec 2009)

a. Papillary
b. Adenocarcinoma
c. Squamous
d. Melanoma

Q22. The most common type of carcinoma gallbladder with gallstones is: (AIIMS Nov 1995)

a. Adenocarcinoma
b. Anaplastic carcinoma
c. Squamous cell carcinoma
d. Transitional cell carcinoma

Q23. The most common association seen in carcinoma gallbladder is: (AIIMS 1991)

a. Peritoneal deposits
b. Duodenal infiltration
c. Secondaries of the liver
d. Cystic node involvement

Q24. Bile is concentrated in the gallbladder to ...... times: (PGI Dec 2006)

a. 5
b. 10
c. 20
d. 50

Q25. Choledochal cyst in intrahepatic biliary tree: (AIIMS Dec 2006)

a. I
b. II
c. IVa
d. IVb

Q26. Caroli's disease is: (AIIMS Dec 2006)

a. Type I choledochal cyst
b. Type III choledochal cyst
c. Type IV choledochal cyst
d. Type V choledochal cyst

Q27. According to Alonso-Lej classification, type IVb is: (JIPMER 2011)

a. Both extra and intrahepatic duct dilatation
b. Extrahepatic duct dilatation
c. Intrahepatic duct dilatation
d. Subhepatic duct dilatation

Q28. Most commonly seen choledochal cyst: (PGI May 2011)

a. Type I
b. Type II
c. Type III
d. Type IVa
e. Type V

Q29. Choledochal cyst: (AIIMS GJS 2003)

a. Resection decreases the incidence of malignancy, but risk persists
b. 80% of cases have stones
c. Treated by Roux-en-Y cystojejunostomy
d. Type IV is most common

Q30. Treatment of choice in choledochal cyst: (AIIMS GJS 2003)

a. Roux-en-Y hepaticojejunostomy
b. Cystojejunostomy
c. Choledochoduodenostomy
d. Choledochojejunostomy

Grade II	***Difficult***

Q1. Lithogenic bile has the following properties: (All India 1996)

a. Above bile and cholesterol ratio
b. Below the bile and cholesterol ratio
c. Equal bile and cholesterol ratio
d. Below cholesterol only

Q2. Incidence of gallstones is high in: (AIIMS Nov 1993)

a. Partial hepatectomy
b. Ileal resection
c. Jejunal resection
d. Subtotal gastrectomy

Q3. True about gallstones: (PGI Dec 2002)

a. More common in females
b. Gallstones, hiatus hernia, and CBD stones from Saint's triad
c. Limey bile precipitated
d. Lithotripsy always done

Q4. Initial investigation of choice for biliary obstruction: (JIPMER 2013)

a. CT abdomen
b. ERCP
c. Magnetic resonance cholangiopancreatography (MRCP)
d. USG

Q5. Not a complication of gallstones: (JIPMER 2010)
a. Mucocele
b. Diverticulosis
c. Acute cholangitis
d. Empyema of the gallbladder

Q6. Under which condition, medical treatment of gallstones is indicated? (All India 1998)
a. Stone is <15 mm in size
b. Radiopaque stone
c. Calcium bilirubinate stone
d. Nonfunctioning gallbladder

Q7. False about gallstone ileus: (AIIMS GIS May 2008)
a. 90% of patients give a history of biliary disease
b. Causes 1% of all small bowel obstruction (SBO); around 25% of cases in >70 years
c. Tumbling obstruction
d. A fistula is mostly formed between the duodenum and the gallbladder

Q8. The treatment of gallstone ileus is: (PGI June 99)
a. Cholecystectomy alone
b. Removal of obstruction
c. Cholecystectomy, closure of fistula, and removal of stone by enterotomy
d. Cholecystectomy with closure of the fistula

Q9. The technique of laparoscopic cholecystectomy was first described by: (AIIMS May 2011)
a. Erich Mühe
b. Phillip Moure
c. Kurt Semm
d. Eddie Reddick

Q10. After surgery, there was 50 mL bile output from abdominal drain on 1st postoperative day. Management is: (JIPMER GIS 2011)
a. Intrabiliary stent
b. Immediate exploration
c. T-tube drainage
d. Observation

Q11. Antegrade cholecystectomy: (PGI Dec 2000)
a. Starts from fundus
b. Starts from cystic duct identification
c. Starts from hilar dissection
d. Considered unsafe

Q12. Features of a healthy gallbladder on laparotomy are: (PGI Dec 2000)
a. Typical "sea-green" colored
b. The wall is thin and elastic.
c. Cannot be emptied
d. Not easily visible

Q13. An otherwise normal female presents with symptoms of flatulent dyspepsia. She was started on proton pump inhibitors, which controlled her symptoms. The next step in management of this condition should be: (All India 2008)
a. Immediate laparoscopic cholecystectomy
b. Laparotomy after 1 or 2 months
c. Wait and watch
d. ERCP

Q14. All are true about acute acalculous cholecystitis, *except*: (AIIMS GIS May 2011)
a. Distended GB is seen in scintigraphy
b. Vascular cause
c. Seen in bedridden patients
d. Rapid course

Q15. Acalculous cholecystitis is caused by: (PGI Dec 2001)
a. Diabetes mellitus
b. Total parenteral nutrition
c. Tuberculosis
d. Anemia
e. Malignancy

Q16. Risk factors for malignant change in an asymptomatic patient with a gallbladder polyp on ultrasound include all of the following, *except*: (AIIMS May 2011)
a. Age >60 years
b. Rapid increase in size of the polyp
c. Size of polyp >5 mm
d. Associated gallstones

Q17. All of the following are risk factors for CA GB, *except*: (JIPMER GIS 2011)
a. Gallstones
b. Adenomyomatosis
c. Porcelain gallbladder
d. Choledochal cyst

Q18. Organism associated with fish consumption and also causes carcinoma gallbladder: (AIIMS Nov 2012)
a. *Gnathostoma*
b. *Angiostrongylus cantonensis*
c. *Clonorchis sinensis*
d. *Hymenolepis diminuta*

Q19. All of the following are risk factors for carcinoma gallbladder, *except*: (AIIMS June 2004)

a. Typhoid carriers
b. Adenomatous gallbladder polyps
c. Choledochal cyst
d. Oral contraceptives

Q20. Laparoscopic cholecystectomy was done, on histopathology, stage was T2. Next line of treatment is: (AIIMS GIS 2003)

a. Observation
b. Extended cholecystectomy
c. Port site excision
d. Chemotherapy

Q21. Regarding carcinoma gallbladder: (PGI June 2002)

a. Squamous cell carcinoma is the most common
b. Present with jaundice
c. Good prognosis
d. Gallstones predispose
e. 65% survival after surgery

Q22. Sphincter of Oddi consists of: (AIIMS May 2011)

a. Two sphincters b. Three sphincters
c. Four sphincters d. Five sphincter

Q23. Endoscopic retrograde cholangiopancreatography is used in all the following, *except*: (AIIMS May 2020)

a. Pancreatitis without features of cholangitis
b. Recurrent pancreatitis
c. Unexplained jaundice
d. Periampullary carcinoma

Q24. True about choledochal cyst is: (AIIMS Sep 1996)

a. Always extrahepatic
b. Treatment is a cystojejunostomy
c. Excision is an ideal treatment
d. Drainage is the treatment of choice

Q25. Not true regarding choledochal cyst: (AIIMS Nov 1995)

a. Epigastric mass
b. Jaundice
c. Pain in the abdomen
d. Cystojejunostomy is the treatment of choice

Q26. Not true about choledochal cyst is: (AIIMS May 2009)

a. Associated with an anomalous junction of the pancreatic and biliary duct
b. Type II is the most common
c. Surgical removal is the treatment of choice
d. If ruptures can cause biliary peritonitis

Q27. All are true about CBD stones, *except*: (AIIMS GIS 2003)

a. Associated with GB stones in 10% of cases
b. Primary stones are usually brown
c. Laboratory values may be normal in one-third cases of choledocholithiasis
d. Retained stones are discovered after 2 years of cholecystectomy

Q28. Treatment of CBD stone includes: (PGI May 2010)

a. Endoscopic papillotomy
b. ERCP
c. Ursodeoxycholic acid
d. Hepaticojejunostomy
e. Choledochotomy

Q29. Most common cause of cholangitis: (AIIMS June 1994)

a. Viral infection b. CBD stone
c. Surgery d. Amebic infection

Q30. What is more appropriate for the diagnosis of CBD stones? (PGI June 1997)

a. Ultrasonography b. ERCP
c. OCG d. IV cholangiography

Grade III ***Most difficult***

Q1. All are true about pigmented stones *except*: (AIIMS GIS Dec 2006)

a. Seen in cholangiohepatitis
b. Secondary CBD stones
c. Primary CBD stones
d. More common in Asians

Q2. Stone formation in gallbladder is enhanced by all, *except*: (All India 1996)

a. Clofibrate therapy
b. Ileal resection
c. Cholestyramine therapy
d. Vagal stimulation

Q3. True statement about gallstones are all, *except*: (AIIMS Nov 1999)

a. Lithogenic bile is required not stone formation
b. May be associated with carcinoma gallbladder
c. Associated with diabetes mellitus
d. More common in males between 30 and 40 years of age

Q4. All are components of Saint's triad, *except*: (AIIMS Nov 1995)

a. Renal stones
b. Hiatus hernia
c. Diverticulosis of colon
d. Gallstones

Q5. Cholesterol gallstones are due to: (JIPMER 1995)

a. Decreased motility of gallbladder
b. Hyposecretion of bile salts
c. Hypercholesterolemia
d. All of the above

Q6. The most common type of gallstone in India is: (MCI March 2009)

a. Cholesterol
b. Pigment
c. Mixed
d. Both a and c

Q7. Which is not required for visualization of the gallbladder in oral cholecystography? (All India 1997)

a. Functioning liver
b. Motor mechanisms of the gallbladder
c. Patency of cystic duct
d. Ability of absorb water

Q8. Investigation of choice for is suspected gallbladder stone is: (MCI March 2010)

a. Ultrasound
b. X-ray
c. Barium study
d. Oral cholecystography

Q9. True about gallstone disease: (PGI SS Dec 2009)

a. Acute cholecystitis presents with GB perforation
b. Acute cholecystitis presents with mucosal ulceration of GB
c. 80% of cases of cholelithiasis are symptomatic
d. Mucocele of the GB contains infected bile

Q10. The most common site of fistula in gallstone ileus is between: (AIIMS GIS Dec 2006)

a. GB and duodenum
b. GB and transverse colon
c. GB and stomach
d. GB and the ileum

Q11. The treatment of choice for a mucocele of the gallbladder is: (AIIMS June 2004)

a. Aspiration of mucus
b. Cholecystectomy
c. Cholecystostomy
d. Antibiotics and observation

Q12. Not an indication for cholecystectomy for asymptomatic gallstones: (AIIMS GIS May 2011)

a. Diabetes
b. Sickle cell anemia
c. Porcelain GB
d. In high-prevalence area of CA GB

Q13. All are indications for cholecystectomy, *except*: (JIPMER GIS 2011)

a. Emphysematous cholecystitis
b. Biliary dyskinesia
c. Perforation of the gallbladder
d. Adenomyomatosis

Q14. Indications of cholecystectomy for gallstone disease is/are: (PGI Nov 2011)

a. Asymptomatic gallstones with DM
b. Porcelain gallbladder
c. Asymptomatic with history of single attack of acute pancreatitis
d. Asymptomatic Gallstone disease
e. Symptomatic cholecystitis

Q15. Which of the following is not an indication for cholecystectomy? (AIIMS May 2005)

a. A 70-year-old male with symptomatic gallstones
b. A 20-year-old male with sickle cell anemia and symptomatic gallstones
c. A 65-year-old female with a large gallbladder polyp
d. A 55-year-old with an asymptomatic gallstone

Q16. A 45-year-old female presents with symptoms of acute cholecystitis. On USG, there is a solitary gallstone of size 1.5 cm. Symptoms are controlled with medical management. Which of the following is the next most appropriate step in the management of this patient? (All India 2008)

a. Regular follow-up
b. IV antibiotics
c. Laparoscopic cholecystectomy immediately
d. Open cholecystectomy immediately

Q17. An 88-year-old male patient presented with end-stage renal disease with coronary artery block, and metastasis in the lungs. Now presenting with acute cholecystitis, the patient's relatives need treatment to do something: (UPPG 2008)

a. Open cholecystectomy
b. Tube cholecystostomy
c. Laparoscopic cholecystectomy
d. Antibiotics, then elective cholecystectomy

Q18. A patient underwent laparoscopic cholecystectomy and was discharged on the same day. On postoperative day 3, he presented himself to the hospital with a fever. Ultrasonography showed a 5 × 5 cm collection in the right subdiaphragmatic region. What will be the management? (AIIMS May 2017)

a. Observe with antibiotic cover
b. Reexplore the wound with T-tube insertion
c. Pigtail insertion and drainage
d. ERCP and proceed

Q19. Which of the following statements about acalculous cholecystitis is incorrect?

a. Manifestation of disturbed microcirculation in a critically ill patient.
b. Prolonged parenteral nutrition can be causative.
c. It is a life-threatening condition.
d. Cholecystectomy is not indicated.

Q20. False about GB polyps: (AIIMS GIS May 2008)

a. Adenomyomatosis <1 cm, pedunculated
b. Cholesterol polyps are most common
c. Symptomatic polyps are an indication for cholecystectomy.
d. A polyp with a stone has an increased risk of malignancy.

Q21. On abdominal ultrasound gallbladder shows diffuse wall thickening with hyperechoic nodules at the neck and comet tail artifacts. The most likely diagnosis will be: (AIIMS May 2011)

a. Adenomyomatosis
b. Adenocarcinoma of the gallbladder
c. Xanthogranulomatous cholecystitis
d. Cholesterol crystals

Q22. Risk factors for cholangiocarcinoma are all, *except*: (AIIMS Nov 2009)

a. Chronic typhoid carrier
b. Chronic ulcerative colitis
c. Parasitic infestation
d. Choledocholithiasis

Q23. Precancerous lesion of gallbladder is: (AIIMS June 1998)

a. Porcelain gallbladder
b. Mirizzi's syndrome
c. Cholesterolosis
d. Acalculous cholecystitis

Q24. Survival in unresectable GB carcinoma is: (AIIMS May 2011)

a. 4–6 months
b. 8–10 months
c. 1 year
d. 12–24 months

Q25. True about CA GB: (PGI SS Dec 2009)

a. Most commonly presents with obstructive jaundice
b. 90% are associated with gallstones
c. 5-year survival is 35%
d. 30% are squamous cell carcinoma

Q26. False regarding CA GB: (PGI SS Dec 2010)

a. T1a: simple cholecystectomy
b. T1b: extended cholecystectomy
c. T1a: extended cholecystectomy if carcinoma in the neck of the gallbladder
d. Excision of port sites improves survival

Q27. A 40-year-old woman has undergone a cholecystectomy. The histopathology reveals that she has a 3 cm adenocarcinoma in the body of the gallbladder, infiltrating up to the serosa. Which of the following further management would you advise her? (AIIMS Nov 2004)

a. Chemotherapy
b. Radiotherapy
c. Radical cholecystectomy
d. Follow-up with regular ultrasound examinations

Q28. In a male after laparoscopic cholecystectomy, the specimen is sent for histopathology, which shows carcinoma gallbladder stage IB. Appropriate management is: (AIIMS Nov 2008)

a. Conservative and follow-up
b. Extended cholecystectomy
c. Excision of all port sites
d. Radiotherapy

Q29. True about cystic duct stump stone are all, *except*: (PGI Nov 2009)

a. The stone cause of postoperative pain
b. Recholecystectomy is the definite treatment of choice
c. ERCP is the investigation of choice to diagnose
d. Basket extraction is the treatment of choice
e. Oral ursodeoxycholic acid relieves symptoms remarkably

Q30. Best treatment modality for common bile duct stone is: (AIIMS Nov 1994)

a. Endoscopic sphincterotomy
b. Observation
c. Chenodeoxycholic acid
d. Percutaneous removal

ANSWERS

Grade I: 1. b; 2. d; 3. a; 4. c; 5. d; 6. c (Sabiston 20/e p1493); 7. c (Schwartz 10/e p1320); 8. c (Sabiston 20/e 1493); 9. d; 10. a; 11. b, e; 12. a; 13. c; 14. a; 15. a (Maingot 11/e p628); 16. a; 17. a (Harrison 20/e p2428), b, c; 18. c; 19. d; 20. a; 21. a; 22. a; 23. c; 24. a, b; 25. c (Sabiston 20/e p1510-1511); 26. d (Sabiston 20/e p1511); 27. b; 28. a; 29. a (Bailey 27/e p1197); 30. a

Grade II: 1. b; 2. b; 3. a; 4. d; 5. b (Sabiston 20/e p1492); 6. a; 7. a; 8. b; 9. a; 10. d; 11. a (Mastery of Surgery 5/e p1128); 12. a; 13. c; 14. a (Schwartz 10/e p1327); 15. a, b; 16. c; 17. b; 18. c; 19. d; 20. b (Blumgart 6/e p797); 21. b; 22. c (Bailey 27/e p1214); 23. a; 24. c; 25. d; 26. b; 27. d; 28. a, b, e; 29. b; 30. b

Grade III: 1. b (Sabiston 20/e p2078); 2. d (Harrison 20/e p2424); 3. d; 4. a; 5. d; 6. b (Bailey 27/e p1198); 7. b (Schwartz 9/e p1141); 8. a; 9. b; 10. a; 11. b (Harrison 20/e p2428); 12. a; 13. d; 14. b, e; 15. d; 16. c; 17. b; 18. c; 19. d; 20. a; 21. a; 22. d; 23. a; 24. a; 25. b; 26. d; 27. c; 28. b; 29. b, e; 30. a

MODEL QUESTIONS

Q1. T2N1 of CA GB represents which stage?

a. IA b. IB
c. II d. III

Ans. d

Q2. All are true about CA GB, *except*:

a. Redo surgery is a radical or extended cholecystectomy that increases a significant survival advantage
b. Interaortocaval node involvement potentially rules out a cure
c. <25% 5-year survival for all stages
d. Pancreaticoduodenectomy has a 5-year survival of 25%

Ans. d

Q3. The most common type of cancer gallbladder in a patient with gallstones:

a. Adenocarcinoma
b. Squamous carcinoma
c. Sarcoma
d. None

Ans. a

Q4. The sentinel node of the gallbladder is:

a. Virchow's nodes b. Iris nodes
c. Cloquet node d. Lymph node of Lund

Ans. d

Q5. "Limey bile" is:

a. Present in the CBD
b. Thin and clear
c. Like toothpaste emulsion in the gallbladder
d. Bacteria rich

Ans. c

Q6. A 60-year-old female presents with increased bowel sounds. X-ray shows dilated bowel loops, with air in the biliary tree. She gives a history of an open hysterectomy done 2 years back. What is the diagnosis?

a. Adhesions
b. Gallstone ileus
c. Mesenteric ischemia
d. Large bowel obstruction

Ans. b

Q7. A patient underwent cholecystectomy and presents to the hospital with bile duct stones after 2 years. What is the name of such stones?

a. Primary stone b. Secondary stone
c. Retained stone d. Missed stone

Ans. a

Q8. A 65-year-old female presented with increased serum glutamic oxaloacetic transaminase (SGOT), serum glutamic pyruvic transaminase (SGPT), bilirubin, and alkaline phosphatase. She has the following findings in USG—sclerotic atrophic gallbladder, large impacted stone in the common bile duct (CBD), distended CBD with dilated intrahepatic radicles. What is the best treatment?

a. Endoscopic retrograde cholangiopancreatography (ERCP)
b. Magnetic resonance cholangiopancreatography (MRCP)
c. Cholecystectomy
d. Observation

Ans. a

Q9. Cholesterol stone is made up of:

a. Amorphous cholesterol monohydrate
b. Crystalline cholesterol monohydrate
c. Cholesterol polyhydrate
d. Cholesterol with calcium palmitate

Ans. b

Q10. A female presents with epigastric pain and right hypochondrial pain radiating to the back with guarding and rigidity in the right hypochondrium. She has had similar episodes past 1 year on and off. Most likely diagnosis is:

a. Acute pancreatitis
b. Acute cholecystitis
c. Hydatid cyst
d. Liver abscess

Ans. b

Q11. By definition, pigment stone contains how much percentage of cholesterol?

a. <10%
b. <20%
c. <30%
d. <60%

Ans. c

Q12. Regarding stones in the gallbladder, the following are true, *except*:

a. Mixed stones are common in the West
b. In Saint's triad, diverticulosis of the colon and hiatus hernia
c. It is a risk factor in the development of GB carcinoma
d. 90% of GB stones are radiopaque
e. A mucocele of the GB is caused by a stone impacted in the Hartmann's pouch

Ans. d

Q13. In gallstone ileus, obstruction is seen at:

a. Jejunum
b. Proximal ileum
c. Distal ileum
d. Colon

Ans. c

Q14. Contraindications for laparoscopic cholecystectomy are all, *except*:

a. Shrunken liver
b. Previous laparotomy
c. Emphysema
d. Obese individual

Ans. a

Q15. A 50-year-old with a history of jaundice in the past has presented with right upper quadrant abdominal pain. Examination and investigations reveal chronic calculous cholecystitis. The liver function tests are within normal limits, and on ultrasound examination, the common bile ducts are not dilated. Which of the following will be the procedure of choice for her?

a. Laparoscopic cholecystectomy
b. Open choledocholithotomy with CBD exploration
c. ERCP + choledocholithotomy followed by laparoscopic cholecystectomy
d. Laparoscopic cholecystectomy followed by ERCP + choledocholithotomy

Ans. a

Q16. Mirizzi syndrome is:

a. GB stone compressing the common hepatic duct
b. GB carcinoma invading the inferior vena cava (IVC)
c. GB stone causing cholecystitis
d. Pancreatic carcinoma

Ans. a

Q17. All of the following are true about porcelain gallbladder, *except*:

a. May be seen on plain X-ray
b. More commonly diagnosed on CT
c. It is an indication for cholecystectomy
d. Always denotes benign etiology

Ans. d

Q18. Sump syndrome occurs most commonly after:

a. Cholecystojejunostomy
b. Choledochoduodenostomy
c. Mirizzi's syndrome
d. Choledochojejunostomy

Ans. b

Q19. A middle-aged patient presents with complaints of right hypochondrial pain. On X-ray, an elevated right hemidiaphragm was seen. All of the following are the possible diagnoses, *except*:

a. Subphrenic abscess
b. Acute cholecystitis
c. Pyogenic live abscess
d. Amoebic liver abscess in the right lobe

Ans. d

Q20. A patient has cholecystectomy presents with intrahepatic biliary radicle dilatation and jaundice. What is the investigation of choice?

a. Magnetic resonance imaging (MRI)
b. CECT
c. PTC
d. USG

Ans. a

Q21. A patient underwent cholecystectomy and had abdominal pain in the postoperative period. The patient had tachycardia. The white blood cell

(WBC) count is 11,000 cells/mm^3. USG done shows a collection 5 × 5 cm in the right hypochondrium. What is the next step?

a. Pig tail drainage USG guided
b. ERCP
c. Reopen the abdomen
d. Observation

Ans. a

Q22. A patient has multiple cholelithiasis with CBD diameter 12 mm. Serum bilirubin 0.8. Alkaline phosphatase is around 380. Gamma-glutamyl transferase (GGT) is normal. What will be the next step for management?

a. ERCP
b. MRCP
c. Lap cholecystectomy
d. CECT abdomen

Ans. b

Q23. A 40-year-old female patient underwent cholecystectomy. Postoperatively, she is complaining of pain in the abdomen. What test is performed to identify a bile leak?

a. Hepatobiliary iminodiacetic acid (HIDA)
b. MRCP
c. ERCP
d. CECT

Ans. c and d

Q24. Bile leak from the aberrant right hepatic duct that is not communicating from the common bile duct comes under which type of Strasberg classification?

a. Type A
b. Type B
c. Type C
d. Type D

Ans. c

Q25. The patient has undergone cholecystectomy a few days back, and now the patient has presented with upper abdominal pain. MRCP was done, which showed the leaking of bile from the cystic duct stump. The patient is hemodynamically stable. Which of the following should be the next line of management?

a. Roux-en-Y hepaticojejunostomy
b. ERCP and stenting
c. Exploratory laparotomy
d. Conservative treatment with antibiotics

Ans. d

Q26. A patient presents with pain in the right hypochondrium. Blood investigations showed AST—221 U/L and ALT—27 IU/L. Serum bilirubin levels—5 mg/dL and also alkaline phosphatase (ALP)—200 mg%. What should be the initial investigation for this patient?

a. USG abdomen
b. CECT abdomen
c. Hepatitis B surface antigen (HBsAg)
d. HIDA scan

Ans. a

SUGGESTED READING

1. Bailey & Love's - Short Practice of Surgery, 27th edition.
2. Depictions of the gallbladder and biliary tree are found in Babylonian models found from 2000 BCE. In: Eachempale SR, Reed RL (Eds). Acute Cholecystitis, 1st edition. Berlin/Heidelberg: Springer; 2015. pp. 1-16.
3. International Journal of Gastroenterology (Volume 9, Issue 1).
4. Schwartz's Principles of Surgery, 18th edition.
5. Tandon RK. Studies on pathogenesis of gallstones in India. Ann Natl Acad Med Sci. 1989;25:213-22.
6. Textbook of Surgery by David Sabiston, 21st edition.

CHAPTER 38

Pancreas

"You rarely hear anyone use the word pancreas in a not-horrible context."

– Christian Finnegan

DEVELOPMENT OF PANCREAS

It develops from the foregut as ventral and dorsal buds. The ventral bud rotates and fuses with the dorsal bud and forms the pancreas. The main duct of the pancreas, the duct of Wirsung, is formed by ventral and dorsal buds, whereas the minor duct, the duct of Santorini, is formed from the dorsal duct only.

The pancreas is divided into the head, body, and tail. The head is 30%, and the body and tail constitute 70% of the pancreas. The uncinate process runs from the head, extending to the left behind the superior mesenteric vein. It weighs around 80 g, and 10–20% is endocrine tissue, and 80–90% is exocrine tissue.

The main duct of the pancreas is called the duct of Wirsung (Johann Georg Wirsung, 1589–1643, Italian anatomist, described in 1642). The accessory duct of the pancreas is known as the duct of Santorini (Giovanni Domenico Santorini, 1681–1737, Italian anatomist).

Groups of endocrine cells called "islets of Langerhans" (Paul Langerhans, 1847–1888, German pathological anatomist, described in 1869) are present all over the world. Pancreatic islets have three types of cells:

1. B cells producing insulin and are 70%.
2. A cells producing glucagon and are 20%.
3. D cells producing somatostatin are the remaining cells **(Figs. 1A and B)**.

Physiological anatomy of the exocrine part of the pancreas:
- The pancreas is a dual-function organ with both exocrine and endocrine functions.
- It consists of blind end pieces (acini/alveoli) with each lined by a single layer of cells containing zymogen granules that possess digestive enzymes.
- The layer surrounds a central globular cavity that is continuous with the lumen of the glandular duct.
- The duct system starts with intercalated ducts, many of which unite to form intralobular ducts, then to interlobular ducts, and finally to the main duct.

Physiology of the exocrine pancreas:
- Secretion of water and electrolytes originates in the centroacinar and intercalated duct cells.
- Pancreatic enzymes originate in the acinar cells.
- Final product is a colorless, odorless, and isosmotic alkaline fluid that contains digestive enzymes (amylase, lipase, and trypsinogen).
- Alkaline pH results from secreted bicarbonate, which serves to neutralize gastric acid and regulates the pH of the intestine.
- Enzymes digest carbohydrates, proteins, and fats.

PHYSIOLOGY OF THE PANCREAS

The pancreas is an organ that has both exocrine and endocrine functions. After a meal, the hormone secretin is released from the duodenal mucosa, which evokes bicarbonate-rich alkaline fluid with digestive enzymes. Cholecystokinin (pancreozymin) is released from duodenal mucosa and is responsible for enzyme release **(Figs. 2A to C)**.

The endocrine part of the pancreas secretes insulin and glucagon and controls and regulates blood sugar.

PANCREATIC FUNCTION TESTS

Exocrine function can be done as in the *Lundh (Goran Lundh, 1926–1999, Swedish surgeon, described in 1962)* test by giving a test meal to see the response.

You may be asked:
Investigations in pancreatic diseases:
- *Serum enzyme levels:* Amylase is the only enzyme that is secreted in active form, and the rest of the enzymes are secreted as proenzymes and activated by trypsin.
- Pancreatic function tests.
- Ultrasonography (USG) and endoscopic ultrasound (EUS)
- CT scan
- MRI
- *Endoscopic retrograde cholangiopancreatography (ERCP):* It can show double duct sign, narrowing of both the pancreatic and bile ducts by a tumor, and chain of lakes sign of chronic pancreatitis, and brush cytology can be done.
- Plain X-ray of abdomen and chest.

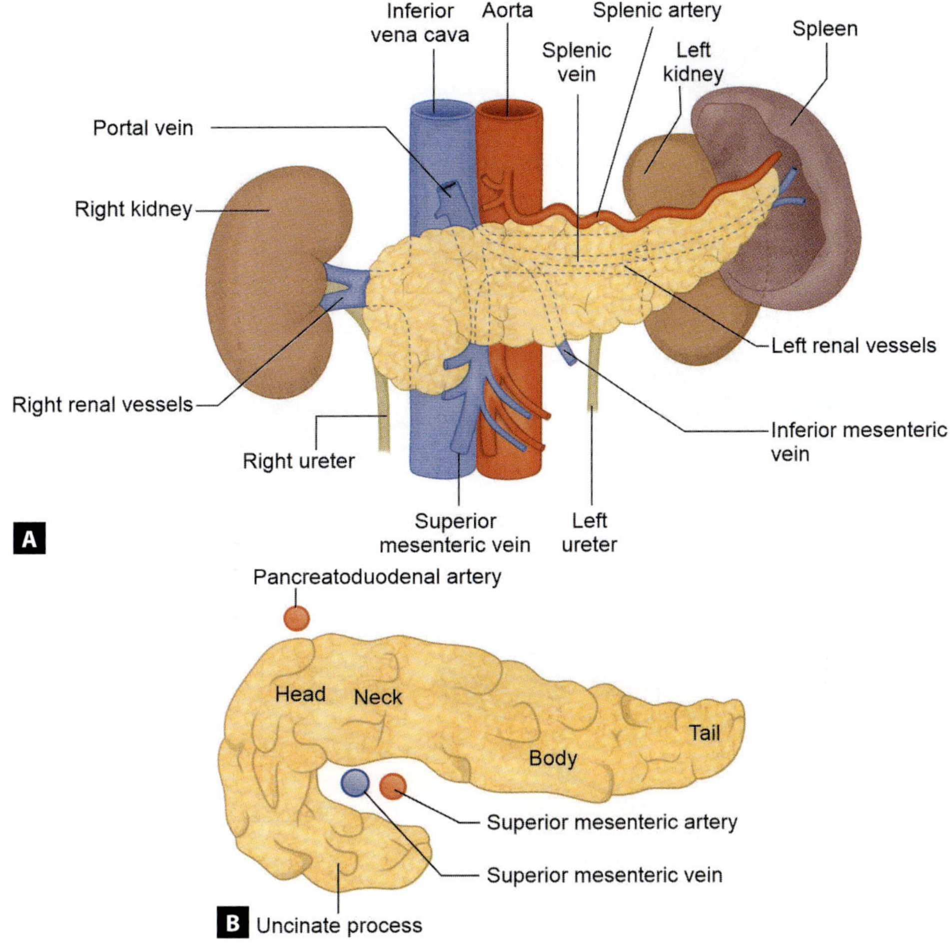

Figs. 1A and B: Anatomy of the pancreas.

Chronic pancreatitis can be classified by the Cambridge criteria by endoscopic retrograde cholangiopancreatography (ERCP) and the Rosemont criteria by endoscopic ultrasound (EUS).

ECTOPIC PANCREAS

Collections of pancreatic tissues are found in the upper gastrointestinal tract (UGIT), most commonly in the duodenum. They are in the submucosa and are functional.

ANNULAR PANCREAS

It is due to the failure of the rotation of the ventral bud during development. So, a ring of pancreatic tissue is formed around the second or third part of the duodenum. Clinical features of gastric outlet obstruction are found. *It is commonly found with Down syndrome and diagnosed by contrast-enhanced computed tomography (CECT).* Duodenoduodenostomy is the treatment **(Figs. 3A and B)**.

PANCREAS DIVISUM

It is due to the failure of the ventral and dorsal buds to join during development. The minor pancreatic duct becomes major. ERCP and magnetic resonance cholangiopancreatography (MRCP) are diagnostic. Main duct sphincterotomy is the treatment.

PANCREATITIS

Inflammation of the pancreas is called pancreatitis, which can be acute and chronic.

Acute Pancreatitis

It is defined as an acute condition presenting with abdominal pain, a threefold or greater rise in the serum levels of the pancreatic enzymes amylase or lipase, and/or characteristic findings of pancreatic inflammation on contrast-enhanced computed tomography (CECT) **(Flowchart 1)**.

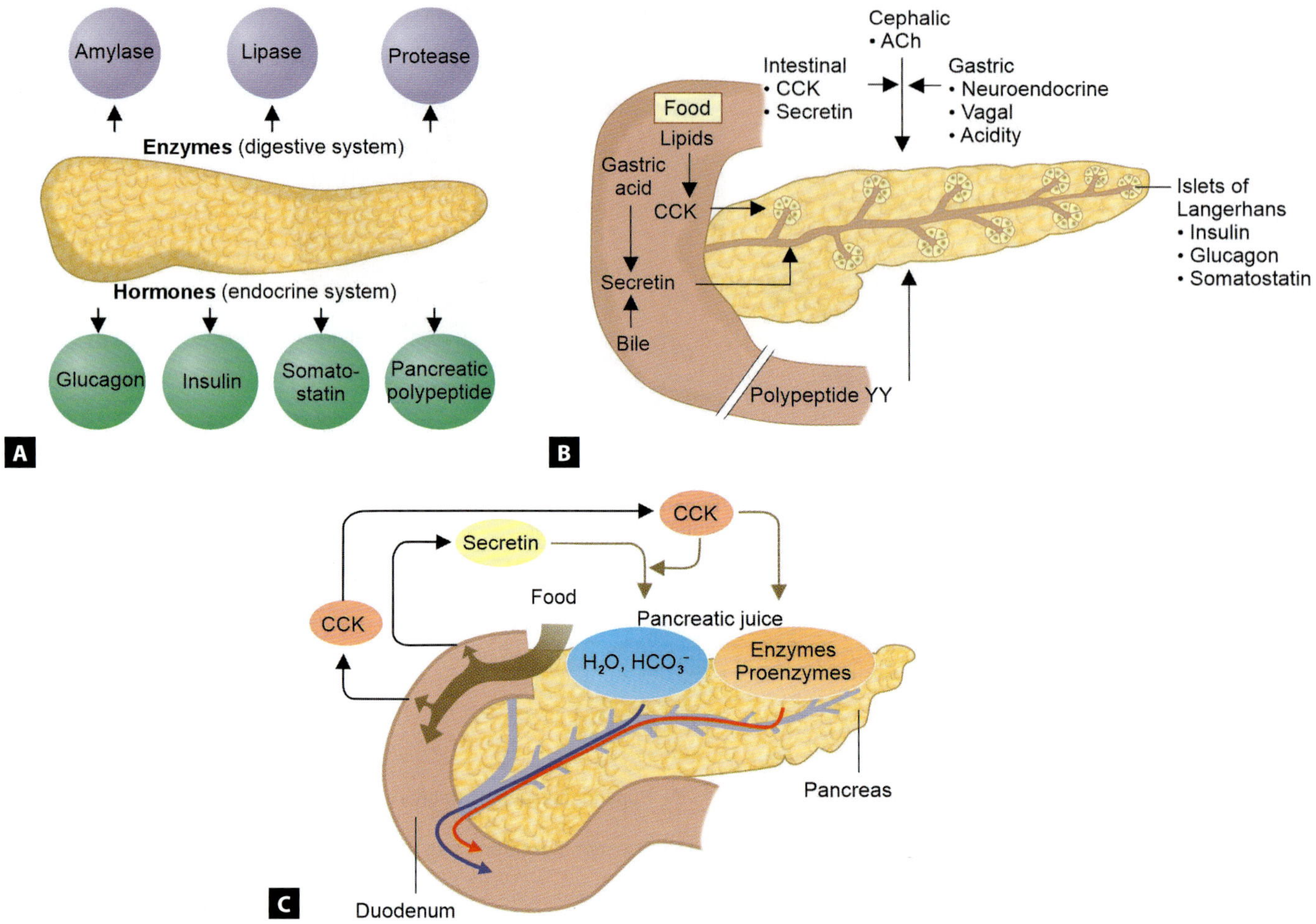

Amylase
Lipase
Protease
Enzymes (digestive system)
Hormones (endocrine system)
Glucagon
Insulin
Somato-statin
Pancreatic polypeptide
A
Cephalic
• ACh
Intestinal
• CCK
• Secretin
Gastric
• Neuroendocrine
• Vagal
• Acidity
Food
Lipids
Gastric acid
CCK
Secretin
Bile
Islets of Langerhans
• Insulin
• Glucagon
• Somatostatin
Polypeptide YY
B
CCK
Secretin
CCK
Food
Pancreatic juice
H2O, HCO3-
Enzymes
Proenzymes
Pancreas
Duodenum
C

Figs. 2A to C: Physiology of the pancreas. (ACh: acetylcholine; CCK: cholecystokinin)

Hepatic duct
Bile duct
Liver
Stomach
Gallbladder
Dorsal pancreas
Annular pancreas
Pancreatic duct
A
Bile duct
Pancreas divisum
Duodenum
Minor sphincter
Papilla of vater
B

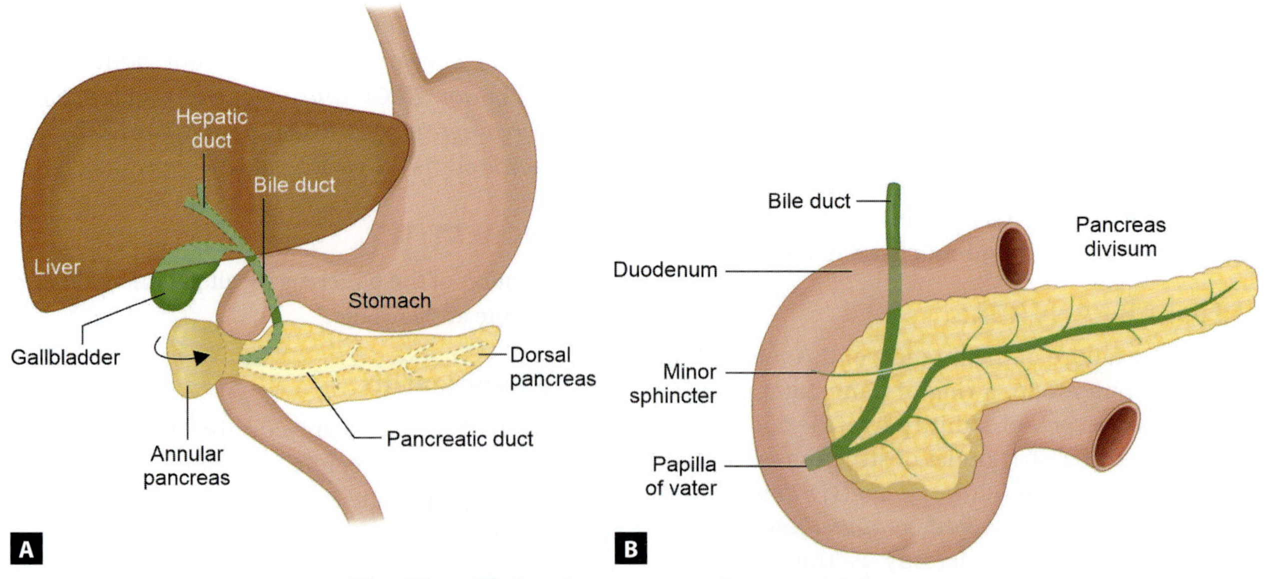

Figs. 3A and B: Annular pancreas and pancreas divisum.

Flowchart 1: Mechanism of acute pancreatitis.

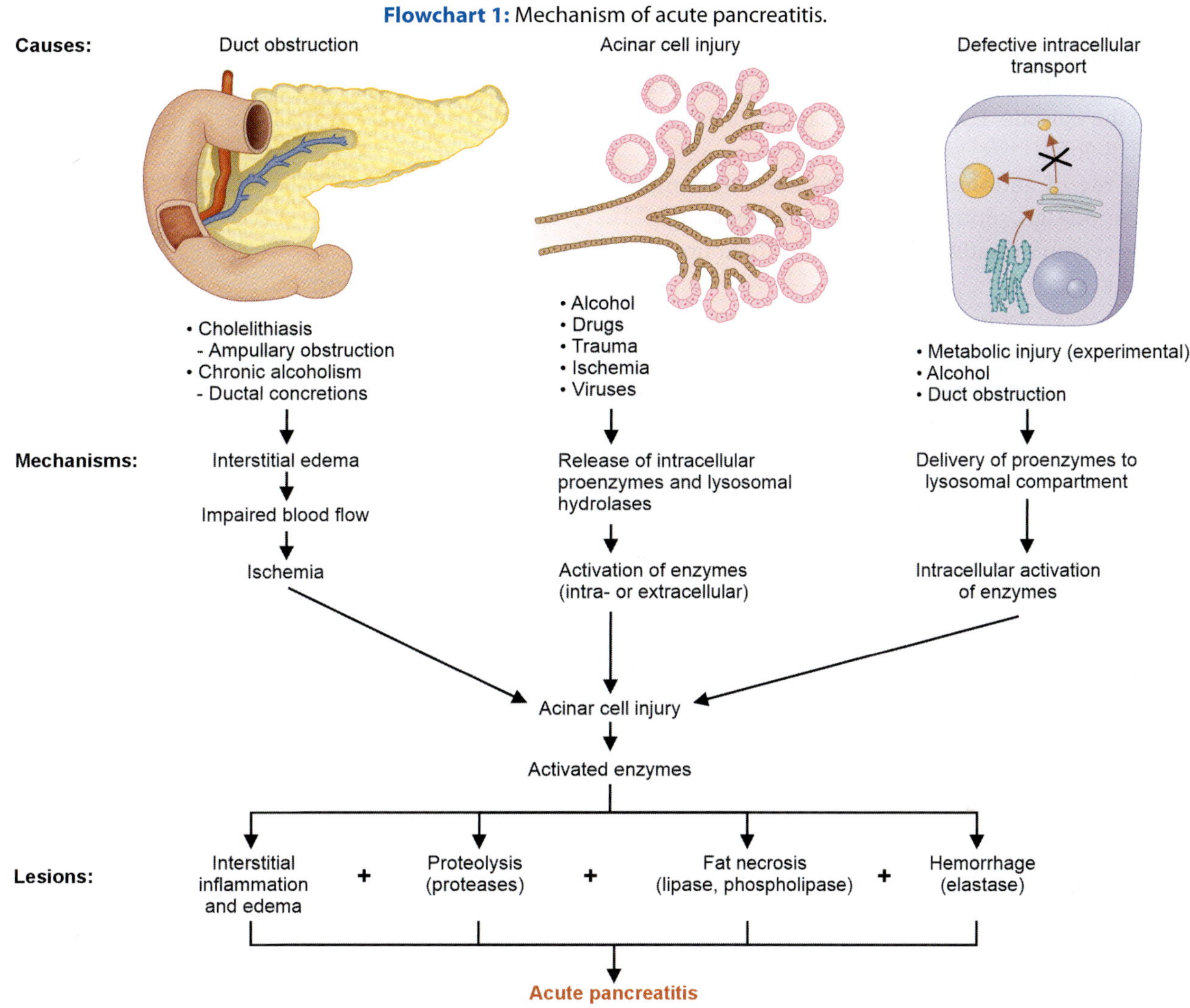

> *Good to remember:*
> *Etiology of acute pancreatitis:*
> *Mn:* ASHAMED GIST
> *A:* Alcohol
> *S:* Steroids
> *H:* Hyperparathyroidism, hyperlipidemia, hypercalcemia
> *A:* Autoimmune diseases as systemic lupus erythematosus (SLE)
> *M:* Mumps
> *E:* ERCP
> *D:* Drugs, azathiaprine, thiazides, and frusemide
> *G:* Gallstones
> *I:* Infections—Cossacks and *Cytomegalovirus* (CMV)
> *S:* Scorpion venom
> *T:* Trauma

Colocalization Hypothesis of Acute Pancreatitis

As per this theory, in the early phase of acute pancreatitis, the zymogens are colocalized and, with the help of other substances, activate trypsinogen to trypsin, and now this trypsin causes cellular injury. Zymogens are proenzymes, which are proteins (enzymes) in an inactive form.

> ### *Clinical Features of Acute Pancreatitis*
>
> Symptoms are pain in the upper abdomen, nausea and vomiting, and forward bending reduces pain.
>
> Signs of acute pancreatitis are tachycardia, jaundice, tachypnea, Cullen's (Thomas Stephen Cullen, 1868–1953, American gynecologist) sign (periumbilical pigmentation), Grey Turner (George Grey Turner, 1877–1951, British surgeon) sign (hemorrhagic discoloration on flanks, ascites, distension of abdomen due to ileus, and Fox sign (chamois at inguinal areas).

Investigations

- Serum amylase and lipase

- Serum lipase is most specific. Serum amylase is also elevated in other diseases such as perforation and intestinal obstruction, and becomes normal after 3 days of the episode. Hyperglycemia and hypocalcemia are also helpful.
- Plain X-ray of abdomen shows baseless abdomen, colon cut-off sign, sentinel loop, and renal halo sign.
- CECT is very informative, but done after 72 hours after the attack.

> *Not to forget:*
> Serum amylase is at times found normal in acute pancreatitis as it returns to normal values, as in severe or total gland destruction by present or past attacks of acute pancreatitis, in hyperlipidemia-induced acute pancreatitis, amylase does not increase. Elevated serum amylase levels also occur in some other diseases than acute pancreatitis: perforation of the intestine, mesenteric infarction, ectopic pregnancy, retroperitoneal hemorrhage, and abdominal organ torsion.

Computed Tomography Severity Index

It is one of the best scoring tools, also called the Balthazar index. It has total points. Disease is severe if the score is 6 or more. It has five grades: 0—normal pancreas, 1—focal or diffuse enlargement, 2—pancreatic gland abnormalities and or peripatetic inflammation, 3—fluid collection in a single location, 4—more than two fluid collections and or gas bubbles in or adjacent to the pancreas. Score can also indicate necrosis of the pancreas: 0—no necrosis, 2 points—1/3 pancreas, 4—1/2 of pancreas, and 6—more than 1/2 of pancreas.

Other scoring systems:

- *Bedside index of severity of acute pancreatitis (BISAP):* Blood urea nitrogen (BUN), impaired mental status, systemic inflammatory response syndrome (SIRS), age above 60 years, and pleural effusion.
- *Ranson score:* It depends upon lactate dehydrogenase (LDH), aspartate aminotransferase (AST), glucose, age above 55 years, total lymphocyte count (TLC) >1,600, base deficit >4 mmol/dL, calcium, hematocrit falls >10%, arterial O_2 saturation, partial pressure of oxygen in the blood (PaO_2) <60 mm Hg, and water sequestration >6 L.
- *Acute Physiology and Chronic Health Evaluation II (APACHE II) scoring:* It is based on 12 factors of general examination, blood levels, and arterial blood gas analysis.
- *RAC classification* is divided into mild, moderate, and severe.

> *Complications of acute pancreatitis:*
> - Acute pancreatitis fluid collection (APFC)
> - Pseudocyst
> - Necrosis
> - Abscess
> - Ascites
> - Pleural effusion
> - Splenic vein thrombosis

Systemic Complications

Systemic complications are shock, gastrointestinal (GI) bleed, renal failure, and acute respiratory distress syndrome (ARDS).

Treatment of Acute Pancreatitis

- Intravenous (IV) fluids, normobaric oxygen (NBO), analgesia, antibiotics, and total parenteral nutrition (TPN).
- ERCP and sphincterotomy for biliary stones.
- Cholecystectomy if gallstones are induced.

> *Pseudocyst of the pancreas:* It is a fluid collection in the lesser sac following acute or chronic pancreatitis. Its symptoms include upper abdominal pain, fullness, and vomiting. Elevated amylase, EUS, and CECT findings are diagnostic. It can get infected, and an abscess develops. Internal drainage by cyst gastronomy is the required treatment.

Chronic Pancreatitis

It is a progressive chronic inflammation with fibrosis and irreversible destruction of pancreatic tissue. It develops diabetes if the destruction of endocrine tissue is >90%, and develops steatorrhea if the exocrine tissue destruction is >90%.

> ### *Etiology of Chronic Pancreatitis*
>
> *TIGARO classification:*
>
> *T:* Toxic or alcohol, it is the most common cause.
> *I:* Idiopathic
> *G:* Genetic, *PRSS, SPINK1,* and *CFTR* gene mutation
> *A:* Autoimmune
> *R:* Recurrent acute pancreatitis
> *O:* Obstructive
>
> Clinical manifestations include severe recurrent pain in the abdomen, diabetes, and steatorrhea.

Investigations in Chronic Pancreatitis

- Fecal measurement of elastase and fat excretion. Steatorrhea is known when fecal fat excretion is >7 g/day.

- CECT is the gold standard for diagnosing chronic pancreatitis.
- ERCP
- EUS

Treatment

The main thing is pain management by analgesics, alcohol block of the celiac plexus, and endoscopic splanchnicectomy. Pancreatic supplements are given for steatorrhea. Diabetes is best managed by insulin.

Surgery for Chronic Pancreatitis

Pancreaticojejunostomy [Frey's (Charles Frederick Frey, American surgeon) procedure] is the procedure of choice, longitudinal, or end-to-end.

Various methods are developed as per the site of lesions: *Beger's (Hans Beger, German surgeon), Puestow's, Izbicki's, and Bern's procedures.*

TUMORS OF PANCREAS

The most common tumor is adenocarcinoma. Endocrine and cystic tumors are less common.

Adenocarcinoma of Pancreas

The tumors are divided according to their site of involvement:

- *Periampullary cancer:* Any tumor within 2 cm of the ampulla is called periampullary.
- It has a good prognosis as it is detected early. Most of these are operable (60%). Intermittent jaundice occurs.
- Carcinoma of the head of the pancreas has pain in the abdomen and jaundice; if diagnosed late, so the prognosis is bad, as only 10% of cases are operable.
- Carcinoma of the body and tail of the pancreas—with the worst prognosis.

Heredity and Genetic Mutation

These include PRSS1, SPINK1, STK11, CFTR, MLH1, FAP, K-ras, P16, P53, and DPC4. K-ras is the earliest and most common mutation to occur in carcinoma of the pancreas. Periampullary carcinoma is usually painless with intermittent jaundice. Others have pain and vomiting. According to Courvoisier's law, the tumor may be palpable.

Tumor Nodes Malignant Classification

Classification includes *T1*—<2 cm, *T2*—2-4 cm, *T3*—>5 cm, *T4*—involvement of superior mesenteric artery (SMA), common hepatic artery (CHA), and celiac artery. Respectable tumor—no infiltration and no metastasis. Borderline—SMA, CHA, and celiac artery involved <180°. Unresectable tumor—involvement of SMA, CHA, celiac artery >180°, and metastasis.

Investigations in Pancreatic Cancer

- CECT investigation of choice
- ERCP
- MRCP
- Barium meal—reverse 3 sign (Epsilon sign) and Frostberg sign
- Biopsy

Management of Carcinoma of the Pancreas

- *Respectable*—surgery
- *Unresectable*—palliative therapy
- Head, respectable tumor—*Whipple operation (pancreaticoduodenectomy)*
- Tumor of the body and tail—*distal pancreatectomy*
- Endocrine tumors
- *Insulinoma:* It arises from B cells and is the most common endocrine tumor of pancreas. It is mostly benign and evenly spread.

Fasting insulin is increased. EUS is best method to localize the tumor.

Treatment

- If the tumor is <2 cm—enucleation.
- If the tumor is >2 cm—wide resection.

GASTRINOMA

The most common site is gastrinoma or Passaro's triangle (boundaries—junction of cystic and common hepatitis duct, junction of head and neck with body of pancreas, and junction of D2 and D3). Contents of Passaro's triangle are: D1, D2 part, head of the pancreas, and lymph nodes. Gastrinoma usually arises from the wall of D1. Extra Passaro's triangle gastrinomas are larger, more aggressive, and have with poor prognosis. It increases gastrin level and HCL production, causing peptic ulcers and diarrhea. They are multiple and recurrent. Commonly metastasizes in the liver. Treated by enucleation if <5 mm and resection if >5 mm.

> *Points to remember:*
> - *Whipple' triad:* Fasting hypoglycemia, low blood glucose levels below 50 mg/dL, rapid resolution when glucose is given.
> - *Zollinger–Ellison triad:* Increased gastrin, increased acid output, and no β-cell tumor.

SOME IMPORTANT QUESTIONS

Q1. The most common functioning neuroendocrine tumor of the pancreas is:

a. Insulinoma
b. Gastrinoma
c. Glucagonoma
d. Pancreatic polypeptidoma (PPoma)

Ans. a

Q2. A 40-year-old alcoholic male presents to the emergency department with acute abdominal pain and distention. A fluid-filled lesion is present in the epigastric region. What is the abnormal investigation seen?

a. Lipase
b. γ-glutamyl transpeptidase (GGT)
c. Bilirubin
d. Carcinoembryonic antigen (CEA)

Ans. a

Q3. What is the most common site of gastrinoma in multiple endocrine neoplasia, type 1 (MEN1) syndrome?

a. Jejunum
b. Ileum
c. Duodenum
d. Stomach

Ans. c

Q4. A patient diagnosed with carcinoma uncinate process presents with sudden abdominal pain for 1 day. The tumor has infiltrated into:

a. Portal vein
b. Superior mesenteric vein (SMV)
c. Spinal muscular atrophy (SMA)
d. Splenic vein

Ans. c

Q5. A patient with acute pancreatitis admitted in the intensive care unit (ICU) suddenly develops tachypnea and respiratory distress. An image of his X-ray is shown below:

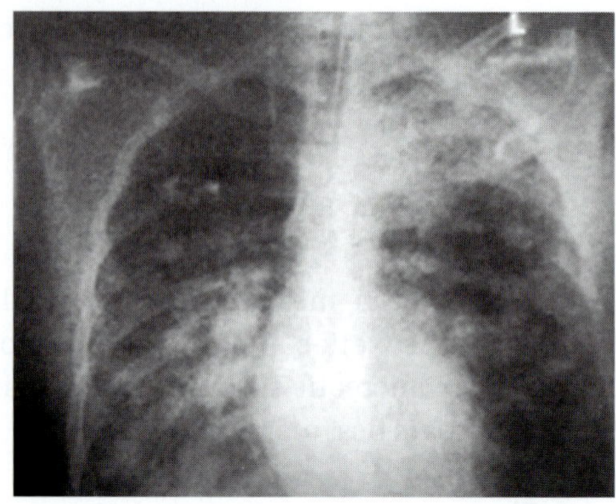

What is your diagnosis?

a. Acute respiratory distress syndrome
b. Pleural effusion
c. Pulmonary embolism
d. Fat embolism

Ans. a

Q6. Best investigation for carcinoma head of the pancreas?

a. Catheter-guided biopsy
b. Fine needle aspiration cytology (FNAC) by endoscopic ultrasound
c. Endoscopic retrograde cholangiopancreatography (ERCP)
d. USG

Ans. b

Q7. Neuroendocrine tumor of the pancreas associated with necrolytic erythema migrans is:

a. Insulinoma
b. Glucagonoma
c. Somatostatinoma
d. Vasoactive intestinal peptide tumors (VIPoma)

Ans. b

Q8. Miss X, a 35-year-old, presented to the emergency department with upper abdominal pain radiating to the back. On X-ray, the colon cutoff sign is seen. Likely diagnosis is:

a. Acute cholecystitis
b. Acute appendicitis
c. Acute pancreatitis
d. Acute cholangitis

Ans. c

Q9. An obese 30-year-old female with the sudden onset of central abdominal pain radiating to the back. What is your diagnosis?

a. Acute cholecystitis
b. Ruptured ectopic
c. Acute pancreatitis
d. Acute appendicitis

Ans. c

Q10. A 25-year-old alcoholic male presents with pain in the epigastric region radiating to the back. What is the likely diagnosis from the image?

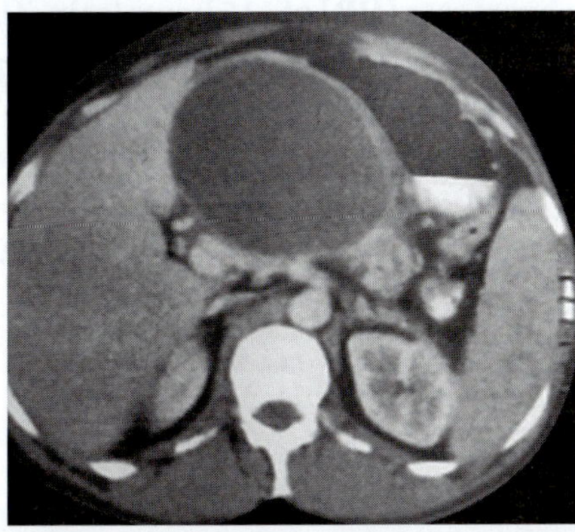

a. Amebic liver abscess
b. Pseudocyst of the pancreas
c. Acute cholecystitis
d. Hydatid cyst

Ans. b

Q11. Which of the following is the most common nonalcoholic cause of acute pancreatitis?

a. Thiazides
b. Hypercalcemia
c. Hyperlipidemia
d. Gallstones

Ans. d

Q12. The most common cause of acute pancreatitis is:

a. Biliary calculi
b. Alcohol abuse
c. Infective
d. Idiopathic

Ans. a

Q13. Postoperative pancreatitis is seen in which type of surgery?

a. Billroth type I
b. Splenectomy
c. Nephrectomy
d. Cardiopulmonary bypass

Ans. b and d

Q14. Which of the following does not cause an increase in serum amylase?

a. Pancreatitis
b. Carcinoma lung
c. Renal failure
d. Cardiac failure

Ans. d

Q15. Which of the following is the most diagnostic investigation for acute pancreatitis?

a. Serum amylase
b. Serum lipase
c. Serum P-isoamylase
d. Serum LDH

Ans. b

Q16. Destruction of fat in acute pancreatitis is due to:

a. Lipase and trypsin
b. Secretin
c. Lipase and elastase
d. Cholecystokinin and trypsin

Ans. a

Q17. All of the following patients presenting with abdominal pain and shock need immediate laparotomy, *except*:

a. Ruptured ectopic pregnancy
b. Hemorrhage pancreatitis
c. Rupture abdominal aortic aneurysm
d. Ruptured liver hemangioma

Ans. b

Q18. Acute pancreatitis is associated with all, *except*:

a. Steatorrhea
b. Epigastric tenderness
c. Upper abdominal pain
d. Cullen's sign

Ans. a

Q19. Which of the following is not a component of the Acute Physiology and Chronic Health Evaluation (APACHE) score?

a. Serum potassium
b. Serum sodium
c. Serum calcium
d. Creatinine

Ans. c

Q20. The computed tomography (CT) severity index is a marker for:

a. Hepatitis
b. Pancreatitis
c. Cerebral trauma
d. Meningitis

Ans. b

MULTIPLE CHOICE QUESTIONS

Grade I	*Simple*

Q1. An alcoholic patient comes to the hospital with severe abdominal pain and vomiting, and severe guarding is seen. X-ray chest was done—looks normal. What is the next investigation to arrive at a diagnosis? (AIIMS May 2019)

a. Serum lipase
b. Upper GI endoscopy
c. CT scan abdomen
d. Alcohol breath test

Q2. Most common (MC) complication after ERCP is: (AIIMS May 2007)

a. Acute pancreatitis
b. Acute cholangitis
c. Acute cholecystitis
d. Duodenal perforation

Q3. Which of the following is not an etiological factor for pancreatitis? (AIIMS May 2014)
- a. Abdominal trauma
- b. Hyperlipidemia
- c. Islet cell hyperplasia
- d. Germline mutations in the cationic trypsinogen gene

Q4. Poor prognosis factor in a patient with acute pancreatitis: (JIPMER 2011)
- a. Leukocytosis >20,000/μL
- b. Decreased serum amylase
- c. Decreased serum lipase
- d. Diastolic blood pressure (BP) >90 mm Hg

Q5. Medical treatment of acute pancreatitis includes: (PGI November 2011)
- a. Calcium
- b. Glucagon
- c. Aprotinin
- d. Cholestyramine
- e. Antibiotics

Q6. Which of the following criteria is/are not included in Ranson's scoring? (PGI November 2011)
- a. WBC >16,000/μL
- b. Serum amylase >350 IU
- c. Age >55 years
- d. Serum lactate dehydrogenase (LDH) >700 IU
- e. Serum aspartate aminotransferase (AST) >250 U/dL

Q7. Hyperamylasemia is seen in all, *except*: (PGI May 2011)
- a. Peritonitis
- b. Acute pancreatitis
- c. Carcinoma of the esophagus
- d. Ruptured ectopic pregnancy
- e. Perforated peptic ulcer

Q8. Ranson's scoring for acute pancreatitis includes: (PGI May 2011)
- a. Age >55 years
- b. WBC >16,000/μL
- c. Sequestration of fluid >6 L
- d. Blood urea nitrogen (BUN) >10 mg/dL
- e. LDH >700 IU

Q9. Which of the following does not correlate with the severity of acute pancreatitis? (AIIMS November 2011)
- a. Serum glucose
- b. Serum amylase
- c. Serum calcium
- d. AST

Q10. A 76-year-old male presents to the emergency department with abdominal pain and an episode of binge drinking in shock with a BP of 70/50 mm Hg and a heart rate (HR) of 115 beats/min. The oxygen saturation of the patient is 70 mm Hg. Serum creatinine level was 2.4 mg/dL. The patient had raised transaminases. What is the likely diagnosis based on the CT image shown below? (AIIMS May 2016)
- a. Liver abscess
- b. Acute pancreatitis
- c. Acute pyelonephritis
- d. Severe acute pancreatitis

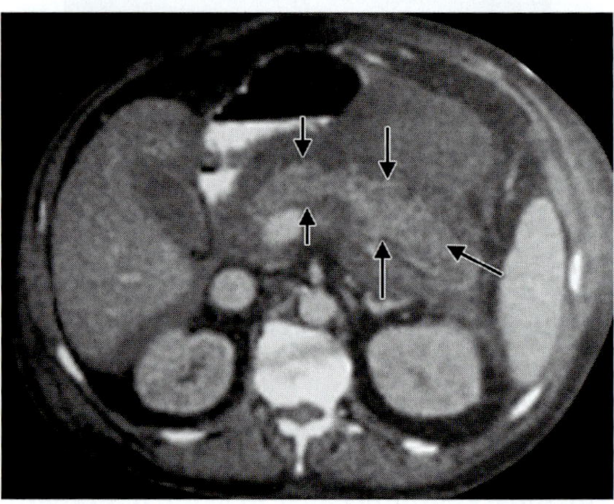

Q11. Gallstones are associated with which neutrophil extracellular trap (NET): (AIIMS GIS December 2010)
- a. Insulinoma
- b. VIPoma
- c. Somatostatinoma
- d. Glucagonoma

Q12. All are true about neuroendocrine tumor of pancreas: (PGI May 2011)
- a. Insulinoma is MC
- b. Vasoactive intestinal peptide (VIP) causes diarrhea
- c. Diarrhea is MC symptom of gastrinoma.
- d. Somatostatinoma causes gallstone formation
- e. Gastrinoma has a high chance of malignancy.

Q13. Treatment of choice for annular pancreas is: (All India 2010)
- a. Division of the pancreas
- b. Duodenoduodenostomy
- c. Duodenojejunostomy
- d. Roux-en-Y loop

Q14. The advantage of bladder drainage over enteric drainage after pancreatic transplantation is better monitoring of: (All India 2009)

a. HbA1c levels
b. Amylase levels
c. Glucose levels
d. Electrolyte levels

Q15. All of the following statements about nesidioblastosis are true, *except*: (All India 2011)

a. Hypoglycemic episodes may be seen.
b. Occurs in adults more than children
c. Histopathology shows hyperplasia of islet cells
d. Diazoxide may be used for treatment.

Q16. All of the following are true about diazoxide, *except*: (AIIMS May 2011)

a. K^+ channel opener
b. Can be used as an antihypertensive agent
c. Causes severe hypoglycemia
d. Used in insulinoma

Q17. Maximum risk of carcinoma pancreas is seen in which of these? (AIIMS May 2017)

a. Hereditary atypical multiple mole melanoma syndrome
b. Hereditary pancreatitis
c. Peutz-Jeghers (PJS) syndrome
d. Familial adenomatous polyposis

Grade II	Difficult

Q1. Grey Turner's sign (flank discoloration) is seen in: (MCI June 2018)

a. Acute pyelonephritis
b. Acute cholecystitis
c. Acute pancreatitis
d. Acute peritonitis

Q2. When to do surgery in pancreatic ascites? (JIPMER May 2018)

a. Symptomatic
b. Recurrent ascites following abdominal drainage
c. Nonresponding to medical therapy
d. Lead from the stented duct

Q3. Cullen's sign is: (UPPG 2007)

a. Bluish discoloration of the flanks
b. Bluish discoloration around the umbilicus
c. Migratory thrombophlebitis
d. Subcutaneous fat necrosis

Q4. Vascular complications of acute pancreatitis include the following, *except*: (UPSE 2007)

a. Splenic vein thrombosis
b. Splenic artery aneurysm
c. Gastroduodenal artery aneurysm
d. Middle colic artery thrombosis

Q5. All are true about acute fluid collection, *except*: (AIIMS GIS May 2008)

a. Not associated with fibrous wall
b. Most are extrapancreatic
c. Commonly associated with hemosuccus pancreaticus
d. Most resolve spontaneously

Q6. Most common metabolic complication of acute pancreatitis is: (AIIMS GIS May 2008)

a. Hyperglycemia
b. Hypocalcemia
c. Hypomagnesemia
d. Hyponatremia

Q7. All are true about chronic pancreatitis, *except*: (JIPMER GIS 2011)

a. Characterized by irregularities of pancreatic ducts, duct structures, and areas of dilatation
b. 60–80% will give a history of acute episodes.
c. CT scan showing pancreatic calcification is diagnostic of chronic pancreatitis.
d. Serum amylase is always raised.

Q8. True regarding chronic pancreatitis is/are: (PGI May 2018)

a. Can present with steatorrhea and malabsorption
b. Present with midepigastric pain radiating to the back
c. Markedly raised levels of amylase and lipase
d. Predisposes to carcinoma
e. Complete pancreatectomy relieves pain in the majority of patients

Q9. Most common symptom of chronic pancreatitis is: (JIPMER GIS 2011)

a. Abdominal pain
b. Cachexia
c. Weight loss
d. Steatorrhea

Q10. Chronic pancreatitis is seen in all, *except*: (PGI December 2011)

a. Chronic renal failure
b. Intraductal mucinous carcinoma
c. Alcohol
d. Gallstones
e. Pancreatic divisum

Q11. Feature of chronic pancreatitis with respect to pancreatic cancer: (PGI May 2011)

a. Smooth pancreatic duct dilatation with an abrupt interruption
b. Calcification
c. Duct penetrating sign
d. Duct/gland width ratio <0.5
e. Dilatation of the bile and pancreatic duct

Q12. Hereditary pancreatitis is characterized by all, *except*: (JIPMER November 2017)

a. 80% penetrance
b. 30% leads to chronic pancreatitis
c. Autosomal recessive inheritance
d. Pancreatic cancer risk is high

Q13. Most common cause of pancreatic pseudocyst is: (JIPMER 2010)

a. Blunt abdominal trauma
b. Pancreatic carcinoma
c. Pancreatitis
d. Postpancreatic surgery

Q14. Most common artery involved in a pancreatic pseudoaneurysm is: (PGI November 2009)

a. Gastroduodenal artery
b. Inferior pancreaticoduodenal artery
c. Gastric artery
d. Splenic artery
e. Hepatic artery

Q15. Regarding intraductal papillary mucinous neoplasms (IPMN), all are true, *except*: (AIIMS GIS May 2011)

a. Treatment is enucleation
b. Can involve either the main or the branch duct
c. Mostly involve the pancreatic head
d. Men and women are equally affected.

Q16. Serous cystadenoma, all are true, *except*: (AIIMS GIS May 2008)

a. 30% are associated with malignancy
b. Mainly microcystic
c. More commonly located in the head
d. Glycogen-rich cells on cytologic examination with a central calcified stellate scar

Q17. Most common mutation in pancreatic adenocarcinoma is: (GB PANT 2010)

a. K-ras
b. P16
c. P53
d. BRAF

Q18. Hereditary pancreatic carcinoma is associated with all, *except*: (AIIMS GIS December 2009)

a. Ataxia telangiectasia
b. PJS syndrome
c. Hereditary pancreatitis
d. Familial adenomatous polyposis (FAP)

Grade III	Most difficult

Q1. What is not autosomal dominant? (AIIMS GIS May 2011)

a. Hereditary nonpolyposis colorectal cancer HNPCC
b. Familial atypical multiple mole melanoma (FAMMM)
c. PJS
d. Ataxia telangiectasia

Q2. In carcinoma head of the pancreas, nausea and vomiting is due to: (JIPMER May 2018)

a. External compression of duodenum
b. Portal vein infiltration
c. Proliferation infiltration of tumor into the duodenum
d. Chemotherapy

Q3. According to the American Joint Committee on Cancer (AJCC) 8th edition, the staging of a 2 cm size pancreatic cancer if it involves the portal vein in is: (JIPMER May 2018)

a. T1
b. T2
c. T3
d. T4

Q4. A 60-year-old chronic smoker presented with progressive jaundice, pruritus, and clay-colored stools for 2 months. The history of waxing and waning of jaundice was present. A CT scan revealed dilated main pancreatic duct and common bile duct. What is the likely diagnosis? (AIIMS November 2015)

a. Carcinoma of the head of the pancreas
b. Periampullary carcinoma
c. Chronic pancreatitis
d. Hilar cholangiocarcinoma

Q5. Which of the following statements is not true about pancreatic carcinoma? (AIIMS May 2011)

a. Mutation in the *p53* gene is associated with 75% of cases.
b. Hereditary pancreatitis significantly increases risk
c. Median survival in locally advanced (stage III) disease is 3–6 months.
d. 5-year survival after curative pancreaticoduodenectomy is 20%.

Q6. All are true about pancreatic carcinoma, *except*: (JIPMER GIS 2011)
a. Ductal adenocarcinoma is the MC type.
b. K-ras mutation and human epidermal growth factor receptor 2 (HER2)-neu overexpression are the earliest changes.
c. Good prognosis
d. Most cases present late

Q7. Asymptomatic, solid 4 cm tumor of the distal pancreas. Treatment is: (PGI SS December 2010)
a. Observation
b. Distal pancreatectomy with splenectomy
c. Near total pancreatectomy with splenectomy
d. Distal pancreatectomy alone

Q8. All are true about pseudopapillary tumors of the pancreas, *except*: (JIPMER GIS 2011)
a. Most commonly occurs in young women
b. Both benign and malignant varieties are seen.
c. These are small tumors.
d. Local resection is usually curative.

Q9. All are true about Frantz tumor, *except*: (AIIMS GIS December 2011)
a. Seen in young females
b. Vimentin and CD56 are positive.
c. Indolent tumor with <15% incidence of metastasis
d. Chromogranin is positive.

Q10. The gold standard test for insulinoma is: (AIIMS May 2011)
a. 72-hour fasting test
b. Plasma insulin levels
c. C-peptide levels
d. Low glucose levels <30 mg/dL

Q11. Which of the following tests is not used in the diagnosis of insulinoma? (All India 2011)
a. Fasting blood glucose
b. Xylose test
c. C-peptide levels
d. Insulin/glucose ratio

Q12. Whipple's triad is seen in: (APPG 2015)
a. Insulinoma
b. Somatostatinoma
c. Glucagonoma
d. Carcinoma of the pancreas

Q13. All are true about gastrinoma, *except*: (GB Pant 2011)
a. Abnormal peptic ulcer location
b. Diarrhea
c. Decreased basal acid output (BAO) and maximal acid output (MAO)
d. Best treatment is omeprazole.

Q14. The least common site of gastrinoma is: (AIIMS GIS May 2008)
a. First part of duodenum
b. Second part of duodenum
c. Third part of duodenum
d. Fourth part of duodenum

Q15. All are true about Zollinger–Ellison syndrome, *except*: (AIIMS GIS December 2011)
a. Recurrent ulceration after acid-reducing surgery
b. Raised gastric levels in all cases
c. Decreased BAO/MAO
d. Diarrhea

Q16. All are true about gastrinoma, *except*: (AIIMS GIS May 2011)
a. 50% are associated with adrenal malignancy
b. Duodenum is the MC site.
c. Diarrhea can be prevented by nasogastric (NG) aspiration.
d. Total gastrectomy should be avoided.

Q17. Which is not true about a nonfunctioning neuroendocrine tumor (NET) of the pancreas? (AIIMS GIS May 2008)
a. Most PPomas are benign.
b. Slow-growing tumors
c. Constitute 30% of all pancreatic NETs
d. The prognosis is better than other exocrine tumors.

ANSWERS

Grade I: 1. a; 2. a (Sabiston 20/e p1526); 3. c; 4. a (Schwartz 10/e p1351-1360); 5. a, e (Harrison 20/e p2443); 6. b, d; 7. None; 8. a, b, c; 9. b; 10. d (Bailey 27/e p1223); 11. c; 12. a, b, d, e; 13. b; 14. b; 15. b; 16. c; 17. c

Grade II: 1. c; 2. d (Schwartz 10/e p1378); 3. b; 4. d (Bailey 27/e p1228); 5. c; 6. b; 7. d (Sabiston 20/e p1531-1536); 8. a, b, d, e; 9. a; 10. None (Harrison 20/e p2445); 11. b, c, e; 12. c; 13. c; 14. d; 15. a; 16. a; 17. a; 18. d

Grade III: 1. d; 2. a (Schwartz 10/e p1395); 3. a; 4. b (Schwartz 10/e p1395); 5. c (Sabiston 20/e p1547); 6. c; 7. b (Sabiston 20/e p1547); 8. c; 9. d; 10. a; 11. b; 12. a; 13. c; 14. d; 15. c; 16. a; 17. a

MODEL QUESTIONS

Q1. Beger's procedure:
a. Duodenum-preserving pancreatic head resection (DPPHR)
b. Lateral pancreaticojejunostomy (LRLPJ)
c. Caudal pancreaticojejunostomy
d. Longitudinal pancreaticojejunostomy

Ans. a

Q2. The operation for chronic pancreatitis is the following, *except*:
a. Beger's procedure
b. Longitudinal pancreatojejunostomy
c. Frey procedure
d. None

Ans. d

Q3. Complications of chronic pancreatitis include all, *except*:
a. Renal artery stenosis
b. Pseudocyst
c. Splenic vein stenosis
d. Fistulae

Ans. a

Q4. All of the following are true about chronic pancreatitis, *except*:
a. Damage to the exocrine part with damage to the endocrine
b. Can lead to malignancy
c. Whipple's procedure can be done
d. Gallbladder stone is the MC cause.

Ans. d

Q5. The treatment of choice for an asymptomatic pseudocyst pancreas is:
a. Marsupialization
b. Conservative
c. Drainage
d. Cystogastrostomy

Ans. b

Q6. The MC complication of pseudocyst of the pancreas is:
a. MC into peritoneum
b. Rupture into the colon
c. Hemorrhage
d. Infection

Ans. d

Q7. Increased amylase, mucin, and carcinoembryonic antigen (CEA) are seen in:
a. Intraductal papillary mucinous neoplasm (IPMN)
b. Mucinous cystadenoma
c. Serous cystadenoma
d. Solid pseudopapillary tumor

Ans. a

Q8. Not a risk factor for carcinoma pancreas:
a. Acute pancreatitis
b. Diabetes
c. Smoking
d. Obesity

Ans. a

Q9. The most likely cause of fluctuating jaundice in a middle-aged or elderly man is:
a. Periampullary carcinoma
b. Liver fluke infestation
c. Choledochal cyst
d. Carcinoma of the head of the pancreas

Ans. a

Q10. Which of the following drugs has been found in increase the survival of locally advanced pancreatic cancer?
a. Doxorubicin
b. Streptozocin
c. Gemcitabine
d. Paclitaxel

Ans. c

Q11. False about carcinoma of the pancreas:
a. The MC site is the head and uncinate process
b. Pain suggests unresectability
c. Two-thirds of patients present with diabetes
d. Acute pancreatitis never occurs in carcinoma of the pancreas

Ans. d

Q12. Localization in insulinoma is best with:
a. Contrast CT
b. Magnetic resonance imaging
c. Somatostatin receptor scintigraphy
d. Selective arteriography

Ans. d

Q13. The investigation of choice to detect gastrinoma <5 mm in size is:
a. Endoscopic ultrasound
b. Octreotide scan
c. CT scan
d. Portal venous sampling

Ans. a

Q14. Which of the following organs is the MC site of origin of the tumor associated with the Zollinger-Ellison syndrome?
a. Duodenum
b. Lymph nodes
c. Spleen
d. Pancreas

Ans. a

Q15. Diarrhea with a nonhealing gastric ulcer with proton pump inhibitors (PPIs) is due to:

a. Multiple endocrine neoplasia type 1 (MEN1) syndrome
b. Zollinger–Ellison syndrome
c. *Helicobacter pylori* infection
d. VIPoma

Ans. b

Q16. The triad of diabetes, gallstones, and steatorrhea is associated with which one of the following tumors?

a. Gastrinomas
b. Somatostatinomas
c. VIPomas
d. Glucagonomas

Ans. b

Q17. Ectopic pancreatic tissue is present in all, *except*:

a. Stomach
b. Meckel's diverticulum
c. Mesentery umbilicus
d. Small intestine

Ans. c

Q18. The Balthazar scoring system is used for:

a. Acute pancreatitis
b. Acute appendicitis
c. Acute cholecystitis
d. Cholangitis

Ans. a

Q19. "Chain of Lakes" appearance seen in:

a. Acute pancreatitis
b. Chronic pancreatitis
c. Carcinoma of the pancreas
d. Strawberry gallbladder

Ans. b

Q20. Gold standard investigation for chronic pancreatitis:

a. Magnetic resonance imaging (MRI)
b. Endoscopic retrograde cholangiopancreatography (ERCP)
c. Pancreatic function tests
d. Fecal fat estimation

Ans. b

SUGGESTED READING

1. Bailey & Love's - Short Practice of Surgery, 27th edition.
2. Schwartz's Principles of Surgery, 18th edition.
3. Textbook of Surgery by David Sabiston, 21st edition.

CHAPTER 39

Small Intestine

"It's like walking through someone's small intestine."

– Cody Lunden

INTRODUCTION

It is about 3–8.5 m in length from the duodenojejunal (DJ) flexure to the ileocecal valve. The first 40% of it is jejunum, and the remaining 6% is ileum, with no visible demarcation, but jejunum is wider with a thicker wall and more prominent folds of mucosa called valvulae conniventes. Ileum, on the other hand, has thicker and fatter mesenteric and more elaborate arterial arcades. The ileum also has more Peyer's patches (lymph nodes). The superior mesenteric artery (SMA) supplies blood, and the superior mesenteric vein (SMV) drains to the portal vein. Lymphatics follow arteries.

Autonomic splanchnic sympathetic nerves are around the SMA and its branches. Referred pain is felt around the umbilicus at T10 distribution.

PHYSIOLOGY OF THE SMALL INTESTINE

The main function of the small intestine is the digestion and absorption of nutrients. Carbohydrates and proteins are disintegrated by pancreatic enzymes and absorbed in the jejunum. Fats are disintegrated by pancreatic lipase, and the products are absorbed in the jejunum. Vitamin B_{12} and bile salts are absorbed in the terminal ileum, whereas all other fluids and salts are absorbed in the jejunum. High-density lipoprotein (HDL), low-density lipoprotein (LDL), and very low-density lipoprotein (VLDL) are synthesized in the small intestine **(Figs. 1 to 3)**.

HISTOLOGY OF THE SMALL INTESTINE

It has four layers: (1) mucosa, (2) submucosa, (3) muscular layer, and (4) serosa. The submucosa is the strongest layer. Cells of absorption are 95% of the whole cell mass, including goblet cells, Paneth cells, and enteroendocrine cells. Paneth cells protect stem cells and also control microbes to keep homeostasis in equilibrium.

INVESTIGATIONS IN INTESTINAL DISEASES

- Plain X-ray of abdomen in erect posture
- Barium meal for stomach and duodenum, and barium meal follow-through for small intestine
- Contrast-enhanced computed tomography (CECT)
- Capsule endoscopy
- Computed tomography (CT) enteroclysis
- Magnetic resonance (MR) enteroclysis

CROHN'S DISEASE (TERMINAL ILEITIS)

Crohn's (Burrill Bernard Crohn, 1884–1983, American gastroenterologist, described in 1932) disease is an inflammatory process of gastrointestinal tract (GIT) and can involve any part from lip to anus and is incurable. *Genetic factors involved are CARD15/NOD2. The most common site is the terminal ileum. Dianna's classification divides into four types: (1) Age, (2) structure, (3) fistula, and (4) site.* Clinically, pains in abdomen, bleeding, diarrhea, fissure, and fistula in anus are common. It can also cause kidney and gallstones, along with arthritis. Contrast-enhanced computed tomography (CECT) shows a comb sign of increased vascularity at the local site. CD can develop complications such as abscess, perforation, fistula, stricture, obstruction, and even cancer. Treatment consists of steroids, aminosalicylates, antibiotics, immunomodulatory drugs, such as azathioprine and cyclosporine, monoclonal antibody therapy, such as infliximab, Salman, vedolizumab, etrolizumab, nutritional supplements, endoscopic dilatation, and surgical treatment for complications.

TYPHOID AND PARATYPHOID

Salmonella typhi causes typhoid fever. Intestinal perforation is common, and surgical excision is done. Typhoid ulcers develop at the terminal ileum along the long axis of the gut.

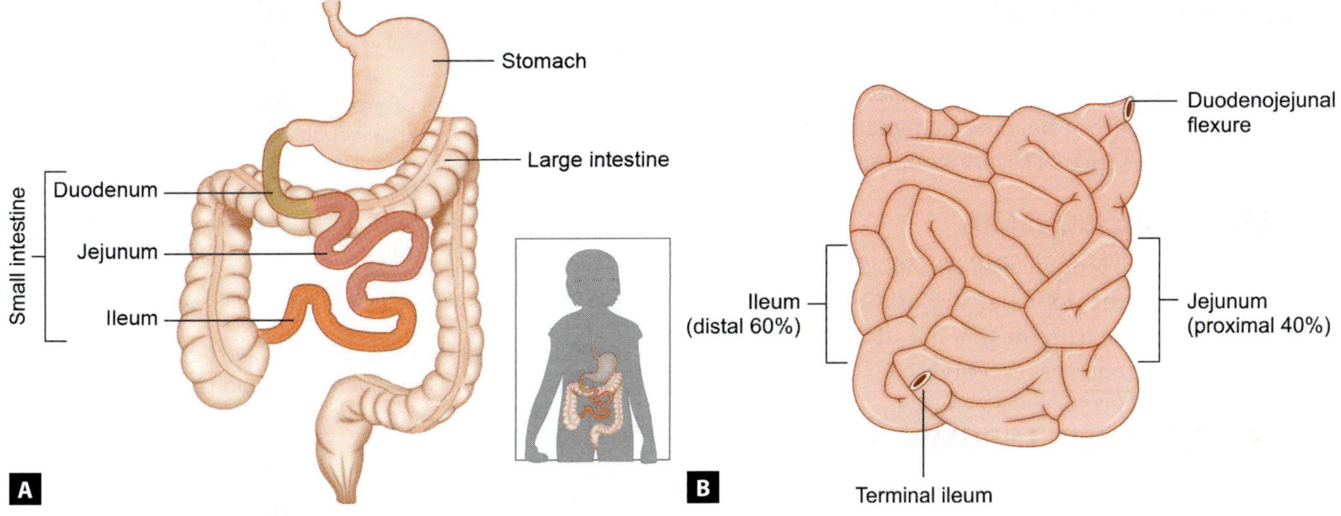

Figs. 1A and B: Anatomy of the small intestine.

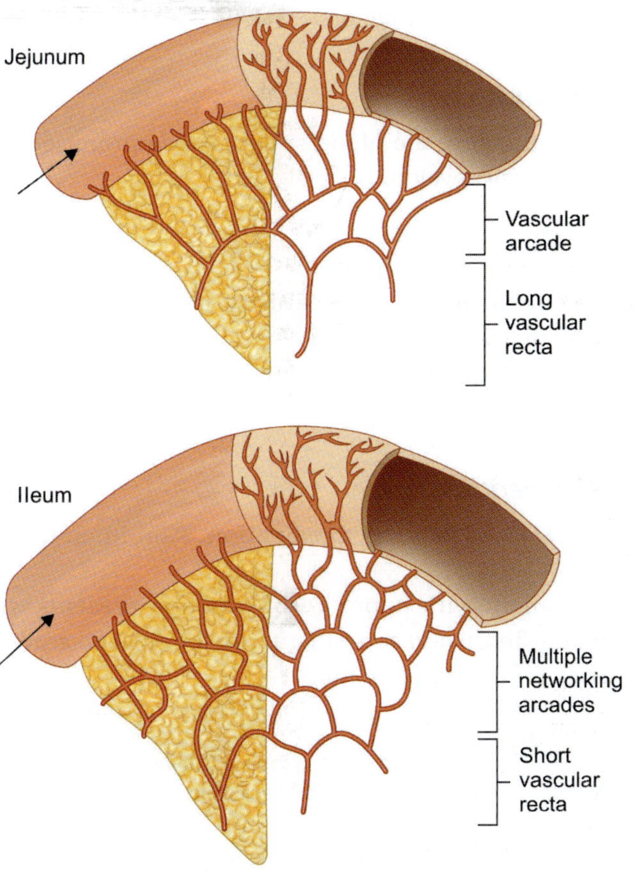

Fig. 2: Arterial arcades of jejunum and ileum.

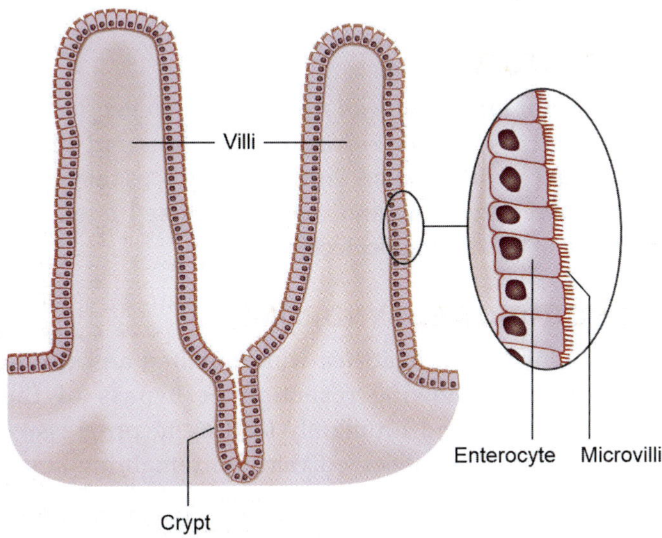

Fig. 3: Intestinal villi.

TUBERCULOSIS OF THE INTESTINE

It occurs in ulcerative form or a hyperplastic type. Treatment is with antituberculosis treatment and surgery for complications.

TUMORS OF THE SMALL INTESTINE

The tumors of the small intestine are rare and mostly benign as lipoma, adenoma, and hemangioma. Malignant tumors are adenocarcinoma, carcinoid tumors, lymphoma, and gastrointestinal stromal tumors (GISTs).

> *Points to remember:*
> *Distention of the proximal to the obstruction is due to the collection of gas and fluid. Gas is produced by aerobic and anaerobic bacteria present in the bowel.* Oxygen and carbon dioxide are absorbed, and nitrogen (90%) with hydrogen sulfide gases remain in the loop.
>
> Strangulation of the bowel is caused by direct pressure on the bowel wall, interrupted mesenteric blood flow, and increased intraluminal pressure.

PEUTZ–JEGHERS SYNDROME

Peutz-Jeghers syndrome is an autosomal dominant disease with perioral melanosis and hamartomatous polyps in the small intestine. Rarely, it become malignant. Resection is rare only in the presence of severe symptoms.

MESENTERIC ISCHEMIA

The most common is acute and chronic SMA ischemia. It is caused by a thrombus at the origin of the SMA. Abdominal pain is at extreme that it leads to gangrene of the bowel, which requires resection.

MESENTERIC VEIN THROMBOSIS

It occurs in hypercoagulable conditions such as pregnancy, dehydration, and deficiency of protein S and C. CT is diagnostic. It is treated by heparin, rehydration, and surgery if gangrene develops.

ILEOSTOMY

It is either a loop or an end ileostomy. Loop ileostomy is done by taking out a loop of the small intestine and is done to function distal intestine. End ileostomy is usually done in subtotal colectomy and may be reversed later, and permanent in panproctocolectomy.

SHORT BOWEL SYNDROME

It is the intractable diarrhea with impaired absorption of nutrients following resection or bypass of the small intestine and ultimately leading to progressive malnutrition. It is observed that the remaining small intestine remains <200 cm caused by acute SMA ischemia, CD, trauma, and necrotizing enterocolitis (NEC).

INTESTINAL OBSTRUCTION

The Road to Health is Paved with Good Intestines.

—Sherry A Rogers

The Fearon and Vogelstein sequence is an order of mutation:
- Normal colon^{APC}—hyperproliferating epithelium^{Kras}—early adenoma^{DCC}—late adenoma^{P53}.
- In order of frequency, intestinal obstruction occurs as adhesions—hernias—malignant tumor—Crohn's disease.
- Partial obstruction allows gas and fluid to reach the distal part.

Intestinal obstruction is most commonly caused by adhesions (approximately), and malignant tumors are the second most common cause about (20%). Hernia (10%) and other causes (10%) are responsible for the rest of the cases.

Intestinal obstruction is of two types:
1. *Dynamic:* It is a mechanical obstruction, and peristalsis acts against it; bowel contractions cause hyperdynamic sounds.
2. *Adynamic:* There is no mechanical obstruction. Bowel sounds are absent as there are no intestinal contractions. So, the abdomen is silent.

Causes of internal obstruction in the case of dynamic obstruction are:
- *Intramural:* Mass, stricture, volvulus, and intussusception.
- *Intraluminal:* Fecal impaction and foreign body.
- *Extramural:* Bands, adhesions, and hernia.

Dynamic obstruction is either paralytic ileus or pseudo-obstruction.

Adhesions are responsible for 40% of obstruction. Obstruction by hernia is around 12%, inflammatory 15%, and the rest by other factors.

Strangulation

In strangulation, the blood supply is compromised. So, ischemia will develop.

Closed Loop Obstruction

- When the intestine is obstructed at both the proximal and distal points.
- *Example:* Malignant stricture of the colon with a competent ileocecal valve.

Clinical Features

Mn: LOAD: Distention, Obstipation, Pain in abdomen, Lump.

A patient with upper GI obstruction presents with vomiting first, whereas a patient with lower GI obstruction presents with distention first.

Not to forget:
Internal hernia is caused when a loop of bowel gets entrapped in a fossa, foramen, or a defect. These hernias are rare and can occur at the following sites:
- Foramen of Winslow
- Defect in the mesentery, transverse mesocolon, and broad ligament
- Diaphragmatic hernia
- Duodenal retroperitoneal fossae (left paraduodenal and right duodenojejunal), appendiceal fossae, and intersigmoid fossa.

PATHOPHYSIOLOGY OF INTESTINAL OBSTRUCTION

Initially, when the obstruction happens, the mortality and contractility of the intestine increase as it tries to push the obstruction entity out to clear the obstruction. It may lead to diarrhea and vomiting. Then the contraction gets less in power and frequency as the bowel gets tired, and it dilates. Water and electrolytes accumulate in the lumen of the bowel and its wall (edema). This third space loss of fluid leads to dehydration and hypovolemia, even hypovolemic shock. With an increase in intraluminal pressure, blood flow in the mucosa and wall of the intestine reduces.

Important Points in Intestinal Obstruction

- Nausea and vomiting are common in proximal intestinal obstruction.
- Abdominal distension and cramps are common distal intestinal obstruction.
- In the early stage of intestinal obstruction, borborygmi increase, but in the late stage, they decrease and gradually disappear.
- *X-ray erect:*
  Three to five air-fluid levels <2.5 cm in length are normal.
  - More than it indicates intestinal obstruction.
- Colicky pain is a feature of mechanical obstruction and not in paralytic ileus.
- Normal period of return of normal activity after operation is, i.e., small intestine (24 hours), gastric (48 hours), and colon (3–5 days).
- Postoperative ileus is more marked in colonic operations.
- The most common rotational abnormality of the small intestine is nonrotation.
- The most common type of intestinal malrotation is incomplete rotation.

ACUTE MESENTERIC ISCHEMIA

- Embolic obstruction is 40–50% of cases of acute mesenteric ischemia (AMI).
- The most common embolism is from the heart secondary to myocardial infarction.
- The most common site of embolic lodgment is SMA.
- Severe, sudden abdominal pain is the most common initial symptom.
- The investigation of choice is mesenteric arteriography.

MALROTATION OF THE INTESTINE

It is of four types:

1. *Nonrotation:* Failure of counterclockwise rotation—cecum on the left side and duodenal C is on right side.
2. *Incomplete rotation:* Arrest at 180° small intestine on right side with flexure to the right of the spine and cecum in midline
3. *Reverse rotation:* Duodenum is anterior and colon posterior
4. *Hyperrotation:* More than 270°, cecum lies in the left hypochondrium. Investigation of choice is an upper GIT contract study.

Investigations

- *Plain X-ray abdomen:*
  - *Erect:* More than three air-fluid levels are the sign of obstruction, and fluid levels increase in number with distal obstruction.
  - *Supine:* It shows the site of obstruction, proximal dilatation, and distal collapse.
- CECT
- *Ultrasound (USG):*
  - More information from plain X-ray.
  - Obstruction in jejunum—complete valvulae, feathery appearance, stepladder pattern.
  - Obstruction in the ileum—featureless.
  - Bowel loop obstruction in the colon can be complete or incomplete. Impending perforation can be told by checking the diameter of the bowel: SI 3 cm, LI 6 cm, and cecum 9 cm.

Management

Start with nil per os (NPO), intravenous (IV) fluids, decompression by Ryle's tube, and IV antibiotics.

Surgery: Exploratory laparotomy on urgent basis.

First, check the cecum, collapsed—small bowel obstruction, distended—large bowel obstruction, then check for viability of the intestine. If viable, then keep the bowel; if not, then resection and anastomosis.

How to check viability?
Mn: CAM
- *C:* Color is dark, both viable or not. Color becomes lighter on waiting if viable. Mesenteric artery pulsations are visible if viable.
- *A:* Appearance—shiny if viable and dull and lusterless if not.
- *M:* If viable, firm and visible peristalsis, if not, then flaccid and no peristalsis.

Intestinal Obstruction by Adhesions and Bands

Any irritation in the peritoneal cavity causes fibrin production, locally causing adhesion between opposite surfaces, leading to fibrous adhesion, which may get vascularized later and may form mature fibrous tissue.

Causes of adhesions:
- *Postoperative:* Most common
- *Others:* Tuberculosis (TB), pelvic inflammatory disease (PID), and Crohn's disease.
- *Investigations:* USG and CT scan.

It is treated by adhesiolysis.

Plain X-ray of the abdomen is the investigation of choice in intestinal obstruction, as dilated loops, multiple air-fluid levels, and no air in the colon. A CT scan is the most important investigation, but it cannot help in biopsy, and it is difficult to diagnose ischemia.

You may be asked:
- *Prevention of adhesions:* Peritoneal adhesions can be prevented by good and neat surgical techniques, saline peritoneal lavage to remove clots, minimizing contact with gauge, covering anastomosis, and raw peritoneal surface.
- *Duodenal atresia:* It commonly occurs in neonates. In Down syndrome, mothers have polyhydramnios, a double-bubble sign on X-ray, and bilious vomiting since birth. Diamond duodenoduodenostomy is a treatment.

INTUSSUSCEPTION

- When one bowel loop enters into other, it has two parts: (1) The receiving or intussuscepiens and (2) the telescopic part of intussusception.
- It is of two varieties: (1) Primary and (2) secondary.
  - Primary type occurs in children below 2 years of age due to hypertrophy of Peyer's patches, and secondary type occurs due to polyps, tumors, or Meckel's diverticulum.
  - In children, it causes red currant jelly stools and signs of Dance—a sausage-shaped mass in the right lumbar region and an empty right iliac fossa (RIF).

Investigations

- Plain X-ray of abdomen
- *USG:* Donut sign—one loop inside the other.
- *Contrast enema:* Claw or pincer sign.
- CECT abdomen.

- A true diverticulum has all the layers of the intestinal wall and false diverticulum has no muscle layer.
- *Hinchey classification of diverticulitis:* Stage I—pericolic abscess, stage II—pelvic abscess, stage III—generalized purulent peritonitis, and stage IV—generalized fecal peritonitis.

Treatment

- Resection and anastomosis, if perforation is expected.
- Reduction by pushing and not by pulling is the first line of treatment.
- Intussusception is most common in children and is of these varieties: Ileoileal, ileocolic, ileoileocolic, colonic, and retrograde.

VOLVULUS

- It is twisting or axial rotation of a portion of bowel about its mesentery.
- Sigmoid volvulus
- *Causes:*
  - Long and narrow mesentery
  - Redundant sigmoid
  - Loaded sigmoid in constipation

Clinically, the signs of obstruction are present. The chances of strangulation are present. It is of two types: (1) Fulminant—sudden onset with severe pain and early vomiting, and (2) indolent—slow, insidious, and late vomiting **(Figs. 4A to D)**.

Investigations in Volvulus

- *X-ray erect and supine:* Coffee bean sign
- CECT abdomen
- *Contrast enema:* Bird's beak and ace of spades signs.

Enteroclysis is done by introducing the contrast media of methylcellulose and barium and air via a nasojejunal tube followed with fluoroscopy to observe details of individual loop.

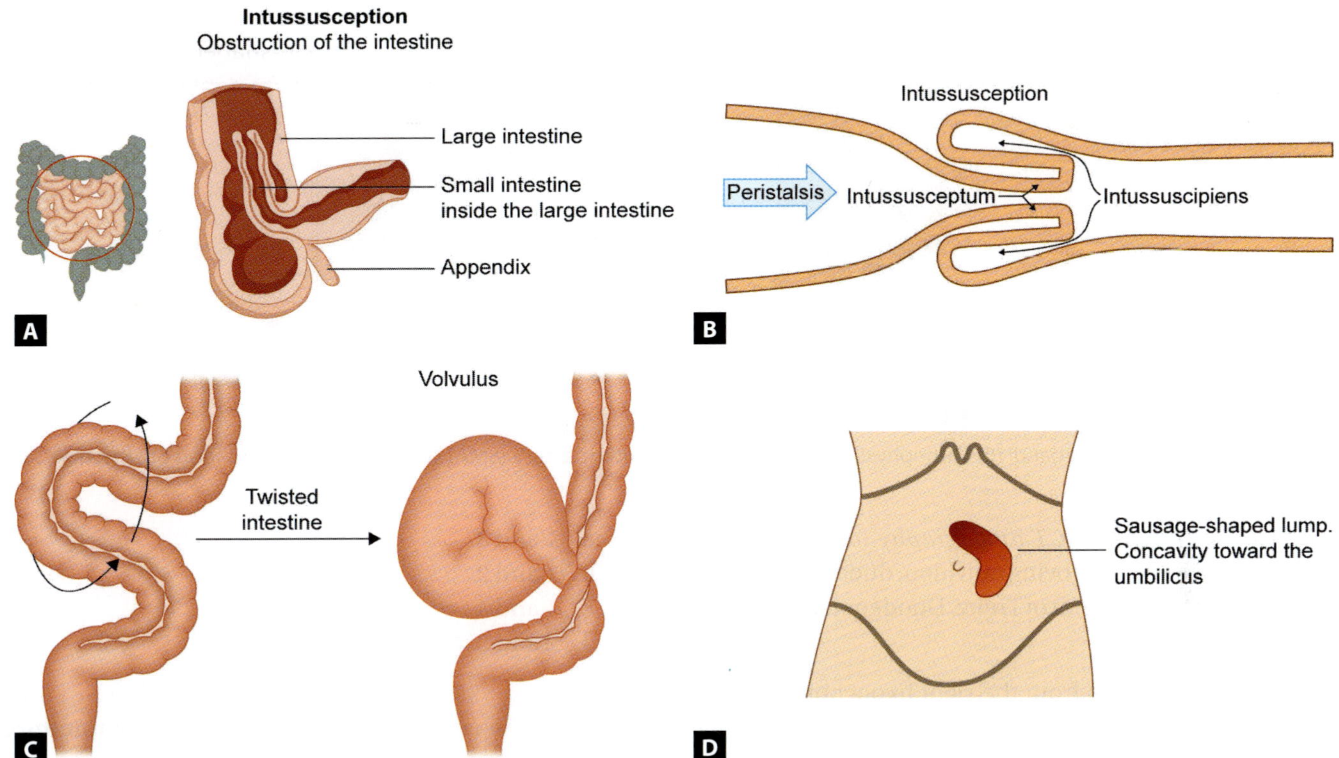

Figs. 4A to D: Mechanism of intussusception and volvulus.

Treatment

Treatment can be detwist volvulus and sigmoidopexy, and sigmoidectomy; decompression is mostly required.

CECAL VOLVULUS

It occurs with mobile cecum, clinically like obstruction, and clockwise rotation of the cecum. It is treated with cecopexy after detonation. Hemicolectomy may be required.

STRICTURE OF THE INTESTINE

- It is caused by cancer, TB, Crohn's disease, and postradiation.
- Clinically, as intestinal obstruction.

Investigations

- Plain X-ray abdomen
- USG
- CECT

How to reduce postoperative paralytic ileus?
- Reduce bowel handling during surgery.
- Avoid extra fluid administration.
- Electrolytes to be corrected.

Treatment

If single or at a distance, strictureplasty—incise longitudinally and suture transversely (Finney's and Heineke–Mikulicz strictureplasty). If multiple, resection and anastomosis.

Good to remember:
- *Jejunal atresia:* It is the noncanalization of jejunum. It shows a triple bubble sign on X-ray and emergency laparotomy is required to do resection and anastomosis.
- TB ulcers in the intestine and give rise to strictures, whereas typhoid ulcers are longitudinal and give rise to perforations.
- *Ogilvie's syndrome:* It is also called colonic pseudo-obstruction.
- It is associated with trauma, psychiatric medications, Alzheimer's disease, and Parkinson's disease. CECT abdomen is diagnostic. It is treated by Catchpole regimen (IV neostigmine after dynamic obstruction is ruled out otherwise perforation can occur. Meteorism is colonic distention 3–4 days after retroperitoneal trauma.

SUPERIOR MESENTERIC ARTERY SYNDROME (CAST/WILKIE SYNDROME)

The third part of the duodenum is caught between the aorta and SMA, forming the SMA aortic angle of 25–45°.

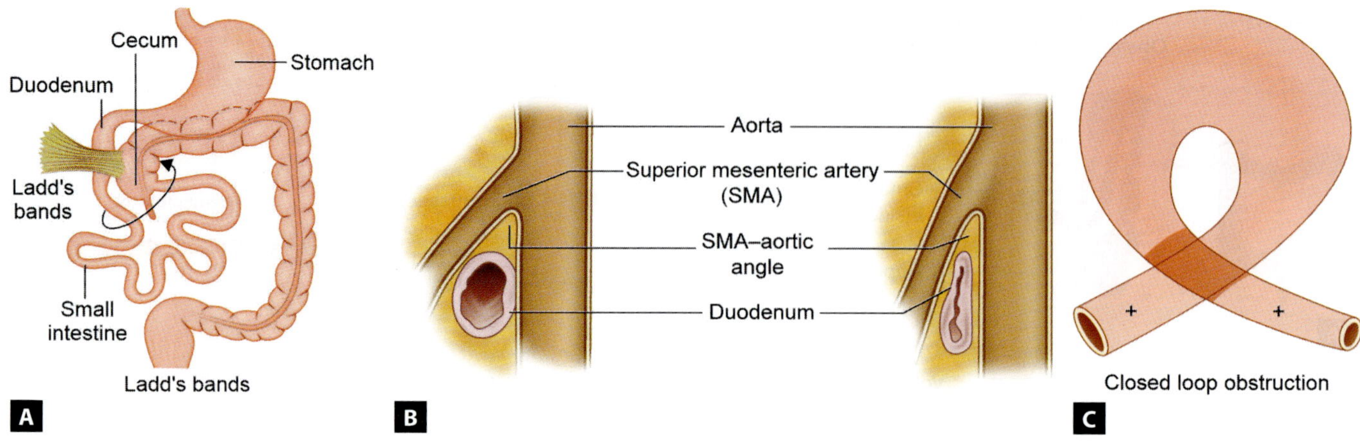

Figs. 5A to C: (A) Ladd's band; (B) Pathophysiology—superior mesenteric artery (SMA) syndrome; (C) Closed-loop obstruction.

Investigation is done by CT angiography to measure the angle. It is treated by improving nutrition, duodenal derotation by cutting the ligament of Treitz. Duodenojejunostomy may be required.

Ladd's band: It extends from the right hypochondrium to the cecum, compressing the duodenum. Bilious vomiting is the main symptom. Clinically, bilious vomiting after food. CECT abdomen is diagnostic. Excision of Ladd's band (Ladd's procedure) is the treatment **(Figs. 5A to C)**.

PARALYTIC ILEUS

Noncontraction (absence of peristalsis) of the bowel happens after a surgery and also after anesthesia, or in hypothyroidism, and hypokalemia. Clinically, as intestinal obstruction. CECT of the abdomen is diagnostic. It is treated by ivermectin fluids and supportive therapy.

SOME IMPORTANT QUESTIONS

Q1. Nutritional complications are more common with which fistula?

a. Pancreatic fistula
b. Duodenal
c. Colonic
d. Distal ileal

Ans. b

Q2. Most common ectopic tissue found in Meckel's diverticulum:

1. Gastric
2. Thyroid
3. Pancreatic
4. Adrenals

a. 1 and 3
b. 1 and 2
c. 1 and 4
d. 2 and 3

Ans. a

Q3. Mark the correct statements about inflammatory bowel disease (IBD):

1. Crohn's disease has skip lesions.
2. Childhood IBD is genetic.
3. Crohn's disease is mucosal, and ulcerative colitis (UC) is transmural.
4. Crohn's disease is curable fully.

a. 2 and 3 are correct.
b. 1 and 2 are correct.
c. 1, 2, and 3 are correct.
d. All are correct.

Ans. b

Q4. A patient who had M/C McBurney's incision is converted to Rutherford Morison incision. What are structures cut?

1. External oblique
2. Internal oblique
3. Transversus abdominis
4. Rectus abdominis

a. 1, 2, and 3
b. 1 and 2
c. 2 and 3
d. 1, 2, 3, and 4

Ans. a

Q5. An infant presents with abdominal pain. Barium enema is done—image shown below, what is your diagnosis?

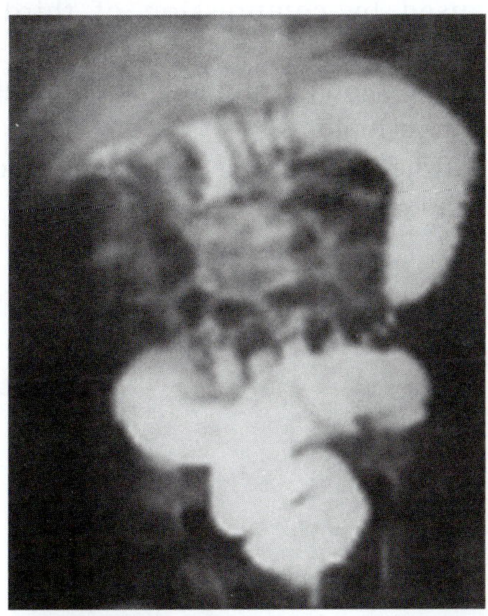

a. Volvulus
b. Malrotation of gut
c. Intussusception
d. Hirschsprung disease

Ans. c

Q6. Which part of the Bowel is shown in the specimen?

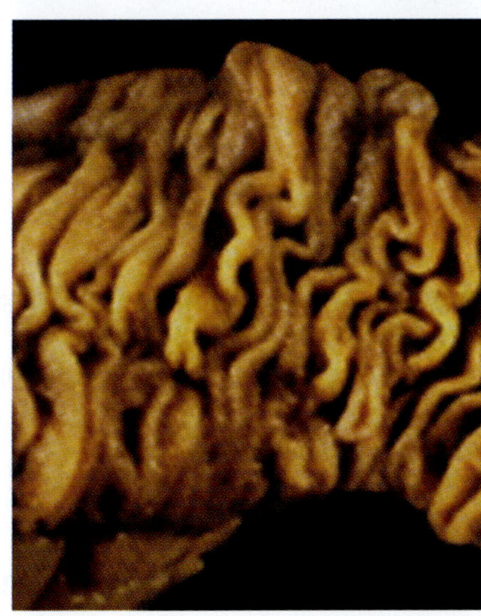

a. Jejunum
b. Ileum
c. Cecum
d. Ascending colon

Ans. a

Q7. A patient presents with abdominal distention features suggestive of intestinal obstruction. Which part of the bowel is distended here in the image?

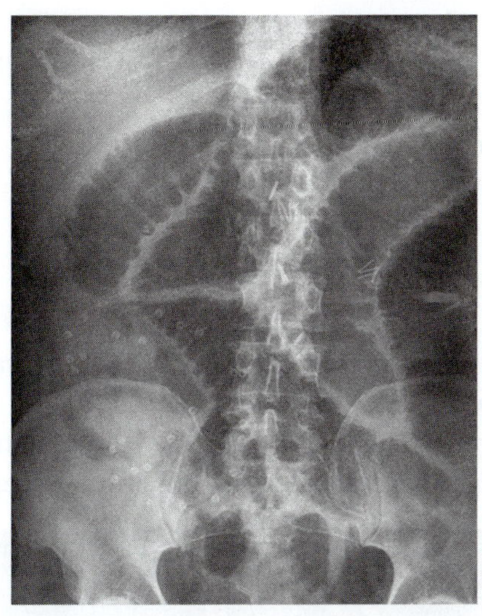

a. Jejunum
b. Ileum
c. Colon
d. Cecum

Ans. a

Q8. What is your diagnosis from the Barium enema image shown below?

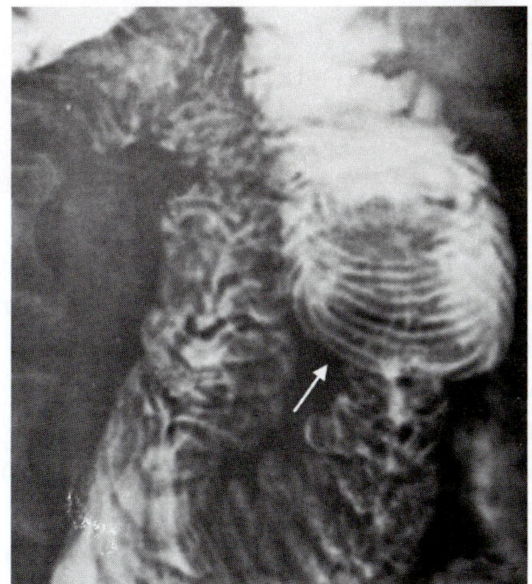

a. Intussusception
b. Sigmoid diverticulum
c. Cancer colon
d. Polyp

Ans. a

Q9. The most common morphological difference between ulcerative colitis and Crohn's disease is:

a. Crypt abscess
b. Diffuse polyps
c. Mucosal edema
d. Lymphoid aggregates

Ans. a

Q10. The most common presenting complication of Meckel's diverticulum is:

a. Hemorrhage
b. Intussusception
c. Meckel's diverticulum
d. Intestinal obstruction

Ans. a

Q11. What does the intraoperative photograph given below depict?

a. Transverse colon
b. Fallopian tube
c. Meckel's diverticulum
d. Intussusception

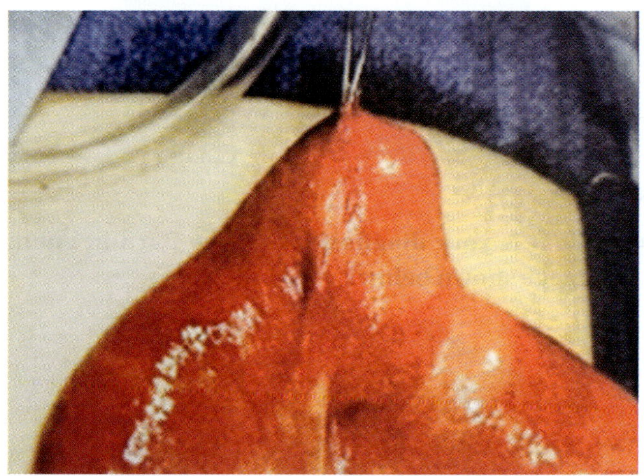

Ans. c

Q12. Which of the following statement is not true about Meckel's diverticulum?

a. Most common congenital anomaly of small intestine
b. Most common is ectopic gastric mucosa.
c. Bleeding may occur from the wall.
d. Wide mouth stapling at the base for nonbleeding cases

Ans. d

Q13. Fleischner sign on barium study is seen in:

a. Ileocecal TB
b. Crohn's disease
c. Small bowel carcinoid
d. Typhoid

Ans. a

Q14. All of the following are true regarding superior mesenteric artery syndrome, *except*:

a. Common in young females.
b. Caused by compression of third part of duodenum.
c. Vomiting and postprandial abdominal pain are typical symptoms.
d. Gastrojejunoscopy is treatment of choice in chronic cases.

Ans. d

Q15. What is the image shown below?

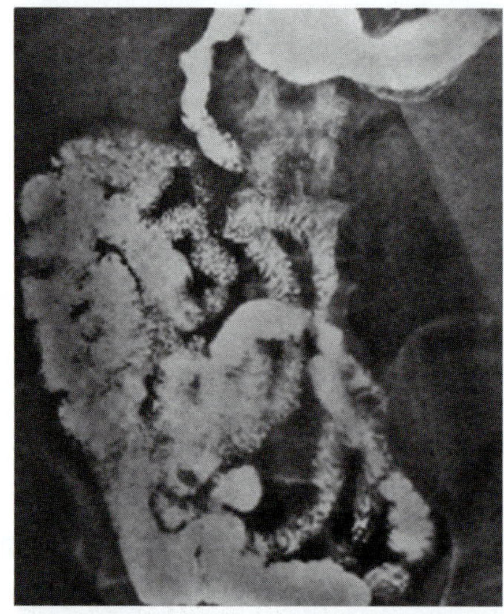

a. Barium enema
b. Barium meal follow through
c. Enteroclysis
d. Barium meal

Ans. b

Q16. Teduglutide is a recently introduced drug for short bowel syndrome. What is it?

a. Glucagon-like peptide-2 (GLP-2) analog
b. GLP antagonist
c. Somatostatin analog
d. H1 blocker

Ans. a

Q17. A patient presented with history of bronchospasm. Tumor was present in the ileum with increased 5-hydroxy indoleacetic acid (5-HIAA) in urine. What is the diagnosis?

a. Carcinoid syndrome
b. Neuroblastoma
c. Pheochromocytoma
d. Leiomyoma

Ans. a

Q18. A 7-day-old infant presents with bilious vomiting and gross abdominal distention with absent of bowel sounds. X-ray abdomen showed multiple gases filled loops. Diagnosis is:

a. Hirschsprung disease
b. Congenital hypertrophic pyloric stenosis
c. Duodenal atresia
d. Malrotation of gut

Ans. d

Q19. Meconium ileus is a presentation seen in which of the following diseases?

a. Mucoviscidosis
b. Hirschsprung disease
c. Ileal atresia
d. Congenital aganglionosis

Ans. a

Q20. Which is false about Crohn's disease?

a. No occurrence after surgery
b. Aphthous ulcer
c. Skip lesions
d. Fistula formation

Ans. a

MULTIPLE CHOICE QUESTIONS

Grade I	*Simple*

Q1. Ectopic mucosa of Meckel's diverticulum is diagnosed by: (AIIMS GIS December 2011)

a. Tc-99 radionuclide scan
b. Angiography
c. Computed tomography (CT)
d. Endoscopy

Q2. All are true about Meckel's diverticulum, *except*: (GB Pant 2011)

a. Congenital
b. True diverticula
c. Develop from the omphalomesenteric duct
d. All incidentally detected Meckel's diverticulum should be resected.

Q3. What is false about Meckel's diverticulitis? (AIIMS November 2015)

a. Present in 3% of the population
b. Presents with periumbilical pain
c. Remnant of the proximal part of the vitellointestinal duct
d. Lies on the antimesenteric border

Q4. All are true about duodenal diverticula, *except*: (AIIMS GIS May 2011)

a. Whenever found, it should be treated due to the increased risk of complications.
b. The most common site is the periampullary region.
c. Can cause acute pancreatitis
d. Most are asymptomatic.

Q5. The feature (s) of jejunal diverticula is/are: (PGI November 2010)

a. Increased folate absorption
b. Decreased ferritin absorption
c. Decreased B_{12} absorption
d. Urea breath test
e. Steatorrhea

Q6. True regarding barium study of ileocecal tuberculosis is: (PGI June 2009)

a. String sign
b. Gooseneck sign
c. Right-sided obstruction
d. Pulled-up cecum
e. Stierlin sign

Q7. Which of the following is wrong regarding superior mesenteric artery syndrome? (AIIMS May 2018)

a. The superior mesenteric artery (SMA) is compressed by a third part of the duodenum at the ligament of Treitz attachment.
b. SMA has a normal angle between 38 and 65° in relation to the duodenum.
c. Strong procedure is corrective surgery in which the ligament of Treitz is divided.
d. SMA syndrome is characterized by an angle <25° due to loss of the intervening mesenteric pad of fat.

Q8. Regarding adhesive intestinal obstruction, the true is: (AIIMS November 1994)

a. Avoid surgery for the initial 48–72 hours
b. Never operate
c. Operate after a minimum of 10 days of conservative treatment.
d. Immediate operation

Q9. Which of the following is most suggestive of neonatal small bowel obstruction? (All India 2003)

a. Generalized abdominal distention
b. Failure to pass meconium in the first 24 hours

c. Bilious vomiting
d. Refusal of feeds

Q10. All statements about adult intussusceptions are true, *except*: (PGI November 2009)
a. Idiopathic and more enteric rather than colonic
b. Lead point present in the majority of cases
c. Resection of the bowel is adequate for large bowel intussusceptions.
d. Hydrostatic reduction with barium or air is done if the bowel is not gangrenous.

Q11. Early sign of intestinal strangulation: (PGI SS June 2001)
a. Continuous pain
b. Abdominal rigidity and shock
c. Abdominal fluid
d. Dilated bowel loops on USG

Q12. While doing emergency laparotomy for an intestinal obstruction, which organ would you first visualize to say whether it is a small bowel or large bowel obstruction? (AIIMS Nov 2018)
a. Ileum
b. Sigmoid colon
c. Cecum
d. Rectum

Q13. The most common cause of intestinal obstruction in a 30-year-old Indian female: (All India 1993)
a. TB stricture
b. Crohn's disease
c. Postoperative adhesions
d. Adenocarcinoma

Q14. Acute intestinal obstruction is characterized by: (PGI Dec 2003)
a. Vomiting is common in duodenal obstruction
b. Pain after each attack of vomiting is characteristic of ileal obstruction
c. In colonic obstruction, distension is common than vomiting
d. X-ray erect posture is diagnostic
e. Colicky pain to steady pain indicates strangulation

Q15. A 30-year-old lady presented with acute abdominal pain, constipation, and vomiting, suspecting acute intestinal obstruction. The investigation of choice for the patient is: (PGI June 2003)
a. X-ray abdomen erect posture
b. Ba enema
c. USG
d. CT scan

Q16. A woman of 35 years comes to the emergency department with symptoms of pain in the abdomen and bilious vomiting, but no distension of the bowel. Abdominal X-ray showed no air-fluid level. Diagnosis is: (AIIMS June 2009)
a. CA rectum
b. Duodenal obstruction
c. Adynamic ileus
d. Pseudo-obstruction

Q17. One of the following will always present with bilious vomiting: (All India 1994)
a. Pyloric stenosis
b. Esophageal atresia
c. Atresia of the third part of the duodenum
d. Malrotation of the gut

Q18. Distended abdomen in intestinal obstruction is mainly due to: (PGI Dec 1998)
a. Diffusion of gas from blood
b. Fermentation of residual food
c. Bacterial action
d. Swallowed air

Q19. In case of a newborn, the commonest cause of intestinal obstruction is: (AIIMS Nov 1995)
a. Annular pancreas
b. Duodenal atresia
c. Jejunal atresia
d. Esophageal atresia

Q20. Water loss is severe if intestinal obstruction occurs at: (JIPMER 1990)
a. First part of duodenum
b. Third part of the duodenum
c. Midjejunum
d. Ileum

Grade II ***Difficult***

Q1. A young, apparently healthy patient presented with air under the bilateral domes of the diaphragm, which is because of: (GB Pant 2011)
a. Pneumatosis cystoides intestinalis
b. Diverticulitis
c. Perforated peptic ulcer
d. Band with Meckel's diverticulum

Q2. True about small bowel resection is: (PGI November 2017)
a. If the jejunum is cut, the ileum can compensate for jejunal function.
b. If ileum is cut, jejunum can compensate ileum function.

c. Ileum resection is generally better tolerated, as the jejunal shows better capacity to compensate.
d. Bile acid malabsorption leads to diarrhea

Q3. Complications of short bowel syndrome are: (GB Pant 2011)

a. Gallstones b. Oxalate renal stones
c. Cirrhosis d. All of the above

Q4. Causes of nonhealing of enterocutaneous fistula are all, *except*: (AIIMS GIS May 2011)

a. Epithelialization of the track
b. Radiation enteritis
c. Acute inflammatory disease
d. Track length >3 cm

Q5. All of the following delay healing of enterocutaneous fistula, *except*: (JIPMER GIS 2011)

a. Radiation b. Foreign body
c. >2 cm fistulous tract d. High output

Q6. The most common tumor of the small bowel in children is: (GB Pant 2011)

a. Lymphoma b. Carcinoma
c. Leiomyosarcoma d. Adenocarcinoma

Q7. In small intestinal malignancy: (PGI SS June 2009)

a. The most common site is the jejunum.
b. The most common site is the ileum.
c. The most common type is adenocarcinoma.
d. Less common due to decreased intestinal transit and increased enzymatic action.

Q8. The most common malignancy of the small bowel is: (PGI SS 2004)

a. Adenocarcinoma b. Carcinoid tumors
c. Lymphoma d. Papilloma

Q9. True about abdominal lymphoma is: (PGI November 2011)

a. GIT lymphoma: Most commonly has a polypoid appearance.
b. *Primary small:* Intestinal lymphomas are most commonly located in the ileum.
c. Lymphoma is the most common primary malignant neoplasm of the spleen.
d. The stomach is the most common site for extranodal lymphoma.
e. Mucosa-associated lymphoid tissue (MALT) lymphoma is associated with *Helicobacter pylori* infection.

Q10. The true about intussusceptions in children is: (PGI November 2010)

a. The most common variety is the ileocolic.
b. Associated with pathological lead point.
c. May be seen after viral infection.
d. Can be relieved by barium enema.
e. Surgery is always indicated.

Q11. Intussusception is frequently associated with: (JIPMER 2014)

a. Submucosal lipoma b. Intramural lipoma
c. Subserosal lipoma d. Subfascial lipoma

Q12. Best way to diagnose lower small intestinal obstruction: (PG 1996)

a. Pain abdomen
b. Abdominal distension
c. Profuse vomiting
d. Multiple air gas shadows on X-ray

Q13. Which of the following is most suggestive of neonatal small bowel obstruction? (All India 2003)

a. Generalized abdominal distension
b. Failure to pass meconium in the first 24 hours
c. Bilious vomiting
d. Refusal of feeds

Q14. A neonate presents with colicky pain and vomiting with a sausage-shaped lump in the abdomen, diagnosis is: (UPPG 2009)

a. Enterocolitis
b. Perforation of the abdomen
c. Intussusception
d. Acute appendicitis

Q15. A previously healthy infant presents with recurrent episodes of abdominal pain. The mother says that the child has been passing altered stool after episodes of pain, but gives no history of vomiting or bleeding per rectum. Which of the following is the most likely diagnosis? (All India 2011)

a. Rectal polyps
b. Intussusception
c. Meckel's diverticulum
d. Necrotizing enterocolitis

Q16. The most common type of intussusception: (MCI June 2018)

a. Ileocolic b. Colocolic
c. Ileoileal d. Retrograde

Q17. A child was operated on for a small intestine mass with intussusception, and after the operation, the tumor was diagnosed in the histological section. Which is the most likely tumor associated? (AIIMS Nov 2012)

a. Carcinoid
b. Villous adenoma
c. Lymphoma
d. Smooth muscle tumor

Q18. A 10-month-old infant presents with acute intestinal obstruction. Contrast enema X-ray shows the intussusceptions. Likely cause is: (All India 2002)

a. Payer's patch hypertrophy
b. Meckel's diverticulum
c. Mucosal polyp
d. Duplication cyst

Q19. Features of intussusceptions are: (PGI June 2001)

a. Pincer sign
b. Target sign
c. Dove sign
d. Coiled spring sign
e. Dance sign

Q20. Recurrent abdominal pain with intestinal obstruction and mass passes per rectum goes in favor of: (PGI Dec 1999)

a. Internal herniation
b. Stricture
c. Strangulated hernia
d. Intussusception

Grade III	*Most difficult*

Q1. The most common primary for small bowel metastasis is: (AIIMS GIS May 2011)

a. Lungs
b. Melanoma
c. Breast
d. Kidney

Q2. False statement regarding a benign small bowel tumor is: (JIPMER 2013)

a. Accidentally discovered during surgeries
b. Most commonly asymptomatic
c. Causes hemorrhage
d. Causes malabsorption

Q3. All are true about carcinoid tumors, *except*: (GB Pant 2011)

a. The small bowel is the least common site.
b. Multifocal in 30% cases
c. Associated with synchronous adenocarcinoma
d. Associated with multiple endocrine neoplasia link type 1 (MEN1) in 10% of cases.

Q4. All of the following statements about carcinoid tumors are true, *except*: (All India 2012)

a. It is the most common malignant tumor of the small intestine.
b. Extensive involvement of the small intestine is associated with a higher probability of lung metastasis.
c. 5-year survival for carcinoid tumors is >60%.
d. Appendiceal are more common in females.

Q5. True about carcinoid syndrome is: (PGI November 2011)

a. Associated with MEN1
b. Serum chromogranin A is elevated.
c. Urinary excretion of 5-hydroxyindoleacetic acid (5-HIAA) is increased.
d. Urinary excretion of 5-HIAA is decreased.
e. Octreotide is used for treatment.

Q6. False about carcinoid syndrome is: (PGI May 2011)

a. Foregut carcinoid—increased serotonin in blood
b. Midgut carcinoid—increased serotonin in blood
c. Foregut carcinoid—increased serotonin in blood
d. Midgut carcinoid—normal urinary 5-HIAA

Q7. Which of the following is true of small bowel carcinoids? (AIIMS November 2006)

a. The most common site is the duodenum.
b. It does not cause endocardial fibroelastosis.
c. Increased risk of carcinoma of the lung.
d. It is the most common malignancy of the small intestine.

Q8. All are true about intestinal transplant, *except*: (JIPMER GIS 2011)

a. The principal barrier to widespread application is vigorous rejection reactions.
b. Severe form of graft-versus-host disease (GVHD) occurs when T cells of the graft respond to foreign human leukocyte antigen (HLA) cells.
c. Uniquely dangerous complication is loss of protective mucosal barrier, bacterial translocation, and severe sepsis.
d. The majority of intestinal grafts are multivisceral grafts.

Q9. Small intestinal biopsy is diagnostic in: (PGI June 2006)

a. Whipple's disease
b. Abetalipoproteinemia

c. Celiac disease
d. Agammaglobulinemia

Q10. Regarding abdominal cocoon, all statements are true, *except*: (PGI November 2009)
a. Common in young girls
b. Associated with liver fibrosis
c. Fibrosis of the small bowel and stomach
d. Chronic peritonitis is seen
e. Seen in tropical and subtropical regions

Q11. Maximum water reabsorption in the gastrointestinal tract occurs in: (All India 2011)
a. Stomach
b. Jejunum
c. Ileum
d. Colon

Q12. On contrast radiography, which among the following is false? (AIIMS May 2011)
a. Ileum is featureless.
b. Colon has haustrations
c. Jejunum is feathery
d. Distal part of the duodenum has a cap.

Q13. Which of the following is the most prominent feature of immunoproliferative small intestine disease? (AIIMS May 2012)
a. Malabsorption
b. Obstruction
c. Bleeding
d. Abdominal pain

Q14. Meconium ileus is associated with: (All India 2000)
a. Fibrocystic disease of the pancreas
b. Liver aplasia
c. Cirrhosis of the liver
d. Malnutrition

Q15. Fluid levels are not visible in: (PGI June 1998)
a. Meconium ileus
b. Intussusception
c. Colon pouch
d. Duodenal obstruction

Q16. A newborn girl has not passed meconium for 48 hours, has abdominal distention, and vomiting. Initial investigation of choice would be: (AIIMS Nov 2007)
a. Manometry
b. Genotyping for cystic fibrosis
c. Lower GI contrast study
d. Serum trypsin immunoblot

Q17. Meconium peritonitis occurs: (PGI June 1999)
a. Just before birth
b. Just after birth
c. Before and after birth
d. Due to birth trauma

Q18. All are true about nonobstructive mesenteric ischemia, *except*: (AIIMS GIS Dec 2006)
a. Vasopressor treatment
b. Cardiac shock
c. Burns
d. Hypercoagulable state

Q19. All are true about acute mesenteric ischemia, *except*: (AIIMS GIS 2003)
a. The branch point of the middle colic artery is the most common location for embolism.
b. Acute venous thrombosis is best judged on CT
c. Nonobstructive mesenteric ischemia has a very good prognosis.
d. The gold standard investigation is angiography.

Q20. All are true about mesenteric ischemia, *except*: (AIIMS GIS 2003)
a. Due to embolism to SMA
b. The most common cause is atrial fibrillation (AF)
c. Embolus gets lodged most commonly at the branching of the SMA from the aorta.
d. A most common cause of small bowel syndrome in adults.

ANSWERS

Grade I: 1. a; 2. d; 3. a; 4. a; 5. c, e; 6. a, b, c, d, e; 7. a; 8. a; 9. c; 10. a; 11. a (Sabiston 20/e p1252); 12. c (Bailey 27/e p1294); 13. c; 14. a, c, d, e (Schwartz 10/e p1147); 15. a; 16. b (Sabiston 20/e p1249); 17. c; 18. d (Schwartz 10/e p1147); 19. b (Bailey 27/e p133, 1293); 20. a

Grade II: 1. a; 2. a, d; 3. d; 4. d; 5. c; 6. a; 7. b; 8. b; 9. b, c, d, e; 10. a, b, c, d; 11. a; 12. d; 13. c; 14. c (Sabiston 20/e p1879); 15. b; 16. a; 17. c (Sabiston 20/e p1879); 18. a; 19. b, d, e; 20. d

Grade III: 1. b; 2. d; 3. a; 4. b; 5. a, c, e; 6. a, d; 7. d; 8. d; 9. a, b, d; 10. b; 11. b; 12. d; 13. a; 14. a (Schwartz 10/e p1617); 15. a; 16. c; 17. a; 18. d (Bailey 27/e p1253); 19. c; 20. c (Sabiston 20/e p1155)

MODEL QUESTIONS

Q1. A 30-year-old man presents with a 4-day history of right iliac fossa pain. The ultrasound (USG) image is shown below. Which is the best management algorithm?

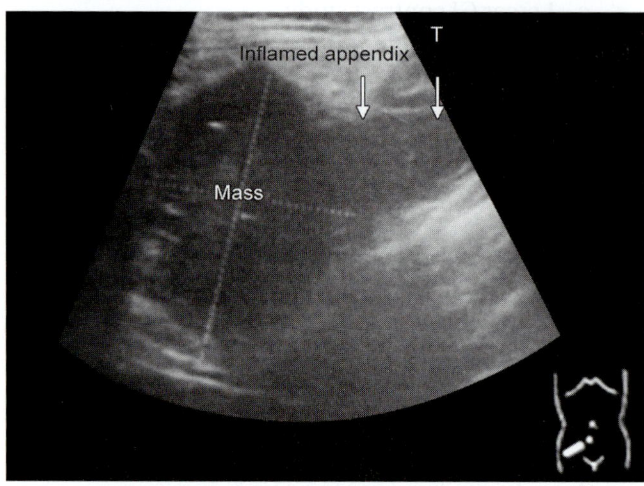

a. Ochsner–Sherren regimen
b. Urgent appendicectomy
c. Extraperitoneal drainage and parenteral antibiotics
d. Per cutaneous drainage and parenteral antibiotics

Ans. a

Q2. Comment on the diagnosis of a film shown below of a 65-year-old man with an acute abdomen.

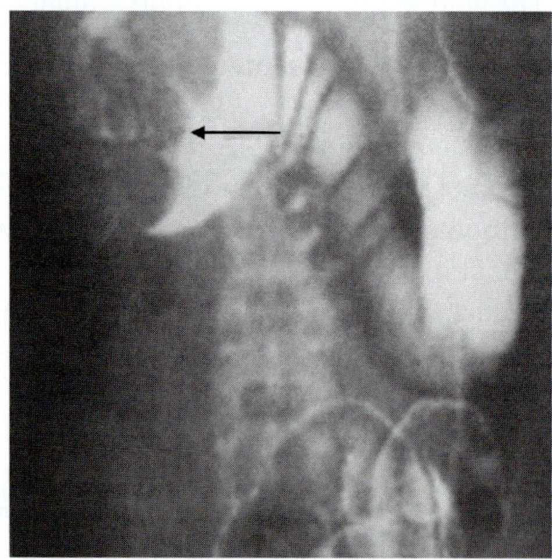

a. Ileocolic intussusceptions
b. Sigmoid volvulus
c. Toxic megacolon
d. Colocolic intussusceptions

Ans. d

Q3. Emergency surgery is indicated in ulcerative colitis in all, *except*:

a. Toxic megacolon
b. Colonic perforation
c. Colonic obstruction
d. Refractory fistula

Ans. d

Q4. Pneumatosis intestinalis in pain abdominal roentgenogram is seen in:

a. Meconium ileus
b. Neonatal necrotizing enterocolitis
c. Duodenal atresia
d. Intestinal obstruction

Ans. b

Q5. Deficiency of which of the following vitamin is most commonly seen in short bowel syndrome with ileal resection?

a. Vitamin B_{12}
b. Vitamin B_1
c. Folic acid
d. Vitamin K

Ans. a

Q6. Favorable features for closure of enterocutaneous fistula are all, *except*:

a. Tract <1 cm
b. No sepsis
c. No underlying bowel disease
d. No distal obstruction

Ans. a

Q7. Sign of Dance is:

a. Empty right iliac fossa in intussusceptions
b. Pincer-shaped appearance in barium enema in intussusceptions
c. Tenderness at the McBurney's point
d. Passing of large quantities of urine in hydronephrosis

Ans. a

Q8. Distal ileum was removed in a 20-year-old girl. Which absorption deficient will be seen?

a. Iron
b. Bile salts
c. Folic acid
d. Copper

Ans. b

Q9. True about Crohn's disease is, *except*:

a. Recurrence is more common.
b. Rectum is involved.
c. Fissures are formed.
d. Transmural

Ans. b

Q10. Alvarado score 2 defines:

a. Temperature
b. Leukocytosis
c. Tenderness in left iliac fossa
d. Migratory pain

Ans. b

Q11. Identify the pathology shown here:

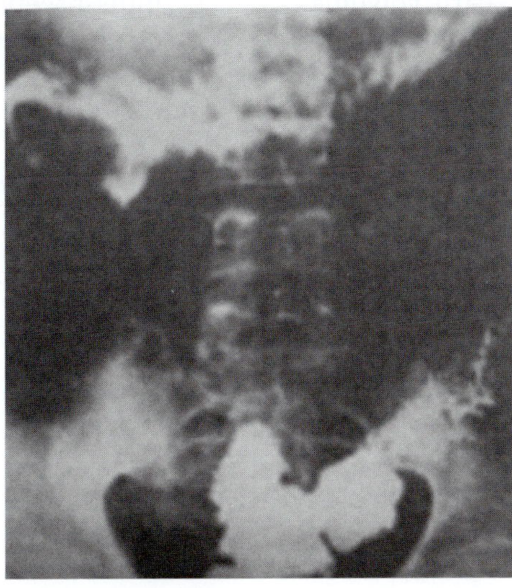

a. Intussusception
b. Ulcerative colitis
c. Cecal cancer
d. Ileocecal tuberculosis (TB)

Ans. a

Q12. An X-ray of the patient after abdominal surgery is shown in the image here. The patient is in a state of ileus. What is the most common cause of this condition?

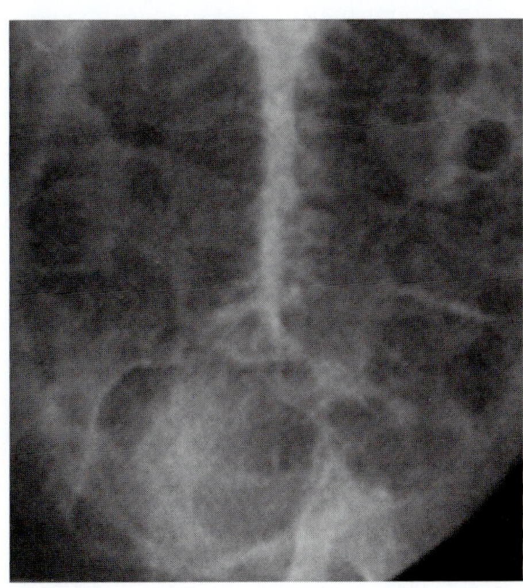

a. Hyponatremia
b. Hypokalemia
c. Hyperkalemia
d. Hypernatremia

Ans. b

Q13. An elderly woman who had not taken food for the past few days now presented with bilious vomiting. Her X-ray is shown below. What is your diagnosis?

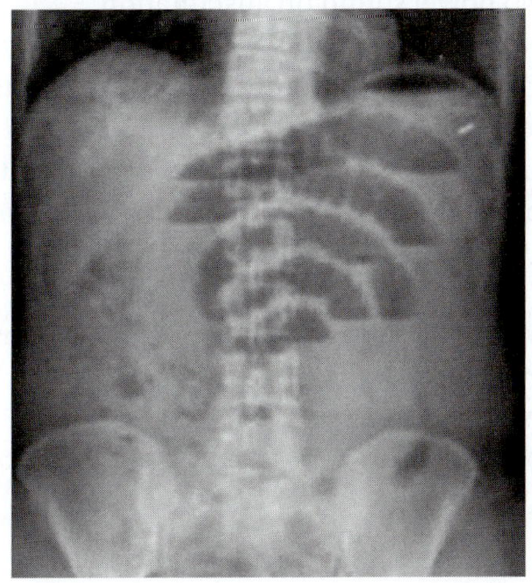

a. Distal obstruction in the small intestine.
b. Proximal obstruction in the small intestine.
c. Pseudo-obstruction
d. Distal colonic obstruction

Ans. a

Q14. Which is the site of maximum pain in acute appendicitis?

a. McBurney's point
b. Left flank
c. Suprapubic region
d. Umbilicus

Ans. a

Q15. Identify the investigation shown here in the image:

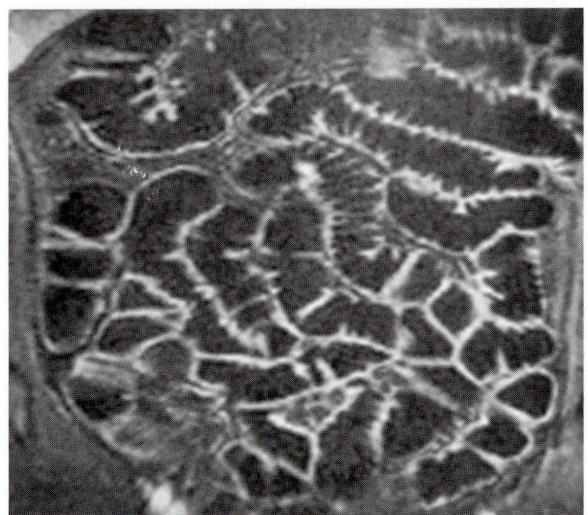

a. Barium meal follow-through
b. Enterography
c. Computed tomography (CT) enteroclysis
d. Magnetic resonance (MR) enteroclysis

Ans. d

Q16. Paralytic ileus is characterized by all, *except*:

a. No bowel sound on auscultation
b. No passage of flatus
c. Gas-filled loops of intestine with multiple fluid levels.
d. Loops of intestine are not seen due to loss of peristalsis.

Ans. d

Q17. Ogilvie's syndrome results from the denervation of the colon distal to the:

a. Hepatic flexure
b. Midtransverse colon
c. Splenic flexure
d. Descending colon

Ans. c

Q18. "Bird of Prey" sign is seen in the radiographic barium examination of:

a. Gastric volvulus
b. Intussusception
c. Sigmoid volvulus
d. Cecal volvulus

Ans. c

SUGGESTED READING

1. Bailey & Love's - Short Practice of Surgery, 27th edition.
2. Schwartz's Principles of Surgery, 18th edition.
3. Textbook of Surgery by David Sabiston, 21st edition.

CHAPTER 40

Large Intestine

"You are not what you eat, you are what you digest and absorb."

– Ashley Koff

INTRODUCTION

It is about 1.5 m long from the ileocecal valve to anus. It consists of the cecum, ascending colon, hepatic flexure, transverse colon, splenic flexure, descending colon, sigmoid colon, and rectum. The colon has a fat-filled sac called appendices epiploicae and three teniae coli, which pull the colon into sacculations called *haustrations* **(Fig. 1)**. These two features differentiate the colon from the small intestine. *Superior mesenteric artery (SMA)* supplies up to the distal transverse colon, and the IMA rest of. Marginal artery of *Drummond (David Drummond, 1852–1932, English physician)* supplies the colon all over, it is made from branches of arteries supplying the colon. Watershed area in the splenic flexure is the junction of the SMA and the *inferior mesenteric artery (IMA)*. Venous and lymphatic drainage follow arteries. Symptomatic splanchnic nerves are around the arteries. Pain from areas supplied by the SMA is in the periumbilical area, and of the IMA is in the Surabhi area.

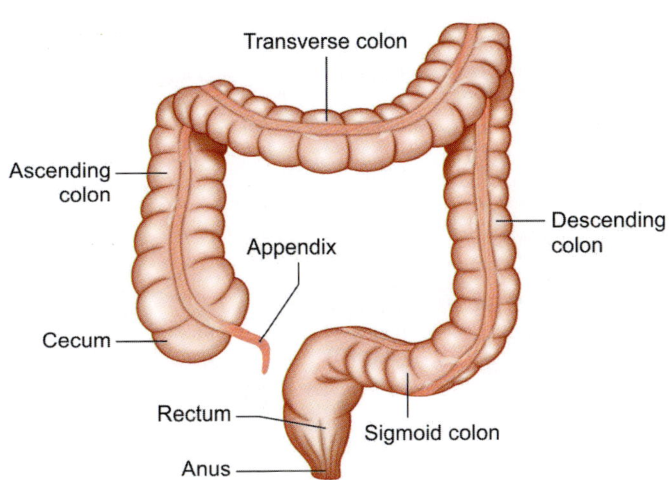

Fig. 1: Anatomy of the large intestine.

Points to remember:

Large intestine:

- Colonic adenoma and adenocarcinoma are similar in various features, but adenocarcinoma patients are about 5 years older.
- Adenoma as well adenocarcinoma distribution is similar; both are common on the left colon, about 70%.
- Adenomas of familial adenomatous polyposis (FAP) are having 100% chance to become malignant.
- Larger adenomas are more likely to be hyperplastic than smaller adenomas.
- Screening programs for screening patients with adenomas, colonoscopy, and polypectomy have reduced the incidence of adenocarcinoma.

PHYSIOLOGY OF THE COLON

Absorption of water, glucose, fatty acids, amino acids, and vitamins. Fecal material reaches the cecum in 4 hours and the rectum in 24 hours after a meal.

Virtual Colonoscopy

It is an imaging procedure with X-rays and computers to produce two- or three-dimensional images of the colon on screen, and the images can be used with the help of CT or MRI, one can pass through the colon through a 3D image, as in a colonoscopy. *It visualizes polyps' diverticulosis and cancer of the colon in detail.* The main disadvantage is that one cannot take a biopsy.

TUMORS OF THE LARGE INTESTINE

Benign

Polyps are protrusions of the mucosa. They are of various types: Inflammatory, hamartomatous, neoplastic, and hyperplastic polyps.

Adenomatous polyps are usually of three types: Tubular, bilious, and tubulovillous. Adenomatous polyps have the risk of malignant change, which increases with an increase in size; therefore, the polyps >5 cm are removed by snare resection or endoscopic mucosal resection.

Familial Adenomatous Polyposis

They are called FAP when colorectal adenomas are >100 in number and also may be associated with duodenal and many extraintestinal manifestations, most of them (80%) are with family history and others are with mutations in *adenomatous polyposis coli* (APC) gene on short arm of chromosome 5. Lifetime risk of cancer is 100% in FAP. *Gardner's (Eldon John Gardner, 1909–1989, American geneticist, described in 1950)* syndrome is associated with epidermoid cysts.

Clinically, FAP is seen on endoscopy from 15 to 30 years, if not then it is not FAP. Blood relatives are to be checked for FAP, malignant changes are rare before 20 years of age, surgery is done after the age of 18 years. Surgery can be ileorectal anastomosis (IRA) with colectomy, restorative proctocolectomy (RPC), and total colectomy.

Lynch syndrome is also called hereditary nonpolyposis colorectal cancer (HNPCC) and is an autosomal dominant mutation genes in most commonly affecting MLH1 and MSH genes. Colorectal, endometrial, gastric, ovarian, and ileal cancer risk is high, and lifetime risk of cancer is 80% in colorectal and 35% in endometrial FAP. Lynch I—only colorectal cancer. Lynch II—BEST PUGO (tumors of brain, endometrial, SI, thyroid, pancreas, urinary tract, gastric, and ovarian). Muir-Torre syndrome—HNPCC with multiple sebaceous cysts. It is diagnosed by Amsterdam II criteria: Three or more family members involved in HNPCC-related cancers, two successive affected generations, at least one diagnosed case of colorectal cancer before 50 years of age. FAP is excluded. Amsterdam criteria I is without cancers of CESUR (colorectal, endometrial, stomach, urinary tract, renal). The Betrhesda criteria include polyps also. Colonoscopy surveillance starts at the age of 20.

Carcinoma of the Colon

The most common site is the rectum **(Figs. 2A to C)**.

Right colon cancer is cauliflower or fungating type, whereas left-sided is stenosis or stricture type. Right-sided cancer presents with right iliac fossa (RIF) lump, melena, anemia, whereas left-sided a change in bowel habit and intestinal obstruction.

Risk factors of carcinoma of the colon:
- Diet-high animal fat, low fiber, and N-nitroso compounds in processed meat.
- Inflammatory bowel disease—ulcerative colitis (UC) and Crohn's disease.
- Smoking
- Alcohol
- Radiotherapy to the large bowel
- Cholecystectomy may increase the risk

Pathology

Cancers from the left colon are more common than right colon. These tumors are: Annular, tubular, ulcer, and fungating or cauliflower types. Colon cancers spread by lymphatics, locally, and by blood to the peritoneum, retroperitoneal, liver, lungs, and, less commonly, ovaries, brain, kidney, and brain.

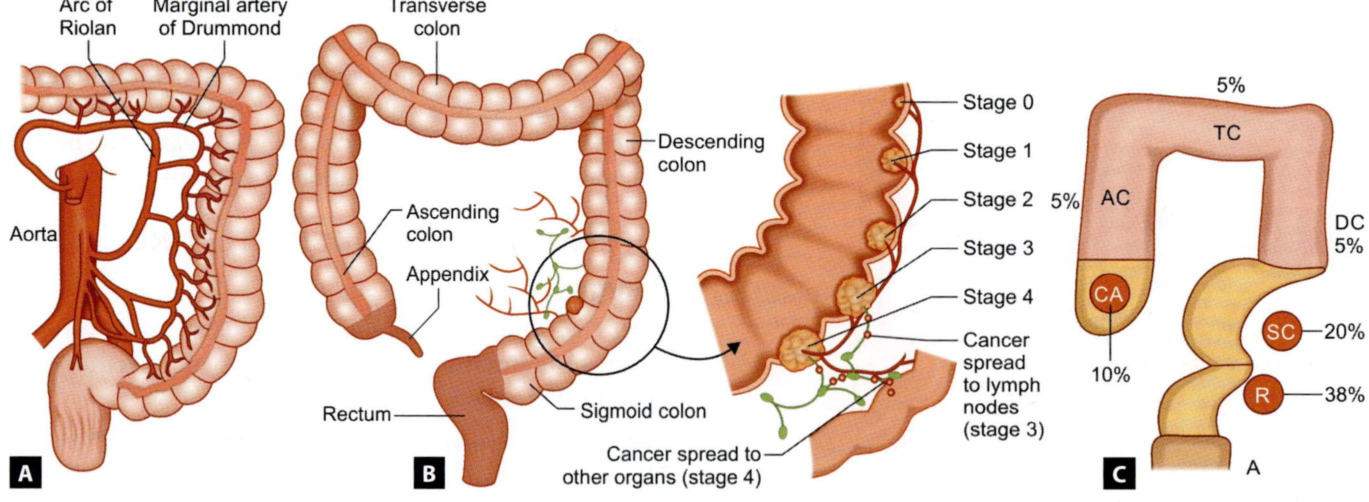

Figs. 2A to C: Carcinoma of the colon.

Staging of Carcinoma of the Colon

Dukes (Cuthbert Esquire Dukes, 1890–1977, English pathologist classified in 1932, he gave only three stages, A to C) staging.

A: Invasion of but not breaching the muscularis

B: Breaching the muscularis properties but not involving lymph nodes (LNs)

C: LNs involved

Tumor, Node, Metastasis Classification

- *T1:* Mucosa and submucosa
- *T2:* Muscularis properties
- *T3:* Pericles tissues, and up to serosa only
- *T4:* Adjacent structures beyond serosa
- *N1:* 1–3 LNs involved
- *N2:* Mets
- *Stage 1:* T1 and T2
- *Stage 2:* T3 and T4
- *Stage 3:* LNs involved
- *Stage 4:* Metastasis present

Prognosis is estimated by two main factors mainly:

1. Depth of invasion
2. LN status

Gardner's Syndrome

It is a subtype of FAP, autosomal dominant variant. It has several polyps in the colon that may become cancerous; nearly every polyp will become malignant if not treated. The triad of Gardner's syndrome is osteomas, polyposis coli, and mesenchymal tumors of skin and soft tissue.

Cowden Syndrome

It is an autosomal dominant inherited condition having hamartomas in the gastrointestinal tract (GIT), and there is a risk of cancer of the breast, thyroid, endometrium, and colon.

Investigations in carcinoma of the colon:

- Tumor, node, metastasis (TNM) staging.
- Contrast-enhanced computed tomography (CECT) abdomen—the most common site of metastasis is the liver.
- Tumor marker—carcinoembryonic antigen (CEA).
- Barium enema—apple core sign
- Colonoscopy with biopsy

Treatment

- Right hemicolectomy
- Extended right hemicolectomy
- Left hemicolectomy
- Total colectomy

You may be asked:

- Diverticular disease of the colon cancer develop some complications, such as Diverticulitis, abscess, bleeding, fistula, obstruction, and peritonitis.
- Hartmann's procedure is the safest operation for emergency surgery for colonic diverticular disease. Hartmann's procedure includes resection of a perforated segment, stoma formation, and reanastomosis once healing takes place.

Extended right hemicolectomy is done up to the splenic flexure for a tumor of the hepatic flexure, transverse colon, and splenic flexure.

Lymph nodes are in four levels, considered while performing hemicolectomy.

Mnemonic is EPIC:

E: Epicolic LNs—on wall of colon

P: Paracolic LNs—on the marginal artery

I: Intermediate LNs—on branches of main arteries

C: Central LNs—on the origin of SMA and IMA

Chemotherapy is only adjuvant, Folfox for six cycles in stage 3, but for stage 4, Folfox for six cycles.

How to do a follow-up for cancer of the colon?

- CEA-3 monthly for 2 years.
- CECT abdomen yearly for 3 years.
- Colonoscopy yearly for 5 years.

Bowel Preparation for Colon Surgery

- Prophylactic antibiotics
- Mechanical preparation—polyethylene glycol (PEG) and sodium phosphate

INFLAMMATORY BOWEL DISEASE

Colitis is the most common problem of UC. It is a disease of the rectum and colon, more common in Western countries than in Asian countries. The cause of UC is not known, but a genetic contribution is indicated.

Pathology

Ulcerative colitis starts in the rectum and then proceeds proximally. Lesions are inflammatory and are diffuse, superficial, involving mucosa and superficial submucosa, coaxing carcinoma possibilities are there. Dome cases have dysplasia-associated lesions or masses (DALMs), which are productive of coexisting carcinoma. Inflammatory cells are found in the lamina propria and crypts of Lieberkühn can cause abscesses in crypts.

Clinically, there is mucus discharge, bloody diarrhea, urgency, anemia, hypoproteinemia, and electrolyte disturbances. UC can be mild (less than four stools per day), moderate (4–6% stools), severe (more than six stools) fulminating (>10 stools). Toxic megacolon is a progressive colonic dilatation of the colon in fulminant colitis, which may lead to colonic perforation if emergency surgery is not done.

Not to forget:
- Principles for UC management are based on medical treatment and prevention of serious complications.
- Patients with colitis are at higher risk of developing malignancy, and especially those who have diffuse or pancolitis for a long time are at an increased risk.
- Plenty of patients are doing well with medication for a long.
- If a patient of UC develops sudden, severe pain in the abdomen, toxic dilatation must be suspected.

Extracolonic manifestations can be arthritis and skin lesions (erythema nodosum and pyoderma gangrenosum).

Investigations

- Endoscopy and biopsy
- Barium enema
- Computed tomography (CT)
- Stool culture

Severe pain development is an indication of suspicion of perforation, which is associated with high mortality. Patients with pangolins of long duration are at maximum risk of developing cancer.

Good to remember!
Left colonic obstruction includes resection, but one should consider the following points before embarking upon resection, and it should be avoided if the patient is very weak, moribund, and macerated, with advanced disease, and also if the operating surgeon is not well-experienced in such procedures.

Medical Treatment

- 5-ASA (amino salicylic acid) derivatives
- Corticosteroids
- Immunosuppressants, such as azathioprine and cyclosporine
- Monoclonal antibodies, Salman, and infliximab
- Surgery

Indications of Surgery

- Fulminant disease not responding to medical treatment
- Chronic disease with anemia
- Steroid dependence
- Neoplastic changes on colonoscopy and biopsy

Surgical procedure in emergency is subtotal colectomy, and as elective proctocolectomy and ileostomy, RPC with ileoanal pouch.

PSEUDOMEMBRANOUS COLITIS

It is caused by antibiotics, watery diarrhea is the main symptom, diagnosed by detecting toxin A (enterotoxin), and treated with metronidazole.

ISCHEMIC COLITIS

It is the most common type of ischemia of the GIT; common sites are the splenic flexure (Griffith point) and sigmoid colon (Sudeck's point). Treated medically, surgery is not required.

STOMAS AND THEIR MANAGEMENT

- Ileostomy—loop or end, protruding as stool is a liquid ileostomy (Brooke's).
- Colostomy—flushed to surface as stool is solid, in LIF (sigmoid colon) or epigastrium (transverse colon). Stoma may be in emergency or elective, temporary or permanent. Stoma can lead to some complications such as: Skin inflammation and excoriation, prolapse (common after loop colostomy), parastomal hernia (common after end colostomy).
- The double mesh technique, known as the Sugarbaker technique, is done for the repair of parastomal hernia.

HIRSCHSPRUNG DISEASE (CONGENITAL MEGACOLON)

There is a failure of migration of neural crest, absence of ganglion cells in Auerbach and Meissner's plexus in the constricted region of the colon, the *RET* oncogene mutation is seen, the constricted part is pathological, but the dilated part is normal. The most common site is the rectum, but it involves the whole colon and can even involve the ileum. Delayed passage of meconium occurs in newborns, but habitual constipation occurs in adults. It is diagnosed by biopsy above the dental line and treated by resection of the ganglion's segment and pull-through operation.

DIVERTICULAR DISEASE OF THE COLON

Investigation of choice for colonic diverticulum is barium enema. Investigation of choice for colonic diverticulitis is a CT scan.

- The sigmoid colon is the most common site of diverticular in the colon.
- *Types*:
  - *True diverticulum*—contains all layers of the intestine
  - *False diverticulum (pseudodiverticulum)*: Not all layer only mucosa
  - Most common are acquired diverticulitis

Pathology

- Herniation of mucosa occurs through the muscularis propria at a point where a nutrient artery penetrates the muscularis propria.
- High intraluminal pressure due to constipation caused by a low fiber diet is an important factor.

Investigation

Barium enema (saw-tooth appearance due to thickening of circular smooth muscle fibers).

Some important points:

- The most common site of Hirschsprung's disease is the rectosigmoid area (75%).
- The most common site of colonic diverticulum is the sigmoid colon.
- The most common colorectal polyp is the hyperplastic polyp.
- The most common type of colorectal hamartoma is a juvenile polyp.
- The most common feature of Cowden's disease is multiple trichilemmomas.
- Left-sided colon cancers are more infiltrative than right-sided.
- The most common site of lower GI bleed is the colon (95%)
- The most common cause of lower GI bleed in India is hemorrhoids.

SOME IMPORTANT QUESTIONS

Q1. In Hirschsprung's disease, an aganglionic segment is:

a. Normal or dilated
b. Normal or contracted
c. Dilated and contracted
d. Always dilated

Ans. a

Q2. True regarding colovesical fistula is:

a. Commonly presents with pneumaturia
b. Barium enema is diagnostic.
c. Common in females
d. May be a surgical complication

Ans. a

Q3. Most common fistula in diverticulosis of colon:

a. Colocutaneous b. Colovaginal
c. Vesicovaginal d. Colovesical

Ans. d

Q4. Massive colonic bleeding in a patient with diverticulosis is from:

a. Inferior mesenteric artery (IMA)
b. Superior mesenteric artery (SMA)
c. Celiac artery
d. Gastroduodenal artery

Ans. b

Q5. The most common site of bleeding diverticula is:

a. Sigmoid colon b. Descending colon
c. Rectum d. Ascending colon

Ans. d

Q6. Hinchey classification is used in cases of:

a. Complicated diverticulitis
b. Complicated pancreatitis
c. Complicated hepatitis
d. Complicated meningitis

Ans. a

Q7. Diagnosis of colonic polyps is best done radiologically using:

a. Barium meal series
b. Double contrast barium enema
c. Instant enema
d. Water-soluble contrast enema

Ans. b

Q8. The polyp associated with the highest risk of malignant transformation is:

a. Juvenile
b. Villous adenoma
c. Tubular adenoma
d. Polyp of Peutz-Jeghers syndrome

Ans. b

Q9. Most common associated cancer in familial adenomatous polyposis (FAP) is:

a. CA pancreas
b. Periampullary carcinoma
c. CA thyroid
d. CA stomach

Ans. b

Q10. Identify the stoma shown in the right iliac fossa:

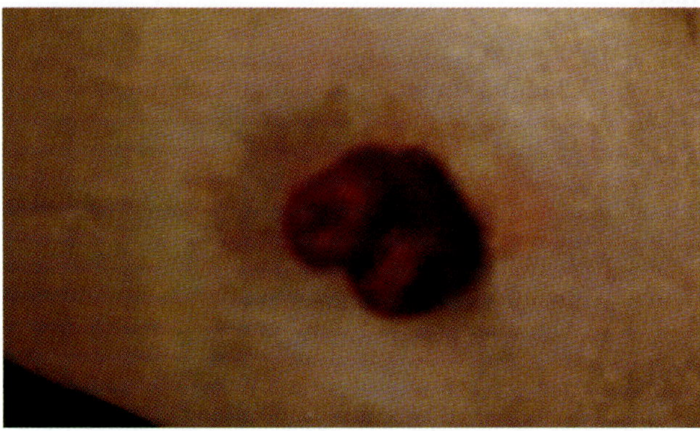

a. Loop colostomy
b. Loop ileostomy
c. End ileostomy
d. End colostomy

Ans. b

Q11. Barium enema image shows:

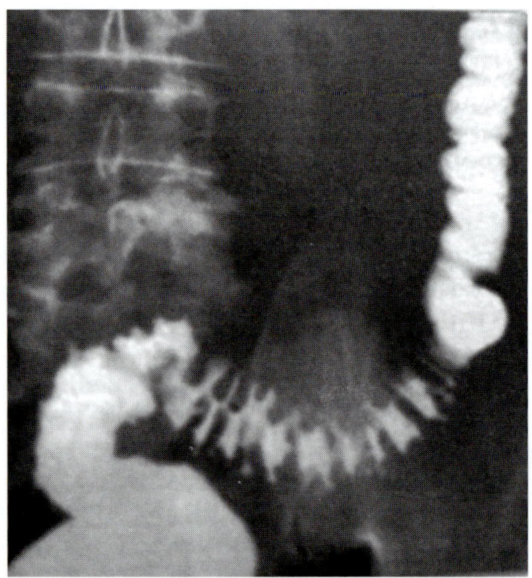

a. Meckel's diverticulum
b. Sigmoid diverticulosis
c. Sigmoid volvulus
d. Colon cancer

Ans. b

Q12. All the following are true regarding familial adenomatous polyposis *except*:

a. It is due to a mutation of the *APC* gene in chromosome 15V.
b. >100 colorectal polyps are present.
c. It is an autosomal dominant disorder.
d. Congenital hypertrophy of retinal pigment epithelium is seen in 50% of patients.

Ans. a

Q13. Lynch syndrome is also known as:

a. FAP
b. PJS
c. Hereditary nonpolyposis colorectal cancer (HNPCC)
d. Cowden's syndrome

Ans. c

Q14. Most common site of colonic carcinoma:

a. Sigmoid
b. Transverse
c. Descending
d. Ascending

Ans. a

Q15. True about enterocutaneous fistula:

a. High output fistula drains 500 mL/day
b. Malignancy is the most common cause
c. Fluid and electrolyte loss can occur
d. No skin damage

Ans. a and c

MULTIPLE CHOICE QUESTIONS

Grade I	Simple

Q1. Not associated with gastrointestinal (GI) malignancy: (GB Pant 2011)

a. Cowden's syndrome
b. Peutz-Jeghers syndrome
c. Juvenile polyposis
d. Gardner's syndrome

Q2. All are true about the risk factors for malignancy in polyps, *except*: (GB Pant 2011)

a. Pedunculated polyp
b. >2 cm
c. Villous polyp
d. Cellular atypical

Q3. All of the following are premalignant, *except*: (AIIMS 2014)

a. Crohn's disease
b. Ulcerative colitis
c. Peutz-Jeghers syndrome
d. Barrett's esophagus

Q4. Which of the following colonic polyps is not premalignant? (AIIMS 2006)
a. Juvenile polyps
b. Hamartomatous polyps associated with Peutz-Jeghers syndrome
c. Villous adenoma
d. Tubular adenoma

Q5. All the following polyps are premalignant, *except*: (AIIMS 2007)
a. Juvenile polyposis syndrome
b. Familial
c. Juvenile polyp
d. Peutz-Jeghers syndrome

Q6. Which of the following is not true about FAP? (JIPMER 2017)
a. Autosomal recessive (AR) inheritance
b. Screening done by sigmoidoscopy
c. Polyps develop in late adulthood
d. Epidermal cysts and osteoma can occur

Q7. Which of the following is true about FAP? (GB Pant 2011)
a. In the stomach, the most common are gastric adenomas.
b. Gastric carcinoma is common.
c. Duodenal carcinoma in 50% of patients.
d. Duodenal adenoma in 60–90% patients.

Q8. A male patient is diagnosed with carcinoma colon. Which of the following gene mutations is likely to be present? (AIIMS 2020)
a. Kara's, APC, DCC
b. APC, Kara's, P53
c. BRCA1, Kara's, APC
d. APC, Kara's, and loss of 10 on myc

Q9. True about familial polyposis colon cancer syndrome, *except*: (JIPMER 2011)
a. Autosomal recessive
b. Associated with fibromyalgia and osteoma
c. Associated with brain tumors
d. 1,100% incidence of colon carcinoma

Q10. True about Hirschsprung's disease: (PGI May 2010)
a. Aganglionic segment is contracted, not dilated
b. Descending colon is the most common site of aganglionosis
c. Barium enema is diagnostic
d. It is seen in infants and children only
e. Barium enema show calcification

Q11. Hirschsprung's disease is best diagnosed by: (AIIMS GIS Dec 2011)
a. Rectal biopsy
b. Anal manometry
c. Computed tomography (CT)
d. Magnetic resonance imaging (MRI)

Q12. Hirschsprung's disease involves which region of the intestine? (MCI March 2008)
a. Colon
b. Rectum
c. Rectosigmoid part
d. Terminal ileum

Q13. Investigation of choice is Hirschsprung's disease is: (AIIMS Nov 2005)
a. Rectal manometry
b. Rectal examination
c. Rectal biopsy
d. Ba enema

Q14. Fecal soiling in children is most commonly due to: (PGI June 1999)
a. Hirschsprung's disease
b. Chronic constipation
c. Rectal atresia
d. None of the above

Q15. Absence of ganglion in myenteric plexus is seen in: (PGI June 1997)
a. Crohn's disease
b. Ulcerative colitis
c. Hirschsprung's disease
d. Intussusception

Q16. Colonic diverticulosis is best diagnosed by: (AIIMS May 2007)
a. Colonoscopy
b. Nuclear scan
c. Barium enema
d. CT scan

Q17. A 17-year-old patient developed intussusception, for which he was operated on and a segment of intestine showing multiple polyps was resected. Microscopy showed the following pathology. What is the likely diagnosis? (AIIMS Nov 2015)
a. Tubulovillous polyps
b. Hamartomatous polyps
c. Inflammatory polyps
d. Adenocarcinoma

Q18. Which polyp has maximum malignant potential? (AIIMS June 1993)
a. Sessile
b. Pedunculated
c. Superficial spreading
d. Any of the above

Q19. All the following statements regarding the malignant potential of colorectal polyps are true, *except*: (AIIMS Nov 2002)

a. Polyps of familial polyposis coli could invariably undergo malignant change.
b. Pseudopolyps of ulcerative colitis have a high risk of malignancy.
c. Villous adenoma is associated with a high risk of malignancy.
d. Juvenile polyps have little or no risk.

Q20. True about neoplastic colorectal polyps: (PGI June 2003)

a. Sessile polyps >1 cm is malignant
b. The MC site is the colon and rectum
c. Adenomatous polyp is premalignant
d. Tubular adenoma is malignant
e. Pseudpolyps are premalignant

Grade II	***Difficult***

Q1. Desmoid tumor is associated with: (JIPMER 2013)

a. Colonic polyps
b. Pancreatic cancer
c. Ovarian cancer
d. Gastric cancer

Q2. Most common extraintestinal malignancy in hereditary nonpolyposis colorectal cancer (HNPCC): (AIIMS 2011)

a. Pancreatic cancer
b. CA stomach
c. Small bowel carcinoma
d. Transitional cell carcinoma

Q3. Colonic disease can be diagnosed by all, *except*: (PGI 2010)

a. Virtual colonoscopy
b. Barium enema
c. Barium swallow
d. Ba follow through
e. Enteroclysis

Q4. Most common site of postischemic stricture is: (JIPMER 2011)

a. Ascending colon
b. Hepatic flexure
c. Splenic flexure
d. Sigmoid colon

Q5. The most common cause of lower GI bleeding is: (UPPG 2007)

a. Diverticulosis
b. Colorectal carcinoma
c. Angiodysplasia
d. Anal fissure

Q6. Agent not used in bowel preparation: (AIIMS 2011)

a. Metronidazole
b. Polymyxin
c. Erythromycin
d. Neomycin

Q7. Which of the following is the terminal group of lymph nodes for colon? (AIIMS 2012)

a. Paracolic
b. Epicolic
c. Pretoria
d. Ileocolic

Q8. All are the features of congenital megacolon *except*: (All India 97)

a. Large bully stools
b. Tight anal ring
c. Pseudodiarrhea
d. Failure to thrive

Q9. All are predisposing factors for colorectal carcinoma, *except*: (AIIMS 2003)

a. Turcot's syndrome
b. Muir/Torre syndrome
c. Cowden's syndrome
d. Juvenile polyposis coli

Q10. Not associated with GI malignancy: (GB Pant 2011)

a. Cowden's syndrome
b. Peutz–Jeghers syndrome
c. Juvenile polyposis
d. Gardner's syndrome

Q11. Strong correlation with colorectal cancer is seen in: (All India 2003)

a. Peutz–Jeghers syndrome
b. Familial polyposis coli
c. Juvenile polyposis
d. Hyperplastic polyp

Q12. Which of the following polyps is not premalignant? (PGI June 2003)

a. Juvenile polyposis syndrome
b. Peutz–Jeghers syndrome
c. Ulcerative colitis
d. Familial polyposis coli
e. Cronkhite–Canada syndrome

Q13. Metabolic abnormality seen in large colorectal villous adenoma: (AIIMS May 2008)

a. Hypokalemic metabolic alkalosis
b. Hypokalemic metabolic acidosis
c. Chlorine-sensitive metabolic acidosis
d. Chlorine-resistant metabolic alkalosis

Q14. On colonoscopy, which of the following is highly malignant? (JIPMER 1998)

a. Single pedunculated polyp
b. Multiple flat polyps about hundreds
c. Multiple pedunculated polyps
d. Solitary flat polyp

Q15. All are true about FAP, *except*: (JIPMER GIS 2011)

a. Gastric and duodenal polyps are most common
b. Most of the gastric polyps represent fundal gland hyperplasia
c. Increased risk of ampullary carcinoma
d. Congenital hypertrophy of the retinal pigment epithelium (CHRPE) can be detected by ophthalmoscopy in 25% of patients

Q16. Recommended treatment of FAP involving sigmoid colon: (AIIMS GIS Dec 2006)

a. Total colectomy with ileorectal anastomosis
b. Total colectomy with IPAA
c. Segmental resection
d. Total proctocolectomy with IPAA

Q17. Are true about FAP, *except*: (AIIMS GIS Dec 2006)

a. >100 polyps for diagnosis
b. Mutation in the *APC* gene
c. Budesonide prevent the CA colon
d. Endometrial carcinoma is a prominent association

Q18. The Amsterdam criteria include, all *except*: (AIIMS GIS Dec 2009)

a. At least three relatives should be affected
b. All three should be first-degree relatives
c. Two successive generations affected
d. FAP excluded

Q19. Microsatellite instability is most common in: (PGI SS June 2005)

a. FAP
b. HNPCC
c. Sporadic colonic carcinoma
d. Juvenile polyposis

Q20. Premalignant conditions is/are: (PGI Dec 2006)

a. Ulcerative colitis
b. Amoebic colitis
c. Familial polyposis coli
d. Juvenile polyp
e. Peutz–Jeghers syndrome

Grade III	Most difficult

Q1. Incidence of malignancy is maximum in: (AIIMS 1997)

a. Villous adenoma
b. Juvenile polyp
c. Hyperplastic polyps
d. Tubular adenoma

Q2. In children, the MC type of polyp is: (PGI 1998)

a. Juvenile polyp
b. Solitary polyp
c. Familial polyposis
d. Multiple adenomatous polyps

Q3. Gardner's syndrome is associated with all, *except*: (PGI 2009)

a. Brain tumor
b. Desmoid tumor
c. Osteoma
d. Abnormal dentition

Q4. Turcot's syndrome is associated with: (PGI 2002)

a. Duodenal polyps
b. Familial adenomatous polyposis
c. Brain tumor
d. Villous adenoma
e. Hyperplastic polyps

Q5. Following genetic counseling in a family for familial polyposis coli, the next screening test is: (MCI 2018)

a. Flexible sigmoidoscopy
b. Colonoscopy
c. Occult blood in stool
d. *APC* gene

Q6. Based on epidemiological studies, which of the following has been found to be most protective against carcinoma colon: (AIIMS 2011)

a. High-fiber diet
b. Low-fat diet
c. Low-selenium diet
d. Low-protein diet

Q7. Genetic abnormality in the case of late adenoma to carcinoma in CA colon is: (AIIMS 2009)

a. APC
b. K-ras
c. DCC
d. p53

Q8. The tendency of colonic carcinoma to metastasis is best assessed by: (AIIMS 2003)

a. Site of tumor
b. Carcinoembryonic antigen (CEA) levels
c. Depth of penetration of bowel wall
d. Proportion of bowel circumference involved

Q9. Antiperistalsis is seen in: (AIIMS 1991)
a. Distal colon b. Jejunum
c. Proxicolon d. Ileum

Q10. Complete bowel preparation is done in a case of: (AIIMS 1999)
a. Colonic carcinoma
b. Hirschsprung's disease
c. Ulcerative colitis
d. Irritable bowel syndrome

Q11. The most common site for ischemic colitis is: (PGI 1997)
a. Hepatic flexure b. Splenic flexure
c. Descending colon d. Ascending colon

Q12. The most common site of perforation during colonoscopy is: (UPSC 2000)
a. Cecum b. Hepatic flexure
c. Splenic flexure d. Sigmoid colon

Q13. Commonly undergoing malignant transformation is/are: (PGI June 2006)
a. FAP b. Crohn's disease
c. Ulcerative colitis d. Enteric colitis
e. Juvenile polyp

Q14. Carcinoma right colon is most commonly of which type? (AIIMS Nov 1994)
a. Stenosing b. Ulcerative
c. Tubular d. Fungating

Q15. True regarding carcinoma colon is: (AIIMS Nov 2000)
a. Lesion on the left side of the colon presents with features of anemia
b. Mucinous carcinoma has a good prognosis
c. Duke's A stage should receive adjuvant chemotherapy
d. Solitary liver metastasis is not a contraindication for surgery

Q16. Colonic metastasis is related with: (AIIMS GIS Dec 2011)
a. Preop CEA level
b. Depth of invasion
c. Size of tumor
d. Circumferential involvement

Q17. Which of the following is true about colon carcinoma? (PGI Dec 2005)
a. Right-sided colon carcinoma associated with young individuals
b. Most common site is sigmoid colon
c. Right-sided colon carcinoma presents as chronic anemia
d. Not resectable in case of metastasis
e. Right-sided colon has a better prognosis than the left-sided colon

Q18. Stage IIIC in colorectal cancer: (GB Pant 2011)
a. T2N0M0 b. T2N2M0
c. T2N1M0 d. T4N1M0

Q19. A 60-year-old man suffering from left colon carcinoma presented with acute left colonic obstruction. The treatment is: (PGI June 2003)
a. Primary resection and Hartman's procedure
b. Defunctioning colostomy
c. Right hemicolectomy
d. Resection of the whole left bowel and end-to-end anastomosis
e. Conservative treatment

Q20. Ramu is a 60-year-old male with CA descending colon who presents with acute intestinal obstruction. In the emergency department, the treatment of choice is: (AIIMS Nov 1999)
a. Defunctioning colostomy
b. Hartman's procedure
c. Total colectomy
d. Left hemicolectomy

ANSWERS

Grade I: 1. a; 2. a; 3. c; 4. a; 5. c; 6. a; 7. d; 8. b; 9. a; 10. a (Sabiston 20/e p1866); 11. a; 12. c; 13. c; 14. b; 15. c; 16. c; 17. b (Schwartz 10/e p1206); 18. a; 19. b; 20. a, b, c

Grade II: 1. a; 2. b; 3. c, d, e; 4. d; 5. a; 6. b; 7. c; 8. a; 9. c; 10. a; 11. b; 12. a, b, c, e (Schwartz 10/e p1206); 13. b (Harrison 19/e p269); 14. b (Sabiston 20/e p1368); 15. d; 16. d; 17. d; 18. b (Schwartz 10/e p292); 19. b; 20. a, c (Schwartz 10/e p291-292)

Grade III: 1. a; 2. b; 3. a; 4. b, c; 5. d; 6. a; 7. d; 8. c; 9. c; 10. a; 11. b; 12. d; 13. a, b, c; 14. d; 15. d (Schwartz 10/e p1293-1294); 16. b (Schwartz 10/e p1209); 17. b, c, e; 18. d; 19. a, b, d; 20. b

MODEL QUESTIONS

Q1. After undergoing surgery for carcinoma of the colon, a patient developed a single liver metastasis of 2 cm. What do you do next?
a. Resection
b. Chemoradiation
c. Acetic acid injection
d. Radiofrequency ablation

Ans. a

Q2. Thumb printing appearance of the colon on barium enema is seen in:
a. Diverticulitis b. Ischemic colitis
c. Ulcerative colitis d. Carcinoma colon

Ans. b

Q3. Which among the following is the drug of choice for *Clostridium* difficult-induced colitis?
a. Gentamycin b. Ciprofloxacin
c. Metronidazole d. Linezolid

Ans. c

Q4. Which of the following is not degraded by colonic flora?
a. Pectin b. Lignin
c. Starch d. Glucose

Ans. b

Q5. Duhamel's operation is done for:
a. Hirschsprung's disease
b. Meconium ileus
c. Annular pancreas
d. Imperforated Anu's

Ans. a

Q6. Acquired diverticula are most commonly seen in:
a. Jejunum/ileum b. Transverse colon
c. Sigmoid colon d. Ascending colon

Ans. c

Q7. Gardner's syndrome has all of the following, *except*:
a. Colonic polyp
b. Multiple epidermal cysts
c. Bony exposes
d. Giant gastric folds

Ans. d

Q8. What is an acceptable screening technique for detecting recurrent colon cancer?
a. Screening sigmoidoscopy
b. Screening the stool for occult blood
c. Stool cytology
d. Measurement of carcinoembryonic antigen (CEA) level

Ans. a

Q9. Functional GI disorders can be differentiated from organic GI disorders by:
a. Abdominal pain b. Diarrhea
c. Tenesmus d. Bleeding P/R

Ans. d

Q10. First investigation to be done in a patient with recurrent occult blood loss:
a. Esophagogastroscopy b. Colonoscopy
c. Barium enema d. Close observation

Ans. b

Q11. Dunking maneuver is used in:
a. Left hemicolectomy
b. Right hemicolectomy
c. Right extended hemicolectomy
d. Anterior resection

Ans. b

Q12. Cattel's maneuver is the mobilization of:
a. Sigmoid colon
b. Descending colon
c. Small bowel
d. Cecum and ascending colon

Ans. d

Q13. Pseudomembranous colitis is associated with:
a. *Campylobacter* b. *Clostridium difficile*
c. *Clostridium* retro d. *Salmonella typhi*

Ans. b

Q14. A constricting type of colonic carcinoma is seen in:
a. Left colon b. Right colon
c. Transverse colon d. Cecum

Ans. a

Q15. The most common cause of lower GI bleed in India is:
a. Benign tumor b. Nonspecific ulcer
c. Cancer rectosigmoid d. Hemorrhoids

Ans. d

SUGGESTED READING

1. Bailey & Love's - Short Practice of Surgery, 27th edition.
2. Schwartz's Principles of Surgery, 18th edition.
3. Textbook of Surgery by David Sabiston, 21st edition.

CHAPTER 41

Vermiform Appendix

"To study the phenomenon of disease without books is to sail an uncharted sea, while to study books without patients is not to go to sea at all."

– Sir William Osler

INTRODUCTION

The word "vermiform appendix" is derived from the Latin words "vermis," meaning "worm," and "forma," meaning "shape," so shaped like a worm, and "appendere" means to "hang upon." The vermiform appendix is a worm-like tubular structure that hangs from the cecum in the abdominal cavity.

Morphologically, the appendix is an undeveloped distal end of the large cecum found in many animals. The appendix was considered a vestigial organ, an organ that becomes rudimentary and functionless in the course of evolution. The vermiform appendix is now considered a specialized part of the gastrointestinal tract and not a vestigial organ. It may be a reservoir for beneficial gut bacteria.

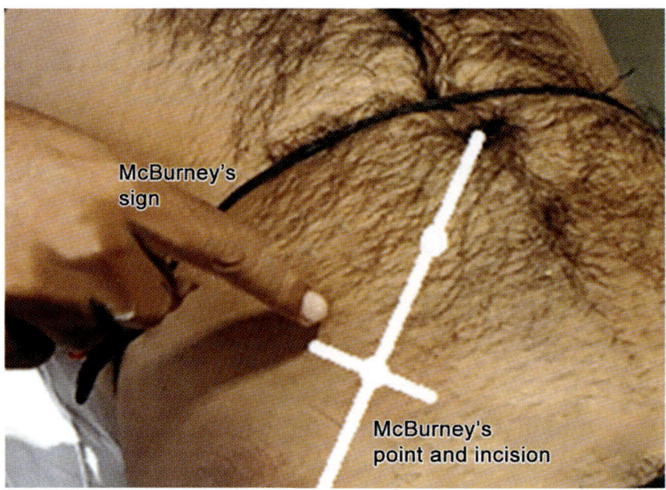

Fig. 1: McBurney's point.

Important milestones:
- In 1736, Claudius Amyand performed the first appendicectomy.
- In 1880, Lawson Tait performed the first appendicectomy, but it was reported in 1890.
- In 1886, Reginald Heber Fitz coined the term "appendicitis."
- In 1886, Krönlein reported the first appendicectomy.
- In 1889, McBurney described McBurney's point **(Fig. 1)**.
- In 1889, McBurney also described Gridiron incision.
- In 1902 Ochsner–Sherren Regimen was given by Ochsner and Sherren.
- In 1982, Kurt Semm performed the first laparoscopic appendicectomy.
- In 2009, the first transvaginal removal of the appendix by Santiago Horgan and Mark A Talamini—a procedure called Natural Orifice Transluminal Endoscopic Surgery (NOTES).

DEVELOPMENT OF APPENDIX (FIG. 2)

The appendix develops as a diverticulum from the wall of the cecum. The appendix appears first as a prominence in the

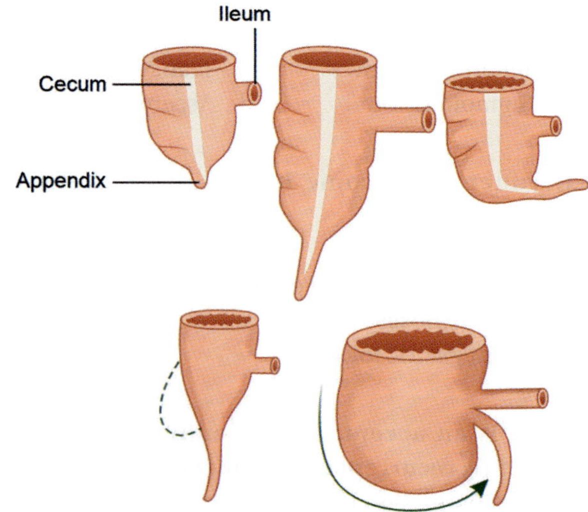

Fig. 2: Development of the appendix.

terminal part of the cecum in the eighth week of intrauterine life, it attains the shape of a tubular structure by about the age of 2 years. In an early embryonic age appendix has the same diameter as the cecum, and it lies in the line of the cecum. The excessive growth of the right and anterior walls of the cecum pushes the appendix to the medial side and posteriorly. In later stages of development, the lumen disparity between the cecum and appendix develops. The lumen of the cecum enlarges and develops fast, but the lumen of the appendix enlarges much more slowly, and the disparity develops. By the fifth month of intrauterine life, the appendix elongates and becomes vermiform in shape. At birth, the appendix is broad and short, then gradually, around 2 years of age, it acquires a tubular shape. *The position of the appendix in relation to the cecum varies greatly, but the relation between the attachment of the base of the appendix and the cecum is always constant.* The base of the appendix is always attached at the same spot as the cecum in relation to the ileocecal valve. The location of the appendix is determined by the location of the cecum. The appendix is devoid of lymphoid tissue before birth, and it appears only after 2 weeks of birth. *The lymphoid tissue increases in amount continuously from birth to puberty, then its amount becomes stationary for 10–12 years, then it starts regressing with age, and by the age of 60 years, again appendix becomes almost devoid of lymphoid tissue. The excessive growth of the right and anterior walls of the cecum pushes the appendix to the medial side and posteriorly.*

SURFACE MARKING OF APPENDIX (FIGS. 3A AND B)

The base of the appendix can be marked on the anterior abdominal wall at a point 2 cm below the point where the transtubercular plane crosses the vertical right lateral plane. McBurney's point is the site of maximum tenderness in acute appendicitis. McBurney's point is situated at the junction of the medial two-thirds and lateral one-third of the imaginary line joining the umbilicus and anterior superior iliac spine (ASIS). The position of the appendix can be marked in relation to the face of a clock (for example, the pelvic position of the appendix is mentioned as a 4 o'clock position). The base of the appendix is fixed as it is attached to the cecum, so it is marked as the center of a clock where the hands of the clock meet. The appendix is marked as the hand of a clock.

POSITION OF APPENDIX

The appendix is situated in the right iliac fossa (RIF). The anatomical position of the appendix in the peritoneal cavity is inconstant. The position of the base of the appendix is always constant in relation to the cecum. However, true but, Howard Atwood Kelly, mentioned in his book, "Appendicitis and Other Diseases of the Vermiform Appendix," that the location of the point of origin depends, entirely upon the topography of the cecum. According to whether the cecal pouch is directed upward or downward, outward, or inward, forward or backward, or whether the colon and cecum have rotated insufficiently or too much around their long axis, the point of origin of the appendix varies in position. It may be found at almost any point of the cecal pouch. The base of the appendix during operation is traced by identifying and following the three taenia coli, especially the anterior taenia coli. The position of the appendix is extremely variable, more so than that of any other organ. As the appendix is attached to the cecum so its position depends upon the position of the cecum. Usually, it is in the RIF, but due to incomplete descent of the cecum, it may be subhepatic. *The cecum may be in the pelvis or even on the left side due to malrotation of the gut*

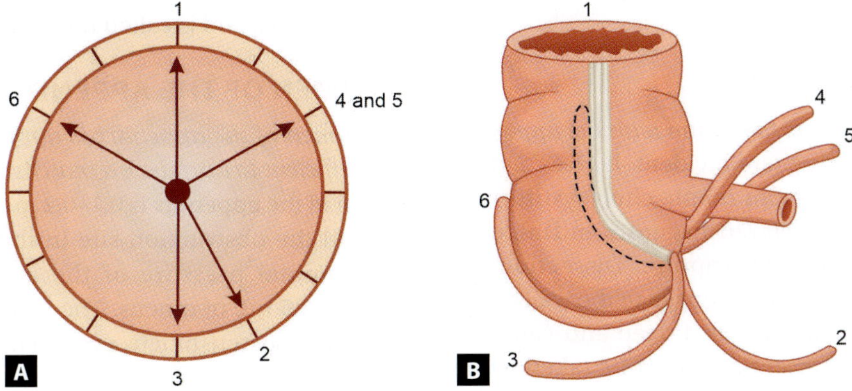

Figs. 3A and B: Positions of the appendix.

or arrest in rotation of the gut. Appendix usually hangs and floats free in the peritoneal cavity and is fixed only in the retrocecal position or when it is inflamed. Appendix can take any of the following positions:

- *Retrocecal (12 o'clock) position (in 70% of persons):* The normal location of the appendix is retrocecal. The appendix lies behind the cecum. It may be embedded in the cecal wall. It is intraperitoneal, but sometimes also extraperitoneal. It may be sometimes difficult to elicit tenderness in RIF, as an inflamed appendix is lying behind the cecum, which is distended with gas. A long retrocecal appendix can mimic cholecystitis if only the tip is inflamed, or it can mimic ureteric colic if it touches the ureter.

- *Pelvic (4 o'clock) position (in 25% of persons):* The appendix hangs down in the pelvis. There may be no tenderness in RIF as the inflamed appendix lies in the pelvis, but deep tenderness may be elicited on digital rectal examination (DRE). The tip of the appendix, if it touches the ureter or bladder patient will have urinary symptoms. When the tip of the appendix touches the rectum patient will have rectal symptoms.
- *Subcecal (6 o'clock) position (in 2% of persons):* The appendix lies just below the cecum.
- *Preileal (2 o'clock) position (in 1% of persons):* The appendix lies in front of the terminal part of the ileum.
- *Postileal (2 o'clock) position (in 1% of persons):* The appendix lies behind the terminal part of the ileum.
- *Paracolic position (in 1% of persons):* It lies just along the lateral wall of the cecum.

Though the retrocecal position of the appendix is the most common, but in some countries, it is different, as in Iran and Bosnia, the pelvic position is most common, with 55.8 and 57.7% occurrence, respectively.

The appendix, ileum, and cecum are depicted in **Figure 4**.

SUBHEPATIC APPENDIX

Malrotation of the gut puts the cecum with the appendix below the liver. It is a very rare incident. It gives a great challenge to diagnosis. It can mimic cholecystitis and liver abscess, may lead to delayed diagnosis, and increase the chances of appendicular rupture. Dissection for subserous appendix can cause damage to the wall of the cecum, which can be dangerous if deep and can lead to fecal fistula, so all precautions must be taken while dealing with appendicectomy for subserous appendix.

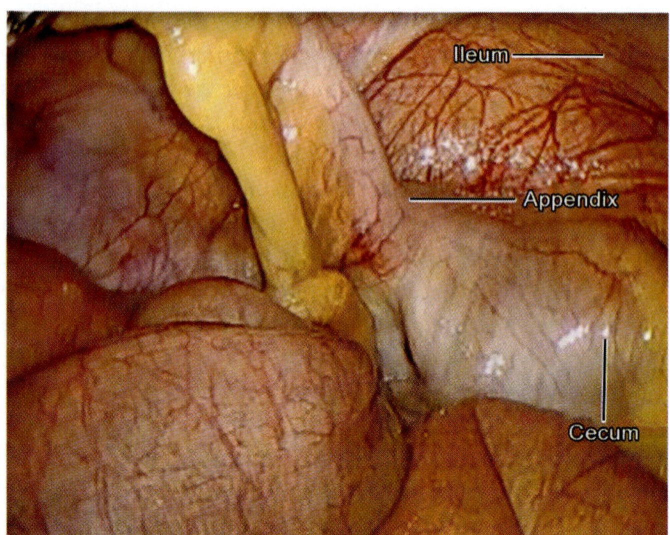

Fig. 4: Appendix, ileum, and cecum.

SIZE OF THE APPENDIX

The size of the appendix varies from person to person. Some studies have indicated a relation between the length of the appendix and with height of a person, but it is not confirmed. The usual length of the appendix is approximately 7.5 cm, but it may vary from 2 to 20 cm. It is longer in children and may atrophy after midadult life. The longest appendix ever removed was 26 cm long. The average length of the appendix is about 8.3 cm or between 3 and 3.5".

APPENDICULAR ORIFICE

It is situated 2 cm below and lateral to the ileocecal orifice at the posteromedial aspect of the cecum. It approximately corresponds to McBurney's point. Often it lies to a point below it. The appendicular orifice is sometimes, but not always, has a semilunar fold of mucus membrane, which acts as a valve and is called the "valve of Gerlach" **(Fig. 5)**.

LUMEN OF THE APPENDIX

The lumen of the appendix is approximately 2 mm wide, just sufficient to introduce a matchstick. The capacity of the lumen of the appendix is 0.1–0.2 mL. The mucus secretion beyond the obstruction site in the lumen can raise the intraluminal pressure of the appendix considerably, even by 0.5 mL of mucus. The capability of appendicular mucosa to secrete mucus even in the presence of raised in intraluminal pressure causes acute appendicitis, which is an important factor **(Fig. 6)**.

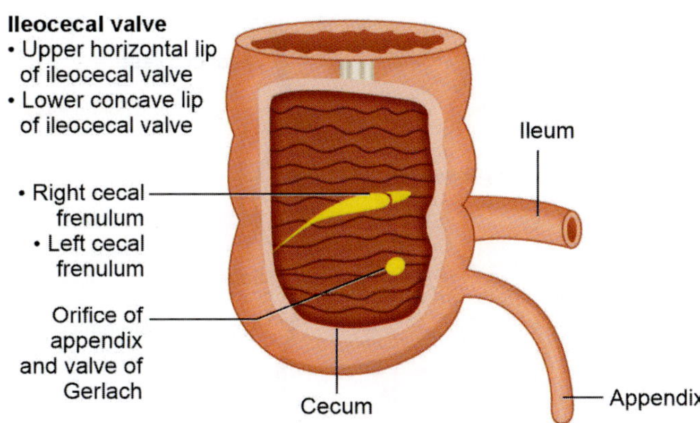

Fig. 5: Appendicular orifice and ileocecal valve.

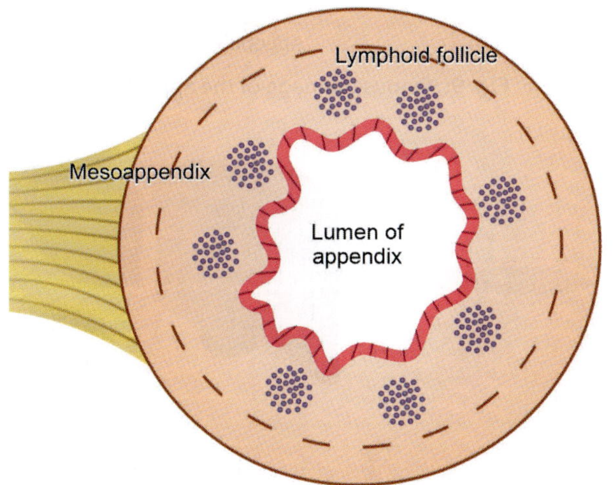

Fig. 6: Lumen and wall of the appendix.

WHY APPENDIX IS PRONE TO INFECTION?

It is due to the following facts:

- It is a long, narrow, blind-ended tube that encourages stasis of contents, which leads to the proliferation of bacteria.
- Lymphoid follicles are present in the wall of the appendix, which catches bacteria.
- The lumen of the appendix has a tendency to be blocked by hard stool (enterolith), which results in stasis.

MESOAPPENDIX OR MESENTERY OF APPENDIX

An appendix has a well-developed mesentery called "mesoappendix." It is continuous with the mesentery of the terminal ileum. It is a triangular fold of the peritoneum. The appendix is suspended in the peritoneal cavity by the mesoappendix. It fuses with the posterior layer of the mesentery of the ileum behind the terminal part of the ileum. The tip of the appendix is not covered by mesoappendix, which is one of the reasons for the early perforation of the tip of the appendix due to the lack of protective covering. The thrombosis of the appendicular artery develops due to inflammation of the appendix as the artery is directly over it. The mesoappendix contains appendicular vessels and nerves. *The mesoappendix in newborns is transparent without any fat deposit, but as we grow, it gradually becomes laden with fat. We identify the vessels in the mesoappendix by seeing them against the light. The fat-laden mesoappendix does not show vessels clearly.*

Appendicular Artery

The appendicular artery is a branch of the lower division of the ileocolic artery. It passes behind the terminal ileum to enter the mesoappendix, a short distance from the base of the appendix from the medial side, and then it runs along the free border of the mesoappendix, but at the tip of the appendix, it lies directly over the wall of the appendix. The appendicular artery gives three to four branches in its course to the appendix in the mesoappendix. The appendicular artery is an end artery, which is why acute appendicitis results in gangrene and perforation once this artery is thrombosed and blocked, causing necrosis of the appendix, which is also known as gangrenous appendicitis. A recurrent branch is given by an appendicular artery near the base of the appendix, which anastomoses with a branch of the posterior cecal artery. While putting a purse-string suture, this artery can be damaged and may cause a big hematoma. The branches of the appendicular artery form two main systems—the superficial in the serous coat, and the deep in the submucosa. From this submucous system, branches run toward the mucosa **(Fig. 7)**.

Accessory Appendicular Artery (Artery of Seshachalam)

It is a branch of the posterior cecal artery. It is quite commonly found. It supplies the base of the appendix. It sometimes bleeds a lot, if not properly ligated during appendicectomy. The tip and antimesenteric border of the appendix have the least blood supply, and therefore, these sites are prone to get gangrene and perforation. T Seshachalam, an Indian surgeon, described this artery in the 1930s **(Fig. 8)**.

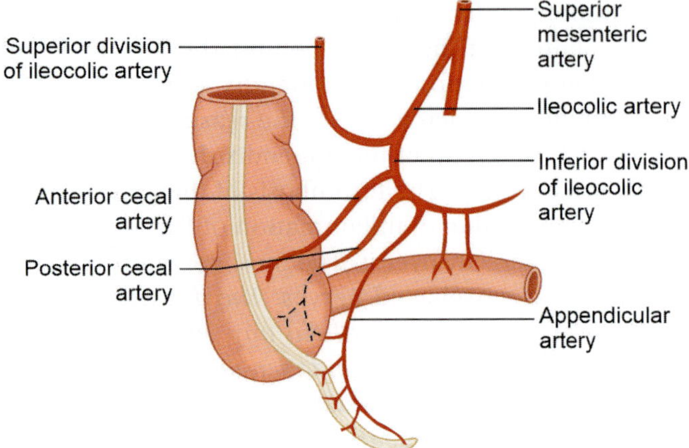

Fig. 7: Appendicular artery.

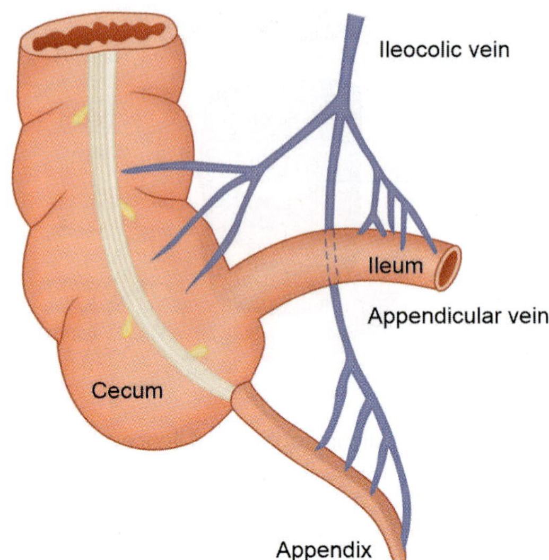

Fig. 9: Venous drainage of the appendix.

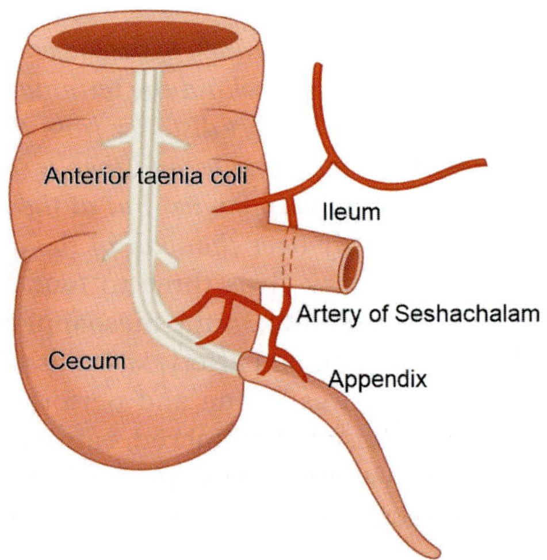

Fig. 8: Accessory appendicular artery of Seshachalam.

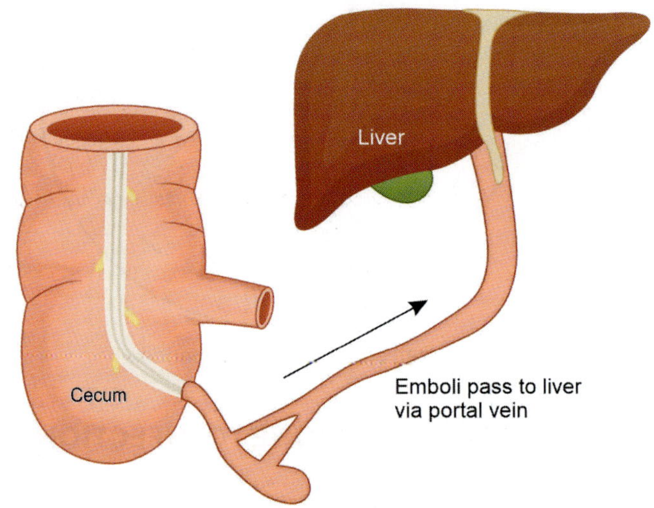

Fig. 10: Emboli passes to the liver via the portal vein.

Venous Drainage of Appendix

The veins draining the blood from the appendix follow the arteries of the appendix ***(Fig. 9)***. The tributaries from the appendix drain into an ileocolic vein, which drains into the superior mesenteric vein, which opens in the portal vein. This is part of the portal circulation. The blood reaches the liver via the portal vein due for this reason, suppurative appendicitis or appendicular abscess can lead to multiple pyemic abscesses in the liver. The veins of the appendix are generally central to the arteries. When we do appendicectomy, we crush the base of the appendix with artery forceps, which blocks the lumen of the veins, and also this avoids sending infected emboli to the portal vein and liver **(Fig. 10)**.

Lymphatic Drainage of Appendix

Lymph is drained from the appendix to the regional lymph nodes by four to six lymphatic channels ***(Fig. 11)****. These channels carry lymph:*

- *Directly to the ileocolic lymph nodes.*
- *Some lymph passes first to the appendicular lymph nodes in the mesoappendix, and then to the ileocecal lymph nodes near the base of the appendix, and then to the ileocolic lymph nodes.* Lymph from the anterior surface of the appendix and cecum reaches via anterior cecal vessels to anterior ileocolic lymph nodes, and lymph

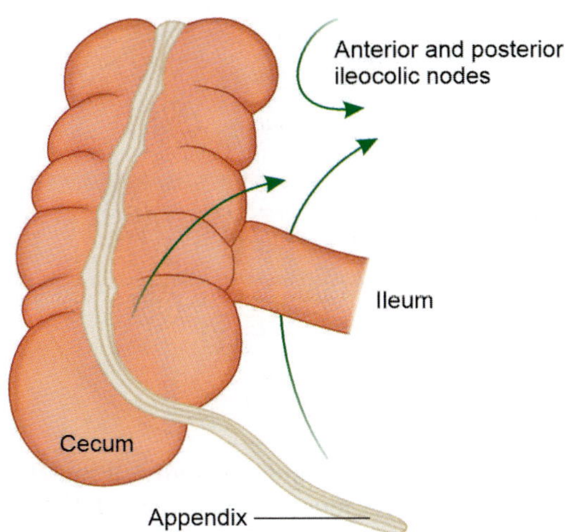

Fig. 11: Lymphatic drainage of the appendix.

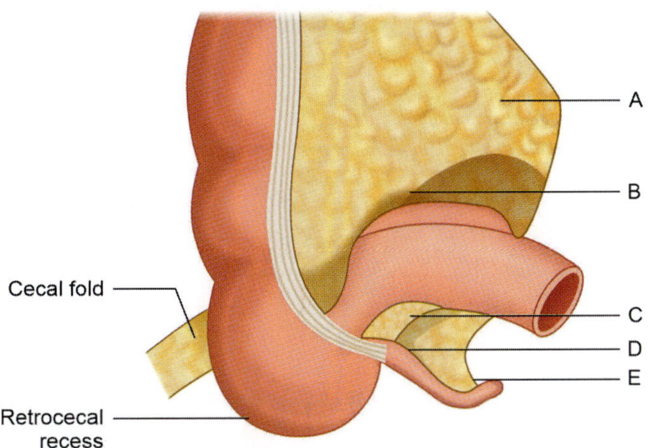

Fig. 12: Folds and recesses in relation to the appendix. (A: vascular fold of cecum; B: superior ileocecal recess; C: inferior ileocecal fold; D: inferior ileocecal recess; E: mesoappendix)

from the posterior surface of the cecum and appendix reaches via posterior cecal vessels to posterior ileocolic lymph nodes. Ultimately, the lymph reaches from the ileocolic lymph nodes to the superior mesenteric lymph nodes. The lymphatics of the appendix run into superficial, middle, and deep groups. Superficial groups lie in the serosa, the middle group is between the muscle coats and submucosa, and the deep group is in the mucosa.

The lowest lymph gland is situated over the posterior cecal pouch and is called the Clades gland or the appendiceal gland. It receives lymph from the cecum and not from the appendix. In a very few instances, it received a small tributary from the cecoappendical angle.

NERVE SUPPLY OF APPENDIX

- Sympathetic nerves come from the thoracic nine (T9) and thoracic ten (T10) segments of the spinal cord through the celiac plexus.
- Parasympathetic nerves come from the vagus nerve. The pain in the initial stage of acute appendicitis is felt at the umbilicus, it is "referred to as pain" as the same segment of the spinal cord (T10), supplies the umbilicus also. It is visceral pain. Later on, the pain shifts to RIF due to irritation and inflammation of the local peritoneum. This pain is due to stimulation of nerve endings of the local peritoneum and is called "somatic pain."

FOLDS AND RECESSES IN RELATION TO THE APPENDIX (FIG. 12)

- Superior ileocecal fold
- Superior ileocecal recess
- Inferior ileocecal fold
- Inferior ileocecal recess

Superior Ileocecal Fold and Recess

It is a commonly seen pair of folds and recesses. The superior ileocecal recess is formed by the superior ileocecal fold, which is a vascular fold present between the terminal ileum and ascending colon. The opening of the recess is directed down and medially.

Inferior Ileocecal Fold and Recess

This fold is a bloodless fold and is also called the "bloodless fold of Treves." It is between the terminal ileum and the base of the appendix. The opening of this recess is downward.

JACKSON'S MEMBRANE

It is a peritoneal fold, attached from the posterior abdominal wall to the anterior surface of the cecum on the lateral side. Sometimes it is required to cut to find out the retrocecal appendix. It is vascular and has blood vessels that run parallel **(Fig. 13)**.

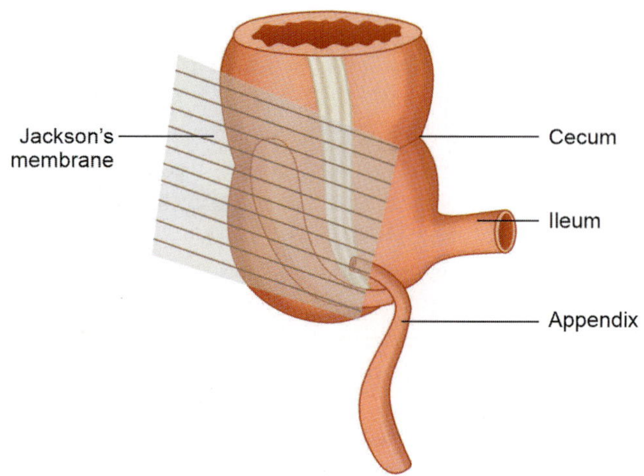

Fig. 13: Jackson's membrane.

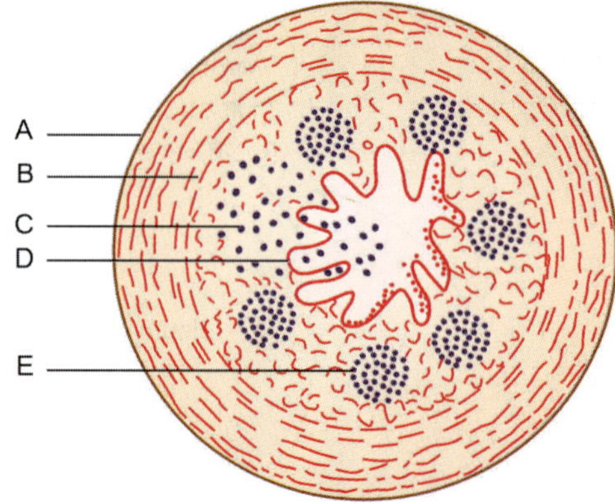

Fig. 14: Cut section of appendix. (A: serosa; B: muscle coat; C: submucosa; D: mucosa; and E: lymph follicle).

Histology of Appendix

Histology, also known as microscopic anatomy or microanatomy, is the branch of biology that studies the microscopic anatomy of biological tissues; whereas, in medicine, histopathology is the branch of histology that includes the microscopic identification and study of diseased tissue. Accurate diagnosis of a sickness sometimes requires histopathological examination of biopsied or resected tissue. Histopathology of the appendix sample after appendicectomy details the correct diagnosis, such as chronic appendicitis, subacute appendicitis, acute appendicitis, gangrene of the appendix, perforation of the appendix, and tumor of the appendix (benign or malignant). Negative appendicectomy is also confirmed by histopathological examination of the appendix sample.

The appendix has the following layers, which are similar to the intestine. These are from outside to inside **(Figs. 14 and 15)**:

- Serosa
- *Muscle coat:*
  - Outer longitudinal muscular coat
  - Inner circular coat
- Submucosa
- Mucosa

It is a complete investment of the appendix, except for a narrow strip along with the mesenteric attachment. There is a subserous layer of connective tissue. The serous layer surrounds the outer surface of the appendix. The *mesoappendix* is the continuation of the mesentery of the ileum, and it wraps the appendix and mixes with the serosa of the appendix.

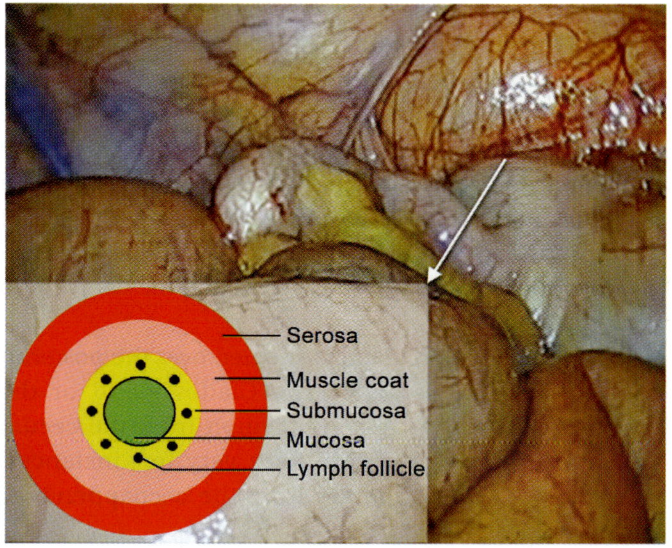

Fig. 15: Structure of the wall of the appendix.

MUSCLE COAT

It has outer longitudinal and inner circular muscle fibers, as in the small intestine, but the muscle fibers in the appendix are weakly developed in comparison to the intestine. They are deficient in some areas where the serosa and submucosa are in contact. These gaps in muscle layers are called "hiatus muscularis." Through these gaps, the infection from the mucosa reaches fast to the serosa and peritoneum quickly. These gaps sometimes act as weak spots, and perforation occurs here due to raised intraluminal pressure. Acquired diverticulum of the appendix occurs through these gaps. The longitudinal muscle layer is thicker near the base of the appendix to form a rudimentary *Taenia,* which is continuous with those of the cecum and colon. The circular muscle layer is separated from the longitudinal muscle layer by connective tissue. The muscularis mucosa is very thin in the appendix.

SUBMUCOSA

It has 20–40 lymphoid follicles in adults. These lymphatic tissues decrease in size as age advances. Follicular and parafollicular zones in the submucosa contain B and T lymphocytes. The lymphoid masses are a local defense against infection. Lymphoid tissues in the appendix are not present at birth but develop at 2 weeks after birth. The number of lymphoid follicles is maximum during 12–20 years of age, 200, then the number of lymphoid follicles reduces with age and almost they disappears by the age of 60 years. This is one of the reasons why acute appendicitis is rare after 60 years of age. Appendicectomy does not cause any change in a person's immune response or cause any cancer. The appendix is also called "abdominal tonsil" due to its rich lymphatic tissue presence.

MUCOSA

The mucosa of the appendix resembles that of the colon. It has several longitudinal folds. The number of crypts in Lieberkühn is less as compared to the colon. *Crypts of Lieberkühn contain Kulchitsky cells or Argentaffin cells.*

The openings of the crypts of Lieberkühn are arranged around certain centers marked by a depression on the surface of the apices of lymph follicles. Nikolai Kulchitsky, first time, described argentaffin cells, which are responsible for tumors. As with the rest of the colon, there are mucus-secreting goblet cells.

The thickness of the longitudinal muscular coat of the appendix varies in different individuals and also in the same specimen from 0.2 to 0.3 mm. The circular muscular coat measures from 0.2 to 0.5 mm in width. The thickness of the submucosa varies greatly in different individuals (0.2 to 0.8 mm or more). It is this layer that gains the most in thickness during the process of obliteration. The submucosa consists of loose, wavy strands of fibrous and elastic tissue that form a framework for the blood, lymph vessels, and nerves. In the interspaces are fat globules. The mucosa is bound to the submucosa by the vestiges of muscularis mucosa. The mucosa presents an irregularly folded appearance, the folds running parallel with the longitudinal axis of the appendix.

Functions of Appendix

The vermiform appendix is a small tubular structure attached to the cecum. Earlier appendix was considered a vestigial organ, serving no function, but now the view has changed. An appendix is found to store and develop body-friendly flora of the intestine that can redevelop after its loss in sicknesses of the digestive tract. An appendix also plays a role in immune function as it contains lymphoid tissue. The appendix has been shown to have an important interaction with the intestinal flora. Though the appendix was considered a vestigial organ but it is found that it is well developed in some animals, which casts doubt on it being as a vestigial organ. In view of its rich vascularity and histological differentiation, the appendix is probably a specialized rather than a degenerate or vestigial organ.

So, it is not considered a vestigial organ and it does not take an active part in the immunity of the body, but:

- *Lymphoid follicles help in the maturation of B-lymphocytes.*
- *Appendix is a part of gut-associated lymphoid tissue (GALT) and forms globulin, which is required for an immune mechanism of the body.* It is proved now proven that appendicectomy does not increase the incidence of carcinoma of the colon, which was doubtful in studies in 1960. The removal of the appendix does not cause a defect in the immunoglobulin system's functioning. So, we can take the following functions of the appendix into consideration.

TO MAINTAIN GUT FLORA

William Parker, Randy Bollinger, and colleagues at Duke University proposed in 2007 that the appendix serves as a haven for useful bacteria when illness flushes the bacteria from the rest of the intestines. This reservoir of bacteria could then serve to repopulate the gut flora in the digestive system following a bout of dysentery or cholera or to boost it following a milder gastrointestinal illness.

IMMUNE FUNCTION

An appendix is an important part of mucosal immune functions through B and T cells to fight off pathogens. Innate lymphoid cells of the gut help the appendix to maintain digestive health.

VESTIGIALITY

Earlier, it was proposed that the human appendix was a vestigial organ, as during evolution, the cecum was thought to have shrunk in size and its remnant was the appendix.

After millions of years, the once necessary cecum degraded to become the appendix of modern humans. Humans have a diet rich in foliates (cellulose-rich plants), but now take easily digestible foods, so a long cecum is not required to host bacteria digesting cellulose.

Though there is no clear role of the appendix in the causation of human disease but studies have shown a correlation between appendicectomy and the development of inflammatory bowel disease (IBD), especially ulcerative colitis. The appendix delays the onset of ulcerative colitis. Association of inflammatory bowel disease is not so clear as in ulcerative colitis.

Diseases of the Appendix

Schnitzler was of the opinion that the so-called chronic appendicitis did not exist. Deaver, on the other hand, believed chronic appendicitis to be a clinical entity and divided it into two distinct types—that which occurs after acute appendicitis and that which has always taken the form of chronic inflammation without acute exacerbation. He felt that there could be a differential diagnosis in these two types of chronic appendicitis. He stated his belief that in cases of chronic peptic ulcer, chronic cholecystitis, ureteric colic, Dietl's crisis, and chronic pelvic inflammatory disease, the appendix is commonly unjustifiably removed.

Congenital Anomalies of the Appendix

According to the World Health Organization (WHO), congenital disorders can be defined as structural or functional anomalies that occur during intrauterine life. Congenital anomalies of the appendix are quite rare—the absence of an appendix, duplication of the appendix, and its diverticulum have been mentioned in the literatures.

AGENESIS OF APPENDIX

Absence of Appendix

It is a very rare occurrence, one in 100,000 cases. Sometimes it is not congenital, but the appendix is autodigested after an attack of acute of appendicitis or appendicular abscess.

DUPLICATION OF APPENDIX

It is also an extremely rare occurrence. A total of 10 cases have been reported in the literature so far. One case reported having one normal appendix, and the other one was inflamed. Maizels G has reported that failure to identify the presence of appendiceal duplicates has resulted in appendectomy being performed twice.

Wallbridge Classification of Duplication of Appendix

- *Type A*: Partial duplication in a single cecum.
- *Type B*: Two separate appendices in a single cecum.
- *Type C*: Double cecum with each one having one appendix.

Appendix in Left Iliac Fossa

It is found in situs inversus viscerum. It occurs in one in 35,000 cases. It also occurs due to malrotation of the gut.

Subhepatic Appendix

It is the most common type of all congenital anomalies of the appendix. It is due to the arrest of the downward migration of the cecum. In this position, it may be close to the gallbladder, so in such a situation, the acute appendicitis mimics acute cholecystitis.

Diverticulum of Appendix

Diverticula of the appendix are rare. They are either congenital or acquired. The wall of the congenital appendicular diverticulum contains all layers. Congenital diverticulum is a rare entity; acquired diverticula occur more frequently. The mucosa of the appendix balloons out from the weak spots in the walls, "Hiatus muscularis." If the appendix with a diverticulum develops appendicitis, then perforation of the appendix occurs early due to a weak wall. The inflammation of the vermiform appendix is called "appendicitis."

TYPES OF APPENDICITIS

Appendicitis can present in the following forms:
- Acute appendicitis
- Subacute appendicitis
- Recurrent appendicitis
- Chronic appendicitis
- Grumbling appendix
- Pseudoappendicitis
- Residual appendicitis
- Appendicitis granulosa
- Appendicitis larvata

Acute Appendicitis

Acute appendicitis is the most common and dangerous type of appendicitis, others are milder versions of acute appendicitis.

Subacute Appendicitis

Subacute appendicitis is actually a milder form of acute appendicitis. If the acute appendicitis subsides before reaching to full-blown appendicitis, it is called subacute appendicitis. The symptoms subside, and the pain disappears. It may recur again. It is treated with appendicectomy, which relieves the pain and prevents future complications.

Recurrent Appendicitis

It is a milder variety of appendicitis that occurs recurrently, there is a symptomatic interval between attacks. It is a common variety of appendicitis. The appendix shows the obliteration of its lumen by fibrosis due to recurrent inflammation. Appendicectomy is the treatment of choice. Recurrent appendicitis occurs with an incidence of 8–14% following the resolution of the acute episode. Out of 142 cases, 92% of the removed appendix showed abnormality, and 95% of these patients were cured.

Chronic Appendicitis

Some researchers say that there is no entity called chronic appendicitis; it is actually recurrent appendicitis. However, recent clinical data document the existence of this uncommon disease. In this type of appendicitis, there is persistent RIF pain. The appendicectomy relieves the pain and other symptoms. Pain lasts longer and is less intense than acute appendicitis. Pain, nausea, anorexia, malaise, and pain with motion are frequent features. The white blood cell (WBC) count and computed tomography (CT) scan are normal. The color of the appendix is reddish with white island areas. The appendix is rigid and bent over itself and is often spiral. The mesoappendix is thickened, shortened, and indurated. The histopathology of the removed appendix shows chronic inflammatory cell infiltration in the wall of the appendix. It may show an old, healed scar of previous inflammation. Appendix may show adhesions, kinks, and nodularity. Appendicectomy is the treatment of choice for chronic appendicitis.

Chronic appendicitis develops either after an acute appendicitis episode or erupts in chronic form. Chronic appendicitis may occur in recurrent form, relapsing form, or in residual form. Recurrent form of chronic appendicitis has repeated attacks of subacute or mild-acute attacks, followed by a disease-free interval. Relapsing form is a continuous form where the patient is never free from symptoms. Residual form of chronic appendicitis is due to residual effects of previous attacks of acute appendicitis, such as adhesions and angulations.

Grumbling Appendix

Recurrent bouts of pain in RIF are sometimes called "grumbling appendix." It is usually a milder recurrent appendicitis. It is common in children. They have been admitted several times in the hospital with pain in the RIF. The grumbling of the appendix is relieved by appendicectomy. It is associated with recurrent pain in RIF, general malaise, tenderness over the appendix, and anorexia.

Pseudoappendicitis

This appendicitis is due to acute ileitis.

It is caused by the following factors:

- Yersinia
- Crohn's ileitis

Residual Appendicitis

Residual deformities of the appendix develop after active inflammation subsides. After the attack of acute or chronic appendicitis, it may be hypertrophy or atrophy, stricture, closure of the lumen, cyst formation, dilation, kink, diverticula, adhesions, or fibrosis. This can cause recurrent pain in RIF. Stump appendicitis is also considered as residual appendicitis, which occurs in the stump of the appendix left after appendicectomy. It is a rare entity. It is difficult to differentiate clinically from acute appendicitis, which delays the diagnosis and treatment. This reminds us to avoid leaving a big stump during appendicectomy.

Appendicitis Granulosa

Riedel believes that acute appendicitis has always had an insidious onset, one of the most important predisposing causes being a chronic primary disease, "appendicitis granulosa". Chronic inflammation of the appendix is essentially a hypertrophic process and produces a characteristic thickening and rigidity of its wall. In rare instances the inflammatory reaction seems to be confined to the mucous membrane, but, as a rule, all the coats are more or less affected.

Note: Alexandre Émile Jean Yersin, 1863–1943, Bacteriologist, Paris, France, discovered the bacillus causing bubonic plague, which was later named after him, "*Yersinia pestis*."

Appendicitis Larvata

The clinical condition described by Lenzmann and by Ewald as appendicitis larvata, acute or chronic appendicitis, exceedingly rarely results in a "restitutio ad integrum" (restoration to original condition). In the mildest cases, there is more or less connective—tissue hyperplasia, and as a consequence, a certain amount of rigidity and enfeebled muscular power persisted. This is also called latent *appendicitis.*

ACUTE APPENDICITIS

Acute appendicitis may be divided into the following groups clinically:
- Catarrhal
- Purulent
- Gangrenous
- Perforative

HISTORICAL BACKGROUND

The acute appendicitis has been reported since 1500 AD, it used to be called "perityphlitis," which they used to meant severe and fatal inflammation of the cecal region of the large intestine. Jean François Fernel, a French physician and astronomer, was the first who reported a case of appendicitis in 1554 when he noted at autopsy the luminal obstruction, necrosis, and perforation of the appendix and cecum. He was the first to describe this disease as "perityphlitis."

Reginald Heber Fitz, Professor of Medicine, Harvard University, Boston, USA, was credited for describing acute appendicitis as a proper clinical entity for the first time. He presented a scientific research paper in the first meeting of the Association of Physicians of America in 1886 entitled. "Perforating inflammation of the vermiform appendix." This paper helped doctors to diagnose more and more cases of acute appendicitis at an early stage of acute appendicitis. He studied 25 patients and found that the appendix was the primary site and source of inflammation in perityphlitis.

French Surgeon Claudius Amyand performed the world's first successful appendicectomy at St George's Hospital, London, on an 11-year-old boy who swallowed a pin. It was a perforated appendix.

In 1889, Charles McBurney, Professor of Surgery, Columbia University College of Physicians and Surgeons, New York, NY, USA, described the clinical manifestation of acute appendicitis, including the point of maximum tenderness in the RIF, which later on was called "McBurney's point." Appendectomy for appendicitis is one of the advancements of surgery. Surgical treatment of appendicitis saves 8 million lives per year in the USA alone.

ACUTE CATARRHAL APPENDICITIS

Catarrhal appendicitis is an inflammatory process affecting only the mucous lining of the appendix throughout the attack, and not involving the deeper layers. In all cases of acute appendicitis, there is probably an early stage in which the reaction is limited to the mucous membrane, but in the majority of cases, this is only momentary, and so speedily gives way to a general involvement of all the coats.

Macroscopically, in acute endoappendicitis, the appendix appears slightly thicker than normal, and owing to more or less general edema, it may be somewhat rigid. The superficial blood vessels, both those immediately beneath the peritoneum and those between the subperitoneal fibrous layer and the muscle, are prominent and tortuous, presenting a characteristic arborescent appearance. There is not, however, the diffuse redness of inflammatory tissue; on sectioning the appendix, its canal is found to be patent, and, as a rule, is of uniform caliber. The mucosa is swollen, edematous, diffusely injected, and granular in appearance.

In the gross specimen, the difference between an inflammation limited to the mucosa and the diffuse process is at once evident. In diffuse inflammation, the appendix shows a notable increase in all of its dimensions, and instead of the normal, pale, flaccid organ, of about the thickness of a goose quill, it may be twice the usual length and is often as thick as the index finger, the tip being frequently slightly clubbed. The appendix is usually tense and rigid, and exceedingly hyperemic, the blood vessels standing out in high relief. Its color is a diffuse bright red or dark mahogany, mottled with subperitoneal extravasations of blood, and often presenting light yellowish or greenish-yellow areas due to localized foci of suppuration or necrosis. Simple catarrhal appendicitis may undergo complete repair, and in cases that presented clinical evidence of repeated attacks, the appendix, when removed in the interval, may appear quite normal.

PURULENT APPENDICITIS

There is no sharp dividing line between purulent and nonpurulent appendicitis, and at any moment, a nonpurulent process may become purulent. The nature of the inflammatory reaction is chiefly due to the virulence of the infection. A mild infection is commonly not suppurative, while a severe infection induces suppuration unless the virulence of the infective material is so great that no migration of leukocytes occurs. In suppuration, there is, first, necrosis of the tissue invaded, and second, the reaction of the tissue, producing cells which form the purulent exudates. Suppuration is evidence of the ability of the tissue to offer resistance to the invasion of the infective agent.

GANGRENOUS APPENDICITIS

This condition is essentially characterized by the death and putrefaction of the tissues and is due to the action of microbes upon tissue. The most important factors, including gangrene are of which act by obstructing circulation, and so producing local ischemia. Interruption to the blood current may occur in one of the small arteries that supply only a limited portion of the appendix, or the main artery may be involved; or, in some instances, both the vein and artery, in which case the entire appendix becomes gangrenous. The obstruction to the circulation may be caused by thromboangiitis, twists, angulations, and compressions by adhesions or by hernial rings. Localized areas of gangrene may also be produced by the pressure of concretions. The pressure of concretion, added to the acute edema that accompanies the early inflammatory changes, compresses the tissue and produces local ischemia with subsequent gangrene. Most frequently, the tip of the appendix is affected, but it is not unusual to find several distinct areas of gangrene both in the proximal and the distal portions of the appendix. The role of bacteria in the production of tissue necrosis is an important one, and in cases where the gangrene of the appendix is partly due to mechanical influences, the heightened virulence of the contained bacteria, in the presence of the lessened vitality of the tissues, undoubtedly promotes the destructive process. The mesoappendix in acute inflammation becomes greatly thickened, due to the dilatation of the blood vessels, and the infiltration of the lax areolar tissue with the serous and cellular exudates. The tissue also becomes exceedingly friable, so that the ligature, although placed with the utmost care, often tears directly through it.

In the appendix, gangrene sometimes occurs only at the proximal part, and it may be due to the presence of a concretion. In this form of gangrene, the appendix remains healthy except for the proximal part connecting with the cecum. In such a form of gangrene, the appendix may lose the attachment to the cecum and fall off into the peritoneal cavity.

PERFORATED APPENDICITIS

Perforation may take place in any variety of acute appendicitis and in any stage of the attack. The rupture may be of pin-hole size, or there may be a wide, ragged aperture through which a large concretion can escape. The factors concerned in the production of a rupture are various; it may follow the eruption of an erosion to the peritoneal surface, the degeneration of the tissue due to purulent infiltration, or it may be the result of thrombosis or embolism. If perforation occurs in the appendix near its base, then it may become completely detached from the cecum and float free in the abscess cavity, as can also occur in gangrene of the appendix. It may get attached to any neighboring organs through adhesions. A tensely distended empyema often terminates in the rupture of the appendix walls, and it is particularly in such cases, where a large amount of highly virulent material empties into the abdominal cavity, that the most fatal forms of peritonitis result. One of the most important causes of rupture is the necrosis of the tissue, induced by the presence of concretions. The favorite location of the perforation is at or near the tip of the appendix, but it is not uncommon to find the perforation directly at the base or at some intermediate point. A perforation at the base may involve the neighboring portion of the cecum and produce a wide opening through which the intestinal contents escape.

Risk factors for perforation of the appendix:

- Extreme of age
- Immunosuppression
- Diabetes mellitus
- Fecolith obstruction
- Pelvic appendix
- Previous abdominal surgery

ETIOLOGY OF ACUTE APPENDICITIS

Common etiological factors of appendicitis:

- Diet
- Familial tendency
- Hereditary factor
- Nationality
- Viral infection
- Lumen of the appendix
- Socioeconomic status
- Obstruction of the lumen of the appendix
- Nonobstructive theory
- Purgatives
- Racial factor
- Epidemic of acute appendicitis
- Seasonal variation of acute appendicitis
- Trauma
- Menstruation

Appendicitis is one of the most common acute problems in medicine, yet we do not know much about its etiology. The real cause of acute appendicitis is still not known. We now understand the process of acute appendicitis well. The important contributing factors are discussed further.

Diet

Burkitt found a higher incidence of appendicitis in the West, and he attributed this to the low-fiber and high-sugar diet. It is found that the incidence of appendicitis is higher in the low-fiber, meat-rich, westernized diet-consuming population than in the high-fiber, vegetarian (cellulose) Indian diet-consuming population. There is an increasing incidence of appendicitis when the diet changes to a low-fiber Western-type diet. However, the role of diet in the etiology of acute appendicitis has not been clarified and the role of dietary fiber is less convincing than was originally thought. The reasons for and against it are:

- *The low-fiber diet-consuming persons have small stools, which take more time to pass through the intestine, and this changes the bacterial flora of the gut.*
- The high-fiber diet increases the bulk of stool, which takes less time to pass through the intestine, and bacterial flora change does not happen.
- *Some people feel that the role of a high-fiber diet in the prevention of acute appendicitis is highly exaggerated.*
- The low-fiber diet reduces the mobility of the intestine, which predisposes for obstruction of the appendix with a fecalith.
- *The incidence of appendicitis is going down in the countries in the West where the intake of dietary fiber is gradually increasing.*
- Appendicitis occurs in newborns and pure vegetarians also, which raises the doubt about the role of fiber-rich vegetarian diet in keeping the incidence of appendicitis low.
- *There is an increase in the incidence of acute appendicitis if high-fiber diet people change to a low-fiber diet.*
- There is also epidemiological evidence indicating that the consumption of green vegetables and tomatoes may be protective against appendicitis, whereas potato consumption appears to be related to the disease. In elderly patients, there is some evidence that chronic intake of nonsteroidal anti-inflammatory drugs (NSAIDs) may increase the risk.

Familial Tendency

Sometimes several members of the same family suffer from appendicitis, which may be a familial tendency (30%), or they are consuming the same diet. It is seen in a long retrocecal appendix (which many members of the same family may have) where the blood supply of the distal part of the appendix tip is diminished which precipitates appendicitis. Genetic factors theory can be explained by the following factors:

- Shared dietary habits
- Genetic resistance to bacterial flora
- Inheritance of fibrous band anomalies in the appendix.

Hereditary Factor

Sometimes, a particular anatomical position of the appendix is found in many members of the same family, which is inherited. The familial anomaly may be the cause of acute appendicitis. A family predisposition is explicable upon the grounds of anatomic peculiarities and constitutional predisposition. It is well known that in some families there is a marked tendency toward affections of the lymphoid tissues. As a rule, the affection appears in the various members of the family at different periods, but there are a considerable number of observations referring to its development in two or more at the same time.

Nationality

Though this factor seems to be of not much importance, but some researchers have found that appendicitis is much less common in colored people (Africans) than white people. Some found it rare to see appendicitis in Africans. Various nations have different incidences of acute appendicitis. Incidence is taken as a number of cases per 100,000 people.

Viral Infection

The relationship of viral infection and acute appendicitis is based on the following factors:

- Appendicitis seems to have seasonal variations, as a viral infection does.
- Raised viral antibodies have also been found during appendicitis.
- Lymphoid hyperplasia in the submucosa of the appendix is commonly seen in histopathology in appendicitis. Viral infection may enlarge the lymphoid

tissue, causing blockage of the lumen of the appendix, leading to appendicitis. Viral infection causes mucosal inflammation, which gets secondarily infected, leading to acute appendicitis. Most commonly, appendicitis is found in association with influenza, leading to catarrhal appendicitis.

Lumen of Appendix

The lumen of the appendix is quite narrow, and so it is prone to getting obstructed. Approximately 60% of inflamed appendix removed during appendicectomy for acute appendicitis show blockage of the lumen. The blockage is most commonly found due to a fecalith, but rarely a neoplasm of the cecum (<1% is also responsible).

> **Socioeconomic Status**
> - *Appendicitis is more common in rich and uppermiddle-class people.* The reason for this is known as probably they tend to take more protein as the main dish and try to ignore vegetables thereby taking a low-fiber diet or high-caloric diet.
> - *The role of personal hygiene and domestic overcrowding is considered as one of the reasons for infection.*

OBSTRUCTION OF THE LUMEN OF THE APPENDIX

Obstruction of the lumen of the appendix is the most common factor in causing acute appendicitis. Wangensteen studied the anatomy of the appendix and postulated that mucosal folds and sphincter-like orientation of muscle fibers at the appendiceal orifice make the appendix susceptible for obstruction. The cause of obstruction of the lumen may be in the lumen, in the wall, or outside the wall of the appendix. Lymphoid hyperplasia and fecalith are the most common factors in appendicular lumen obstruction; 60% of obstruction in teens is due to submucous lymphoid hyperplasia, and 35% in older adults and children.

Causes of Obstruction

- *In lumen:*
  - Fecalith
  - Worm
  - Foreign body, i.e., seeds of fruits
- *In the wall:*
  - Hyperplasia of lymphoid follicles
  - Fibrosis and stricture due to previous appendicitis—if a normal appendix get adherent to a neighboring organ or a previous operation scar, it becomes prone to inflammation.
  - Neoplasm
  - Crohn's disease
  - Distal colonic obstruction
- *Outside the wall:*
  - Adhesions
  - Kinks
  - Bands
- *Fecalith: It is a mass of inspissated fecal material, and it is made up of:*
  - Fecal material
  - Calcium phosphate
  - Bacteria
  - Epithelial debris
  - *Foreign body:* Foreign bodies causing appendicitis are rare, but Fitz, in 1886, found foreign bodies in 12% of cases of perforative appendicitis. Gallstones are also found as enterolith inside the appendix. The clinical evidence in some of these cases so strongly supports the gallstone theory as to leave no doubt in the mind of the observer. Global distribution of appendicitis varies according to various factors, such as geographic site, eating habits, and environmental factors. Fecaliths are the most common cause of appendicitis. They are found in 40% of cases of acute appendicitis, 65% of cases of purulent appendicitis with rupture, and nearly 90% of cases of gangrenous appendicitis with rupture. It is also found that a histologically normal appendix having fecalith and appendicitis may show no fecalith obstruction. A fecalith in combination of localized right lower quadrant (RLQ) pain is highly diagnostic of appendicitis. The fecalith is also called an enterolith.

> *Worms*: Usual parasites found in the appendix are the following:
> - Pin worm (Oxyuris vermicularis)
> - *Ascaris lumbricoides*
> - *Enterobius vermicularis*
> - *Strongyloides stercoralis*
> - *Echinococcus granulosus*
> - *Entamoeba histolytica*
>
> *The most common intestinal parasite causing obstruction of the appendix lumen is pinworm (Oxyuris vermicularis).* Careful examination of stools for worms and ova is important. The presence of parasites in the lumen of the appendix sometimes produces difficulty in ligation or stapling of the base of the appendix. All such cases must be given deworming treatment post appendicectomy, and cases of amebiasis with antiamoebic therapy.

Nonobstructive Theory

This is due to bacterial infection in the wall of the appendix without obstruction of its lumen. It is due to the following factors:

- Hematogenous spread of generalized infection.
- Vascular occlusion
- Diet with low roughage
- *Disorders of digestion:* Many persons suffering with appendicitis have a history of indigestion or constipation or diarrhea.

Purgatives

Acute appendicitis sometimes is precipitated by the administration of purgatives, and it can cause perforation of the appendix in a patient suffering from acute appendicitis. That is why purgative is contraindicated in RIF pain as generally it is said "purgation means perforation."

Racial Factor

It is seen that appendicitis is most common in white Westerners than in dark-colored Asians and Africans.

Epidemic of Acute Appendicitis

The epidemic of acute appendicitis is also reported. It usually occurs in institutionalized children.

Seasonal Variation of Acute Appendicitis

In Europe, it has been observed that between May and August, more cases of acute appendicitis are reported in hospitals. In some Western countries, a link between viral infection and appendicitis is found which also explains the seasonal variation.

Menstruation

The intimate relationship existing between menstrual periods and appendicitis has been frequently noted, not only when the appendix is situated in the pelvis, but also when it is retrocecal. The probable explanation lies in the fact that the congestion of the whole splanchnic area which accompanies the lowered blood pressure (BP) of the peripheral circulation during menstruation creates a favorable soil for the activities of the microorganisms contained in the appendix. I have observed this association in several instances, in some of which the recurrent appendiceal attacks invariably occurred during the menstrual period.

PATHOLOGY OF ACUTE APPENDICITIS

Acute appendicitis starts as inflammation and then converts to infection of the appendix. The infection in the appendix develops from the bacteria contained in the contents of the appendix. No single organism is found responsible for acute appendicitis. Usually, it is a mixed infection with aerobic and anaerobic bacteria. The obstruction of the lumen accelerates the process of infection as the contents become stagnant and bacteria multiply fast. The bacteria gain access to the wall of the appendix through a breach in the continuity of the mucosa of the appendix.

The infection and inflammation spread in the wall of the appendix from inside to outside (from mucus membrane to the serosa) which is why sometimes at an early stage of appendicitis appendix looks normal from the outside but on exploration it is found inflamed from the inside, it is called "macroscopic normal appendix" but microscopically it is diseased.

Bacteriology

The infection in an appendix is a mixed infection by anaerobic and aerobic organisms. In 85% of cases, the organism responsible is Escherichia coli.

The appendiceal flora remains constant throughout life except *Porphyromonas gingivalis* which is seen only in adults. *Porphyromonas* is a gram-negative, rod-shaped, anaerobic, pathogenic bacterium. It is found in periodontal disease, the gastrointestinal tract, and the respiratory tract.

- Peritoneal fluid cultures show bacteria in <50% of cases of nonperforated appendicitis and in >85% of cases of perforated or gangrenous appendicitis.
- It is usually caused by organisms normally residing in an appendix.
- *Enterococcus* is also responsible for appendicitis infection in a large number of cases.
- In 1938, Altemeier demonstrated the polymicrobial nature of perforated appendicitis. Now due to this, the routine peritoneal culture in perforated appendicitis is questioned.
- The bacteria commonly contained in an appendix in acute appendicitis are given below.

COMMON ORGANISMS SEEN IN PATIENTS WITH ACUTE APPENDICITIS

Foul-smelling odor in a perforated appendix is not due to *E. coli* or anaerobic bacilli, as it is commonly and wrongly believed, but is due to anaerobic streptococci.

TABLE 1: Common organisms seen in acute appendicitis.

Aerobic and facultative	*Anaerobic*
Gram-negative bacilli	Gram-negative bacilli
Escherichia coli	*Bacteroides fragilis*
Pseudomonas aeruginosa	*Bacteroides* species
Klebsiella species	*Fusobacterium* species
Gram-positive cocci	Gram-positive cocci
Streptococcus species	*Peptostreptococcus* species
Streptococcus species	Gram-positive bacilli
Enterococcus species	*Clostridium* species

Routine culture of intraperitoneal samples in patients with either perforated or nonperforated appendicitis is questionable, the peritoneal fluid culture should be reserved for immunosuppressed patients and those who developed abscess after appendicitis **(Table 1)**.

Obstructive Acute Appendicitis

In most of cases of acute appendicitis, the obstruction of its lumen is the main and essential reason. Obstruction is found in 50–80% of cases of acute appendicitis. Gangrene and perforation of the appendix usually do not occur if the appendix is not obstructed. When obstruction happens due to lymphoid hyperplasia or other obstructing agents, the intraluminal pressure in the appendix increases due to continuous mucus secretion and inflammatory exudate formation, and a closed-loop obstruction is produced. Secretion of even 0.5 mL of fluid distal to obstruction raises intraluminal pressure to quite a high level. Rapid distension of the appendix ensues because of its small luminal capacity, and intraluminal pressure can reach 50–65 mm Hg. The distension of the appendix stimulates nerve endings of visceral afferent nerve fibers, producing dull, vague, diffuse pain in midabdomen or lower epigastrium, it also causes reflex nausea and vomiting. The raised intraluminal pressure does not decrease or stop further mucus secretion. The raised intraluminal pressure obstructs the lymphatic drainage from the wall of the appendix, which leads to the edema of the wall. The high intraluminal pressure and edema cause superficial ulcerations in the wall, which become a port of entry for the bacteria to the wall of the appendix from the luminal contents. The further increase in intraluminal pressure causes venous obstruction, which further increases the edema of the wall. Now, the increased intraluminal pressure, venous obstruction, and increasing edema of the wall cause compromise of arterial blood flow, which leads to ischemia of the wall. Further bacterial invasion causes full-blown acute appendicitis.

TYPES OF ACUTE APPENDICITIS

Acute appendicitis is of two types:

1. Obstructive acute appendicitis
2. Nonobstructive acute appendicitis

The further development leads to acute gangrenous appendicitis and then the further increase in intraluminal pressure causes perforation of the wall of the appendix, leading to local or general peritonitis. The body tries to limit the damage and tries to prevent the spread of infection to other parts of peritoneal cavity. So, loops of the small intestine, greater omentum, and cecum come close and become adherent to wall-off the appendicular lesion to avoid peritoneal contamination. This leads to the formation of an appendicular mass or lump. The omentum is therefore called "abdominal policeman," as it helps to contain the problem. Rarely, the obstructed appendix become a mucus-filled sac called "mucocele of appendix" when infection subsides and sometimes it becomes "empyema of the appendix," when the obstructed appendix becomes filled with frank pus. The most dreaded complication of appendicitis is perforation of a gangrenous appendix leading to generalized peritonitis. *Sir David Wilkie, Professor of Surgery, Edinburgh, Scotland (1882–1938) stated that close examination of gangrenous appendicitis directly after their removal shows conclusively that they usually belong to the obstructive group.* Usually, the perforation occurs at the tip of the appendix due to poor vascularity or at the site of obstruction due to pressure necrosis, or at the antimesenteric border. The fate of appendicitis can lead to resolution, operation, perforation, peritonitis, fecal fistula, appendicular mass, abscess. This appendicular condition leads to enlargement of cecum due to cecal localized ileus, caused by the inflammatory process. The cecal content is stored and is not conducted to the right colon. The presence of fecal loading inside a large cecum is identified in the plain abdominal radiography as a specific sign of acute appendicitis.

Nonobstructive Appendicitis (Catarrhal Appendicitis)

The infection occurs in the wall of the appendix from the mucosa and the process of inflammation is slow. Nonobstructive appendicitis is usually a catarrhal type of appendicitis. Generalized peritonitis is not a common finding with nonobstructive appendicitis but it can occur. It occurs due to:

- Transmigration of bacteria to the peritoneal cavity through the wall of the appendix.
- Rarely due to perforation of the appendix.

Macroscopic Changes

In a normal-looking appendix, only the mucosa is inflamed, so every normal-looking appendix must be opened to see the mucosa.

- Early stage of acute inflammation—the appendix is swollen with hyperemic serosa.
- Late stage of acute inflammation—the surface is coated with fibrinopurulent exudates with prominent vessels. In later stages, edema, necrosis, and gangrene develop.

Microscopic Changes

- Neutrophilic infiltration of the muscularis mucosa is characteristic of acute appendicitis.
- Congestion, edema, microabscesses, immobilized blood vessels, necrosis, and gangrene may be seen.
- The cause of obstruction is also confirmed. Many patients, who are forced to undergo an operation with acute appendicitis, give a history of previous similar, but less severe, attacks of RLQ pain.
- Pathologic examination of the appendices removed from these patients often reveals thickening and scarring, suggesting old, healed, and acute inflammation.

CLINICAL FEATURES OF ACUTE APPENDICITIS

Incidence

The lifetime incidence of acute appendicitis is 6.7–20%, with a lifetime risk of appendectomy of 12% for men and 23% for women. Acute appendicitis represents about 17% of all cases of acute abdominal pain presented to the hospital. Acute appendicitis is the most common emergency in surgery, where a general surgeon is called. It is the most common cause of acute abdomen in young adults. It is more common in Western countries than in India, probably due to diet, which is more vegetarian and with high roughage content. By adulthood, one in six people will have undergone the removal of this appendix. Nowadays, the disease is increasing in the developing areas of the world, but decreasing in Western countries, probably due to changing food habits. The incidence of acute appendicitis in the population is most frequently seen from the second to fourth decades, with a mean age of 31.3 years and a median age of 22 years.

- Appendicectomy is one of the most common operations performed in general surgery.
- The lifetime rate of appendicectomy is 7% for the Population, it is 12% for men, and 25% for women.
- The rate of appendicectomy for appendicitis is 10 per 10,000 patients per year and is constant.
- The rate of misdiagnosis of appendicitis is 15.3%, higher in women (22.2%) than in men (9.3%).
- Negative appendicectomy rate for females, if fertile age is 23.1%, and is highest in females above 80 years.

Age

The maximum incidence occurs in the second and third decades, the mean age is 31.3 years.

Acute appendicitis is rare in infancy; it is uncommon before the age of 2 years, but no age is exempted from it. The incidence of acute appendicitis gradually decreases after middle age. *The peak incidence occurs between 20 and 30 years, and the median age is 22 years.* This is also the age of peak increase in size and number of lymphoid follicles. This indicates the relation between the incidence of acute appendicitis and amount and number of lymphoid follicles. The incidence of acute appendicitis becomes very low after 60 years of age, almost a rarity; 70% of appendicitis occurs <30 years of age.

The mortality rate of acute appendicitis is 0.8%; such patients are either very young or very old.

The incidence of acute appendicitis in males and females is age-related. Before puberty, it is equal among both sexes. In the second and third decades, the male and female ratio is 3:2. After the third decade, the incidence among males declines and becomes equal gradually. Acute appendicitis is more common in teenage girls. The highest incidence of appendicitis in males is at early years, whereas in females it is later years. The association between menstruation and appendicitis is frequently noted. Some researchers indicate that the probable explanation lies in the fact that the condition of the whole splanchnic area, which accompanies the lowered BP of the peripheral circulation during menstruation, creates a favorable soil for the activities of the microorganisms contained in the appendix *(Howard A Kelly).*

Symptoms

Important symptoms of acute appendicitis **(Fig. 16):**

- Pain
- Nausea
- Vomiting
- Anorexia
- Fever
- Murphy's syndrome
- Constipation or diarrhea

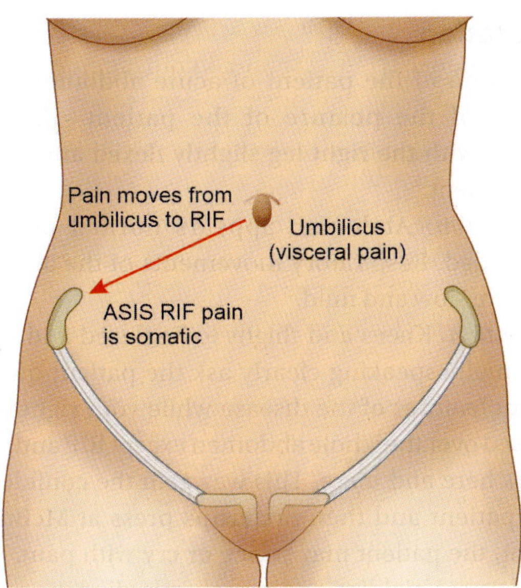

Fig. 16: Migratory pain in acute appendicitis.

Pain

Pain in acute appendicitis usually starts in the early morning. The patient sleeps well in night, and the pain wakes him up in the early morning. The pain in appendicitis is produced by distension of its lumen or spasm of the muscle due to stimulation of visceral nerve endings responsible for pain. First, the pain is felt at the umbilicus. It is referred to as pain, as both the umbilicus and the appendix receive their nerve supply from the thoracic tenth (T10) segment of the spinal cord. Appendix receives its sympathetic nerve supply from T10 via the celiac plexus and the umbilicus by somatic nerves via the vagus nerve. This is referred to as pain and is vague pain. The explanation of referred pain is that the nerve fibers from the diseased organ and the area where the referred pain is felt (here the umbilicus) ascend to the cerebral cortex and the cerebral cortex sometimes becomes incapable of differentiating between the causative site and referred site, which is why some patients complain of umbilical pain. This umbilical pain is seen in appendicitis irrespective of the position of the appendix. One can explain this visceral pain by midline radiation of delta nonmyelinated fibers that have very poor localization. The pain increases gradually as the inflammation increases. The pain later migrates to the RIF. This shift of pain is due to the involvement of the parietal peritoneum by inflammation over the appendix. As the inflammation increases, pain spreads. The visceral layer of the peritoneum is insensitive to pain, but the parietal peritoneum is sensitive to pain, which is why in the early stage of inflammation, when the parietal peritoneum is not involved, the pain is not felt in RIF and is only felt at the umbilicus. When the parietal peritoneum is involved, the pain is conveyed by alpha fibers at the RIF.

> Initial pain is visceral pain, which is felt at the umbilicus, and later on, pain is somatic pain, which is in the RIF. It is called the "shifting pain" of acute appendicitis. The history of shifting pain from the umbilicus to RIF, if present, is a very important symptom to diagnose acute appendicitis. The visceral pain in acute appendicitis is dull, diffuse, and vague in the umbilical, paraumbilical, and lower epigastrium region. 25% of patients have no visceral pain and present with localized pain. Sudden movement or coughing increases the pain, and even walking increases the pain. The diminution of pain is not always good news. In acute appendicitis sudden disappearance of pain may be due to perforation of a gangrenous appendix or obstructive appendicitis. In pelvic appendicitis, the pain is aggravated when the right obturator internus muscle is stretched by flexion and medial rotation of the right thigh. It is due to the fact that the inflamed appendix is touching the obturator internus muscle. Pain severity and associated nausea and vomiting depend upon the degree of distension of the appendix.

In retrocecal appendicitis pain is aggravated or even caused when the psoas major muscle of right side is stretched by extension of right hip joint. This is not often seen in obese patients. The distension of lumen of appendix also stimulates the peristalsis in appendix which produces cramp-like pain as in acute gastroenteritis or in ureteric colic so the visceral pain may be cramp-like pain super imposed on dull pain.

Anorexia

It is a constant feature in every patient with acute appendicitis. It is more marked in infants and children than adults. It is difficult to find a case of acute appendicitis without anorexia. If anorexia is absent, the diagnosis of acute appendicitis is reconsidered. Hiccoughs are rare but are present in generalized peritonitis due to irritation of the peritoneal surface of the diaphragm.

> *Anorexia is a reliable and permanent feature of acute appendicitis, usually, it is the first sign. If anorexia is not present, then the diagnosis of acute appendicitis may be deferred.*

Nausea

It is a common symptom in both types of obstructive and nonobstructive appendicitis. Nausea and vomiting occur in 70% patients of with appendicitis.

Vomiting

It occurs due to reflex pylorospasm which is protective as the body does not want food to reach the site of inflammation, i.e., the appendix. It is more marked in obstructive appendicitis than nonobstructive appendicitis. It follows abdominal pain. It is more marked in children than adults. Vomiting is not persistent; it subsides when the stomach becomes empty. If vomiting precedes the pain, the diagnosis of acute appendicitis should be questioned.

Fever

It is due to bacterial infection and is of low grade (<100°F). Fever is the last symptom after pain and vomiting. So, it is not present in the initial sickness. In 20% of patients, there is no fever. A higher fever indicates that a complication has occurred or that another diagnosis should be considered. High and persistent temperature relates to the severity of infection and local or metastatic collection of pus.

> **Murphy's Syndrome**
>
> *Pain first, followed by vomiting and then by fever, is called "Murphy's triad of acute appendicitis" or "Murphy's syndrome" after John Benjamin Murphy.* He used to say that "If vomiting precedes the pain, probably you are not dealing with acute appendicitis." It is not a must to find Murphy's triad in every case of acute appendicitis.

Constipation or Diarrhea

Constipation is a common feature in acute appendicitis except in pre- and postileal appendicitis where diarrhea occurs due to irritation of the ileum. In pelvic appendicitis patient may have "tenesmus" (ineffectual straining at defecation with passage of mucus and blood only). Due to irritation of the rectum diarrhea occurs in 10% patients of with acute appendicitis, causing doubt about acute gastroenteritis and delay in diagnosis of acute appendicitis and appendicectomy.

Hematuria

It is not a common finding and when occurs it is due to irritation of the right ureter, especially in retrocecal appendicitis. Patients may feel strangury (painful and frequent attempts at micturition passing only a small quantity of urine) if the appendix is touching the urinary bladder or ureter in pelvic appendicitis or retrocecal appendicitis.

Examination

Examination of the patient of acute abdomen attracts attention of the posture of the patient—the dorsal decubitus with the right leg slightly flexed and avoiding any movement.

- *Inspection:* Abdomen appears normal or slightly distended. Respiratory movements of the abdominal wall are slow and mild.
- *Palpation:* Knees and thighs to be flexed and relaxed. Gradually speaking clearly ask the patient questions about features of the disease while your right hand is passed over the whole abdomen except RIF and slightly press here and there. This way gain the confidence of the patient and then fingertips press at McBurney's point, the patient may wince or cry with pain, feeling tenderness, rigidity, and muscle guarding.

Note: John Benjamin Murphy (1857–1916), Professor of Surgery, Northwestern University, Chicago II, USA. He described this syndrome in 1903.

- *Percussion:* It shows normal tympany but dullness if an appendicular mass or abscess is present.
- *Auscultation:* It shows a reduction or absence of bowel sounds if ileus is present. In the olden days an instrument called "piezometer" was used to measure the amount of pressure required to produce pain. It has become obsolete now.

Signs

> Important signs of acute appendicitis:
> - Cough sign (Dunphy's sign)
> - Rovsing sign
> - Hyperesthesia in Sherren's triangle
> - Cope's psoas test
> - Cope's obturator test
> - Bed shaking test of Bapat
> - Baldwin's test
> - Tenderness on DRE
> - Bastedo's sign
> - Markle sign or jar tenderness

Pyrexia

Usually, the patient looks unwell with low-grade pyrexia. The temperature is not very high, but in children, the temperature may be high. It is between 90 and 100°F. The temperature may be normal in uncomplicated and early appendicitis. When generalized peritonitis occurs temperature goes up to 102–103°F. It must be remembered that pyrexia is not an early sign of acute appendicitis. In acute appendicitis, pyrexia comes after pain and vomiting, so it is the last sign of the three, i.e., pain, vomiting, and fever (Murphy's syndrome).

Tachycardia

It is a good diagnostic guide for acute appendicitis. Sometimes, when the pain is not severe and the patient cannot locate the abdominal pain properly, the pulse plays an important role in suspecting acute appendicitis. The pulse rate is usually slightly elevated between 80 and 90 beats/min. Temperature and pulse rate are usually not elevated in the first 4–6 hours, the pulse increases in proportion to the temperature rise. *Osborne Joby Dunphy (1898–1989), a British American physician, observed this sign for the first time.*

> A high tachycardia or very rapid pulse is not a good sign, it may be a grave sign. Tachycardia out of proportion to fever is also a grave sign.

Coated and Dry Tongue

Rough, brownish-coated, and dry tongue-it indicates toxemia. Even in early acute appendicitis tongue may be thickly coated and dry, as the patient might have vomited several times and is dehydrated.

Limited Respiratory Movements

Movement of the abdominal wall during respiration may be limited in RIF in acute appendicitis due to localized irritation of the peritoneum from the inflammation. The vigorous respiratory movements will shake the inflamed parietal peritoneum and will cause pain, so the movement of the abdominal wall is limited. It is also a protective phenomenon.

Pointing Test

This test confirms RIF inflammatory pathology, the patient is asked to indicate the site of pain by the tip of a finger, and indicates toward RIF. If the pain is diffuse, then the patient will use his whole hand instead of one finger to point toward the site of pain.

Method of test:

- Ask the patient to lie down.
- Ask to indicate the site of maximum pain.

If it is also the point of maximum tenderness, this is the site of the inflamed organ.

Tenderness

In acute appendicitis, the RIF is tender. The maximum tenderness is elicited at McBurney's point. The tenderness can be best elicited in the left lateral position when coils of a small intestine shift to the left, exposing the appendix directly to palpation. The abdominal wall also becomes relaxed in this position. Tenderness persists even after cessation of pain till the inflammatory process is present.

> *Tenderness on pressing RIF is one of the most important signs of acute appendicitis.* It is very significant that if it is absent surgeon is doubtful of the diagnosis of acute appendicitis.

In acute appendicitis, the site of muscle guarding varies according to the position of the appendix.

- In paracecal appendicitis, guarding is in RIF.
- In retrocecal appendicitis, it may be present over the flank and even on the back muscle and may be RIF totally free. In pelvic appendicitis, there may not be any rigidity in the anterior abdominal wall. In preileal and postileal appendicitis, guarding may be near the umbilicus.
- Muscle guarding is an indication of irritation of the parietal peritoneum. It is a protective mechanism for inflamed organs not to get hurt. It is important to differentiate the involuntary muscle rigidity of acute appendicitis from voluntary muscle guarding. Involuntary muscle rigidity indicates local parietal peritonitis due to an underlying inflamed appendix. Voluntary muscle guarding is brought by the patient himself due to fear of being hurt. In every case of acute appendicitis, there is some degree of voluntary muscle guarding. It is more so in children. To elicit muscle guarding, the patient's confidence must be gained by your polite manners and behavior.

> ### Rebound Tenderness (Blumberg's Sign)
>
> *The RIF is palpated with flat of the right hand. With each expiration hand on the abdomen is gradually pressed down the abdomen.* Then the hand is suddenly withdrawn completely, so the abdominal musculature springs back suddenly to its original position, and the patient will cry or will wince due to pain. This pain is due to the sudden movement of the inflamed parietal peritoneum.

Muscle Guarding

Spasm or rigidity is the involuntary tightening of the abdominal musculature that occurs in response to underlying inflammation. This stiffness can be felt when

CLINICAL FEATURES ACCORDING TO THE TYPE OF APPENDICITIS

Not to forget:
- Appendicitis is common in 20–30-year-olds of age.
- Gangrene and perforation of the appendix are common in obstructive appendicitis and rare in nonobstructive or catarrhal appendicitis.
- Pneumoperitoneum is uncommon in appendicular perforation, but common in duodenal perforation.
- Appendicitis in a child <2 years is uncommon, but if it happens, then perforation, peritonitis, and poor prognosis are common.
- Appendicitis is found in LIF in a case of situs inversus and mimics acute diverticulitis.
- The mortality rate in appendicitis is <1%.
- If a normal appendix is found on the operation is called "Lilly White Appendix." If the appendix is found directly on the introduction of the laparoscope in the abdomen, it is called "handshake appendix."

OBSTRUCTIVE APPENDICITIS

- The onset of symptoms is abrupt, and then symptoms progress fast.
- Pain is severe.
- Pain is of a colicky nature.
- Vomiting is common.
- Temperature may be normal.
- The patient immediately goes to bed as they cannot perform their usual day-to-day duty due to tiredness and pain.
- Tenderness is more.
- It is a more dangerous variety.
- The obstruction makes the appendix a closed loop, so the contents stagnate and the walls get infected fast, and it rapidly progresses to perforation and gangrene.
- It may mimic acute intestinal obstruction.

NONOBSTRUCTIVE APPENDICITIS

It is also called "acute catarrhal appendicitis."

- The onset and progress are slow and not so abrupt as in acute obstructive appendicitis.
- Pain is less and of a dull type or constant burning pain rather than colic.
- Vomiting is not much and may be absent.
- Fever is usually present, which may be normal in obstructive appendicitis.
- Patient carries out his usually day-to-day duties but with discomfort in the abdomen, nausea, vomiting, and anorexia. He is not very sick.
- Tenderness is not much.
- It is not so dangerous a variety as acute obstructive appendicitis.
- Usually does not lead to gangrene and perforation.
- Does not mimic acute intestinal obstruction.
- Inflammation spreads from the mucosa to the serosa slowly, and the appendix becomes congested.
- The inflammation ends in:
  - Resolution
  - Fibrosis
  - Suppurate
  - Gangrene
- Nonobstructive appendicitis can be acute, subacute, chronic, or recurrent.

CLINICAL FEATURES ACCORDING TO THE POSITION OF THE APPENDIX

Characteristic features in different anatomical positions of the appendix in acute appendicitis:
- Retrocecal appendicitis—silent
- Pelvic appendicitis—diarrhea
- Preileal and postileal—diarrhea
- Subhepatic—pain above RIF, as in cholecystitis, and RIF is pain-free.

RETROCECAL APPENDICITIS

This may be silent without any tenderness and rigidity in the RIF, which is why called a "silent appendix." It is due to a distended cecum with gas lying anterior to the appendix, so the pressure exerted cannot pass up to the appendix. In such cases, deep tenderness may be present in the loin, and muscles of the loin (i.e., quadratus lumborum) may be found in spasm. Here, the inflamed appendix lies over the psoas major muscle, so it may be in spasm, causing flexion of the hip joint, and the extension of the hip joint causes pain. If the irritation of the psoas major muscle is not much, then instead of extension, hyperextension of the hip may cause pain, as extension may not cause sufficient stretching of the psoas muscle.

In retrocecal appendicitis, if the appendix is totally and completely retroperitoneal, then there is no rigidity and tenderness in the anterior abdominal wall. There may be tenderness and rigidity in the right flank and more posteriorly. To elicit such tenderness patient has to be rolled to the left side. If the appendix is in direct contact with the right ureter, a patient may feel pain radiating from the loin to the groin and may have hematuria.

This may confuse the surgeon with ureteric colic, but an initial history of pain around the umbilicus, Rovsing sign, psoas test, and examination in the left lateral position will diagnose the appendicitis. One has to be very careful in history taking and examination to not to miss appendicitis.

Pouch of Douglas is named after James Douglas (1675–1742), an anatomist and male midwife who practiced in London, England.

PELVIC APPENDICITIS

It can produce diarrhea instead of constipation if the inflamed appendix is in contact with the rectum. If the inflamed appendix is in contact with the urinary bladder, then it may cause frequency of micturition, leading to the doubt of urinary tract infection.

> Per-rectal examination in males and bimanual examination in females by putting one hand over the lower abdomen and a finger in the vagina is necessary to not to miss pelvic appendicitis.

Tenderness and abdominal muscle rigidity may be altogether absent, and DRE may reveal tenderness in a pouch of Douglas (Rectovesical pouch). The inflamed pelvic appendix may touch the psoas muscle or internal obturator muscle and cause spasms of these muscles, causing flexion of the hip joint or flexion and internal rotation of the thigh.

- *Postileal and preileal appendicitis:* It causes diarrhea, and one may miss appendicitis and be diagnosed as acute gastroenteritis. So, it is called a "missed appendix." Tenderness may be present just on the right side of the umbilicus.
- *Subhepatic appendicitis:* The pain is present above the RIF. It may mimic acute cholecystitis.

INVESTIGATIONS FOR APPENDICITIS

The acute appendicitis is diagnosed clinically only, but investigations are done to avoid the removal of a normal appendix. Approximately 20% of appendices removed on appendicectomy are found normal on histopathological examination. The most important criteria in the diagnosis of acute appendicitis are given here.

> *Important preoperative investigations in acute appendicitis*:
> - Complete blood count
> - Urine analysis
> - Pregnancy test
> - Urea, creatinine, and electrolytes
> - C-reactive protein
> - Radiography
> - Barium meal or enema
> - Ultrasound
> - Contrast-enhanced computerized tomography (CECT) scan of the abdomen
> - Diagnostic laparoscopy
> - Alvarado scoring system
> - Nigam's Scoring System (NSS)

COMPLETE BLOOD COUNT

More than 90% of patients suffering from acute appendicitis have some leukocytosis. The total leukocyte count (TLC) is usually above 10,000/mm^3 (12,000–18,000/mm^3). There is a shift toward the left means polymorph nuclear cells predominance. In perforated appendicitis, the count may be >18,000 mm^3. Serial WBC measurement improves diagnostic accuracy, with a rising value over time commonly seen in patients with appendicitis.

As a matter of fact, the total number of leukocytes is subject to fairly wide variations even under normal conditions, so the conclusion drawn from an absolute count alone may prove entirely erroneous. While on the one hand in the majority of individuals, an absolute count from 5,000 to 7,500 is the rule, on the other hand in a lower state of nutrition than an average, lower values are also normally present (3,000–5,000), while higher figures (up to 10,000) may be found in unusually vigorous and well-nourished persons. It, thus, becomes clear that an absolute count of 8,000–10,000 in a poorly developed and ill-nourished individual might really indicate a decided hyperleukocytosis. reliance upon the absolute count alone may here give rise to disastrous consequences.

High value, it is true, indicates in a general way that the disease is active, and increasing values—where repeated examinations are made—that the decrease is progressive. Low count or falling values, on the other hand, may indicate either that the disease is abating, or that the infection is unusually severe, or that the perforation with general peritonitis has developed. In these cases, again, the differential leukocyte count will tell the true story. Eosinophil count is a "septic factor" in infective states, such as appendicitis.

URINE EXAMINATION

Dehydration is caused due to repeated vomiting. So, the urine shows high specific gravity. Urine may also show RBCs and WBCs if the appendix touches the urinary bladder or ureter in pelvic or retrocecal appendicitis. If urine shows >20 WBC per high power field or shows >30 WBC per high power field, it indicates urinary tract infection (UTI).

Bacteriuria in a catheterized patient is not generally seen with acute appendicitis. Failure to find blood or pus cells in the urine is not a certainty of exclusion of right renal or ureteric problem but the diagnosis of a renal problem is less likely, especially in the presence of peritoneal signs.

PREGNANCY TEST

The negative pregnancy test will rule out RIF pain due to ectopic gestation.

BLOOD UREA, CREATININE, AND ELECTROLYTES (SODIUM, POTASSIUM, AND CALCIUM)

Vomiting can cause raised blood urea and abnormal serum electrolytes. The estimation of urea, creatinine, and electrolytes also helps to assess the renal function of the patient, which also helps the anesthetist with anesthesia for the operation.

C-REACTIVE PROTEIN

C-reactive protein (CRP) estimation is found helpful in the diagnosis of acute appendicitis, CRP is produced by the liver when infection occurs in any part of the body, it increases rapidly within the first 12 hours and then within the next 12 hours comes to a normal level.

C-reactive protein levels above 1 mg/dL are found in acute appendicitis, and very high level of CRP with leukocytosis indicates advanced or gangrenous appendicitis. The high level of CRP in blood shows inflammation. The CRP value comes to normal once the infection is controlled. It is not very useful. Clinically as it is nonspecific and cannot distinguish between sites of infection.

RADIOGRAPHY

X-ray neither confirms acute appendicitis nor excludes it. It can be of benefit to exclude other pathologies, such as calculus in the ureter. There is no classical sign of acute appendicitis on plain X-ray. Plain X-ray of the abdomen is not a very important investigation in acute appendicitis, except in perforation of the appendix. Avoid doing radiographs if a patient is pregnant. Acute appendicitis is quite common in young females, so keep in mind the pregnancy when X-ray is advised.

The following findings may help to support the diagnosis of acute appendicitis in association with clinical signs:

- *Sentinel loops of bowel:* These are seen as gas shadows due to localized ileus due to inflammation.
- *Calcified fecaliths:* Approximately 15% of cases of acute appendicitis show calcified fecaliths on X-ray. A fecalith shows a laminated shadow. The presence of fecaliths in X-ray in RIF pain is suggestive of appendicitis.
- *Mass effect around the appendix:* The bowel loops are displaced away from an appendicular lump.
- The presence of free gas under the diaphragm is a sure sign of perforation of the appendix, but it is not always seen, so the absence of this sign does not rule out the diagnosis of appendicitis or perforation of the appendix.
- Scoliosis of the spine with concavity toward the right side due to spasm of the psoas muscle due to irritation by an inflamed appendix is rarely seen on X-ray.
- The psoas muscle margin of the right side is lost due to the superimposed inflamed appendix.
- Retained barium from previous studies is to be noted. It is noted that inspissated barium from earlier barium enema or meal can rarely cause acute obstructive appendicitis.
- Blurring of preperitoneal fat on the flank is also an important sign on plain X-ray of abdomen. Gas in the appendix is not a sign specific for appendicitis and should not mandate laparotomy for appendicitis.

ULTRASOUND OF ABDOMEN

Ultrasound cannot visualize a healthy normal appendix. It may not be very helpful in early acute appendicitis. It is more useful in excluding gynecological causes of RIF pain. Ultrasound is highly operator-dependent which is the main limitation of ultrasound in the diagnosis of acute appendicitis, frequently unable to visualize the normal appendix.

A blind-ended tubular structure, easily compared possible and <6 mm in diameter is the feature of a normal appendix and if it is found then appendicitis is excluded from the diagnosis.

Ultrasound findings in acute appendicitis are:

- Probe tenderness at McBurney's point.

- A blind-ending, tubular structure with a thick wall, without peristalsis and noncompressible originating from the cecum, is detected in RIF. It is seen, especially when the lumen is >6 mm in diameter.
- Appendicolith may be present.
- Intussusception
- Periappendicular fluid collection.

If an ultrasound of the abdomen shows an abscess cavity in an appendicular mass, then drain the abscess.

Nowadays with better ultrasound machines and advanced probes, the full fledged acute appendicitis can be diagnosed in >90% of cases. In most of hospitals, now ultrasound is used as a routine investigation of RIF pain. It is helpful in diagnosing appendicular lumps and abscess.

Ultrasound can diagnose approximately 86% of appendicitis cases. However, the ultrasound is usually not used as a tool to diagnose acute appendicitis than to rule out other causes of such pain or when the diagnosis is uncertain or in females of childbearing age. Tzanakis et al. proposed the use of ultrasound as it is more readily available than a CT scan.

Graded Compression Sonography

It is recommended as an accurate way to establish the diagnosis of appendicitis. The diameter of the appendix is measured in anteroposterior dimension with maximal compression. The presence of appendicolith establishes the diagnosis. Thickening of the appendicular wall and periappendicular fluid are highly suggestive signs on ultrasound. The sonographic diagnosis of acute appendicitis has a specificity of 85–98%.

Normal appendix demonstration on sonography is as easily compressible as a blind-ending tubular structure 6 mm or less in diameter, which excludes the diagnosis of acute appendicitis. Transvaginal ultrasound alone or a combination of transabdominal scans is a must in a female of reproductive age with RIF pain to diagnose acute appendicitis. It reveals pelvic pathology and fluid in a pouch of Douglas.

Advantages of Graded Compression Ultrasonography

- Reduced negative appendicectomies from 37 to 13%.
- Reduces preoperative time.
- Improves the diagnosis of acute appendicitis diagnosed on physical examination.

COMPUTED TOMOGRAPHY SCAN OF ABDOMEN

It is not used as a routine investigation. Selective use of CT is required as a standard approach. CT scans used in acute appendicitis can be focused and nonfocused or enhanced and nonenhanced. CECT of the abdomen is a better option than NCCT (noncontrast CT).

Computed tomography scans with oral contrast medium or rectal Gastrografin enema may help in the diagnosis of appendicitis.

- When patient scores 6 or <6 in Alvarado Scoring System.
- *Particularly useful in elderly patients as it rules out intestinal obstruction, neoplasm, and diverticulitis, and diagnoses acute appendicitis in the absence of signs.*

Contrast-enhanced computed tomography reduces the chances of removal of a normal appendix.

Computed tomography scans can diagnose acute appendicitis in approximately 98% of cases, i.e., 92–97% sensitivity, 85–94% specificity, 90–98% accuracy, and 75–95% positive and 95–99% negative predictive values. A CT scan is good for patients who come late, after 48 hours, with appendicitis as a mass or abscess.

Indications of Computed Tomography Scan in Acute Appendicitis

- *Suspected case of acute appendicitis where the diagnosis is not confirmed by ultrasound and other investigations.*
- Appendicular abscess
- Pelvic abscess

Disadvantages of Computed Tomography Scan

- Expensive
- Radiation
- Cannot be used during pregnancy.
- Some patients may develop an allergy to the dye used in CECT.
- Some patients cannot take oral dye due to nausea and vomiting.
- Optimal CT technique requires complete small bowel opacification (CECT).

Advantages of Computed Tomography Scan

- A study by Rao and colleagues showed that CT scans have reduced the incidence of negative appendectomies from 20 to 7%, it is confirmed by others too.

- Decreased perforation rate from 22 to 14%.
- Established an alternative diagnosis in 50% of cases
- Saved unnecessary appendicectomies
- Saved inpatient hospital stay days
- Lowered per-patient costs by $ 447.

Improved image resolution to a 0.5–1.0 cm range which has improved the accuracy of CT scanning.

DIAGNOSTIC LAPAROSCOPY

Diagnostic laparoscopy is particularly helpful in obese patients and females of childbearing age to exclude acute gynecological pathology. It can help in 30–40% of negative appendicectomies, some surgeons routinely do diagnostic laparoscopy in all ovulating women with suspected acute appendicitis to avoid delay and negative appendicectomies.

It is useful in the following cases: Infants, elderly, and female patients.

SCORING SYSTEMS

Alvarado (MANTRELS) Scoring System

It is a system developed to diagnose acute appendicitis more precisely to avoid negative appendicectomies **(Table 2)**.

Alfredo Alvarado, Contemporary Surgeon, Plantation, FL, USA, gave this scoring system, which is most widely used globally. A score of 7 or more is strongly indicative of acute appendicitis. Score <5: Not sure of diagnosis of acute appendicitis, *score 5–6:* Compatible with acute appendicitis, *score 7–9:* Probably acute appendicitis, *score 10:* Confirmed acute appendicitis, if score is 7 or more, admit the patient for urgent appendicectomy, if score is 5–6, further investigations are required to reach to a diagnosis. Any patient with a score of <6 cannot have a perforated appendix.

TABLE 2: Alvarado (MANTRELS) scoring system.

Features	*Score*	
Symptoms	Migrating RIF pain	1
Anorexia	1	
Nausea, vomiting	1	
Signs	Tenderness RIF	2
Rebound tenderness	1	
Elevated temperature	1	
Laboratory	Leukocytosis ($>10 \times 1{,}000$ cells/mm^3)	2
Shift to the left (segmental neutrophils) (>75%)	1	
Total	10	

Raja Isteri Pengiran Anak Saleha Appendicitis Scoring System

It is similar to the Alvarado scoring system. It typically provides a quantitative value for a clinician's clinical score for appendicitis.

Nigam's Scoring System

It is invented to deal with the drawbacks of the Alvarado scoring system and improve accuracy. Nigam's scoring system (NSS) has 17 scoring points. This scoring system can be divided into three parts, 6 and below 6, 7–10, and 11 and above. If NSS comes to 6 or below, probably we are not dealing with acute appendicitis. If the score is between 7 and 10 probably diagnosis of appendicitis cannot be ruled out. If the score is 11 or more, we are dealing with a case of appendicitis. The higher the score after 11, severe is the inflammation, from acute appendicitis to impending perforation or gangrene. The scoring by NSS decides about the management of the case also. Patients with scores <6 are advised outpatient department (OPD) treatment. Patients with scores 7–10 are admitted to the hospital for observation and scores 11 or above are operated. The diagnosis of acute appendicitis by NSS was compared with the ultrasonography findings, operation findings, and histopathological results.

We have to confirm the diagnosis of acute appendicitis before doing an appendectomy otherwise there is a chance of a negative appendectomy. NSS confirmed the diagnosis of acute appendicitis in all cases before appendectomy. The diagnosis was based on NSS which was compatible to the operative and histopathological findings in all cases. There was not a single case of negative appendectomy among 34 operated cases. The negative appendectomy rate was zero. Out of 34 patients diagnosed as appendicitis by NSS all patients underwent appendectomy, and appendicitis was confirmed in all cases by operative and histopathological findings. Four patients had perforation and these all patients had leukocytosis above 15,000 and tenderness in RIF was severe. Nigam's scoring system has better accuracy than Alvarado's scoring system in diagnosing acute appendicitis [*Source*: Nigam VK, Nigam S. Nigam's scoring system for acute appendicitis with high accuracy surpassing Alvarado scoring system. Int Surg J. 2022;9(4):835-40]. NSS is an easy, economical, simple, accurate, fast, and dependable scoring system. NSS is best suited for small hospitals that lack advanced investigative techniques such as ultrasound, CT scan, and magnetic resonance imaging (MRI).

NUCLEAR MEDICINE INVESTIGATIONS

Two types of nuclear imaging are done for appendicitis diagnosis:

1. Radiolabeled WBCs (Tc-99m WBC)
2. Immunoglobulin G (Tc-99m Igl)

The localization of Tc-99 labeled WBCs, and Igl is done with the use of scintigraphy. Their value lies only in cases with negative ultrasound and CT scans.

These are highly sensitive and highly specific, but the procedure is time-consuming and not widely available, and not useful in emergency conditions.

VAGINAL EXAMINATION

Look for tenderness in the movement of the cervix if present then appendicitis is less likely, young women about the age of 20 years have the highest incidence of a normal appendix on operation and persistence of symptoms thereafter.

URINARY 5-HYDROXYINDOLEACETIC ACID

Few studies have shown the estimation of *urinary 5-hydroxyindoleacetic acid (U5-HIAA)* can be of help in the diagnosis of acute appendicitis due to the presence of a large amount of serotonin-secreting cells in an appendix. The level of U5-HIAA increases with the development of acute appendicitis and reduces with the development of gangrene or necrosis.

DIAGNOSIS OF ACUTE APPENDICITIS

One has to diagnose acute appendicitis in case of acute abdomen by excluding other causes.

Common causes of RIF pain:
- Acute gastroenteritis
- Mesenteric lymphadenitis
- Right ureteric colic
- Ruptured ovarian follicle (Mittelschmerz)
- Acute salpingitis
- Ruptured ectopic pregnancy
- Torsion of an ovarian cyst
- Meckel's diverticulitis
- Regional ileitis (Crohn's disease)
- Acute pyelonephritis
- Perforated duodenal ulcer (DU)
- Acute cholecystitis
- Acute pancreatitis
- Acute intestinal obstruction

PROBLEMS OF ACUTE APPENDICITIS AT DIFFERENT AGES AND STAGES

In Infancy and Childhood

Acute appendicitis is usually underdiagnosed. Tere are some special problems with younger age.

- *Appendicitis is seen in neonates associated with aganglionosis and neonatal necrotizing enterocolitis.*
- Infants and children are more sensitive to examination, so it is not easy to do a proper examination. Children <5 years of age have a negative appendicectomy rate of 25% and a perforation rate of 45%, whereas children >5 years of age have rates of negative appendectomy and perforation of 10 and 20%, respectively.
- *Most infants and children are uncooperative due to apprehension.*
- Infants, especially, cannot complain correctly.
- *The clinician has to win the confidence of the infant and child before proceeding for the examination.*

Differences between the appendix of the child and adult:
- Size of the appendix.
- Thickness of appendicular walls.
- Cecoappendicular junction Appendix in children is larger than in adults as compared to the size of the body and the gastro-intestinal tract (GIT). The coats of the walls of the appendix are more delicate than in adults. Cecoappendicular junction is often funnel-shaped when the cecum and appendix are in the same line. Valves at the cecal junction of the appendix do not close as in adults; this makes fecal contents easier to enter into the lumen of the appendix and renders its expulsion also easy.

- The omentum is not well developed in infants and children. Omentum is like a "Bib" in children but an "Apron" in adults. So appendicular lump does not develop and perforation occurs earlier.
- Eliciting tenderness in infants and children is not an easy task, and you cannot do without it also. So, palpate the abdomen of a child with your own hand. The child will try not to touch the tender area, or he will pull his hand.
- Constitutional disturbances are more common in children.

- Temperature and pulse are high.
- Tere is a complete dislike for the food.
- There is diarrhea and vomiting instead of constipation, so it mimics acute gastroenteritis, and this is the main confusing factor in the diagnosis of acute appendicitis at this age.
- "Hunger Sign" if the child is being hungry, then for sure he is not suffering from acute appendicitis (AA).
- In the early stage, the bowel sounds may be absent.
- Appendicular lump is rarely seen due to short omentum and poor inflammatory response.
- Early perforation is quite common in children, so diagnosis at a very early stage is essential to avoid perforation. Diagnosis is often delayed in children and infants.
- Vomiting is a common feature of appendicitis in children. It is rare to find acute appendicitis in children without vomiting.
- Approximately, there are 80% chances of perforation with 50% mortality in infancy when acute appendicitis develops.
- The child should be asked to stand on their right leg and hip. If he can probably, he does not have acute appendicitis.

Perforation of the appendix occurs so frequently in children that one has to follow the rule that "Every child having RIF pain with diarrhea and vomiting should be suspected as suffering with acute appendicitis unless proven otherwise."

In children, worms such as pinworms and roundworms have been considered one of the etiological factors. Sometimes deworming relieves from mild appendicitis symptoms.

The mortality in infants and children due to acute appendicitis is higher than in adults. It is due to:

- The omentum is underdeveloped, so it cannot reach RIF and so cannot seal and limit or wall off the infection.
    - Difficulty in diagnosis due to its resemblance to enteritis.
    - Diagnostic laparoscopy is of great help for children as laparoscopy is an effective form of treatment in children.

Trauma

Blows, falls, and exertions in children occur due to running and playing and can also be considered as one of the etiological factors of appendicitis. Rectal examination in children must not be omitted. The adult finger is longer for a child's rectum, and this can reach high in the pelvis, avoiding not finding pelvic appendicitis.

Acute Appendicitis in Old Age

There are some special situations in old age due to acute appendicitis in old age has become a serious problem.

- A total of 5–10% of cases of acute appendicitis occur in old age, lower than in younger patients, but the morbidity and mortality are higher due to more rapid progression to perforation. In patients older than 80 years of age, perforation rates of 49% and mortality rates of 21% have been reported, and some workers have reported perforation as high as 50%.
- The clinical signs are not well marked at this age.
- The abdomen is lax due to muscle wasting or weakness, so the muscle guard or rigidity is not prominent.
- Tere is atherosclerosis in an appendicular artery at this age and is responsible for the rapid development of gangrene and perforation.
- The distension of the abdomen, lack of rigidity, vomiting, and constipation make the picture mimic acute intestinal obstruction. Sometimes this may lead to the introduction of an enema, which can perforate the appendix in acute appendicitis.
- Recently, it has been observed that the incidence of acute appendicitis is decreasing in young adults and increasing in older age in spite of recent advances in imaging and laparoscopy.
- Mortality rate in old age >65 years of age is 4.6%.
- Gangrene and perforation occur more frequently in old age due to poor vascularity.
- *Mortality is high due to:*
    - Early gangrene and perforation.
    - Delayed diagnosis
    - Associated old age medical diseases

Acute Appendicitis in Pregnancy

- Acute appendicitis is the most common extra-uterine disease requiring operation during pregnancy; the incidence is one in 2,000 pregnancies.
- Acute appendicitis occurs most commonly in the first and second trimesters.
- In normal pregnancy, TLC may be between 15,000 and 20,000, and in acute appendicitis, it can go higher; in 10% of cases, it may be normal.
- There is a chance of abortion if appendicectomy is done, but one has to weigh the risk.
- Mortality increases considerably by appendicectomy in the third trimester.
- In the first trimester, the nausea and vomiting of appendicitis is taken wrongly as morning sickness,

which delays the diagnosis and treatment, but nausea and vomiting after the first trimester must raise doubt of acute appendicitis.

- Rebound tenderness and muscle guarding are less marked due to a lax abdomen.
- Marked leukocytosis and ultrasonography may help to reach the diagnosis.
- Mortality in both mother and fetus increases with trimester and delay in diagnosis. In third-trimester fetuses, the mortality rate is 20%, whereas the maternal mortality rate is 9%. RB Parker was of the view that after 6 months, the mortality is 20%—10 times greater than in the first 3 months.
- Laparoscopic surgery becomes technically difficult after 26 weeks of pregnancy.
- Appendicectomy is the treatment of choice in all trimesters of pregnancy as soon as it is diagnosed.
- The enlarged uterus causes upward displacement of the cecum and appendix during the second and third trimesters of pregnancy, which may cause confusion in diagnosing appendicitis with acute cholecystitis.
- Visceral and parietal peritoneum are separated due to an enlarged uterus, so the somatic component of pain decreases.
- Sometimes necrobiosis of uterine fibroids or concealed accidental hemorrhage may cause similar pain as that of acute appendicitis.
- Careful history and positive Rovsing sign help to diagnose acute appendicitis.
- Put the patient in a supine position and mark the most tender spot with a marker, and then put the patient in the left lateral position. In acute appendicitis, the maximum tender spot will not shift, but in a uterine pathology, it will shift.
- Pyelitis, pyelonephritis, and cystitis are common during pregnancy. Pyelitis or pyelonephritis may mimic acute appendicitis. So, one should keep in mind these conditions during pregnancy.
- Appendicectomy during pregnancy carries a 10–15% risk of premature labor, and it increases to 30% in the presence of perforation.
- Intrauterine fetal death occurs in 3–5% of cases of acute appendicitis and 35% in perforation of the gangrenous appendix.
- Acute appendicitis is evenly distributed among all trimesters, but the maximum incidence of perforation occurs during the third trimester.

Appendicitis in Young Females

A lot of gynecological problems mimic acute appendicitis, so every young female going for appendicectomy must undergo gynecological examination by a gynecologist and lower abdominal, pelvic, and endovaginal ultrasound to avoid negative appendicectomies.

STUMP APPENDICITIS

It is defined as "appendicitis in the remaining appendicular stump after appendectomy." Surgeons must also remember that a previous appendectomy does not definitely exclude the diagnosis of appendicitis, as 'stump appendicitis,' although rare but has been described. RLQ tenderness is always present.

DIFFERENTIAL DIAGNOSIS OF ACUTE APPENDICITIS

Different diagnosis is a process of differentiating between the conditions that show similar signs and symptoms, so mimic the real disease. The process is based on symptoms, science, laboratory results, history, and physical examination. The aim of *differential diagnosis (DDX)* is to arrive at the correct diagnosis by excluding other provisional diagnoses. Similarly, acute appendicitis is diagnosed in a suspected case.

Meckel's Diverticulitis

- Johann Friedrich Meckel* described the diverticulum in 1809.
- Clinically it cannot be differentiated from acute appendicitis.
- Sometimes pain in Meckel's diverticulitis is more central or to the left than in acute appendicitis.
- *Tere may be intermittent lower gastrointestinal bleeding.*

Johann Friedrich Meckel (1781–1833), Professor of Anatomy and Surgery, Halle, Germany* **(Fig. 17).

Rule of 2 of Meckel's diverticulum

Meckel's diverticulum occurs in 2% children at the age of 2 years, it usually measures 2 inches in size, it arises at about 2 feet distance from ileocecal junction, can have two types of tissues, i.e., gastric and pancreatic, and it has a gender ratio of 1:2 in females and males.

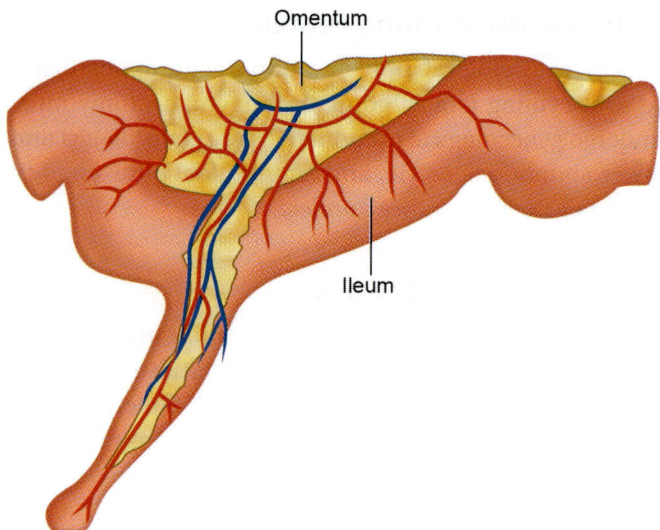

Fig. 17: Meckel's diverticulitis.

IN CHILDREN

Acute Mesenteric Lymphadenitis

- It is the most commonly confused disease with acute appendicitis in children.
- Recent history of upper respiratory tract infection is present.
- The pain is colicky in nature, and lasts for a few minutes.
- Vomiting is less marked than in acute appendicitis.
- Cervical lymph nodes may be enlarged.
- Shifting tenderness may be present if the child is placed in a left lateral position.
- True muscle rigidity is rare.
- Relative lymphocytosis may be present.
- It is a self-limiting disease.
- If the diagnosis is in doubt, then urgent exploration is the safest action.

Acute Gastroenteritis

- It usually presents as intestinal colic with vomiting and diarrhea.
- Tenderness is less localized and even may be no tenderness at all.
- Other members of the family are also affected at the same time.
- Laboratory values may be normal.
- In viral gastroenteritis stool is watery and profuse.
- In typhoid fever diagnosis is made by prostration, maculopapular rash, leukopenia, and culture of *Salmonella typhi* from stool and blood, 1% of patients develop terminal ileum perforation requiring urgent surgical interference.

Intussusception

Intussusception is most common at the age of 18 months, whereas acute appendicitis is rare before the age of 2 years.

A sausage-shaped lump is palpable in the lower abdomen, usually in the right side, and the RLQ feels empty.

- It occurs in well-nourished children.
- Colicky pain occurs, and the child doubles up, but in between colics, the child appears well.
- After several hours of pain, stool mixed with mucus and blood is passed.

> *If the intussusceptions is large as the bowel enters the distal bowel, it can be seen or felt at the anus. Rectal examination may find a polyp-like mass in the rectum.* So, the rectal examination in acute abdomen in children must not be omitted. In intussusceptions, the invagination may be partial or complete or the appendix with cecum can invaginate into the colon.

Henoch–Schönlein Purpura

- Henoch described this form of purpura in 1886. Johann Lukas Schönlein described this form of purpura in 1837.
- Preceded by sore throat or respiratory infection.
- Abdominal pain can be very severe.
- Ecchymotic rash on external surfaces of limbs and buttocks.
- Microscopic hematuria is common.
- Platelet count and bleeding time are normal.
- Joint pain and nephritis may be present.

Lobar Pneumonia

- Pain of pleurisy and lobar pneumonia at the right base may mimic acute appendicitis pain.
- There is minimal or absent abdominal tenderness and muscle guarding.
- Pleural friction—rub or altered breath sounds are present.
- Tere is marked pyrexia.
- X-ray of the chest is diagnostic.

---

*Eduard Heinrich Henoch (1820–1910), Professor of Diseases of Children, Berlin, Germany.

**Johann Lucas Schönlein (1793–1864), Physician, Charity Hospital, Berlin, Germany.

IN ADULT MALE

Ureteric Colic

- If a stone is lodged in the ureter near the site of the appendix it mimics acute appendicitis.
- Pain radiates from the loin to the groin.
- Cough test is negative but positive in acute appendicitis.
- Urine examination will reveal red blood cells (RBCs).
- Ultrasound, CT scan, and intravenous urography (IVU) are diagnostic.

Regional Enteritis (Regional Ileitis or Crohn's Disease)

- History of abdominal cramps, diarrhea, and weight loss.
- Doughy, vague, tender lump in RIF with fever, RLQ pain, and leukocytosis is present.
- The mesenteric lymph node may be palpable.
- Small bowel enema will show the "string sign of Kantor."
- Pain is very severe, much more than what happens in acute appendicitis.

Torsion of Testis

- Torsion of the undescended testis causes similar pain, but the scrotum is found empty.
- Usually occurs in a young adult male.
- Scrotal examination is diagnostic.
- Color Doppler or an ultrasound of the scrotum will confirm the diagnosis.

Acute Pancreatitis

- Epigastric pain that radiates to the back by penetrating directly to the back.
- Referred pain of acute appendicitis in the epigastrium is of much less severity.
- A high level of serum amylase, >1,000 IU, is diagnostic of acute pancreatitis.
- History of alcohol intake or gallbladder disease is present.

Rectus Sheath Hematoma

- It is due to rupture of the inferior epigastric artery, usually after a violent attack of cough or strenuous exercise.
- It is a rare entity.
- Acute pain and tenderness in RIF after an episode of strenuous physical exercise.
- Localized pain without gastrointestinal upset is the rule.
- Elderly patients on anticoagulant therapy may get it after minor and trivial trauma.

Right-sided Acute Pyelonephritis

- There is an increased frequency of micturition
- The tenderness in the loin is accompanied by fever, rigors, bacteriuria, and pyuria.

It is difficult to differentiate between acute pyelonephritis and acute appendicitis during pregnancy as the appendix is lifted up by the uterus and comes at the level of the kidney.

Amebic Typhlitis

- It is characterized by diarrhea and blood-mixed mucus.
- There is tenderness at the "Manson–Bahr amebic point" in LIF, Sir Philip Manson Bahr gave this point corresponding to McBurney's point in LIF. In amebiasis, there are two tender spots, one over the cecum at McBurney's point in RIF and the other over the sigmoid colon over Manson Bahr* point in LIF.

Valentino Appendix

It is also called Valentino syndrome or Valentino appendicitis. In a perforated duodenal ulcer, the contents and bile from the ulcer hole pass down through the right paracolic gutter in RIF, causing local peritonitis and hyperemia of the appendix, resembling appendicitis. Clinical features resemble acute appendicitis, as happened in this case. It is named after a famous film director, Rudolph Valentino, who suffered like this. In 1926, Valentino collapsed in a New York City hotel and underwent surgery for presumed appendicitis at New York Polytechnic Hospital. At the time, he was found to have a perforated ulcer. Postoperatively, he developed peritonitis, multiple organ system dysfunctions, and died several days later (Valentino loses battle with death: Greatest of screen lovers fought valiantly for life.

Yersinia Ileitis (Pseudoappendicitis)

- About 6% of cases of acute mesenteric lymphadenitis and 5% of cases of acute appendicitis are caused by *Yersinia* infection.

---

*Sir Philip Henry Manson-Bahr (1881-1966), English Zoologist and Physician.

- It is a condition that mimics acute appendicitis. It is caused by the *Yersinia pseudotuberculosis* organism. The terminal ileum looks red, edematous, and inflamed.
- It subsides by itself.
- It does not require any treatment.

IN ADULT FEMALE

Inflammatory diseases of the right uterine adnexa more frequently mimic appendicitis than other parts. Some genital tract ailments in a female of childbearing age mimic acute appendicitis. A careful history of menstrual cycle, vaginal discharge, and pregnancy may help to reach to diagnosis.

After the expulsion of the fetus uterus suddenly contracts, and it can cause the rupture of appendicular or periappendicular abscess, leading to a grave situation.

Mittelschmerz

The typical midcycle lower abdominal or pelvic pain is indicative of Mittelschmerz. It is the rupture of a midcycle follicular cyst with bleeding. Mittelschmerz's name is given to this condition as pain occurs at the midpoint of the menstrual cycle.

- Usually, no GIT symptoms.
- Patient is not looking sick or toxic.
- Pregnancy test is negative.
- Usually not many signs are present.
- Leukocytosis and fever are absent or minimal.
- Diagnostic laparoscopy may be required.

Pelvic Inflammatory Disease

It is a common condition and includes the following conditions:

- Salpingitis
- Endometriosis
- Tubo-ovarian sepsis
- Every young female should be suspected of pelvic inflammatory disease (PID) in lower abdominal pain. It is very common.
- History of purulent vaginal discharge, dysmenorrhea, and burning pain during micturition are important features.
- Anorexia, nausea, and vomiting are absent.
- Pain is felt on both sides and lower than in appendicitis.
- The pain is typically bilateral.
- Pain starts within 7 days of menstruation and stays for >2 days.
- On vaginal examination the cervical and bilateral adnexa are found tender.
- Transvaginal ultrasound is of help in reaching to diagnosis.
- Diagnostic laparoscopy may be of help to diagnose it in difficult situations.
- Thorough examination and keeping in mind PID can 15% reduce negative appendectomies.

Pyelonephritis

- Patients of pyelonephritis have a dull pain in the lumbar region.
- Patients usually have high fever associated with rigors.

Ectopic Pregnancy

When a fertilized egg implants outside the uterus, most commonly it happens in fallopian tube.

Torsion of an Ovarian Cyst

- Torsion or hemorrhage in ovarian cysts may cause sudden severe pain in the abdomen.
- May be low-grade fever with vomiting present.
- A mass is felt on RIF if the cyst is big.
- Pelvic ultrasound and CT scan are diagnostic.

Endometriosis

Endometriosis in RQL can mimic AA as the endometrial tissue can get deposited over the right ovary, right fallopian tube, and the appendix.

Gallstone Colic

Gallstone colic can mimic acute appendicitis, but the pain will be located in or near the right hypochondrium and may radiate to the back, whereas the acute appendicitis pain is in the RIF.

IN ELDERLY

Appendix in old age progressively atrophies.

Diverticulitis

Diverticulitis develops due to inflammation of a colonic diverticulum. A CT scan is a diagnostic investigation for diverticulitis.

Acute Intestinal Obstruction

- Acute appendicitis is uncommon in the elderly, and intestinal obstruction is common.

- The diagnosis of intestinal obstruction is easy, as an X-ray abdomen and an ultrasound are diagnostic.
- Early decision for surgery is important.

Carcinoma of Colon

Acute appendicitis can be a sign of cancer of the colon, as the growth may obstruct the lumen of the appendix.

Torsion of Appendix Epiploica or Epiploic Appendicitis

It is an infarction of the appendix epiploica due to its torsion. Appendices epiploicae are small peritoneal sacs filled with fat and are attached to the colon. Pain may be mild or severe and last for a few days.

- The site of pain is the colon area.
- There is no anorexia, sequence of symptoms, and shifting pain of appendicitis.
- The patient does not look ill.
- Nausea and vomiting are uncommon.
- Recurrence of pain occurs.
- Local signs of tenderness and rebound tenderness are present.

Mesenteric Infraction

It causes interruption of the blood supply to varying portions of the small intestine. Mortality is approximately 50%. Early diagnosis and surgical treatment are of utmost importance. In a case where *acute mesenteric ischemia (AMI) is suspected, urgent computed tomography angiography (CTA)* should be performed.

Leaking Aortic Aneurysm

It causes sudden and severe pain in the abdomen, and 80% of patients die before reaching hospital.

RARE DIFFERENTIAL DIAGNOSIS

Amebic Typhlitis

Amebic typhlitis can present as appendicitis, as it is the inflammation of the cecum, which harbors the appendix.

Spinal Conditions

- Tuberculosis of the spine or Pott's spine is a common condition. It causes nerve root compression, which may appear as appendicitis pain if T10 or T11 are affected.
- Lumbar spine rigidity may be present.
- Movement aggravates pain.
- No intestinal symptoms

Preherpetic Pain

- Preherpetic pain especially of 10th and 11th dorsal nerves, which occurs over the same area of appendicitis.
- Tere is marked hyperesthesia.
- Pain is not shifting.
- Tere is no muscle rigidity or guarding.
- A herpetic eruption will develop after a few hours.

Tabetic Crisis

It is rare nowadays.

Abdominal Crisis of Diabetes Mellitus

- History of diabetes mellitus
- No abdominal rigidity
- Abdominal crisis of porphyria
- Severe attacks of intestinal colic occur.
- Urine is of an orange color, which changes to a high color when exposed to sunlight.
- It is precipitated by barbiturates.

Leukemic Ileocecal Syndrome

- It is rare.
- It occurs in immunosuppressed patients.
- Gram-negative septicemia (*Clostridium septicum*) occurs.

Primary Peritonitis

It occurs in the following conditions:

- Nephrotic syndrome
- Cirrhosis
- Immunosuppression

It is diagnosed by peritoneal aspiration showing only gram-positive cocci.

Sigmoid Diverticulitis

- It has almost identical findings such as appendicitis on the left side, but if the sigmoid colon loop is big and lies right to the midline, then it becomes clinically impossible to differentiate acute sigmoid diverticulitis from acute appendicitis.
- A CT scan of the abdomen is of value to differentiate acute sigmoid diverticulitis from acute appendicitis.
- Ultrasound is not of much value.

Carcinoma of the Cecum

- Sometimes carcinoma of the cecum may mimic acute appendicitis, especially when it is perforated.
- History of change of bowel habits and anemia with a palpable mass is diagnostic of carcinoma of the cecum.
- Contrast CT scan is an important diagnostic tool.

COMPLICATIONS OF APPENDICITIS

In 1886, Fitz reported the associated mortality rate of appendicitis to be 67% without surgical therapy. Currently, the mortality rate of acute appendicitis is reported to be <1%. Elderly patients have a higher rate of complications.

Complications of Appendicitis

- Perforation of the appendix
- General peritonitis
- Appendicular abscess
- Appendicular lump or mass
- Septicemia
- Portal pyemia
- Infertility
- Recurrent appendicitis
- Obliteration of the appendix
- Intestinal obstruction
- Appendicular cysts
- Vascular infections as complications of appendicitis

PERFORATION OF APPENDIX

Urgent appendicectomy is the treatment of choice for acute appendicitis, which prevents the risk of perforation. The average rate of perforation of the appendix in acute appendicitis is 25.8%. Children younger than 5 years and patients older than 65 years have the highest rate of perforation (45% and 51%, respectively). Nonoperative treatment exposes the patient to perforation.

Perforation usually occurs due to increased intraluminal pressure, which occurs in obstructive appendicitis. Patients having nonobstructive appendicitis rarely get perforation, if at all, and it is usually late. Perforation is uncommon within the first 12 hours.

The accuracy in diagnosing acute appendicitis does not change the rate of perforation. Surprisingly, the diagnosis accuracy diminishes, but the appendicectomy rate increases. Usually, a perforated appendix is brought from home, it is rare to happen in admitted hospital patients. Hospital-admitted patients can be diagnosed after some time if he/she is not diagnosed early.

Overall, about 20% of all patients with acute appendicitis have perforation at the time of operation. At the extremes of age (<5 years and >60 years) the rate of perforation is in the region of 60%.

Promoting factors of general peritonitis due to perforation of the appendix are:

- Extremes of age—too young or too aged.
- Diabetes mellitus
- Poor nutritional state of the patient
- Other debilitating conditions
- Immunosuppression
- Previous abdominal surgery—which reduces the ability of the greater omentum to wall off the infection.
- Pelvic appendix—it hangs freely in the pelvis without protection.
- Obstruction of the appendix lumen, e.g., finding a fecalith in the lumen of an appendix on exploratory laparotomy for any other reason, is an indication of appendicectomy to prevent future acute appendicitis and generalized peritonitis.

When to Suspect Perforation?

Perforation of the appendix in a case of acute appendicitis should be suspected in the following conditions:

- Fever higher than 102°F
- WBC count >18,000/mm^3
- Sudden increase of pain in RIF with localized rebound tenderness
- Generalized peritonitis

When to Suspect General Peritonitis?

When perforation of the appendix leads to general peritonitis, you will find:

- Patient looks toxic
- Tenderness all over the abdomen
- Initial board-like rigidity of the abdomen, later distension of the abdomen
- Vomiting
- Absolute constipation
- High fever
- No bowel sounds, silent abdomen

Treatment

- *If it presents as a small abscess:* Incision and drainage is done extraperitoneally, and after a 6-week interval, appendicectomy is advised.

- *If generalized peritonitis is present:* Laparotomy is done. Appendicectomy is done if the appendix is easily accessible.
- *If the appendix is inaccessible:* If the appendix is found inaccessible and cannot be removed, then interval appendicectomy is recommended after 6 weeks.

GENERAL PERITONITIS

It develops after perforation of the appendix when the protective phenomenon of the body tries to seal it off from other parts of the peritoneal cavity by omentum and loops of the small bowel, but fails. The pain, fever, tenderness, and rigidity increase. At this stage or later, the abdomen should be opened, a midline or right paramedian incision. Peritoneal lavage with normal saline should be performed.

Some researchers believe that, as per exudate in the peritoneal cavity after perforation of the appendix following types of peritonitis can happen:

- Acute fibrinous peritonitis
- Acute serofibrinous peritonitis
- Acute fibrinopurulent peritonitis
- Acute purulent peritonitis
- Acute dry or septic peritonitis

APPENDICULAR ABSCESS

The first reported case of the appendicular abscess was reported in 1848 and operated by Henry Hancock, Surgeon, Charring Cross Hospital, London. There is a tender mass in RIF with high fever, which may be associated with chills. Ultrasound and CT scans are diagnostic.

Causes of Appendicular Abscess Open Surgical Repair

- Appendicular mass does not resolve with *open surgical repair (OSR)* and converts to an abscess.
- Acute appendicitis leads to abscess formation.

The appendicular abscess should be drained. If appendicectomy can easily be performed, do it; otherwise, do not do blind dissection. Interval appendicectomy is done after 6–8 weeks. Usually, the appendicular abscess develops from the appendicular mass, which fails to resolve.

Important features of appendicular abscess are:

- Hot and tender mass in RIF.
- High pyrexia with chills and rigors
- High TLC (>14,000)
- Increase the size of the appendicular mass
- Shift to the left, polymorphs increase
- Tachycardia

Subphrenic Abscess

It may occur between the diaphragm and liver which is the most common site for a subphrenic abscess. It may occur in one of the three following ways:

1. As a part of general systemic infection
2. As a localized abscess from general purulent appendicitis
3. Direct extension from infected appendix by lymphatics.

Subphrenic abscess may occur even after recovery from acute appendicitis.

Rupture of Appendicular Abscess

Appendicular abscess can rupture and can cause:

- *Fistulae between*:
  - Appendix and urinary bladder
  - Appendix and small bowel
  - Appendix and sigmoid colon
  - Appendix and rectum
- *Intraperitoneal residual abscesses*:
  - Pelvic abscess
  - In between coil of small bowel
  - Paracolic abscess
  - Subdiaphragmatic abscess
  - Subhepatic abscess

Resolution of Appendicular Abscess

Appendicular abscess can be resolute in the following ways:

- Resolution by rupture of an abscess—it produces tissue necrosis due to pressure and abscess walls give way at a point of least resistance.
- Resolution by absorption of its contents—it may be partial or complete. Sometimes only the liquid part of the abscess gets absorbed and the solid part forms a mass.

Role of Interval Appendicectomy after Appendicular Abscess

In most of cases of appendicular abscess, the appendix is destroyed by necrosis and gangrene so appendicectomy should be performed only if symptoms recur, otherwise you may not be able to find the appendix.

APPENDICULAR LUMP OR MASS (PHLEGMON)

Appendicular mass can develop in any case of acute appendicitis if appendectomy is not done. A total of 2–5% of patients with appendicitis present with a palpable mass in RLQ. Usually, appendicular mass develops on the third day from the start of the attack of acute appendicitis. When the infection goes beyond the wall of the appendix, or the appendix becomes gangrenous then small bowel loops and omentum come near the appendix and try to limit the spread of infection. The omentum that is why called the "policeman of the abdomen." It is nature's attempt to limit and prevent the spreading of infection causing generalized peritonitis. If an appendicular mass develops in a patient whose age is 50 years or above must go to CECT abdomen or barium enema and meal study after the resolution of the appendicular mass to rule out malignancy.

Constituents of Appendicular Lump

An appendicular lump consists of:

- Inflamed appendix in the center of the lump
- Cecum
- Loops of small bowel
- Omentum
- Maybe some pus, usually there is no pus. There is a tender lump in RIF. Usually, the appendicular mass resolves after conservative treatment. Appendicular mass is a tender, from well-circumscribed, localized mass, and smooth lump. It is nonmobile, does not move with respiration, and is resonant on percussion.

Mortality from Appendicitis

- Mortality from appendicitis is reducing. It was 9.9 deaths per 100,000 in 1939 and 0.2 per 100,000 in 1986.
- In ruptured appendix mortality increases up to 3%—a 50-fold increase, in the elderly it goes up to 15%.

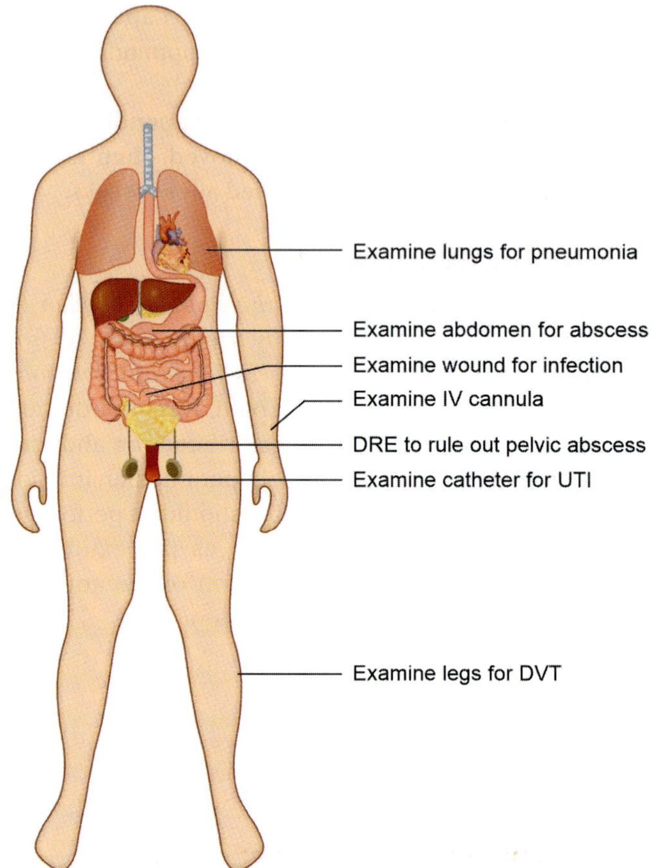

Fig. 18: Postappendectomy pyrexia. (DVT: deep vein thrombosis; IV: intravenous; UTI: urinary tract infection)

Postappendicectomy Pyrexia (Fig. 18)

What to look in postappendicectomy pyrexia?

- Wound for infection. Look for hyperemia, cellulitis, or pus discharge.
- Examine lungs for atelectasis or pneumonia.
- Examine legs to rule out deep vein thrombosis (DVT).
- DRE to rule out pelvic abscess.
- Keep in mind intraperitoneal abscess, i.e., "when pus is somewhere, pus is nowhere, and pus is under the diaphragm." Remember this saying so you will not forget to examine the extra RIF sites of pus collection: Extra RIF sites of pus are:
    - Subdiaphragmatic abscess
    - Subhepatic abscess
    - Paracolic abscess
    - Interloop small bowel abscess
    - Pelvic abscess
    - Abscess at an operative site
- See the IV cannula site for thrombophlebitis; change it every third day.
- Catheter for UTI. UTI is one of the main causes of postappendicectomy pyrexia as the organism colonizes here and causes inflammation.
- Examine eyes—for jaundice—as pyrexia may be due to hepatitis.
- Examine urine for pyelonephritis.
- In children, look for tonsils for tonsillitis and the ear for otitis media.

Causes of Mortality

- Uncontrolled sepsis, i.e., septicemia, peritonitis, and intraperitoneal abscess.
- Pulmonary embolism

Differential Diagnosis of Appendicular Mass

- Carcinoma of the cecum
- Ileocecal hyperplastic tuberculosis
- Crohn's disease
- Actinomycosis
- Ovarian carcinoma
- Ilial lymphadenitis
- Parametritis
- Amebic typhlitis
- Twisted ovarian cyst

Treatment

The regimen of treatment is called the "**Ochsner–Sherren regimen**."*

Principle of Ochsner–Sherren Regimen

The inflammatory process of acute appendicitis is localized. Appendicular mass formation is nature's protective phenomenon. The operative search for the appendix may prove difficult and dangerous due to edema of the cecum and surrounding tissue, a fecal fistula can develop. Ochsner–Sherren regimen is a preparation for operation and not a postponement of appendicectomy.

Ochsner–Sherren regimen:
- Bed rest
- Nil orally
- Nasogastric aspiration
- Observation chart for pulse/temperature/size of mass
  - Intravenous (IV) fluids
  - IV antibiotic

The OSR consists of:
- Bed rest
- The head end of the bed is kept 30° up.
- Patient is kept nil orally. Gradually, orally water started at 30 mL hourly, then 60 mL.
- First oral fluids are given, then gradually semisolids, and then solids are started in 3–4 days.
- Observation chart is maintained. Pulse and temperature recorded 4 hourly.
- Daily abdomen examined and reexamined.
  - The limits of the lump is marked with a skin marker to see whether the lump increases or decreases.
- Intake and output chart is maintained.
- Hourly nasogastric aspiration by Ryle's tube** is done. Aspirate is collected, measured, color noted, and shown to a surgeon.
- IV fluid intake record is kept.
- IV antibiotics—a third-generation cephalosporin and metronidazole are given, targeting aerobic, gram-negative, and anaerobic organisms.
- After 48 hours, clinical improvement should be seen.
- Oral hygiene is maintained by 8 hourly mouthwashes.
- Deterioration in condition after 48 hours indicates the development of peritonitis.
- If a patient has not passed stool for 4–5 days, then a glycerin suppository is given.
- Desire for food occurs on the fourth to fifth day, which is a good sign.
- Usually an appendicular mass takes 2–6 weeks to resolve.

Contraindications of Ochsner–Sherren Regimen

- When one cannot make a definite diagnosis between acute appendicitis and any other cause of acute abdomen which needs urgent operation, e.g., rupture of ectopic gestation.
- Infection is still limited to the appendix and appendicectomy can be done.
- When the patient is an infant or child, perforation occurs early.
- If a patient is >60 years of age when perforation and peritonitis occur without much sign.

Fate of Appendicular Lump

- Resolution
- Appendicular abscess

In 9–15% of cases of appendicular lump, OSR fails, requiring operative intervention. Percutaneous or operative drainage of the abscess is not considered a failure. 40% of patients require appendicectomy before the planned time of interval appendicectomy, 6–10 weeks.

*Albert John Ochsner, Surgeon (1896-1981), and James Sherren, Physician.

** John Alfred Ryle (1889–1950), Professor of Physics at the University of Cambridge and Professor of Social Medicine at the University of Oxford, England; developed Ryle's tube in 1921.

Future Plan

Interval appendicectomy is advised after complete resolution of the appendicular mass. The full resolution of appendicular mass takes 6–8 weeks. So, interval appendicectomy should be done after 6–8 weeks.

How do You Assess Improvement by the Ochsner–Sherren Regimen?

- Pain is diminishing and localizing.
- The size of the lump is reducing.
- Temperature is becoming normal
- Pulse rate returning to normal
- No vomiting and nasogastric aspiration is reducing in quantity. The patient is discharged only when he/she is taking a normal diet and passing normal stools.

When to Stop Ochsner–Sherren Regimen?

- Rising pulse rate
- Increasing and spreading abdominal pain
- Increase in size of the appendicular mass
- Increase in nasogastric aspiration amount or vomiting
- Diarrhea with infection, mucus in stool: This shows that the patient is not getting controlled by nature and treatment anymore, and peritonitis is setting in, so urgent operation is required.

SEPTICEMIA

It can occur at any stage of acute appendicitis but is commonly seen in perforation and peritonitis.

PORTAL PYEMIA OR SUPPURATIVE PYLEPHLEBITIS AND PYEMIC ABSCESSES

Pus emboli from suppurative appendicitis enter tributaries of the mesenteric vein and reach the liver, causing multiple abscesses. These are caused by *E. coli* present with high fever and jaundice. Now it is not commonly seen due to good antibiotics.

- Portal pyemia is a rare entity now. It is a form of septic portal system thrombosis and causes septicemia, which is a dangerous entity, and that is why it carries a poor prognosis. It is common in immunosuppressed patients.
- Portal pyemia causes a tender and enlarged liver with jaundice.
- It is treated by IV fluids and antibiotics.

Abscess can also develop due to portal pyemia in the kidneys, lungs, brain, spleen, etc. Pyrexia is accompanied with chills, rigors, fever, and excessive sweating. Fever is intermittent with periods of pyrexia. It may even run for months.

INFERTILITY

In a young girl perforated appendix can cause a frozen pelvis, due to extensive chronic inflammation in the pelvis, leading to infertility.

OBLITERATION OF THE APPENDIX

An obliterated appendix appears as thick and rigid, or it may become a thin fibrous strand or band. The whole appendix may be obliterated or only the tip gets affected, resulting in a clubbed appearance. If the middle of the appendix is affected and atrophies, then the appendix appears as a dumbbell. The color of the appendix becomes pale in the obliteration of the appendix, but if only the tip is involved, then the rest of the appendix is pink as a normal appendix. On cross-section, the appendicular wall consists only of two layers, the outer muscular layer and the inner or central layer of fibrous tissue.

INTESTINAL OBSTRUCTION

Usually, intestinal obstruction develops as a late complication of acute appendicitis. It develops when a patient recovers fully from an attack of acute appendicitis, it may also develop in the course of chronic appendicitis. The cause of intestinal obstruction is usually bands, or sharp flexures and adhesions developed due to an earlier attack.

APPENDICULAR CYSTS

Retention cysts of the appendix are produced in appendicitis if a portion of the lumen of the appendix distal to the obstruction remains patent, the normal secretion is accumulated, and a retention cyst develops. Sometimes the appendicular luminal tube is occluded at more than one site, and then multiple cysts develop. Usually, the contents of the retention cysts are clear.

VASCULAR INFECTIONS AS A COMPLICATION OF APPENDICITIS

Infection can spread far by circulation from the infected appendix and can cause the following complications:

- Thrombotic and embolic processes
- Erosion hemorrhage can occur in the stomach and intestine in acute appendicitis.

- Gangrene by embolus blocking an artery.
- Lymphatic spread can lead to subphrenic abscess or lymphadenitis.

TREATMENT OF ACUTE APPENDICITIS

General Principles

The goal of the treatment of acute appendicitis is threefold:

- Early diagnosis
- Urgent appendicectomy
- Prevention of complications

Urgent appendicectomy is the golden rule—it is done by open, conventional, or by laparoscopic method.

The aim of doing an appendicectomy is to prevent the complications of appendicitis, so there should not be a delay in removing the inflamed appendix.

On the other hand, the normal appendix should not be removed unnecessarily. Early diagnosis and early appendicectomy reduce the incidence of complications, morbidity, and mortality.

The discomfort and risk associated with the operation of appendicitis cannot be compared with the discomfort and risk (morbidity and mortality) associated with perforation of the appendix and peritonitis.

Appendicectomy is the treatment of choice for acute appendicitis.

Appendicectomy can be performed by two methods.

1. Open or conventional appendicectomy
2. Laparoscopic appendicectomy

PROGNOSIS OF ACUTE APPENDICITIS

- If appendicectomy is done properly and early, then recovery is fast, and the patient goes home without any long-term effects.
- The mortality in uncomplicated cases of acute appendicitis is <0.1%.
- The mortality in a perforated appendix with peritonitis is <1%.
- The mortality in perforated appendix in elderly patients is up to 15–20%.
- *The mortality rate of the acute appendix is nowadays falling due to:*
    - Early diagnosis
    - Early appendicectomy when the infection is limited to the appendix.
    - Increasing awareness of the public.

SOME GOLDEN RULES IN ACUTE APPENDICITIS

- Rectal examination must be done in every patient with RIF pain.
- Gynecological examination is necessary for every child-bearing age female, especially 13–25 years suffering with RIF pain.
- There is no harm in removing a normal appendix, but there is big harm in not removing an inflamed appendix.
- Always examine external genitals in a young male with RIF pain.
- Take a decision immediately and not to postpone it for the next morning as hours matter in acute appendicitis, not days.
- When you go for a ward round, always examine the pulse of the patient yourself.

SOME IMPORTANT AND PRACTICAL HINTS TO THE BEGINNERS

- Do not rely solely on laboratory investigations, e.g., TLC and urine examination, which can be normal.
- If you cannot diagnose for sure and have doubts, then do not commit but reexamine the patient.
- The laparoscopy may be helpful in both diagnosis and treatment.
- Ultrasound of the abdomen cannot diagnose 100% in an early stage of acute appendicitis and it may be deceptive. So, depends more upon signs and symptoms than on ultrasound. A normal ultrasound is not a contraindication for appendicectomy.
- Localized abscess can be aspirated by CT-guided process under local anesthesia, which reduces the morbidity.
- Do not try medical therapy, e.g., antibiotics, once you have made the diagnosis of appendicitis; always advise urgent appendicectomy.
- With laparoscopy, several time-honored rituals have been proven unnecessary.
- Josef E Fischer, Editor of Master of Surgery, says, "We currently do not oversee the appendiceal stump or cauterize the mucosa after using a stapler."
- If you cannot decide, call some more experienced surgeon; remember your timely decision can prevent your patient's morbidity and mortality.
- Various studies have shown that during pregnancy, laparoscopic appendectomy can be done with a low

incidence of fetal loss. But it should be done with caution. An open approach should be used after the first trimester.

SOLUTION

- Incision should not be >3 cm medial to ASIS.
- Give more importance to the situation of the appendix than cosmetic reasons.
- Do not hesitate to enlarge the incision if you require more space.
- Do not hesitate to open the rectus sheath medially if you feel the space is less and a lot of retraction is required. The junction of the internal oblique muscle and rectus sheath is the thinnest part, so incise here.
- The best way to gain more space is to enlarge the incision by cutting deep muscles in the line of skin incision and converting a muscle splitting to muscle cutting, incision, and catching the bleeders.

OTHER CONDITIONS OF APPENDIX

- Mucocele of the appendix.
- Pyocele of the appendix or empyema of the appendix.
- Intussusception of appendix.
- Diverticulum of the appendix.
- Cyst of the appendix.

MUCOCELE OF APPENDIX

Mucocele of the appendix is a retention cyst of the appendix. It is of four types:

1. Retention cyst
2. Mucosal hyperplasia
3. Cystadenoma
4. Cystadenocarcinoma

Sometimes obstruction of the lumen of the appendix happens without the development of infection, it leads to mucocele of the appendix as mucus secretion continues in spite of obstruction of the lumen of the appendix. The mucus gets collected in the appendix. It should be differentiated from cystadenocarcinoma of the appendix.

The symptoms of mucocele of the appendix are like mild recurrent appendicitis. If infection occurs, then it turns to empyema of the appendix. It is diagnosed by ultrasound and CT scan.

Treatment of mucocele of the appendix is appendicectomy.

Malignant Mucocele

It is a mucous papillary adenocarcinoma grade I of the appendix.

PYOCELE OF APPENDIX OR EMPYEMA OF APPENDIX

- Distention of the appendix with pus is called "empyema or pyocele" of the appendix.
- Mucocele of the appendix may convert to empyema due to infection and pus formation.
- Rupture of empyema of the appendix causes generalized peritonitis.
- Treatment of empyema of the appendix is appendicectomy.

INTUSSUSCEPTION OF APPENDIX

It is a rare condition and usually occurs in children. It is diagnosed only when an operation is done for acute appendicitis.

Clinical Features

Its symptoms are of subacute appendicitis.

Complications

- Appendicocecal or appendiculocecocolic intussusception.
- Appendix may slough out and be treated as agenesis of the appendix later on.

Treatment: Appendicectomy

Diverticulum of Appendix

It is a rare entity.

The diverticulum of the appendix is of two types:

1. Congenital or true diverticulum. It has all the layers of the wall of the appendix.
2. Acquired or false diverticulum.

It has only a mucus membrane and no muscle layer. It occurs due to the rise of pressure inside the lumen of the appendix as in mucocele. The mucosa is pushed out of weak spots in the muscle layer, "Hiatus muscularis."

The diverticula of the appendix can also occur by external traction by adhesions. When the lumen of the appendix gets blocked at a place cystic distension of the appendix occurs which follows the development of the diverticulum. It is more common when the muscular walls of the appendix are weakened. Appendicular diverticula may be single or multiple. Most of the diverticula in an appendix developed between the folds of the mesoappendix.

Diverticula of the appendix can occur at any site in the appendix but are commonly found at the tip of the appendix.

TUMORS OF APPENDIX

Tumors of the appendix:
- *Benign tumors:* Lymphoma, fibroma, myxoma, angioma, myoma, and endometriosis.
- *Malignant tumors:* Carcinoid tumor, adenocarcinoma, and pseudomyxoma peritonei.

These are extremely rare tumors. Mostly the tumors of the appendix are malignant, benign tumors are rarer than malignant tumors.

Benign Tumors of the Appendix

Following benign tumors of the appendix are reported but are extremely rare:
- Lymphoma
- Fibroma
- Myxoma
- Angioma
- Myoma
- Endometriosis

Endometriosis

The endometrium of the appendix is not an extremely rare entity. It causes pain in RIF which becomes monthly and is associated with melena.

Treatment: Appendicectomy

MALIGNANT TUMORS OF THE APPENDIX

- Carcinoid tumor or argentaffinoma of appendix
- Adenocarcinoma of appendix
- Pseudomyxoma peritonei

Carcinoid Tumor or Argentaffinoma of Appendix

It is found in one case in 400 appendix specimens subjected to histopathology after appendicectomy in acute appendicitis. One study has shown mean age of carcinoid of the appendix is 42.2 years and predominance in females.

Origin

- Kulchitsky cells of crypts of Lieberkühn (Johann Nathanael Lieberkühn, 1711–1756, physician and anatomist, Berlin, Germany).
- It is the most common tumor of the appendix.
- The most common site of carcinoid tumors is the appendix.

Site

- It can be found at the tip, base, or body of the appendix.
- Most commonly it is found near the tip of the appendix, (70% of cases).

Pathology

- It is yellow, from and small tumor.
- It is situated between the mucosa and peritoneal coat of the appendix.
- Tumor cells are typically arranged in small nests.
- Carcinoid tumor of the appendix very rarely gives metastasis, only in 2% of cases. One unique carcinoid tumor is the "Goblet cell carcinoid" (adenocarcinoid). The histological behavior of the tumor is between the carcinoid tumor and the adenocarcinoma of the appendix.
- This tumor arises from argentaffin or enterochromaffin cells. Argentaffin cells are present among the cells lining the wall appendix. The cytoplasmic granules of these cells strain black with silver salts so-called "Argentaffin" and brown with chromium salts so-called "Enterochromaffin" cells. *They are classified as a type of Amine Precursor Uptake and Decarboxylation (APUD) cells.*

Treatment

The malignant potential of the tumor is related to its size.
- Appendicectomy is the treatment of choice if the tumor is <2 cm in size.
- *Right hemicolectomy is done if:*
  - Tumor is >2 cm in size.
  - Cecal wall is involved.
  - Regional lymph nodes are enlarged.

Carcinoid Syndrome

It is due to chemicals in carcinoid tumors. These chemicals are:
- 5-HT (5-hydroxytryptamine or serotonin)
- 5-hydroxytryptophan
- 5-HIAA
- Histamine
- Kallikrein
- Bradykinin

Clinical Features of Carcinoid Syndrome

Carcinoid tumors that metastasize to the liver are sometimes associated with a symptom complex called carcinoid syndrome which is characterized by mnemonic (Mn)—DABAR.

D: Diarrhea

A: Attack of bronchial asthma due to histamine.

B: Increased borborygmi

A: Attack of flushing of the face is induced by alcohol.

R: Reddish blue hue (cyanosis) due to histamine.

Carcinoid syndrome is rarely associated with appendix carcinoid unless widespread metastases are present, which occur in 2.9% of cases. Symptoms due to carcinoid are rare, although tumors can obstruct the appendix lumen and result in acute appendicitis.

Adenocarcinoma of Appendix

The most common presentation of carcinoma of the appendix is acute appendicitis.

- It is a very rare tumor.
- Usually, the tumors are diagnosed late.
- Neoplasm occurs in three major histologic subtypes.
  - Mucinous adenocarcinoma
  - Colonic adenocarcinoma
  - Adenocarcinoid
- Mucus-secreting adenocarcinoma of the appendix can rupture and disseminate malignant cells in the peritoneal cavity and cause pseudomyxoma peritonei.
- *10% of patients have dissemination at the time of operation.*

Malignant mucocele: It is a mucus-secreting papillary adenocarcinoma where the appendix gets distended with mucoid secretion.

Treatment

- Right hemicolectomy.
- If pseudomyxoma peritonei, then resection of the involved peritoneum is also done, and then chemotherapy is given.

Pseudomyxoma Peritonei

Recent studies suggest that the appendix is the site of origin for most of the cases of pseudomyxoma and not the ovary. Mucin-secreting adenoma (mucinous cyst adenoma) and adenocarcinoma (mucinous cyst adenocarcinoma) invade through the wall of the appendix and produce intraperitoneal seedlings and spread to the whole peritoneal cavity. The abdomen is filled with yellow-colored jelly. It is a locally malignant condition. It does not give extraperitoneal metastasis. Diagnosis is made by ultrasound and CT scan. It is three times more common in females than males.

Treatment

Debulking surgery is done with appendicectomy. The jelly is scoped out. Recurrence is common but takes years to develop.

Resection of the peritoneum and intraperitoneal chemotherapy helps some patients.

OPERATIVE SURGERY OF APPENDIX

Introduction

Since the first appendicectomy was done by Claudius Amyand in 1735 on a boy, it is the treatment of choice for appendicitis. Appendicitis is a common problem, and the gold standard treatment of appendicitis is appendicectomy. There is a possibility of developing complications in the inflamed appendix if there is a delay in appendicectomy. Complications can be serious like perforation of the appendix and general peritonitis and therefore, the appendicectomy for inflamed appendicectomy is considered a medical emergency.

ANATOMY OF RIGHT ILIAC FOSSA IN RELATION TO APPENDIX SURGERY

The anterior abdominal wall has the following features:

Skin

The skin of the anterior abdominal wall has an enormous capacity for stretching as during pregnancy.

Superficial Fascia

It has two layers below the level of the umbilicus and one layer above the umbilicus.

The two layers of superficial fascia are:

1. Camper's fascia superficial fatty layer.
2. Scarpa's fascia, deep membranous layer.

Cutaneous Nerves

Cutaneous nerves are derived from the lower five intercostal nerves, subcostal nerves, and iliohypogastric nerves.

Cutaneous Arteries

These are branches of arteries that accompany nerves:

- Superior epigastric artery
- Inferior epigastric artery
- Lower intercostal arteries

Cutaneous Veins

- Accompany arteries
- Veins radiate from the umbilicus, veins above the umbilicus drain to the superior vena cava, and veins from below the umbilicus drain to the inferior vein cava.

MUSCLES OF ANTERIOR ABDOMINAL WALL

There are four muscles on either side of midline:

1. External oblique muscle
2. Internal oblique muscle
3. Transversus abdominis muscle
4. Rectus abdominis muscle

External Oblique Muscle

- It originates from lower eight ribs.
- It inserts in xiphoid process, linea alba, pubic symphysis, pubic crest, and pectineal line.

Direction of Fibers

- Medially
- Downward
- *Forward:* Fleshy fibers of muscle are laterally present and tough and whitish aponeurosis is situated medially.

The junction of fleshy fibers and aponeurosis of the external oblique muscle is approximately medial to a line drawn down from the tip of the ninth costal cartilage; medial to this line is aponeurosis, and lateral are fleshy muscle fibers.

Internal Oblique Muscle

- It originates from the inguinal ligament, iliac crest, and thoracolumbar fascia.
- It inserts as an aponeurosis to the lower four costal cartilages, xiphoid process, linea alba, pubic crest, and pectineal line.

Direction of Fibers

- Medially
- Upward
- Forward
- The aponeurosis of the internal oblique muscle is in the medial part. Internal oblique aponeurosis takes part in the formation of the rectus sheath. It forms two layers, anterior and posterior, above the point midway between the umbilicus and the pubic symphysis; below this point, it forms only an anterior layer. The posterior layer of internal oblique aponeurosis ends at a point midway between the umbilicus and pubic symphysis and is called "arcuate line" or "fold of Douglas" or "linea semilunaris."

Transversus Abdominis Muscle

- Originates from the inguinal ligament, iliac crest, thoracolumbar fascia, and lower six costal cartilages.
- Inserts at the xiphoid process, linea alba, pubic crest, and pectineal line.

Direction of Fibers

- Medially
- Horizontally
- Forward
- The neurovascular plane of an anterior abdominal wall lies between the internal oblique and transversus abdominis muscle. Various nerves and vessels run in this plane so while splitting or cutting this muscle taking care of nerves and blood vessels sometimes bleeding from here can be annoying.

Rectus Abdominis Muscle

- Rectus abdominis muscle runs vertically, originating as two heads from pubic crest and anterior pubic ligament.
- Inserts at xiphoid process and seventh, sixth, and fifth costal cartilages.
- Tere are three tendinous intersections in rectus abdominis muscle which divide the muscle in smaller parts at three levels:
  1. Xiphoid process
  2. Umbilicus
  3. Between xiphoid process and umbilicus
- Fascia transversalis lines the transversus abdominis muscle and is separated from peritoneum by connective tissue.

INFERIOR EPIGASTRIC ARTERY

It arises from external iliac artery, it runs upward and medially in extraperitoneal connective tissue, reaches rectus sheath, and divides in upper and lower branch.

> Important point to remember is that neurovascular bundle runs between the internal oblique and transversus abdominis muscle. Iliohypogastric nerve pierces the internal oblique muscle about 2.5 cm in front of ASIS and then runs medially and forwards and pierces external oblique fascia 2.5 cm above inguinal ligament. This nerve can be damaged in big incision for appendicectomy and can cause right inguinal hernia.

- The ilioinguinal nerve pierces the internal oblique muscle and runs below the iliohypogastric nerve and external oblique muscle, and runs with the spermatic cord in the inguinal canal and emerges from the superficial inguinal ring.

PREOPERATIVE PREPARATION FOR APPENDICECTOMY

Shaving of the part is done in a ward before surgery. It is done from the nipples to the midthigh level. Nowadays, shaving one night before an operation is avoided if possible, to reduce the chance of postoperative infection, as skin abrasions will act as ports of entry for bacteria and will give them time to multiply.

- Patient is told to pass urine before going to the operating theater (OT).
- *Nil per os (NPO = Nil Per Oral, nothing by mouth)—6-hour fasting is required, but in an emergency, appendicectomy can be done in a shorter essential period for preoperative preparation.*
- IV fluid is to be given to avoid dehydration and to maintain normal urinary output.
- Antibiotics and IV antibiotics have been shown to significantly reduce the incidence of postoperative wound infection and intra-abdominal abscess formation. Antibiotics should be administered 30 minutes prior to incision to achieve the required tissue level of antibiotics. Antibiotics alone have been used in rare situations, such as with sailors on long submarine tours and long-distance travelers. IV antibiotics are given to cover gram-negative and anaerobic organisms. *The commonly used such antibiotics are:*
    - Cephalosporin
    - Metronidazole
    - Amikacin or another aminoglycoside
- Some doctors prefer a 1 g metronidazole suppository before the operation.
- A nasogastric tube should be introduced if you suspect perforation or peritonitis, or if the patient is profusely vomiting.
- If a patient has a fever, then cold sponging is done to reduce the temperature.
- Preanesthetic medicines are given according to the anesthetist's advice.
- Patient's anxiety and apprehension are reduced by properly explaining about the anesthesia and operative procedure.
- An indwelling Foley catheter is passed in patients with generalized peritonitis.

APPENDICECTOMY OR APPENDECTOMY

Appendicectomy

- In 1736, Claudius Amyand (1685–1740, Surgeon, St George's Hospital, London, England) successfully removed an acutely inflamed appendix from the hernial sac of a boy.

Appendicitis is the most common indication of appendicectomy, including its complicated entities.

- Lawson Tait (1845–1899, Surgeon, Hospital for Diseases of Women, Birmingham, England) was the first surgeon to perform the first planned appendicectomy in May 1880, but he did not report it till 1890.
- Thomas Morton (1835–1903, Surgeon, Philadelphia, PA, USA) was the first to diagnose appendicitis, drain the abscess, remove the appendix, and publish in 1887.

Definition

Removal of the appendix is called appendicectomy or appendectomy (in British English, it is called *appendicectomy* and in American English, appendectomy).

> *Types of appendicectomy*:
> - *Appendicectomy:*
>   - Open or conventional appendicectomy
>   - Laparoscopic appendicectomy
> - Interval appendicectomy
> - Incidental appendicectomy
> - Retrograde appendicectomy
> - Inversion appendicectomy

Indications of Appendicectomy

- Acute appendicitis
- *Appendicular tumor:*

- Carcinoma of the appendix involving only the mucosa but not the base of the appendix
- Small carcinoid tumor <2 cm in size and at the body or tip of the appendix

- Subacute appendicitis
- Chronic appendicitis
- Recurrent appendicitis
- Interval appendicectomy after appendicular mass
- Mucocele of appendix.
- Empyema of the appendix
- *Endometriosis of the appendix*
- Diverticulum of the appendix—the acquired diverticulum of the appendix perforates early if appendicitis develops.

Open or Conventional Appendicectomy

Anesthesia

- Usually, the anesthetist decides during the preanesthesia checkup (PAC) about the kind of anesthesia is required.
- General anesthesia is preferred.
- Spinal anesthesia is also used.
- Local anesthesia with sedation and IV analgesics can be tried in very sick patients with other serious systemic ailments, and or where other forms of anesthesia are contraindicated.

Steps of Appendicectomy

Steps of Open Appendicectomy

- Incision
- Identification and isolation of the appendix
- Cutting of mesoappendix
- Removal of the appendix
- Inspection of the operative site, cecum, terminal ileum, and pelvic organs
- Closure of the wound

INCISIONS

Common incisions for appendicectomy ***(Fig. 19)****:*
- Gridiron incision (McBurney's incision)
- Lanz or crease incision
- Rutherford Morison's muscle cutting incision
- Lower right paramedical incision
- Lower midline incision
- Medial muscle cutting incision (Fowler–Weir approach)
- Battle's pararectus incision
- Rockey–Davis incision

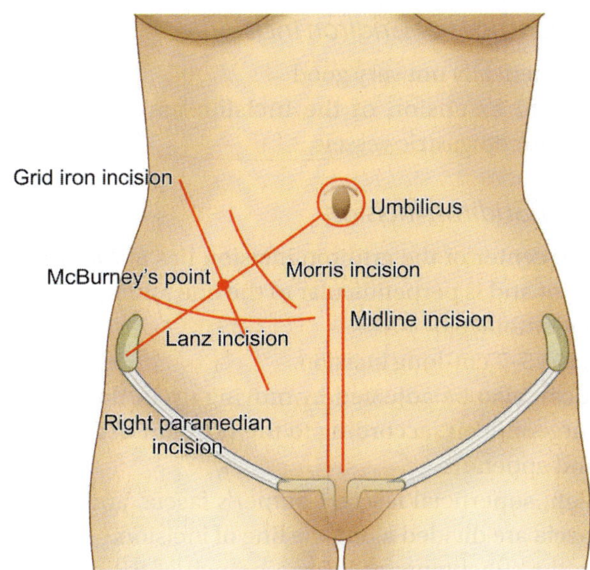

Fig. 19: Incisions for appendectomy.

Antibiotics should be administered 30 minutes prior to incision to achieve adequate tissue levels. IV antibiotics have been shown to significantly reduce the incidents of postoperative wound infection and intra-abdominal abscess.

Source: Andersen BR, Kallehave FL, Andersen HK. Antibiotics versus placebo for prevention of postoperative infection after appendicectomy. Cochrane Database Syst Rev. 2003;(2): CD001439.

The most commonly used incision in appendicectomy is the gridiron incision. A gridiron is a frame of crossbeams. It is used to support a ship during repairs.

Gridiron Incision

Gridiron incision was first described by Lewis Linn McArthur (1858–1934, Surgeon, St Luke's Hospital, Chicago, IL, USA). It is also called McBurney's gridiron incision.

Principle: It is a muscle-splitting incision. It is used to cause rapid healing and the least damage to the anatomy of the anterior abdominal wall. The incision was made in the abdominal wall in cases of appendicitis, with a description of a new method of operating.

Advantages of Gridiron Incision

- No nerve injury
- It heals fast
- Lowest mortality rate
- No muscle damage
- Less time-consuming compared to muscle-cutting incisions.

Disadvantages of Gridiron Incision

- Cosmetically not very good
- Medial extension of the incision can damage the inferior epigastric vessels.

Steps of Gridiron Incision

- The center of the gridiron incision lies at McBurney's point and is perpendicular to the line joining ASIS and the umbilicus.
- It is a 5–7 cm-long incision.
- It can also be adjusted by moving up or down as the surgeon feels, according to the position of the cecum and appendix.
- Skin, superficial fascia, Camper's fascia, and Scarpa's fascia are divided along the line of incision.
- In the subcutaneous layer, a branch of the superficial circumflex artery is caught and cauterized or ligated.
- The external oblique aponeurosis is divided into the line of its fibers, which is in the same line as the incision. The external oblique fibers are kept separated by retraction with Czerney's retractors.
- Mayo's scissors or artery forceps are inserted and opened between the fibers of the internal oblique muscle and the transversus abdominis muscle, which splits the fibers of the muscles. Now, two index fingers are introduced and pulled apart to enlarge the space.
- Now the peritoneum is visible.
- Peritoneum is exposed by retraction.
- Two Langenbeck's retractors are inserted deep into the muscles, and the peritoneum is exposed. The peritoneum is incised between two artery forceps. First, the peritoneum is picked up by the surgeon by artery forceps. The peritoneum is now picked up by the assistant by artery forceps in front of the surgeon's artery forceps. Now surgeon leaves the peritoneum and again catches the fold of the peritoneum to avoid injury to the underlying bowel. Now the surgeon feels the fold of the peritoneum between his thumb and index finger to confirm that the bowel is not caught between artery forceps. Now he cuts the peritoneum fold with a knife. Do not cut by scissors as scissors can cut the bowel within the peritoneum fold.
- *As soon as the peritoneum is opened air sucks in, and intestinal loops fall back then the small cut is extended with scissors.*
- Gridiron incision can be converted to Rutherford Morison incision and can be extended up or down by cutting the muscle fibers if the exposure is not sufficient.

Closure of Incision

- The closure is done in layers.
- First the peritoneum and fascia transversalis are sutured with 2/0 Vicryl.
- Secondly, the fibers of the internal oblique and transversus abdominis are sutured together.
- Thirdly aponeurotic layer of the external oblique is sutured.
- Fourthly, the subcutaneous tissue and skin are approximated by staples or 3/0 Prolene, or subcuticular sutures. Even in advanced appendicitis or perforation, primary closure is cost-effective and without a high risk of wound infection, with proper use of antibiotics.

Lanz or Crease Incision

Otto Lanz (1865–1935, Surgeon, Amsterdam, the Netherlands) started this incision.

Principle: It is a cosmetic incision as it is a transverse incision in the skin crease, i.e., Langer's lines, which heals well and gives the scar in the skin crease.

Rutherford Morison's Muscle-Cutting Incision

James Rutherford Morison (1853–1939, Professor of Surgery, Durham, England) describes it for the first time.

Principle: It is an oblique muscle-cutting incision.

Details of incision: It starts at McBurney's point and goes up laterally.

- It cuts external oblique aponeurosis, internal oblique and transverses abdominis muscle in same line.
- Further steps are like gridiron incision.

Indications of Rutherford Morison's Incision

- Appendicectomy
- To expose ureter
- To expose external iliac vessels

Disadvantages of Rutherford Morison's Incision

- The chances of postoperative hernia are more due to nerve injury and local muscle cutting.
- Incisional hernia is also seen if the wound is not well-repaired.
- More chances of wound infection than other incisions due to more bleeding.
- The chances of postoperative hematoma are higher.

Lower Midline or Right Paramedian Incision

- A lower midline incision is preferred over a lower right paramedian incision.
- *Indication:* It is used when in doubt about the diagnosis of perforation and peritonitis.

Advantages of Lower Midline Incision

- Midline incision is easy to extend upward if there is a perforated duodenal ulcer.
- It gives good access to the pelvic cavity as well as the abdominal cavity.
- Easy to close.
- Less damaging to the tissues, so it heals early.

Advantages of Right Paramedian Incision

- It gives good access to pelvic organs.
- It can be extended up if a perforated duodenal ulcer is present.

Disadvantages of Lower Midline or Right Paramedian Incision

- A lot of retraction is required to expose the appendix and cecum. It gives poor access in retrocecal appendicitis.
- The chances of postoperative hematoma and infection are higher with this incision as it behaves as a trapdoor for infection.
- It can contaminate the peritoneal cavity.

Fowler–Weir Approach

Similar to Battle's incisions, but the muscles are cut medially over the rectus muscle.

- Not used nowadays.

Battle's Pararectal Incision

William Henry Battle, 1855-1936, started this incision. Battle WH modified the incision for the removal of the vermiform appendix. (Br Med J. 1895;2:1360)

It is not used nowadays.

Indications of Battle's pararectal incision:

- Appendicectomy
- Gynecologic operations

Rockey–Davis Incision

It is similar to the Lanz incision. It is a transverse muscle-splitting incision. It is extended up to the rectus sheath for better exposure.

Identification of Cecum

- One retractor is placed on the medial side of the wound.
- If pus is present, take a swab for culture and sensitivity before removing it by suction.
- *Identify the cecum by:*
  - Anterior taenia coli
  - It is whitish-pale in color, whereas ileal loops are pinkish
  - Absence of appendices epiploicae

Delivering the Cecum and the Appendix

Hold the cecum with a swab by thumb and index finger and bring it out in wound by pulling it down and medially.

Identification and Isolation of Appendix

- *Appendix is caught with Babcock forceps near its tip encircling it and not crushing. Now it is pulled so as to see the mesentery and base of the appendix clearly.*
- The loops of the ileum are returned back to the peritoneal cavity.
- The abdominal pack is put around to wall of the peritoneal cavity from the wound.
- One can easily reach the cecum by following the peritoneal reflection from the abdomen wall.
- Sometimes, even the sigmoid colon and transverse colon could be present in RIF. The transverse colon has an omentum attached to it, and the sigmoid colon is identified by its mesocolon, whereas the cecum has no mesocolon or omentum.
- A word of caution—do not use cautery near the bowel as thermal injury may cause necrosis later on, which can form a fecal fistula.
- The right index finger is introduced into the wound to help in the gentle delivery of the appendix by hooking, but must be done under vision. Now the cecum is given to the assistant to hold.

Cutting of Mesoappendix

Mesoappendix is made tense by holding and pulling the appendix with Babcock forceps, or the mesoappendix is caught with curved artery forceps.

- One-pointed and curved mosquito artery forceps is introduced in the mesoappendix near its base near the appendicular artery. The 4-0 Vicryl ligature passes in this hole, and the appendicular artery is ligated. Gradually, in the same manner, the whole mesoappendix is ligated close to the appendix.

- Accessory appendicular artery is also ligated.

In most of cases, vessels are clearly divided at the base of the appendix and in such cases, ligature can be applied high enough to have perfect control of all vessels. In some cases, the cecal artery also supplies the base of the appendix.

Here, one has to be cautious against bleeding after amputation of the appendix.

Removal of Appendix

Crush the base of the appendix with straight artery forceps, which crushes only the mucus membrane and muscle coat but does not crush the serosa. The crushed mucosa and muscle coat block the lumen. Ligate the appendix base at the crush site with 3/0 Vicryl.

When the Base of the Appendix is Not Crushed?

- If the appendix is gangrenous.
- If there is a perforation at the base of the appendix.
- If the base of the appendix and cecum are edematous.

Occasionally, in certain cases, the appendiceal inflammation extends to the base of the appendix or beyond to the cecum. The division of the appendix through inflamed, infected tissue leaves the potential for leakage of cecal contents with a residual abscess or fistula—Poole GV (Am Surg. 1993;59:624-5)

A purse string suture or 'N' shape suture with 3/0 Vicryl is applied ***(Fig. 20)****. It is applied on the wall of the cecum around the base of the appendix. Take care of not injuring any blood vessels while taking a purse-string suture, as it may become a big hematoma in the wall of the cecum. It is a seromucosal suture. Take taenia coli in it to give strength to this ligature.*

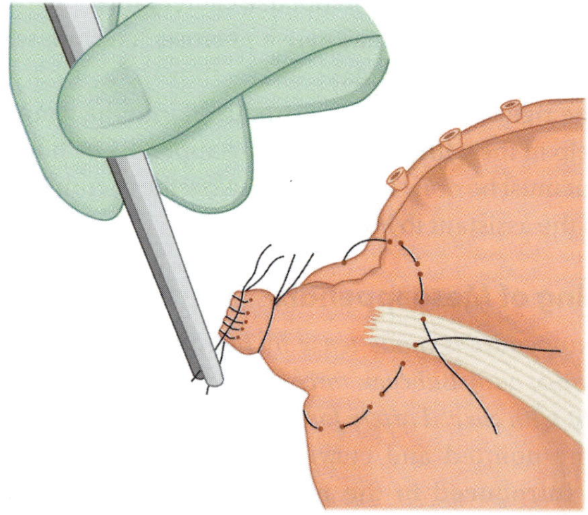

Fig. 20: Purse string suture.

Clamp the base of the appendix with an artery forceps 5 mm away from the ligature.

Before putting the clamp on the appendix milk, the intervening portion of the appendix between the ligature and the artery forceps by sliding with the artery forceps, to avoid soiling of the operation site when the appendix is cut.

- Now the appendix is cut flushed with artery forceps by a knife.
- Place a swab behind the appendix base to avoid spillage.
- Cut the ligature of the appendix stump.
- The cut stump of the appendix is touched with phenol or betadine solution or spirit or cauterized by diathermy to avoid contamination.

Burying the Base of the Appendix

Recent prospective studies show no advantages to appendiceal stump inversion.

Inversion may also have the deleterious effect of deforming the cecal wall, which could be misinterpreted as a cecal mass on future contrast radiographs. Furthermore, the long-standing notion that stump inversion reduces postoperative adhesion was discredited by Strut and colleagues. Now, the general opinion is to avoid the burying of the base of the appendix.

Invaginate the stump with pursue string suture or "figure of Z or N" suture by holding the stump base near the knot of a purse-string suture with a straight toothless dissecting forceps while pushing the stump of appendix in cecum the purse string suture is tied then cut this ligature 5 mm from the knot.

COMPLICATED SITUATIONS DURING APPENDECTOMY

The main purpose here is how to avoid injury to the intestine and other organs while doing an appendectomy in complicated situations.

- When the tip of the appendix is densely adherent then first do amputation of the appendix at the base and then free the tip by careful dissection. It is easier than when both ends are fixed.

- If the whole appendix is fixed by dense adhesions, then there is a risk of bleeding and injuring other structures by dissecting deep in adhesions. First, free the base of the appendix then give traction by applying artery forceps at this end of the appendix, cut the peritoneal covering over the appendix on its direction, and the appendix can be stripped.
- When omentum is adherent strongly with the appendix then it is better to tie and excise the omentum with the appendix.
- When the appendix is totally concealed and cannot be identified then utilize various landmarks, especially the cecum. Examine minutely cecum to find the base of the appendix. If you directly attempt to enucleate the mass, you may land up with disaster.

LAPAROSCOPIC APPENDICECTOMY

Historical Background

In 1982, Kurt Semm, a German Gynecologist, performed the first successful laparoscopic appendicectomy, several years before laparoscopic cholecystectomy **(Fig. 21)**.

Two meta-analyses have confirmed the benefits of the laparoscopic approach—this is at the expense of slightly longer operating time and a trend to higher incidence of intra-abdominal abscesses [*Source:* Sauerland et al. Kargar, Basil, 1998:109-14. Golub R, Siddiqui F, Pohl D. Laparoscopic versus open appendectomy: a metaanalysis. J Am Coll Surg. 1998;186(5):545-53].

Chronic or Subacute or Recurrent Appendicitis and Grumbling Appendix

Advantages of laparoscopic appendicectomy over open or conventional appendicectomy:

- A large meta-analysis comparing open to laparoscopic approach showed that the duration of surgery and operation costs are higher with laparoscopic appendicectomy.
- Faster convalescence, early mobility, shorter hospital stays, and early return to work.
- Less pain
- Better scar, so cosmetic
- Access to pelvic organs is better.
- Postoperative wound infection is less than open procedure.
- Exploration of the peritoneal cavity is possible.

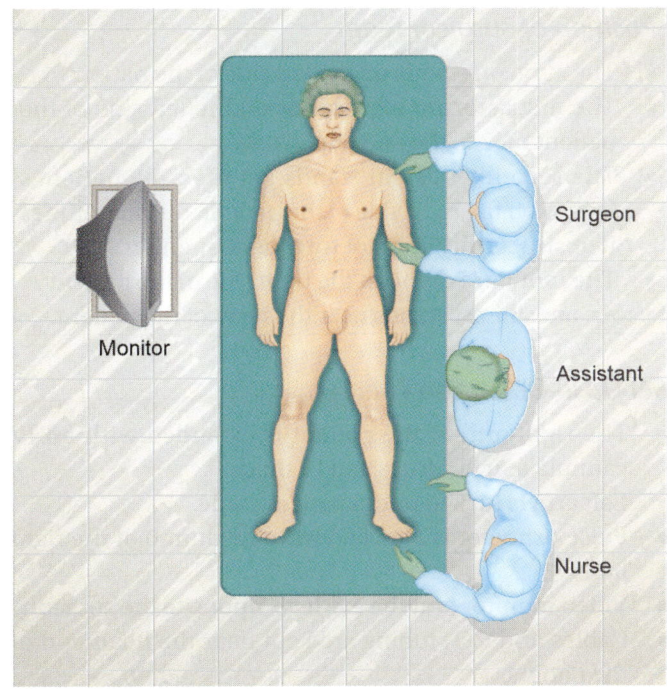

Fig. 21: Laparoscopic setup for appendicectomy.

- Treatment of other causes of RIF pain is possible.
- Unnecessary laparotomy is avoided.
- Better in obese patients as there is less risk of wound infection in fat patients. Wound infections were about as likely (Peto or Position: Supine in 15° Trendelenburg position with rotation of the table to the left side. 15–20°, right side up.

Indications

Acute Appendicitis

- In suspected cases where the diagnosis is not clear.
- In females of childbearing age.
- In obese appendicitis patients, the laparoscopic technique proved to be superior to an open technique in criteria such as perioperative-postoperative complications, operation time, etc. In open appendectomy in obese patients, sometimes incisions are required to be enlarged, extra time is required, and the risk of wound complications is higher.

In the first trimester of pregnancy.

- Incidental appendicectomy when the appendix is found inflamed during laparoscopy for other ailments.

Position of Surgical Team

- The surgeon stands on the left side of the patient.
- The first assistant also stands on the left side of the patient next to the surgeon.
- The second assistant stands between the patient's legs or on the right side of the patient, but sometimes it obstructs the vision of surgeon to monitor.
- The monitor is kept on the right side of the patient.
- An anesthetist stands near the head of the patient.

Set Up in Operation Theater

- The right arm of the patient is extended with an IV cannula in it for drugs and IV fluids.
- Left arm is tucked under patient's side.
- Pulse oximeter is attached with the thumb of the right hand.
- Video monitor is at the eye level opposite the surgeon.
- Cables and CO_2 tubing are kept near the head end of the patient.
- The instrument tray is kept near the foot end of the patient.

Relative Contraindications

- Inexperienced surgeon
- Suspicion of malignancy
- Pregnancy
- Previous lower abdominal surgery
- PID
- Severe systemic medical disease as congestive heart failure (CHF)

Preoperative Preparation

A Foley's catheter is passed to evacuate the urinary bladder and monitor urinary output before sending the patient to OT, which can be removed after the operation in the OT itself. A nasogastric tube should be passed to decompress the stomach.

Anesthesia: General anesthesia.

Steps of laparoscopic appendicectomy:
- Introduction of instruments by three ports
- Division of mesoappendix
- Extraction of the appendix

Procedure

It is usually done with their ports. The fourth port is sometimes used in the retrocecal appendix to mobilize it.

Pneumoperitoneum

- A stab wound is made at the umbilicus with a No. 11 blade, and the Veress needle is passed through it to produce pneumoperitoneum.
- Nowadays, some surgeons use the open technique by using Hasson's cannula rather than the Veress needle to produce pneumoperitoneum.

Trocar Placement

- A 5 mm or 10 mm telescope is passed through the umbilical A port and the peritoneal cavity is surveyed in all four quadrants.
- Safe access to the peritoneal cavity is by Hasson's trocar, a 3 cm incision is given infraumbilically in midline up to linea alba, and Hasson trocar is bound to the abdominal wall. It is fixed with 2-0 Vicryl with fascia.
- Under the vision of the telescope the abdominal wall is transilluminated between the umbilicus and pubic symphysis then another 1-cm incision is made in the skin just above the pubic symphysis without damaging any vessel which is visible in transillumination, and a 10 mm port is introduced. Some surgeons prefer the port at McBurney's point in LIF to avoid the swording of instruments (collision of instruments).
- Another 10 mm post is introduced in LIF lateral to the inferior epigastric artery.
- Intraperitoneal pressure is kept at 12 mm Hg and a maximum to 14. In children, the pressure equals the age.
- Trocars should be inserted in a slightly oblique direction to prevent incisional hernia.
- Placement of trocars through the rectus muscle is avoided to avoid injury to inferior epigastric vessels.
- The table is tilted in the Trendelenburg position with the right side up by 25°. By this maneuver, the omentum and the coil of the small bowel fall away from the cecum and appendix.

Exploration

Sometimes, as you introduce a laparoscope in the peritoneal cavity, you find an appendix lying in front. It is called "handshake appendix" or "how do you do the appendix." When the appendix is found shining and normal, it is called the Lilly white appendix."

- First, the abdomen is thoroughly explored to exclude any other pathology.

- Now the search for the appendix is started first identifying the cecum by the taenia coli. Follow the anterior taenia coli to find the appendix.
- If the appendix is found normal, then search for other causes of RIF pain, e.g., Meckel's diverticulitis, Crohn's ileitis, Port placement in laparoscopic appendices-salpingitis, and tuboovarian pathology.
- If the appendix cannot be found or cannot be exposed well then do not hesitate to convert the laparoscopy operation to an open operation.
- The appendix is caught near the tip with Babcock's forceps, and the mesoappendix is then visualized.
- A window is created in the mesoappendix near the base of the appendix, mesoappendix and base of the appendix are dealt with separately between clamps or staples.
- The mesoappendix is divided between two staples.

Removal of Appendix

- Two staples are applied at base of the appendix then the appendix is divided between two staples. Some surgeons prefer using endoloop at stump of the appendix.
- If the appendix appears gangrenous, then catch it with Babcock's forceps to avoid perforation.
- The base of the appendix is not inverted or buried.
- The appendix is put into the endobag, and the endobag is retrieved from the 10 mm port.
- The area of the appendix and cecum can be irrigated with saline if the site is soiled with pus or seropurulent fluid.
- Inspect the stump of the appendix and mesentery for any hemorrhage.
- RLQ may be irrigated if there is spillage.

Closure

- Remove all ports under vision so any bleeding from the abdominal wall can be seen and stopped.
- Skin staples are used at a 10 mm port site.
- At the 5 mm post site adhesive band-aid is applied.
- Drain is put in if there was generalized peritonitis.
- It is advised to locally infiltrate long-acting local anesthetic at three port sites for relief of postoperative pain.
- Some surgeons feel that in the case of a perforated appendix, the CO_2 pneumoperitoneum enhances the bacteremia and toxemia, though it is not confirmed.

Various inflammatory stages of the appendix in appendicitis and how to deal:
- *If the appendix is normal*: Look for other sources of abdominal pain; if it is not found, then proceed for appendicectomy.
- *If the appendix is mildly inflamed without the involvement of mesoappendix:* The appendix can be held with a grasper gently and without fear of perforation; it can be removed by putting it in a 10 mm trocar and removing the trocar and appendix together, protecting the abdominal wall from contamination.
- *Highly inflamed appendix with thickened mesoappendix:* Be gentle and do not move the appendix too much unnecessarily. A fourth port, if required, should be introduced to facilitate the dissection. The appendix must be removed on a retrieval bag to avoid spillage in the peritoneal cavity. Adhesions can be relieved by gentle traction on the appendix. A pretied ligature may be used to elevate the grossly inflamed appendix with minimal trauma.

Needlescopic Approach

- In laparoscopic approach two 10 mm ports and one 5 mm port are used.
- In needlescopic approach one 10 mm and two 2 mm ports are used.

Postoperative Care

- Foley's catheter is removed in the postoperative period.
- The rest of the care is the same as in the open procedure.
- Patient is discharged on the second postoperative day.
- Two recent meta-analyses have confirmed the benefit of the laparoscopic approach in relation to less pain, faster recovery, and a lower incidence of wound infection. But a Cochrane database systematic review of over 4,000 patients suggested that there was a threefold increase in intra-abdominal abscesses and a longer operating time (16 minutes) in those patients undergoing laparoscopic procedures.

Interval Appendicectomy

Interval appendicectomy is defined as "an elective appendicectomy in the interval" between attacks of appendicitis. It is the easiest appendicectomy. It is usually done 6–10 weeks after the resolution of the appendicular mass.

Incidental Appendicectomy

Incidental appendicectomy is an appendicectomy for a normal appendix during laparotomy or laparoscopy for another condition.

Inversion Appendicectomy

Indication

It is done when an incidental appendicectomy is performed.

Aim

- To avoid the risk of sepsis in otherwise clean laparotomy.
- In appendicectomy the bowel is opened, and bacterial soiling of peritoneum may happen.

Postoperative Complications of Open Appendicectomy

Age and perforation of the appendix significantly increase the complications; one study showed the rate of complications 3% in nonperforated appendicitis and 47% in perforate cases.

> **Complications of Appendicectomy**
> - Wound infection
> - Hemorrhage
> - Intraperitoneal abscesses
> - Paralytic ileus
> - Fecal fistula
> - Portal pyemia (pylephlebitis)
> - Postoperative adhesions
> - Acute intestinal obstruction
> - Right inguinal hernia
> - Pelvic abscess

Wound Infection

It is the most common postoperative complication. It occurs in <10% of cases; it increases with perforated appendicitis to 15–20% and is highest with diffuse peritonitis (35%). It is usually seen at home on the fourth or fifth postoperative day. Infection is most commonly found in subcutaneous tissue.

- Wound infection is almost always confined to subcutaneous tissue and responds to simple drainage.
- Wound infection can cause dehiscence or burst abdomen in laparotomy wounds but not in gridiron incisions.

> Postoperative sequelae after appendectomy are early, intermediate, and late. Early sequelae are due to anesthesia or operations, such as hemorrhage, infection, and peritonitis continues. Intermediate sequelae develop within a few days to a few weeks, such as abscess, ileus, phlebitis, and embolus lodgment. Late sequelae arise after months or years, such as hernia and intestinal obstruction.

Hemorrhage

Slipping of the ligature of the appendicular artery or the accessory appendicular artery is usually the cause of reactionary hemorrhage. Take the patient to OT and open the wound and ligate the bleeding vessel.

Intraperitoneal Abscesses

The incidence of intraperitoneal abscesses has gone down due to preoperative and perioperative antibiotics. Locally increased pain, tenderness, and high fever suggest an intraabdominal abscess. A CT scan of the abdomen is diagnostic. The abscess can be in the following forms:

- Appendix fossa abscess
- Right paracolic gutter abscess
- Pelvic abscess
- Pouch of Douglas abscess
- Subphrenic abscess
- Subhepatic abscess
- Inter small bowel loop abscess, usually multiple

Paralytic Ileus

It happens after every appendicectomy but usually stays longer in the gangrenous, perforated appendix and generalized peritonitis.

Fecal Fistula

Nowadays, fecal fistula is rare due to the regular use of pre-, peri-, and postoperative antibiotics. It is an annoying but not a dangerous complication. The causes of the development of fecal fistula after appendicectomy are:

- Cecal wall edema with inflammation and sloughing of part of the cecum inside the purse string suture.
- Attempted appendicectomy in appendicular mass.
- Leakage from the appendicular stump due to slipping of the ligature in a noninvaginated stump.
- Appendicectomy in Crohn's disease, tuberculosis, actinomycosis, and carcinoma of the cecum.
- Tight and deep purse-string suture sometimes causes necrosis and leakage.
- Erosion of the cecum by a drain.
- When carcinoma of the appendix is the cause of appendicitis.
- By necrosis of the cecum from an abscess. All fecal fistulae close spontaneously in a few days unless there is distal obstruction.

> Fecal fistula formation is most common when the appendectomy is performed for gangrene or perforation of the appendix.

- *Clinical features:*
  - Features of infection are present as fever, erythema over the drain site or operation incision.
  - Foul-smelling, feculent discharge from the operation wound site or the drain site.
  - The skin around the fistula becomes excoriated.
- *Investigations*:
  - CT scan abdomen to look for other pathology.
  - CT fistulogram.
- *Treatment:* Conservative treatments are—antibiotics, IV fluids, dressing, and protective cream on the skin around the fistula, such as Lacto Calamine or zinc oxide cream. If the fistula does not close within 6 weeks, then consider resection and anastomosis of the ileocecal region.

Portal Pyemia (Pylephlebitis)

- It is rare nowadays due to the use of antibiotics.
- *It is characterized by:*
  - High fever
  - Chills and rigors
  - Jaundice
- It is due to the spread of suppuration to the portal vein via the superior mesentery vein. It may lead to multiple liver abscesses.

Postoperative Adhesions

It is a late complication of appendicectomy. Diagnostic laparoscopy is required to diagnose. It causes:

- Persistent pain in RIF
- Intestinal obstruction

Acute Intestinal Obstruction

It can occur after appendicectomy due to adhesions. Initially may be paralytic, but later on may become mechanical. Obstruction may occur due to band development, but it is much less common than adhesions. It is seen in some studies occurring within 6 months and in 1% of cases.

Right Inguinal Hernia

It is a direct inguinal hernia. The incidence of hernia is three times greater than in a normal person. It occurs more in a lower right paramedian incision. It can be caused by injury to an iliohypogastric nerve or an ilioinguinal nerve, especially in the Rutherford Morison incision.

Pelvic Abscess

Nowadays it is reducing due to antibiotic coverage. It is characterized by:

- High spiking pyrexia.
- Tenesmus or discomfort at defecation
- Loose stools
- Tender mass on DRE
- Ultrasound and CT scans are diagnostic

Prophylaxis is, which is the best safeguard against hernia the small incision whenever it can be employed with equal safety and in the separation of the muscular layers without cutting them (McBurney).

Treatment

- If left untreated leads to generalized peritonitis.
- Transrectal drainage of pelvic abscess—DRE is done, and then push the closed sinus forceps in the pelvic abscess and the abscess is drained.

Mortality

In a survey of 8,651 appendectomies done in England and Wales in 1992, the mortality rate was 0.24%, and morbidity was 8%.

Postoperative Complications After Laparoscopic Appendicectomy

Inferior Epigastric Artery

It begins as a branch of the external iliac artery and ascends medially along the medial margin of the deep inguinal ring, pierces the fascia transversalis, and crosses the arcuate line, entering the rectus sheath and running upward between the rectus abdominis muscle and the posterior rectus sheath. To avoid injuring to these vessels, the trocars should be either in midline or lateral to the left rectus muscle.

Ascending Branch of Deep Circumflex Iliac Artery

The deep circumflex iliac artery arises as a branch of the external iliac artery opposite the origin of an inferior epigastric artery. It runs up and laterally near ASIS, it gives an ascending branch that runs upward between the internal oblique and transversus muscles, to avoid its injury to the tracer should be one finger breadth above ASIS.

Bleeding

Aggressive dissection of the mesoappendix is usually responsible for bleeding. Careful and minimal dissection prevents bleeding. An additional trocar may be required to identify and grasp the bleeding vessel.

Leakage of Pus or Fecolith

It occurs when the appendix is distended with pus and inflamed; careful dissection and removal in an endobag prevents it. Remove the fecolith or pus immediately and irrigate and suck the field after removal of the appendix.

Big Stump is Left or Appendix is Incompletely Removed

It can cause recurrent appendicitis, so remove it.

Postoperative Abdominal Abscesses

Intra-abdominal abscess formation is three times more common after laparoscopic appendicectomy than after open appendicectomy.

POSTOPERATIVE CARE

The person in charge of the case should give instructions, and these should be followed. Not many people of the unit treat the patient. The postoperative care instructions should be written clearly. Any change in treatment should also be written and not be verbal. A surgeon must explain nurse on duty everything in detail.

- Nil orally for 24 hours, but sips of water can be given from the same evening.
- IV fluids for 24 hours.
- Oral fluid intake allowed by the next morning if no complication develops.
- Patient is allowed to be out of bed the same evening so as not to get deep vein thrombosis.
- Gastric suction is not advised in uncomplicated cases of acute appendicitis after smooth appendicectomy.
- A soft diet is started from the second postoperative day.
- In case of perforated appendicitis with generalized peritonitis, oral intake takes more time, so nasogastric suction is done till bowel sounds appear.
- *Antibiotic:*
  - In case of nonperforated acute appendicitis, antibiotic coverage is given for 36–48 hours after appendicectomy
  - In perforated appendicitis with or without generalized peritonitis, antibiotic coverage is given for 7–10 days. IV antibiotics are given until:
    - Patient becomes afebrile for 24 hours
    - While the blood count becomes normal
  - Peritoneal culture is not of much use, as by the time the culture reports come, the patient has recovered. Peritoneal culture is of use in the following conditions:
    - In an immunosuppressed patient
    - A patient who develops an abscess.

Postappendectomy checklist if the patient is unwell:
- Examine the wound for infection or abscess
- Per-rectal examination to rule out pelvic abscess
- Examine lungs to rule out lobar pneumonia
- Rule out pylephlebitis, liver abscess, subphrenic abscess, and pyelonephritis.

MNEMONICS

Introduction

The word "Mnemonic' is derived from the ancient Greek word, "Mnemonikos," meaning "of memory" or "relating to memory." It is also related to the Greek goddess of memory, "Mnemosyne." The mnemonic word was discovered by a Greek poet, Simonides, in 447 BC. According to the Oxford Dictionary mnemonic can be defined as a word, sentence, or poem used to help remember a rule, name, etc. Mnemonics help our memory to retain information and make it easy to remember. Mnemonics are used in medicine as instruments to remember medical knowledge for the long term. Various medical terms and facts that are difficult to remember can be remembered for a long time with the help of mnemonics. A mnemonic couplet to help students learn the names of cranial nerves has been in use in the United States since the mid-19th century.

- *Murphy's triad:*
  - *Mnemonic (Mn)*: PVP
    - P = Pain in abdomen
    - V = Vomiting
    - P = Pyrexia
- *Etiology of appendicitis (common causes)*:
  - *Mn:* DR SODA
    - D = Diet
    - R = Racial, familial, and geographical factors
    - S = Socioeconomical level
    - O = Obstruction of the appendix by fecalith and worms
    - D = Diseases of the cecum: Cancer, Crohn's disease, and tuberculosis
    - A = Abuse of purgative

- *Alvarado scoring*:
  - M = Migrating RIF pain
  - A = Anorexia
  - N = Nausea, vomiting
  - T = Tenderness RIF
  - R = Rebound tenderness
  - E = Elevated temperature (>37.3°C)
  - L = Leukocytosis (>10 × 1,037.3 cells)
  - S = Shift to left (segmental neutrophils) (>75%)

- *Ochsner–Sherren regimen*:
  - *A* = Aspiration—Ryle's tube
  - *B* = Bowel care—no purgatives
  - *C* = Charts for pulse/temperature/BP/size of mass
  - *D* = Drugs, antibiotics
  - *E* = Exploration is avoided in the appendicular mass
  - *F* = Fluids, IV
- *Common differential diagnosis of acute appendicitis*:
  - *Mn*: PUNAM TRIPS MRCP
    - P = Perforated peptic ulcer
    - U = Ureteric colic
    - N = Nonspecific mesenteric lymphadenitis
    - A = Acute gastroenteritis
    - M = Mittelschmerz
    - T = Torsion of ovarian cyst
    - R = Regional ileitis
    - I = Intestinal obstruction
    - P = Pancreatitis
    - S = Salpingitis
    - M = Meckel's diverticulitis
    - R = Ruptured ectopic gestation
    - C = Cholecystitis, acute
    - P = Pyelonephritis, acute
- *Clinical features of carcinoid syndrome*:
  - *Mn:* DABAR
    - D = Diarrhea
    - A = Attack of bronchial asthma due to histamine
    - B = Increased borborygmi
    - A = Attack of flushing of the face, induced by alcohol
    - R = Reddish blue hue (cyanosis) due to histamine

- *Differential diagnosis of appendicular mass:*
  - *Mn:* TIC-T-TAC
    - T = TB (Ileocecal TB)
    - I = Ilial lymphadenitis
    - C = Crohn's disease
    - T = Tumor, carcinoma of cecum
    - T = Tumor, carcinoma of the ovary
    - A = Amoebic typhlitis, actinomycosis
    - C = Twisted ovarian cyst

- *Complications of appendicectomy:*
  - *Mn:* 2 PACIF
    - P = Portal pyemia
    - P = Paralytic ileus
    - A = Abscess, pelvic and intraperitoneal
    - A = Adhesions, postoperative
    - C = Complication of any operation, wound infection
    - C = Complication of any operation, hemorrhage
    - I = Intestinal obstruction, acute
    - I = Inguinal hernia, right
    - F = Fecal fistula

- Important signs of acute appendicitis:
  - *Mn:* Remember Best Teachers Certify MCH 2 2 2 2
    - R = Rebound tenderness
    - R = Rovsing sign
    - B = Bed shaking test of Bapat
    - B = Baldwin's test
    - T = Tenderness in RIF
    - T = Tenderness in DRE
    - C = Cope's psoas test
    - C = Cope's obturator test
    - M = Muscle guarding
    - C = Cough sign
    - H = Hyperesthesia in Sherren's triangle
- *Complications of acute appendicitis*:
  - *Mn:* GAPSAP
    - G = Generalized peritonitis
    - A = Appendicular abscess
    - P = Perforated appendix
    - S = Septicemia
    - A = Appendicular lump
    - P = Portal pyemia
- *Important tumors of the appendix*:
  - *Mn:* CAP
    - C = Carcinoid tumor
    - A = Adenocarcinoma
    - P = Pseudomyxoma peritonei (PMP)
- *Two layers of subcutaneous tissue in RIF*:
  - c *Mn:* CS (C comes before S as an alphabet)
    - C = Camper's superficial fatty layer
    - S = Scarpa's deep membranous layer
- *Names of three taenia coli*:
  - *Mn:* MOL
    - M = Taenia mesocolica
    - O = Taenia omentalis
    - L = Taenia libera

Key points

Remember MAO Mnemonics, Murphy's triad, Alvarado scoring, and Ochsner–Sherren regimen.

SOME IMPORTANT QUESTIONS

Q1. All are true about the appendicular artery, *except*:
a. Supplies only appendix
b. Supplies the terminal ileum also
c. Is an end artery
d. Branch of the lower division of the ileocolic artery

Ans. b

Q2. The fold of Treves is:
a. The fold of mucous membrane projecting into the lumen to the rectum
b. The ilio-appendicular fold of the peritoneum
c. The fold of the mucous membrane around the papilla of water
d. The fold of the peritoneum over the inferior mesenteric vein

Ans. b

Q3. Diffuse peritonitis following appendicitis is usually seen:
a. When appendicular perforation occurs early (within 24 hours)
b. When perforation occurs late (after 24 hours)
c. Particularly in nonobstructive appendicitis
d. When antibiotics are withheld

Ans. a

Q4. "Ten horn" sign is a feature of:
a. Rectus muscle hematoma
b. Acute pancreatitis
c. Choledocholithiasis
d. Acute appendicitis

Ans. d

Q5. Which one of the following is a muscle-splitting incision?
a. Kocher's
b. Rutherford–Morrison
c. Pfannenstiel
d. Lanz

Ans. d

Q6. The most dangerous position of the appendix is:
a. Retrocecal
b. Paracolic
c. Pelvic
d. Retroperitoneal

Ans. c

Q7. Diffuse peritonitis following appendicitis is usually seen:
a. When appendicular perforation occurs early (within 24 hours)
b. When perforation occurs late (after 24 hours)
c. Particularly in nonobstructive appendicitis
d. When antibiotics are withheld

Ans. a

Q8. A 26-year-old male presented with a 4-day history of pain in the right-sided lower abdomen with frequent vomiting. The patient's general condition is fair, and clinically, a tender lump was felt in the right iliac fossa (RIF). The most appropriate management for this case would be:
a. Exploratory laparotomy
b. Immediate appendectomy
c. Ochsner–Sherren regimen
d. External drainage

Ans. c

Q9. The most common tumor occurring in the appendix:
a. Melanoma
b. Carcinoid tumor
c. Adenocarcinoma
d. Mucinous carcinoma

Ans. b

Q10. Grid-iron incision was first described by:
a. McArthur
b. Rutherford Morrison
c. Hamilton Bailey
d. Lanz

Ans. a

Q11. During appendectomy, if it is noticed that the base of the appendix is inflamed, then a further line of treatment is:
a. No appendectomy
b. No burying of stump
c. Hemicolectomy
d. Cecal resection

Ans. b

Q12. The recurrent appendicular artery is a branch of:
a. Ileocolic artery
b. Right colic artery
c. Middle colic artery
d. Posterior cecal artery

Ans. d

Q13. The appendicular artery is a branch of:
a. Ileocolic artery
b. Right colic artery
c. Middle colic artery
d. Posterior cecal artery

Ans. a

Q14. The most common site of the appendix:
a. Retrocecal
b. Preileal
c. Paracecal
d. Postileal

Ans. a

Q15. The earliest symptom in acute appendicitis is:

a. Pain
b. Fever
c. Vomiting
d. Rise in pulse rate

Ans. a

Q16. McBurney's point:

a. Lies in the middle of the right spine umbilical line
b. At the junction of the lateral two-thirds and medial one-third of line
c. At the junction of the lateral one-third and the medial two-thirds of line
d. Lies at the umbilicus-liver junction

Ans. c

Q17. The following signs are not seen in acute appendicitis, *except*:

a. Rovsing's sign
b. Murphy's sign
c. Boa's sign
d. Macewen's sign

Ans. a

Q18. Rovsing's sign is seen in:

a. Acute appendicitis
b. Acute cholecystitis
c. Pancreatitis
d. None of the above

Ans. a

Q19. The pointing index sign is seen in:

a. Acute appendicitis
b. Acute pancreatitis
c. Perforated duodenal ulcer
d. Acute cholecystitis

Ans. a

Q20. A gridiron incision becomes a Rutherford–Morrison incision when the incision is extended by:

a. Splitting the muscle laterally
b. Cutting the muscles laterally
c. Cutting the muscles medially into the rectus sheath
d. Incising vertically along the rectus muscle

Ans. b

Q21. The most common initiating factor in acute appendicitis is: (JIPMER GIS 2011)

a. Luminal obstruction
b. Bacterial infection
c. Lymphoid hyperplasia
d. Perforation

Ans. a

Q22. All of the following signs are not seen in acute appendicitis, *except*:

a. Rovsing's
b. Murphy's
c. Boa's sign
d. Macewen's sign

Ans. a

Q23. False about appendicitis in children:

a. Localized pain is the single most important symptom
b. Vomiting precedes abdominal pain
c. Perforation occurs in 80% of cases <5 years
d. 60% of perforation occurs within 48 hours

Ans. b

Q24. Which of the following statements is not true of McBurney's incision?

a. Most suitable if the diagnosis of appendicitis is definite
b. It is it converted into a muscle-cutting incision, it is called Rutherford Morrison's incision
c. Inguinal hernia is a sequelae of the incision
d. The incision can be extended upwards and downwards

Ans. d

Q25. Treatment of choice for mucinous adenocarcinoma of the appendix:

a. Right hemicolectomy
b. Appendicectomy
c. Percutaneous aspiration
d. Total colectomy

Ans. a

Q26. When the rectum is inflated with air through a rectal tube, pain, and tenderness occur in the RIF in case of appendicitis. This is known as:

a. Aaron's sign
b. Battle's sign
c. Bastedo sign
d. McBurney's sign

Ans. c

Q27. The frequent mechanism in perforation of the appendix is:

a. Impacted fecolith
b. Tension gangrene due to the accumulating secretions
c. Necrosis of the lymphoid patch
d. Retrocecal infection

Ans. b

Q28. Aaron's sign is seen in:

a. Achalasia cardia
b. Hiatus hernia
c. Mediastinum emphysema
d. Acute appendicitis

Ans. d

Q29. Regarding appendicitis in pregnancy, false is:

a. Most common cause of acute abdomen in the first trimester
b. Pregnancy does not increase the risk
c. Conservative management by antibiotics should be tried
d. After rupture, fetal mortality is around 30–40%

Ans. c

Q30. Treatment of choice for mucinous adenocarcinoma of the appendix:

a. Right hemicolectomy
b. Appendectomy
c. Percutaneous aspiration
d. Total colectomy

Ans. a

Q31. Mark the correct statement about inflammatory bowel disease (IBD):

1. Crohn's disease has skip lesions
2. Childhood IBD is genetic
3. Crohn is mucosal and ulcerative colitis (UC) is transmural
4. Crohn is curable fully

a. 2, 3 are correct
b. 1 and 2 are correct
c. 1, 2, 3 are correct
d. All are correct

Ans. b

Q32. Which of the following statements is not true of McBurney's incision?

a. Most suitable if the diagnosis of appendicitis is definite.
b. If it is converted into a muscle-cutting incision, it is called Rutherford–Morrison incision.
c. Inguinal hernia is a sequelae of the incision.
d. The incision can be extended upward or downward.

Ans. c

Q33. All are true about appendicular rupture, *except*:

a. Common in low socioeconomic status people
b. Common in extremes of age
c. Early antibiotics prevent perforation
d. Appendicectomy done even in the presence of rupture

Ans. d

Q34. All of the following are early complications arising after appendicectomy for acute appendicitis, *except*:

a. Ileus
b. Sterility
c. Intestinal obstruction
d. Pulmonary complications

Ans. b

Q35. Ochsner–Sherren regimen is used in the management of:

a. Appendicular abscess
b. Chronic appendicitis
c. Appendicular mass
d. Acute appendicitis

Ans. c

Q36. Mucocele of the appendix is:

a. Benign tumor
b. Low-grade malignancy
c. Retention cyst
d. Infective process

Ans. c

Q37. The most common site of carcinoids is:

a. Ileum
b. Liver
c. Rectum
d. Appendix

Ans. d

Q38. Carcinoid of which site is least likely to be malignant?

a. Appendix
b. Stomach
c. Small intestine
d. Lung

Ans. a

Q39. The most common tumor of the appendix is:

a. Argentaffinoma
b. Lymphoma
c. Leiomyosarcoma
d. Adenocarcinoma

Ans. a

Q40. Surgery for carcinoid tumor of the appendix:

a. Right hemicolectomy
b. Appendicectomy
c. Limited resection of the right colon
d. Right hemicolectomy with removal of inches of the ileum also

Ans. b

Q41. What is "peritoneal mice"?

a. Pseudomyxoma peritonei
b. Appendices epiploicae
c. Peritoneal seedings of the tumor
d. Endometriosis

Ans. b

Q42. Epidemic appendicitis is due to:

a. Fecalith
b. Worms of the ileocecal region
c. Streptococcal infections
d. Abuse of purgatives
e. None of the above

Ans. c

Q43. The frequent mechanism in the perforation of the appendix is:

a. Impacted fecalith
b. Tension gangrene due to accumulated secretions
c. Necrosis of lymphoid tissue
d. Carcinoid tumor

Ans. b

MULTIPLE CHOICE QUESTIONS

Grade I	Simple

Q1. Most common organism isolated from perforated appendicitis: (AIIMS GIS May 2008)

a. *E. coli* b. *Pseudomonas*
c. *Klebsiella* d. *Enterococcus*

Q2. When acute appendicitis is suspected, it can be confirmed by: (PGI JUNE 2002)

a. Clinical examination
b. Ultrasound (USG)
c. Computed tomography (CT) scan
d. Blood counts
e. Upper gastrointestinal (GI) endoscopy

Q3. A patient with Crohn's disease was opened for and an inflamed appendix was found. The treatment of choice is: (PGI 1988)

a. Appendicectomy
b. Ileocolic resection and anastomosis
c. Close the abdomen and start medical treatment
d. None of the above

Q4. The most common neoplasm of the appendix is: (AIIMS NOV 1993)

a. Lymphoma b. Adenocarcinoma
c. Leiomyosarcoma d. Argentaffinoma

Q5. Mucocele of the appendix is: (All India 1989)

a. Benign tumor b. Low-grade malignancy
c. Retention cyst d. Infective process

Q6. In the case of retrocecal appendicitis, which movement aggravates pain? (AIIMS Nov 2007)

a. Flexion b. Fever
c. Medical rotation d. Lateral rotation

Q7. Acute appendicitis is due to: (AIIMS 1990)

a. Fecolith
b. Worms of the ileocecal region
c. Streptococcal infections
d. Abuse of purgative
e. None of the above

Q8. Which of the following is a muscle-splitting incision? (AIIMS Nov 2016)

a. Kocker's incision
b. Lanz incision
c. Rutherford-Morrison incision
d. Pfannenstiel incision

Q9. The commonest anatomical position of the appendix is: (Karnataka 2013)

a. Retrocecal b. Pelvic
c. Paracecal d. Prelieal

Q10. Rovsing sign is seen in: (PGI 1995)

a. Acute appendicitis b. Acute cholecystitis
c. Pancreatitis d. None

Grade II	Difficult

Q1. True statement about appendix: (PGI June 2006)

a. Does not have mesentery
b. Has taenia coli
c. Develops from midgut
d. Supplied by an appendicular branch of the ileocolic artery

Q2. Appendicitis is diagnosed by: (PGI JUNE 2003)

a. Total leukocyte count (TLC) and differential leukocyte count (DLC)
b. X-ray abdomen
c. USG
d. Color Doppler
e. Ba enema

Q3. True about appendicular rupture is A/E: (PGI DEC 1999)

a. Common in extremes of age
b. Common in people with fecalith obstruction

c. Early antibiotics prevent rupture
d. Appendicectomy is done always in the presence of a rupture

Q4. In a case of retrocecal appendicitis, which movement aggravates pain: (AIIMS NOV 2007)

a. Flexion b. Extension
c. Medial rotation d. Lateral rotation

Q5. A 26-year-old male presented with a 4-day history of pain in the right-sided lower abdomen with frequent vomiting. Patient's general condition is fare and clinically a tender lump was felt in the RIF. Most appropriate management for this case would be: (MCI March 2010)

a. Exploratory laparotomy
b. Immediate appendectomy
c. Ochsner–Sherren regimen
d. External drainage

Q6. The most common tumor occurring in the appendix: (JIPMER 2010)

a. Melanoma b. Carcinoid tumor
c. Adenocarcinoma d. Mucinous carcinoma

Q7. A pregnant female presents with pain in the abdomen on examination, tenderness is found in the right lumbar region. TLC is 12,000/mm^3, and urine examination is normal, for diagnosis further tests done is: (AIIMS June 1999)

a. Chest X-ray with abdominal shield
b. Ultrasound abdomen
c. Noncontract CT abdomen
d. Laparoscopy

Q8. Investigation of choice for acute appendicitis in children: (AIIMS May 2015)

a. CT scan b. MRI
c. USG d. X-ray

Q9. What is the treatment of a patient with a carcinoid tumor of the appendix of size >2 cm? (AIIMS June 1999)

a. Right hemicolectomy
b. Appendectomy
c. Appendectomy + Abdominal CT scan
d. Appendectomy + 24-hour urinary 5-hydroxyindoleacetic acid (HIAA)

Q10. The nerve commonly damaged during McBurney's incision is: (All India 2003)

a. Subcostal b. Iliohypogastric
c. 11th thoracic d. 10th thoracic

Grade III	*Most difficult*

Q1. During appendectomy, if it is noticed that the base of the appendix is inflamed, then a further line of treatment is: (PGI 1996)

a. No appendicectomy
b. No burying of stump
c. Hemicolectomy
d. Cecal resection

Q2. What is the T/t of patient with a carcinoid tumor of the appendix of size >2 cm? (AIIMS JUNE 1999)

a. Right hemicolectomy
b. Appendicectomy
c. Appendicectomy + abdominal CT scan
d. Appendicectomy + 24 hours urinary HIAA

Q3. Treatment of an incidentally detected appendicular carcinoid measuring 2.5 cm is: (MCI March 2009)

a. Right hemicolectomy
b. Limits the resection of the right colon
c. Total colectomy
d. Appendectomy

Q4. A young boy presented to the casualty with a history of fever, abdominal pain, and vomiting. On examination, he was febrile with a pulse rate of 104/min. The resident was eliciting the sign shown below. Identify the sign. (AIIMS May 2017)

a. Rovsing's sign
b. Balance sign
c. McBurney's point tenderness
d. Psoas sign

Q5. All are useful in acute appendicitis, *except*: (Kerala 1994)

a. Antibiotics b. Analgesics
c. Intravenous (IV) fluids d. Purgation

Q6. All are to be done in case of a 20-year-old female coming to casualty with right iliac fossa pain, with local guarding and tenderness, *except*: (AIIMS Nov 1999)

a. IV glucose
b. Pethidine 100 mg intramuscular (IM)
c. Nil orally
d. X-ray abdomen

Q7. False about appendicitis in children: (JIPMER 2011)

a. Localized pain is the single most important symptom

b. Vomiting precedes abdominal pain
c. Perforation occurs in 80% of cases <5 years
d. 60% perforation occurs within 48 hours

Q8. Most common occurrence before appendicitis: (PGI Nov 2011)
a. Blockage of the lumen b. Ileitis
c. Gastroenteritis d. Perforation

Q9. A pregnant female presents with pain in the abdomen on examination, tenderness is found in the right lumbar region. TLC is 12,000/mm^3, and urine examination is normal. For diagnosis, further tests are done is: (AIIMS June 1999)
a. Chest X-ray with abdominal shield
b. Ultrasound abdomen
c. Noncontrast CT abdomen
d. Laparoscopy

Q10. A 25-year-old patient presented with a mass in the right iliac fossa, which, after laparotomy, was found to be a carcinoid of 2.5 cm in diameter. What will be the next step in management? (AIIMS Nov 2000)
a. Segmental resection
b. Appendectomy
c. Right hemicolectomy
d. Do a yearly 5-HIAA assay

ANSWERS

Grade I: 1. a; 2. a, b, c, d (Bailey 27/e p1307); 3. a (Bailey 27/e p1308); 4. b (Bailey 26/e p1213); 5. a, b, c (Sabiston 20/e p1308); 6. b (Bailey 27/e p1304); 7. a; 8 b; 9. a; 10. a

Grade II: 1. c (Sabiston 20/e p1296); 2. a, c (Bailey 27/e p1307); 3. c (Schwartz 10/e p1250-51); 4. b (Bailey 27/e p1304); 5. c; 6. d; 7. b; 8. c; 9. a; 10. b (Bailey 25/e p1213)

Grade III: 1. b (Sabiston 20/e p1300); 2. a; 3. a; 4. c (Schwartz 10/e p1244); 5. d (Bailey 27/e p1308); 6. None (Harrison 16/e p84); 7. b (Bailey 27/e p1303); 8. a; 9. b; 10. c (Bailey 27/e p1315)

MODEL QUESTIONS

Q1. The earliest symptoms in acute appendicitis are:
a. Pain b. Fever
c. Vomiting d. Rise of pulse rate

Ans. a

Q2. A patient with Crohn's disease was opened, and an inflamed appendix was found. The treatment of choice is:
a. Appendectomy
b. Ileocolic resection and anastomosis
c. Close the abdomen and start medical treatment
d. None of the above

Ans. a

Q3. The most common organism isolated from perforated appendicitis:
a. *Escherichia coli* b. *Pseudomonas*
c. *Klebsiella* d. *Enterococcus*

Ans. a

Q4. A 15-year-old boy is admitted with a history and physical finding consistent with appendicitis. Which of the following findings is most likely to be positive?
a. Pelvic crepts b. Iliopsoas sign
c. Murphy's Sign d. Flank ecchymosis

Ans. b

Q5. In appendicitis, the initial periumbilical pain is eventually localized to the right iliac fossa because of:
a. Peritoneum b. Iliopsoas
c. Colon d. Cecum

Ans. a

Q6. Which of the following organisms produces signs and symptoms that mimic acute appendicitis?
a. Enteropathic *Escherichia coli*
b. *Enterobius vermicularis*
c. *Trichomonas hominis*
d. *Yersinia enterocolitica*

Ans. d (Sabiston 20/e p1105)

Q7. The Alvarado score consists of:
a. Leucopenia
b. Anorexia
c. Diarrhea
d. Periumbilical pain

Ans. b

Q8. The most common differential diagnosis for appendicitis:

a. Gastroenteritis
b. Mesenteric lymphadenopathy
c. Intussusception
d. Meckel's diverticulitis

Ans. b

Q9. Which is the best test for the diagnosis of acute appendicitis in a pregnant female?

a. Alder's test
b. Aaron's test
c. Angell's test
d. McBurney's test

Ans. a

Q10. Which of the following is true about the appendicular mass is all, *except*?

a. Ochsner-Sherren regimen followed
b. Develops after 72 hours
c. Fever is present
d. Operation is to be done immediately

Ans. d

Q11. Grid-iron incision was first described by:

a. McArthur
b. Rutherford Morrison
c. Hamilton Bailey
d. Lanz

Ans. a (Bailey 27/e p1309)

Q12. Which of the following statements is now true of McBurney's incision?

a. Most suitable if the diagnosis of appendicitis is definite
b. If it is converted into a muscle-cutting incision, it is called Rutherford's Morison's incision
c. Inguinal hernia is a sequele of the incision
d. The incision can be extended upwards or downwards

Ans. d (Bailey 27/e p1309)

Q13. A Gridiron incision becomes a Rutherford Morison's incision is extended by:

a. Splitting the muscles laterally
b. Cutting the muscles laterally
c. Cutting the muscles medially into the rectus sheath
d. Incising vertically along the rectus muscle

Ans. b

Q14. Which one of the following is a muscle-splitting incision?

a. Kocher's
b. Rutherford-Morrison
c. Pfannenstiel
d. Lanz

Ans. d

Q15. An appendicular fistula is least likely to heal if:

a. The stump was sutured with Vicryl
b. There is stenosis/narrowing of the sigmoid colon
c. Superadded infection
d. None

Ans. b (Sabiston 20/e p1287)

Q16. Fecal fistula after appendectomy may occur due to:

a. Adhesions
b. Gangrenous appendicitis
c. Undiagnosed ileocecal disease
d. Postoperative infection

Ans. c (Bailey 27/e p1314)

Q17. Incision at McBurney's point corresponds to:

a. Tip of the appendix
b. Base of appendix
c. Midpoint of the appendix
d. Base of the cecum

Ans. b

Q18. All are true about the appendicular artery, *except*:

a. Supplies only appendix
b. Supplies the terminal ileum also
c. Is an end artery
d. Branch of the lower division of the ileocolic artery

Ans. b (Sabiston 20/e p1296)

Q19. The fold of Treves is:

a. The fold of the mucous membrane projecting into the lumen of the rectum.
b. The ilio-appendicular fold of the peritoneum.
c. The fold of the mucus membrane around the papilla of water.
d. The fold of peritoneum over the inferior mesenteric vein.

Ans. b (Sabiston 20/e p1296)

Q20. The Malone procedure is used in:

a. Anorectal incontinence
b. Urinary incontinence

c. Neurogenic bladder
d. Gastroesophageal reflux disease (GERD)

Ans. a (Bailey 27/e p137)

Q21. The most common anatomical position of the appendix is:

a. Retrocecal
b. Pelvic
c. Paracecal
d. Preileal

Ans. a

Q22. The frequent mechanism in perforation of the appendix is:

a. Impacted fecolith
b. Tension gangrene due to the accumulating secretions
c. Necrosis of the lymphoid patch
d. Retrocecal infection

Ans. b

Q23. Acute appendicitis is characterized by all of the following, *except*:

a. Anorexia
b. Rovsing's sign
c. Fever >42°C
d. Periumbilical colic

Ans. c

Q24. A 15-year-old boy is admitted with a history and physical finding consistent with appendicitis. Which of the following findings is most likely to be positive?

a. Pelvic crepts
b. Iliopsoas sign
c. Murphy's sign
d. Flank ecchymosis

Ans. b

Q25. True about the appendicular mass is all, *except*:

a. Ochsner–Sherren regime followed
b. Develops after 72 hours
c. Fever is present
d. Operation is to be done immediately

Ans. d

Q26. A Gridiron incision becomes a Rutherford Morison's incision is extended by:

(Karnataka 1994)

a. Splitting the muscle laterally
b. Cutting the muscle laterally
c. Cutting the muscle medially into the rectus sheath
d. Incising vertically along the rectus muscle

Ans. b

Q27. A 25-year-old patient presented with a mass in the RIF. Which, after laparotomy, was found to be a carcinoid of 2.5 cm in diameter. What will be the next step in management?

a. Segmental resection
b. Appendectomy
c. Right hemicolectomy
d. Do a yearly 5-HIAA assay

Ans. c

Q28. A 25-year-old man presents with a 3-day history of pain in the right lower abdomen and vomiting. The patient's general condition is satisfactory, and clinical examination reveals a tender lump in the RIF. The most appropriate management in this case would be:

a. Immediate appendectomy
b. Exploratory laparotomy
c. Ochsner–Sherren regimen
d. External drainage

Ans. c

Q29. Best treatment option for appendicular lymphoma:

a. Right hemicolectomy
b. Chemotherapy
c. Right hemicolectomy + chemotherapy
d. None

Ans. c

Q30. ALVARADO score 2 defines:

a. Temperature
b. Leukocytosis
c. Tenderness in LIF
d. Migratory pain

Ans. b

Q31. A 25-year-old female who had pain in the RIF with vomiting was managed conservatively. He was stable for 2 days, after which he had worsening of symptoms, for which extraperitoneal drainage was done by USG guidance. What is the diagnosis?

a. Perinephric abscess
b. Appendicular abscess
c. Ruptured ectopic
d. Acute cholecystitis

Ans. b

Q32. The lady is in the first trimester of pregnancy and presents to the ER with acute abdominal pain. She is diagnosed with acute appendicitis. The next step in the management will be:

a. Terminate the pregnancy
b. Give antibiotics and wait till the second trimester
c. Do appendectomy
d. Wait and watch

Ans. c

Q33. What do you do for a 2.5 cm carcinoid in the appendix?
a. Right hemicolectomy
b. Appendicectomy with yearly CT scan
c. Total colectomy with ileoanal pouch anastomosis
d. Limited colonic resection with adjuvant chemotherapy

Ans. a

Q34. In an incidental diagnosis of carcinoid of the appendix covering an area of 2.5 cm, the line of action will be:
a. Appendicectomy
b. Appendicectomy with yearly follow-up of 24 hours, estimation of HIAA
c. Appendicectomy along with right hemicolectomy
d. Appendicectomy and annual CT scan

Ans. c

Q35. When the rectum is inflated with air through a rectal tube, pain, and tenderness occur in RIF in case of appendicitis. This is known as:
a. Aaron's sign
b. Battle sign
c. Bastede's sign
d. McBurney's sign

Ans. c

Q36. All of the following are parts of prolonged antibiotic therapy in intra-abdominal sepsis, *except*:
a. Masking of general signs
b. Subacute intestinal obstruction
c. Malignant change
d. Frozen pelvis

Ans. c

Q37. Odorless peritoneal fluid is noticed in:
a. Perforated peptic ulcer
b. Perforated ileum
c. Perforated appendix
d. Tuberculosis (TB) peritonitis

Ans. a

Q38. All are useful in acute appendicitis, *except*:
a. Antibiotics
b. Analgesics
c. IV fluids
d. Purgative

Ans. d

SUGGESTED READING

1. A handbook of Appendix, Vinod Kumar Nigam, Siddharth Nigam, 1st edition.
2. Bailey & Love's - Short Practice of Surgery, 27th edition.
3. Schwartz's Principles of Surgery, 18th edition.

CHAPTER 42

Rectum

"Do not ignore the feeling of incomplete evacuation after defecation, as it may prove to be serious."

– **Vinod Kumar Nigam**

RECTUM

It starts at the level of the sacral promontory from the sigmoid colon and runs in the curve of the sacrum, ending at the anorectal junction. The puborectalis muscle encircles the rectum anteriorly and laterally, pulling it back, making an angle of 120° **(Figs. 1A to C)**.

The rectum is about 16 cm long and has three parts: The upper one-third, which is covered by peritoneum anteriorly and laterally, the middle one-third, which is covered by peritoneum anteriorly and partly laterally, and the lower one-third is not covered by peritoneum as it is below the peritoneal reflection.

Rectum is separated anteriorly from prostate/vagina by Denonvilliers (Charles Pierre Denonvilliers, 1808–1872, French anatomist) fascia and posterity from lower sacrum and coccyx by Waldeyer's (Heinrich Wilhelm Gottfried Waldeyer-Hartz, 1836–1921, German anatomist) fascia. The rectum has three lateral curves: The upper and lower are on the right side, and the middle is on the left side. These curves appear as semicircular folds when looked

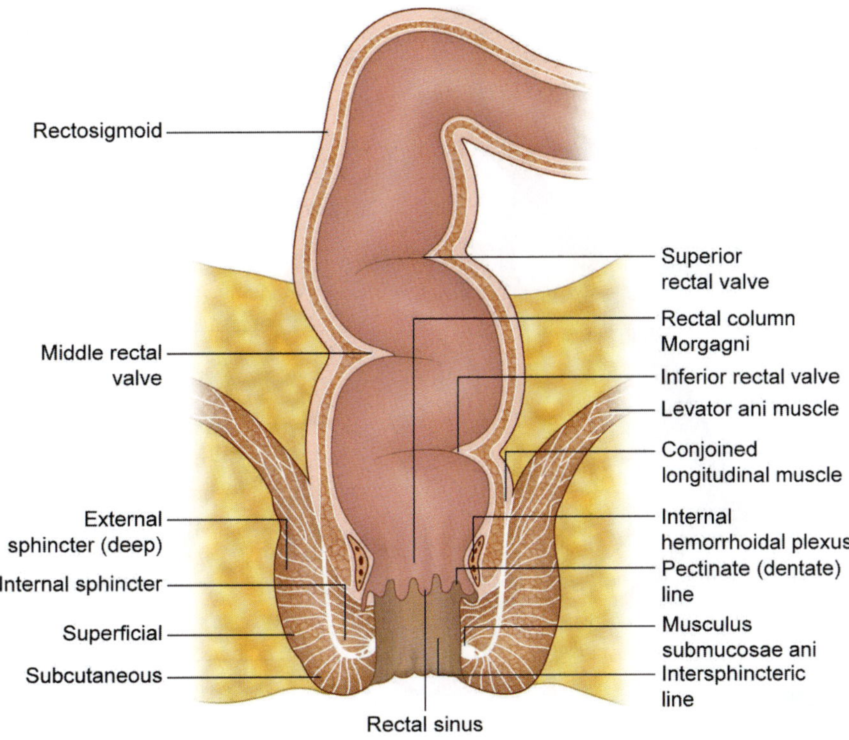

Fig. 1A

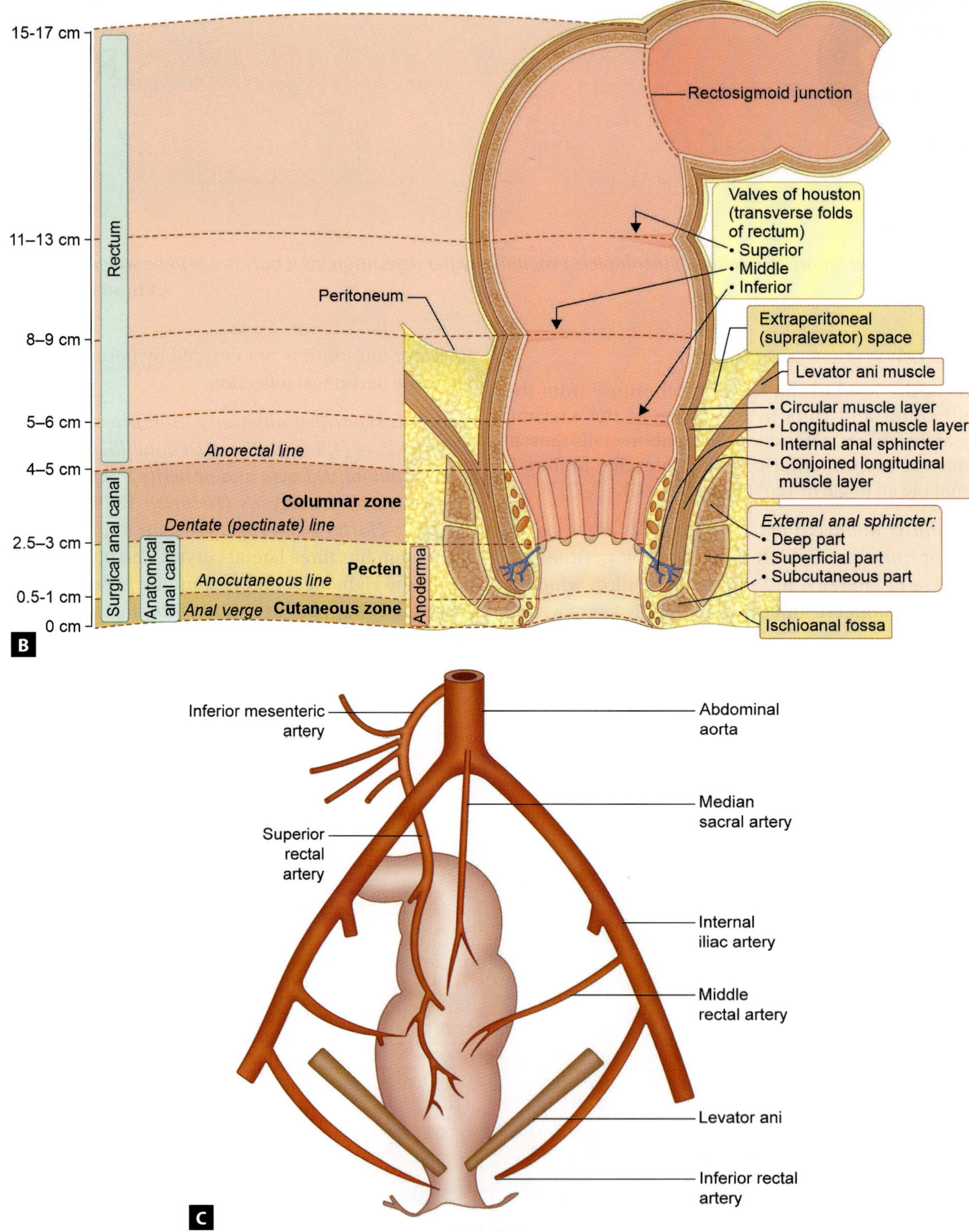

Figs. 1B and C

Figs. 1A to C: Anatomy of the rectum and anal canal.

from the lumen, called *Houston's (John Houston, 1802–1845, English physician) valves.*

> *Points to remember:*
> *Solitary rectal ulcer syndrome (SRUS)*: It is situated in the anterior or anterolateral wall of the rectum. It is more common in women, and only half of the patients have a real ulcer; and others have only erythema. It is caused by increased intraluminal rectal pressure, seen in intense cases and polyps. Mucosal hyperplasia is common. It is common in young woman who strains on defecation and has rectal bleeding. Defecography diagnoses it and is treated by dedicated training and a high-fiber diet.

Blood supply to the rectum is from the superior rectal artery direct continuation of the inferior mesenteric artery (IMA), the middle rectal artery, arising from an internal iliac artery, and the inferior rectal artery from an internal pudendal artery, which runs on the inferior surface of the levator ani muscle. Most of the blood supply is from the superior rectal arteries. The part of the rectum above the dentate line is drained by the superior hemorrhoidal vein to the portal system via the inferior mesenteric vein (IMV). Lymphatic drainage is mostly upward to lymph nodes (LNs) around the superior rectal artery **(Figs. 2A to C)**.

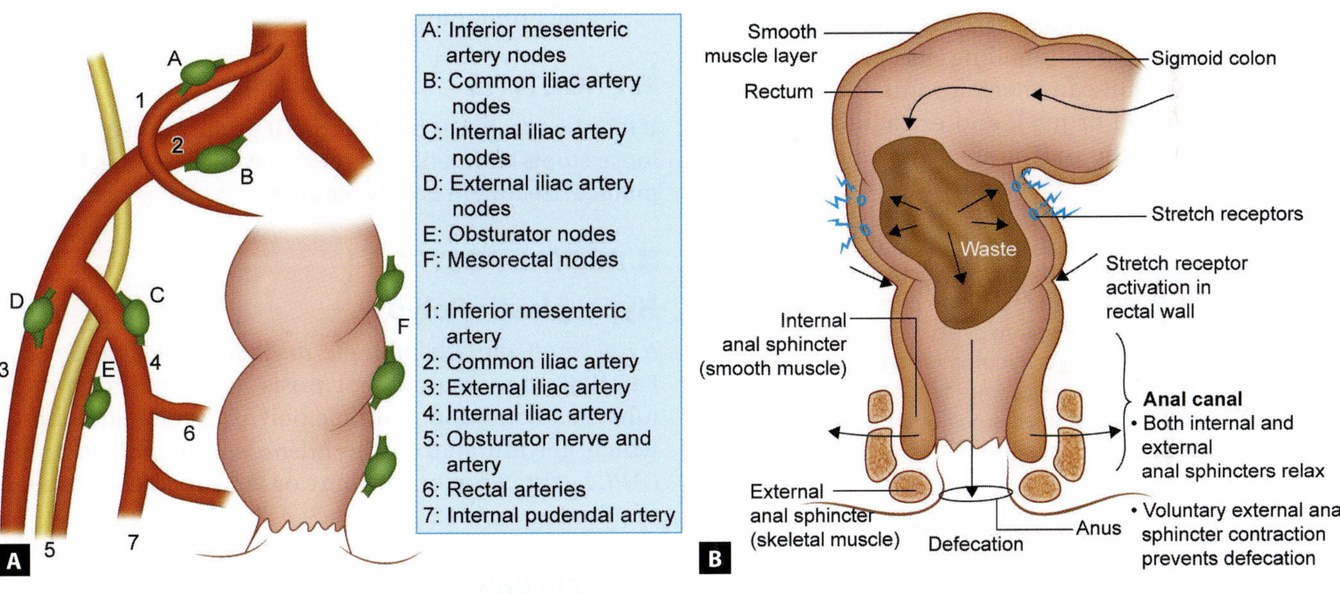

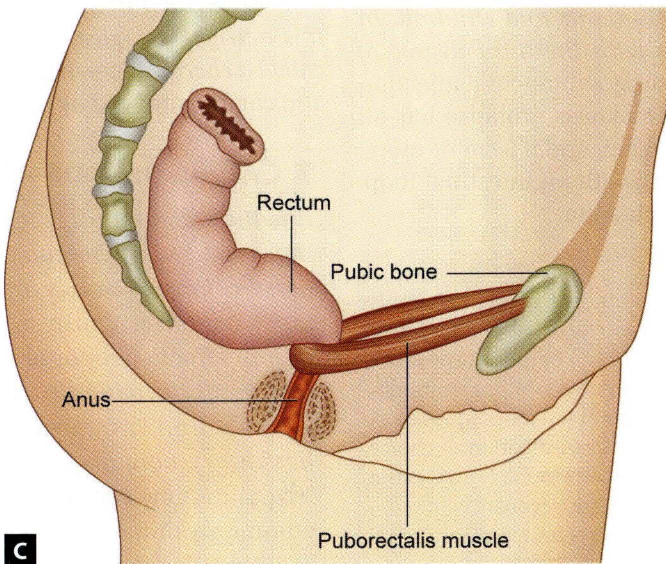

Figs. 2A to C: Lymphatic drainage of the rectum and the mechanism of defecation.

Clinical symptoms of rectal disease:
- Altered bowel habits, i.e., constipation
- Pain (proctalgia)
- Bleeding per rectum—it is fresh blood
- Prolapse
- Mucus discharges
- Tenesmus

TENESMUS

Tenesmus is the feeling of incomplete evacuation, which is an important symptom in cancer of the rectum. Proctalgia is episodic pain due to the spasm of the levator ani muscle. Examination of rectum is done in left lateral position of *Sims (James Marion Sims, 1813–1883, American gynecological surgeon)* by digital rectal examination (DRE), inspection of anal and surrounding area, proctoscopy, and sigmoidoscopy. DRE can check for intramural (tumor), intraluminal (blood or pus), and extramural (prostate) lesions. Lesions of the wall of the rectum can be fixed or mobile.

Not to forget:
Sense of incomplete evacuation: The patient feels that the rectum is not emptied completely, and he has to pass more stool. It is a very important and early symptom of a tumor of the rectum and is almost always present in carcinoma of the lower part of the rectum. The patient goes several times to the toilet to pass stool, and sometimes a blood-stained small quantity is passed only with flatus (bloody slime).

RECTAL MUCOSAL PROLAPSE

It is usually up to 1–4 cm in length, has mucosa and submucosa, and is common in infants and children. In adults, it is mostly associated with the third degree of hemorrhoids. Treatment is banding, submucosal injection of phenol, and excision. Full thickness prolapse has all layers of the rectal wall and is >4 cm, and if 5 cm or more, then it contains a peritoneal sac with an intestinal loop. Complete prolapse is called procidentia.

You may be asked:
The most common symptom of carcinoma of the rectum is bleeding per rectum, the most common site of lymphatic spread is inguinal LNs, and the most common site of metastasis is the lung. Weight loss is a feature of liver metastasis. Most commonly, the symptoms of carcinoma of the rectum are misdiagnosed as hemorrhoids. Sigmoidoscopy is the first investigation of choice in carcinoma of the rectum. Transrectal ultrasound (TRUS) is the best test for diagnosing T staging. Magnetic resonance imaging (MRI), specifically the endorectal coil type, is best to diagnose LN involvement.

Treatment

Treatment of rectal prolapse can be done by:
- Thiersch (Karl Thiersch, 1822–1895, German surgeon) operation—a sting of steel wire nylon is applied
- Delorme's (Edmond Delorme, 1847–1929, French surgeon) operation—rectal mucosa is stripped over prolapse, and the underlying muscle is plicated, and the mucosa is sutured.
- Altemeier's (William Altemeier, 1910–1983, American surgeon) operation–the prolapse is excised, and continuity is maintained by stapling or suturing.
- Abdominal rectopexy—a mesh is anchored with the anterior surface of the rectum and suspended from the sacral promontory by sutures.

PROCTITIS

It may be specific or nonspecific. It usually causes frequent loose stools with tenesmus and may be bleeding. Usually, medical treatment is only required.

RECTAL POLYPS

Hyperplastic Polyp

It is a small, pinkish, multiple, and usually harmless polyp. Familial adenomatous polyposis-autosomal dominant inherited condition, multiple polyps develop at puberty, which get mutated in the *adenomatous polyposis coli (APC)* gene. Proctocolectomy or panproctocolectomy is required.

Juvenile Polyp

It is a bright red, glistening tumor in children and infants called a cherry tumor. It has almost no malignant tendency and can be removed by snare.

CARCINOMA OF RECTUM

It is the second most common malignancy worldwide, the second most common cancer in women, the third most common cancer among men, and the fourth most common cause of death by cancer. It commonly affects people older than 70 years of age and commonly originates from premalignant lesions of the rectum. The most common hereditary type is *hereditary nonpolyposis colorectal cancer (HNPCC)*. The mutations can be congenital or acquired, and the commonly mutated gene is *APC*. Mutations in the gene *TP53* are also common.

Clinical Features

- Bleeding is the most common and earliest symptom.
- Tenesmus
- Alteration of bowel habits—early morning bloody diarrhea
- Pain is a late symptom.
- Weight loss is also a late symptom.

Investigations

- Abdominal examination may show distension due to stricture.
- DRE
- Sigmoidoscopy
- Colonoscopy
- Computed tomography (CT) scan

Spread

- *Local*: It is more common in circumferential than longitudinal way.
- *Lymphatic*: It mostly goes up to LNs around main arteries.
- Venous—to liver, lung, etc.
- Peritoneal dissemination

Stages

Dukes Staging

- Limited to the rectal wall, prognosis is excellent, and >90% 5-year survival
- Extension to extrarectal tissue but no metastasis in regional LNs—70% 5-year survival
- LNs are involved, C1—local pararectal LNs only, C2—LNs + distant metastasis, 40% survival 5 years

Tumor, Node, and Metastasis or Radiological Staging

Magnetic resonance imaging is the best tool to stage: Tx, T0, Tis, T1, T2, T3, T4a, T4b, Nx, N0, N1, N2, M0, M1, M1a, and M1b.

> *Good to remember*:
> Low anterior resection, which is a sphincter-saving operation in carcinoma of the rectum, is advised for tumors in the proximal two-thirds of the rectum. The tumor must be located at least 5 cm above anal verge whereas *abdominoperineal resection (APR)* is advised for lower 5 cm of rectum. *Hartmann's procedure is good for elderly patients who are unable to tolerate anterior resection or APR.*

Histological Grading

- Well differentiated—less aggressive
- Undifferentiated—more aggressive

Treatment

It is based on physical fitness for operation and the extent of spread of the tumor. Radical excision of the rectum and associated LNs should be the principle. Anterior resection (Hartmann's procedure) is now done with sphincter-saving surgery. Transanal total mesorectal excision (taTME) is done to reduce the trauma of anterior resection.

Abdominal Excision of the Rectum

Abdominal excision (APR)—Miles operation: Usually, two surgeons operate simultaneously, one on the abdomen and the other at the perineum. Nowadays, the first abdominal part is done, then the perineal part. The first position of the patient is in *Lloyd-Davies (Oswald Vaughan Lloyd-Davies, 1905-1987, British surgeon),* then in the jack-knife position, the Trendelenburg (Friedrich Trendelenburg, 1844–1924, German surgeon, described in 1885) position is used for the abdominal part of surgery also. Liver resection of secondaries is now done with low morbidity and mortality.

Radiotherapy

Adjuvant radiotherapy is given pre- and postoperatively.

Chemotherapy

It is given alone postoperatively to reduce dissemination and also in combination with radiotherapy-chemoradiotherapy.

Some important points:

- The most common symptom of carcinoma of the rectum is bleeding per rectum.
- The earliest symptom of carcinoma of the rectum is bleeding per rectum.
- The most common site of colorectal carcinoma is the rectum.
- The most common variety of carcinoma of the rectum is adenocarcinoma.
- The most common organ for distant metastasis in carcinoma of the rectum is the liver.
- Features of incomplete evacuation are tenesmus, spurious diarrhea, and bloody slime (passage of blood-stained mucus with flatus).
- Backache indicates a tumor invading the sacral plexus.

- Weight loss indicates liver metastasis.
- Investigation of choice for carcinoma of the rectum is sigmoidoscopy.
- The best investigation to check metastasis is contrast-enhanced computed tomography (CECT).

SOME IMPORTANT QUESTIONS

Q1. Regarding villous adenoma, all are true, *except*:

a. Dysentery
b. Watery diarrhea
c. Hypokalemia
d. Constipation

Ans. a

Q2. Rectal polyps usually present with:

a. Obstruction
b. Perforation
c. Bleeding
d. Malignant change

Ans. c

Q3. Dukes' A stage of rectal carcinoma is managed by:

a. Surgical resection only
b. Surgical resection + selective adjuvant chemotherapy
c. Surgical resection + routine adjuvant chemotherapy
d. Chemotherapy primarily

Ans. a

Q4. A patient with carcinoma of rectum which is 5 cm from anal verge, which procedure you will prefer to perform?

a. Anterior resection
b. Abdominoperineal resection
c. Hartman's procedure
d. Defunctioning colostomy

Ans. b

Q5. Which of the following is more aggressive rectal carcinoma?

a. Adenocarcinoma
b. Secondary mucoid carcinoma
c. Signet ring carcinoma
d. Squamous cell carcinoma

Ans. c

Q6. All are true regarding solitary rectal ulcer syndrome, *except*:

a. Usually in the anterior wall
b. Associated with rectal prolapse
c. Usually malignant
d. Bowel training helps a lot

Ans. c

Q7. Rectal prolapse is common in:

a. 1–3 months
b. 3–5 months
c. 5–8 months
d. 8–12 months

Ans. d

Q8. Delorme's procedure is used for:

a. Rectal prolapse
b. Solitary rectal ulcer
c. Rectal bilharziasis
d. Proctalgia fugax

Ans. a

MULTIPLE CHOICE QUESTIONS

Grade I	Simple

Q1. Rectal adenoma is associated with: **(JIPMER 2003)**

a. *Familial polyposis coli*
b. Hypokalemia
c. Intussusception
d. Hemorrhoids

Q2. A toddler has a few drops of blood coming out of the rectum. Probable diagnosis is: **(AIIMS May 2013)**

a. Juvenile rectal polyp
b. Adenomatous polyposis cell
c. Rectal ulcer
d. Piles

Q3. Local excision in cancer (CA) of the rectum is done in all *except*: **(AIIMS GIS Dec 2009)**

a. Within 6 cm of anal verge
b. Lesion <4 cm
c. Involvement of <40% circumference
d. T1 and T2 cancer with or without lymph node involvement

Q4. In rectal carcinoma, the distal margin should be at least: **(PGI SS June 2001)**

a. 2 cm
b. 3 cm
c. 4 cm
d. 5 cm

Q5. True about surgical treatment of rectal cancer: **(PGI SS December 2009)**

a. Irrigation of divided bowel ends with cytotoxic solution may reduce local true recurrence.
b. Intramural spread is commonly >4 cm.
c. A minimum of 5 cm distal resection margin is required.
d. The mesorectum is devoid of lymph nodes.

Q6. Which of the following is the investigation of choice for assessment of depth of penetration and perirectal nodes in rectal cancer? (AIIMS November 2004)

a. Transrectal ultrasound
b. Computed tomography (CT) scan pelvis
c. Magnetic resonance imaging (MRI) scan
d. Double contrast barium enema

Q7. Vimal, a 70-year-old male, presents with a history of lower gastrointestinal (GI) bleed for the last 6 months. Sigmoidoscopic examination shows a mass of 4 cm about 3.5 cm above the anal verge. The treatment of choice is: (AIIMS June 2001)

a. Colostomy
b. Anterior resection
c. Abdominoperineal resection
d. Defunctioning anastomosis

Q8. The most common presentation of CA rectum is: (JIMPER 2012)

a. Diarrhea
b. Constipation
c. Bleeding per rectum (P/R)
d. Feeling of incomplete defecation

Q9. Sphincter-saving surgery for rectal malignancy is not done in: (PGI December 2001)

a. Age over 50 years
b. Lymph node involvement
c. Infiltration of lamina propria
d. >4 cm from and verge
e. High-grade tumor

Q10. In which case anterior resection is the method of treatment? (AIIMS February 1997)

a. CA sigmoid colon
b. CA rectum
c. CA colon
d. CA anal canal

Grade II	*Difficult*

Q1. Prognosis for carcinoma rectum is best assessed by: (AIIMS 1987)

a. Site of tumor
b. Histological grading
c. Size of tumors
d. Duration of the symptoms

Q2. The best procedure in midrectal carcinoma is: (AIIMS 1992)

a. Abdominoperineal resection
b. Anterior resection
c. Perineal loop
d. Transverse colostomy

Q3. Ideal management in an old and frail patient presenting with a mass situated 15 cm away from anal orifice: (MCI March 2005)

a. Abdominoperineal resection
b. Colonoscopic removal
c. Hartmann's operation
d. Anterior resection

Q4. Aim of surgery in carcinoma rectum is: (MCI March 2010)

a. Limited excision of the rectum
b. Sacrificing gastrointestinal continuity
c. Preserving the anal sphincter
d. Preserving mesorectum

Q5. Colitis cystic profunda is seen in case of: (AIIMS GIS December 2009)

a. SRUS
b. Rectal carcinoma
c. Rectocele
d. Fissure

Q6. Most common site of solitary rectal ulcer syndrome (SRUS): (GB Pant 2011)

a. Posterior, 7–10 cm from anal verge
b. Anterior, 7–10 cm from anal verge
c. Posterior, 2–3 cm from anal verge
d. Anterior, 2–3 cm from anal verge

Q7. Treatment of solitary rectal ulcer are all, *except*: (PGI December 2007)

a. Laxatives
b. Rectopexy
c. Banding
d. Sclerosant injection
e. Enema

Q8. Treatment of rectal prolapse in childhood is: (AIIMS June 1994)

a. Lahaut's operation
b. Incision of prolapsed mucosa
c. Thiersch wiring
d. Ripstein operation

Q9. A 30-year-old male presents with complete rectal prolapse. Which of the following procedures is associated with the lowest risk of recurrence? (All India 2012)

a. Delorme's procedure
b. Thiersch procedure
c. Abdominal rectopexy
d. Altemeier's procedure

Q10. All are true about TME for CA rectum, *except*: (AIIMS GIS Dec 2009)

a. Decreases local recurrence
b. Decreases the incidence of impotence
c. Decreases incidence of bladder dysfunction
d. Decreases survival

Grade III	*Most difficult*

Q1. Resting tone of rectum is decreased in all, *except*: (All India 1991)

a. Micturition
b. Retained feces in the rectum
c. Prolapse rectum
d. Trauma involving the perineum

Q2. Which of the following statements about the valves of Houston is true? (All India 2012)

a. The middle valve corresponds to the middle convex fold to the right.
b. The upper valve corresponds to the peritoneal reflection
c. The valve contains all three layers of muscle wall
d. Valves disappear after the mobilization of the rectum

Q3. In an adult male, on per rectal examination, the following structures can be felt anteriorly, *except*: (All India 2005)

a. Internal iliac lymph nodes
b. Bulb of the penis
c. Prostate
d. Seminal vesicle, when enlarged

Q4. The following are important in the maintenance of normal fecal continence *except*: (All India 1995)

a. Anorectal angulation
b. Rectal innervations
c. Internal sphincter
d. Haustral valve

Q5. Which of the following is not a component of the anorectal ring? (AIIMS May 2013)

a. External anal sphincter
b. Puborectalis
c. Anococcygeal raphe
d. Internal and sphincter

Q6. External anal sphincter is innervated by: (AIIMS November 2013)

a. S2, S3, S4
b. S2, S3
c. L5, S1
d. L2, L3

Q7. Bleeding per rectum is present in all, *except*: (AIIMS June 1994)

a. Meckel's diverticulum
b. Sigmoid volvulus
c. Carcinoma rectum
d. Ulcerative colitis

Q8. In the CA rectum, preoperatively: (AIIMS GIS Dec 2009)

a. Only RT is given
b. Only chemotherapy is given
c. Chemoradiation is given
d. Chemoradiation is given postoperatively only

Q9. All are true about rectal cancer, *except*: (JIPMER GIS 2011)

a. The most common symptom is hematochezia.
b. The precise location of the tumor is done with rigid proctosigmoidoscopy.
c. Dissection lateral to the endopelvic fascia investing the mesorectum causes local recurrence
d. Radiation dose is 60 Gray

Q10. False about an indication of local resection in CA rectum: (AIIMS GIS 2003)

a. T2N0, T1N1
b. <10 cm from anal verge
c. <4 cm or <40% of circumference involved
d. Well differentiated with no LN involvement

ANSWERS

Grade I: 1. b; 2. a; 3. b, c, d (Sabiston 20/e p1379); 4. a (Schwartz 9/r p1050); 5. a (Bailey 25/e p1236); 6. c (Sabiston 20/e p1378); 7. c; 8. c; 9. d; 10. b

Grade II: 1. b (Sabiston 20/e p1377); 2. b; 3. c; 4. c; 5. a (Bailey 27/e p1324); 6. b; 7. c, d; 8. c; 9. c; 10. d (Schwartz 10/e p1203-1216)

Grade III: 1. b; 2. d (Sabiston 20/e p1394); 3. a; 4. d (Bailey 27/e p1339); 5. c; 6. a; 7. b; 8. c (Bailey 27/e p1337); 9. c; 10. a

MODEL QUESTIONS

Q1. The most common cause of anorectal abscess is:
- a. Inflammation of anal gland
- b. Folliculitis
- c. Inflammation of the rectal mucosa
- d. Rectum

Ans. a

Q2. The length of a standard proctoscope is:
- a. 4″
- b. 6″
- c. 8″
- d. 3″

Ans. a

Q3. The internal sphincter of the rectum is formed by:
- a. Levator ani
- b. Puborectalis
- c. Longitudinal muscle fibers condensation
- d. Circular muscle fiber condensation

Ans. d

Q4. What is false regarding the dentate line?
- a. Glands of Morgagni open below the line
- b. Anal glands open at the line
- c. The dentate line lies 2 cm above the anal verge
- d. The transitional epithelium lies above the dentate line

Ans. d

Q5. True statement about the upper half of anal canal is:
- a. Insensitive to pain
- b. Drained by superficial inguinal lymph node
- c. Lined by squamous epithelium
- d. Supplied by the superior mesenteric artery

Ans. a

Q6. A patient with external hemorrhoids develops pain while passing stools. The nerve mediating this pain is:
- a. Hypogastric nerve
- b. Pudendal nerve
- c. Splanchnic visceral nerve
- d. Sympathetic plexus

Ans. b

Q7. Dentate line measurement from anal margin:
- a. 1 cm
- b. 1.5 cm
- c. 2 cm
- d. 2.5 cm

Ans. c

Q8. Hemangioma of the rectum:
- a. Common tumor
- b. Fetal hemorrhage seen
- c. Ulcerative colitis-like symptoms seen
- d. None

Ans. b and c

SUGGESTED READING

1. Bailey & Love's - Short Practice of Surgery, 27th edition.
2. Schwartz's Principles of Surgery, 18th edition.
3. Textbook of Surgery by David Sabiston, 21st edition.

CHAPTER 43

Anus and Anal Canal

"Clinton Mitchell of Illinois, USA, was the first to use carbolic acid for injecting hemorrhoids."
– **Bailey & Love** *(Short Practice of Surgery, 27th Edition)*

ANUS AND ANAL CANAL

Anal canal is approximately 4 cm in length, starting from where the rectum passes through the pelvic diaphragm, the anorectal junction to anal verge. The anorectal ring can be palpated as a thick ring.

ANORECTAL RING

It is made by amalgamating the four structures:

- Puborectalis muscle
- Deep external sphincter
- Conjoined longitudinal muscle
- The highest part of the internal sphincter

Puborectalis Muscle

It is a part of the pelvic diaphragm and makes an angle between the all canal and rectum, so it plays a role in the process of continence mechanism. The external sphincter is actually a single muscle but is divided into deep, superficial, and subcutaneous divisions by laterals from the longitudinal muscle layer. Some of its fibers from the posterior are attached to the coccyx, and some anteriorly with the perineal muscles. It is a skeletal muscle and is underrated by the pudendal nerve (**Figs. 1A to C**).

Internal Sphincter

It is a continuation of the circular muscle of the rectum. It is an involuntary muscle that starts from where the rectum passes through pelvic diaphragm to above anal verge. Its lower border is palpable at the intersphincteric groove. It is pearly white in color, innervated by the autonomic nervous system, and receives intrinsic nonadrenogenic and noncholinergic fibers (NANCs), which, if stimulated, cause release of neurotransmitter nitric oxide and cause internal sphincter relaxation.

Points to remember:
The intersphincteric plane is a potential space between external anal sphincter and longitudinal muscle. It is important as it contains anal glands, which are the source of pus when get infected and pus travels up, down, and laterally causing perineal, ischiorectal, and supralevator abscesses. During defecation, the contraction of the longitudinal muscle of rectum and anal canal widens anal canal, flattens anal cushions, shortens anal canal, and everts anal margin, and relaxation allows the anal cushions to distend to make an airtight seal. The pink mucous membrane of the rectum goes down and becomes red. The dentate line is an important landmark as it is the site of proradium and the postallantoic gut. Columns of Morgagni and anal sinuses end here with anal crypts, which are at lower ends of columns of Morgagni as pockets for anal duct openings.

BLOOD SUPPLY

It is through the superior, middle, and inferior rectal arteries. The superior rectal artery divides into right and left branches. The right branch further down divides into anterior and posterior branches; the left branch does not divide and continues down. These three arteries depict the sites of three primary hemorrhoids, at 3, 7, and 11 o'clock positions. The venous drainage is by the superior, middle, and inferior rectal veins. Lymphatic drainage of the upper half goes to parasitic lymph nodes (LNs).

PHYSIOLOGY OF ANUS AND ANAL CANAL

Anal continence is a complex process, with the combined efforts of nerves (cerebral, autonomic, and enteric nerves), gastrointestinal tract (GIT), pelvic floor and sphincters **(Flowchart 1) (Figs. 2A and B)**. Sphincters provide vital help in maintaining continence and defecation, which can be tested by an enrolment ultrasound. Conduction velocity through the pudendal nerve can be estimated for neuromuscular function. Dynamics of defecation can be assessed radiologically by evacuation proctography **(Figs. 3A to C)**.

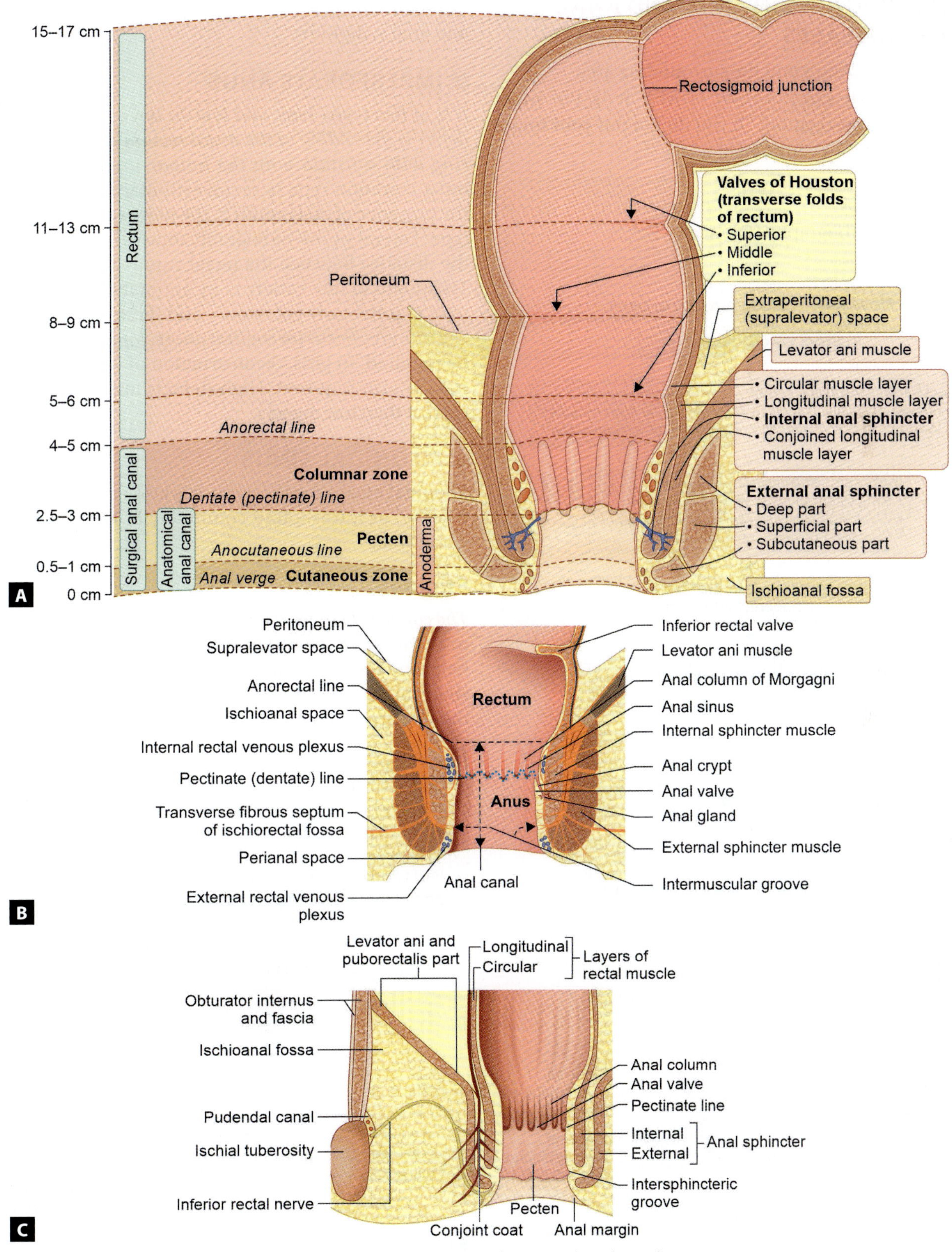

Figs. 1A to C: Anatomy of anus and anal canal.

INVESTIGATIONS IN ANUS AND ANAL CANAL DISEASES

- Inspection of Anu's and the surrounding area
- *Digital rectal examination (DRE):* It is the most important investigation. "If you do not put your finger in, you might put your foot in it."
- Proctoscopy
- Sigmoidoscopy
- Computed tomography (CT) scan

Flowchart 1: Algorithm of anal canal.

Stool enters the rectum

↓

Rectoanal inhibitory reflex
- Closure of glottis and contraction of pelvic floor muscles
- Contraction of diaphragm and abdominal wall muscles

↓

Increased abdominal pressure
- Relaxation of internal anal sphincter
- Contraction of external anal sphincter
- Sampling of anal canal contents

↓

Increased anorectal angle
Relaxation of puborectalis muscle

↓

Anal canal widening
Relaxation of puborectalis and external anal sphincter muscles

↓

Pelvic floor descent (<2 cm)

↓

Evacuation of contents

↓

Closing reflex
- Pelvic floor rises
- Rebound sphincter contraction occurs

Sigmoidoscopy must be done in every case of rectal and anal symptoms.

IMPERFORATE ANUS

It is of two types, high and low. In boys, the most common defect is the ending of the distal rectum at the puborectalis ring with a fistula with the bulbar urethra. In girls, the most common type is rectovestibular fistula. Clinically, the presence of meconium in the perineum indicates a low type. Lateral prone radiograph shows the air, which gives the distance between the rectal stump and the perineum. Treatment of low variety is by anomaly. Complex variety may require early colostomy and definitive surgery after 7–8 months. *Posterior sagittal anorectoplasty (PSARP)* may be required. In girls, reconstruction of vagina and urinary tract is also required. High defects are more difficult to correct than low defects.

PILONIDAL SINUS

Pilonidal means nest of hairs, it is also called "jeep driver's disease" as it was found commonly in Jeep drivers in the world wall.

Etiology

The congenital theory has been rejected now and confirmed as an acquired condition. The buttock friction breaks the hairs and they get collected there, and the buttock friction, shearing strain, and so created negative pressure drills these sharp hairs through the skin.

> *Not to forget*:
> Proctoscopy can examine lower 8–10 cm of rectum and anal canal, flexible sigmoidoscopy 60 cm, and colonoscopy 160 cm.
> Parts of anal canal above and below dentate line are different in various ways:
> - Parts above the dentate line are derived from the primitive anorectal canal, and parts below from the proctodeum.

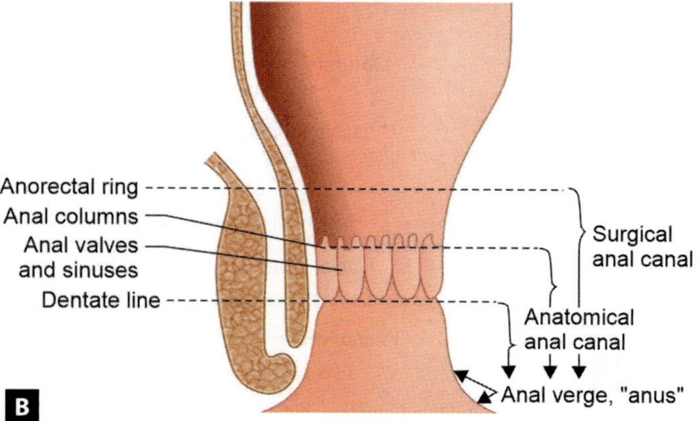

Figs. 2A and B: Anatomy, physiology, and types of anal canal.

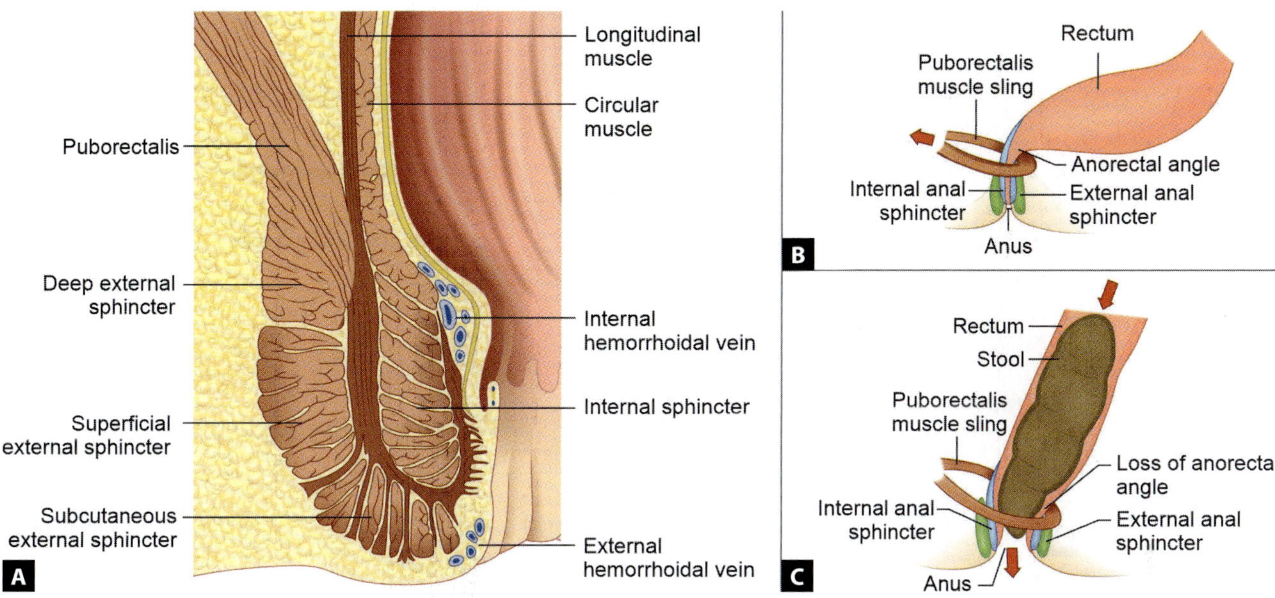

Figs. 3A to C: Physiology of defecation.

- Parts above receive autonomic nerve supply, and parts below by somatic (inferior rectal nerves).
- Blood supply from the superior rectal artery for parts above the line and by the inferior rectal artery parts below the line
- Lymphatic drainage to internal iliac LNs from above and to superficial inguinal LNs from below the line
- Lesions are painful above the line and painless below the line.

Clinical Features

Intermittent painful swelling, which ruptures with discharge, is the history from the patient.

Treatment

The open method removes all sinus tracks, and the wound is left open to heal, to avoid recurrence, which is common. In the close method, after removal of sinus tracks, the wound is closed in several layers to avoid recurrence.

ANAL INCONTINENCE

It can happen due to old age or after injury or surgery (abdominal, spinal, and pelvic) commonly, but various causes can be there: Congenital, cardiovascular system (CVS), diabetes, psychological issues, certain drugs, and Parkinson's disease. Treatment can be done by operations to strengthen the sphincter or unite the divided sphincter.

Fissure-In-Ano or Anal Fissure

It is a longitudinal ulcer or split in the anoderm extending from anal verge to up but not beyond dentate line. It is caused by trauma from hard stool in constipation. Clinically, a patient has severe pain during defecation and may be bleeding. Posterior fissures are more common than anterior fissures, and anterior fissures are more common in women. Treatment requires laxatives to avoid constipation and analgesics with *glyceryl trinitrate (GTN)* cream to reduce spasm, pain, and promote healing by increasing vascular perfusion, duties cream 2% is used twice a day. Lateral sphincterotomy or anal advancement flap is required as surgical procedure.

HEMORRHOIDS

The word hemorrhoid is taken from the Greek and Latin languages, haima = blood, rhoos = flowing from Greek, and oils = a ball for piles from Latin. Hemorrhoids are internal and external, external from inferior hemorrhoids plexus deep in the skin around anal verge and these are not true hemorrhoids **(Figs. 4A and B)**.

Causes of Hemorrhoids

- Constipation is the main culprit, especially habitual.
- Hypotonic anal sphincter.
- Pelvic problems as gravity uterus, big fibroids, and ovarian cancer.
- Neurological disorders as paraplegia and multiple sclerosis.

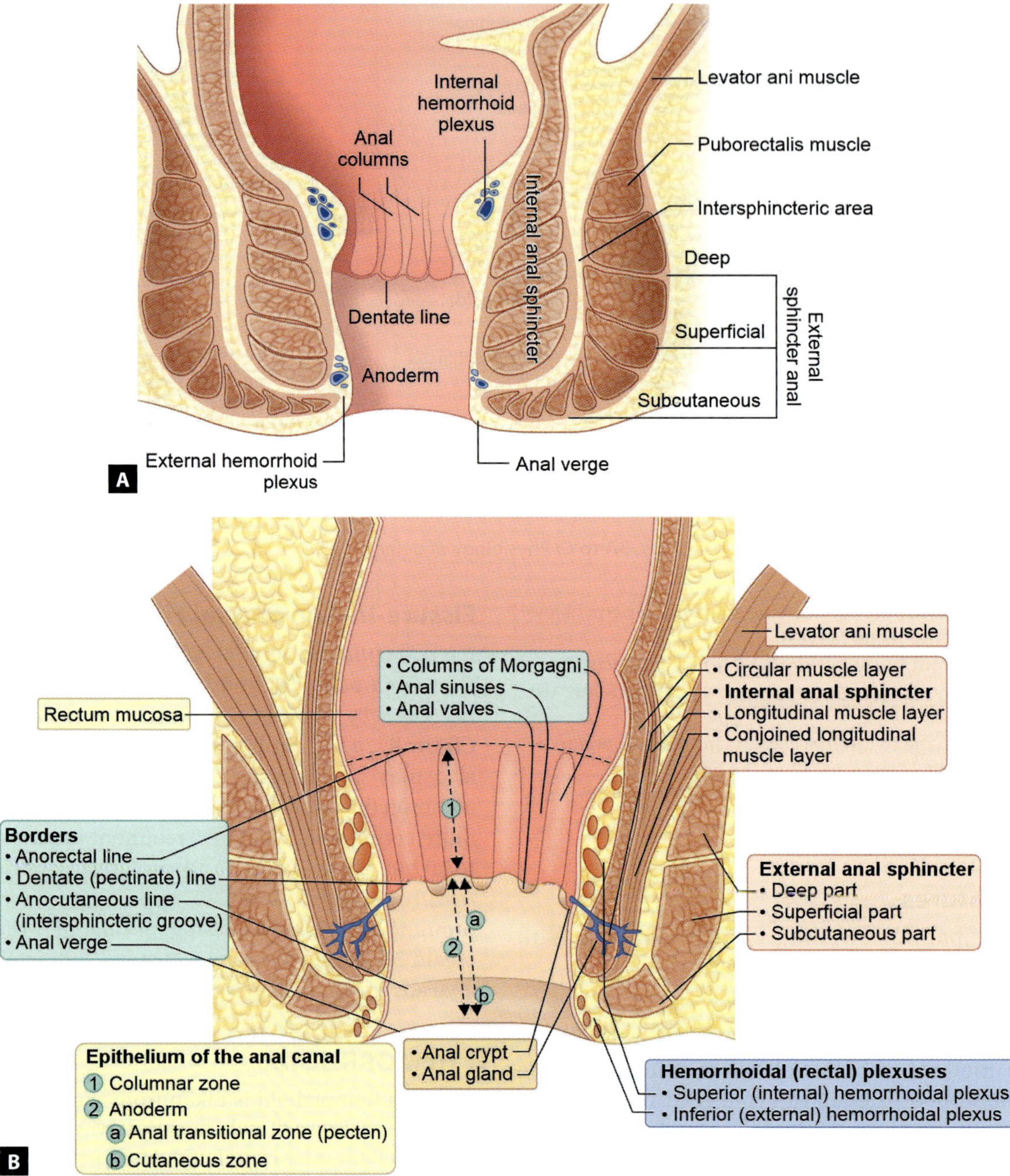

Figs. 4A and B: Anatomy and physiology of anal canal and hemorrhoids.

You may be asked:
Pruritus ani:

- It is severe itching around anus.
- Skin becomes reddened, moist, and cracked. Causes are: lack of personal hygiene and cleanliness, fissures and fistula, discharge anal or personal, parasites, allergy, infection, psychological problems, and diabetes. It is treated by hygiene correction and local application of antiallergic and hydrocortisone cream. The most common site of fissure in ano is the 6 o'clock position in midline posteriorly, but during pregnancy, on anteriorly, while in Crohn's disease, it may occur laterally. The chronic fissures have a protective anal tag, hypertrophied anal papilla, and deep canoe-shaped ulcer. The most common site of colorectal carcinoma is the rectum, the most common type is adenocarcinoma, and the most common site of metastasis is the liver.

Clinical Features

They are asymptomatic or symptomatic and occur when intraluminal pressure is raised, as in constipation and pregnancy. They are present at 3, 7, and 11 o' clock positions; with bright red painless bleeding, they can prolapse and look as lumps at anal verge.

Hemorrhoids are of four degrees:
- *First degree*—bleeding only without any prolapse.
- *Second degree*—prolapse but gets reduced by itself spontaneously.
- *Third degree*—prolapse is there, but the hemorrhoid has to be reduced manually.
- *Fourth degree*—prolapsed permanently and cannot be reduced.

Complications

- Thrombosis
- Strangulation
- Ulcerations
- Gangrene
- Fibrosis
- Portal pyemia

Conservative Treatment

- Conservative treatment includes training for normalization of bowel habits and defecation and laxatives.
- Phenol injection in hemorrhoids.

Stapled hemorrhoidopexy—Antonio Longo, Italian surgeon, developed this technique of preserving anal cushions but getting relief with a stapling gum.

Hemorrhoidectomy—open or close? In the close method, the wound is covered with mucosa.

- Open technique is called the Milligan-Morgan technique, and the close technique is called the Ferguson technique.

Good to remember:
Paget's disease of anal canal: It is one of the common sites of extramammary Paget's disease, common in females of about 65 years age, in females common in vulva and usually found in hair bearing areas. It clinically looks like pruritic, erythematous plaques, with ulcerations and serous discharge. Treatment is a wide excision. The endorectal coil magnetic resonance imaging (MRI) is a good predictor of LN involvement and overall staging. It identifies the involvement of LNs due to their characteristic features on MRI. In colorectal carcinoma, the size of the tumor, duration of symptoms, and whether endophytic or exophytic do not influence the prognosis. Dentate line is situated between upper and middle parts of anal canal.

A white line of Hilton lies between the middle and lower parts. Valves of Houston have no specific function. Full surgical mobilization of the rectum can gain 5 cm in length. Resting pressure due to the internal sphincter is 90 cmH_2O. The contraction of external anal sphincter and puborectalis muscle cause squeeze pressure. The pressure difference between pressure in rectum and anal canal helps maintain continence. Anorectal angle acts like a flap valve or a sphincter.

Complications of Hemorrhoidectomy

- Pain
- Bleeding
- Urinary retention
- Incontinence
- Fissure
- Stricture

ANORECTAL ABSCESSES

According to a cryptoglandular theory, the intersphincteric anal glands get infected, and pus is formed which travels down to form perianal abscess and travelling laterally forms ischiorectal abscess and if travels up then forms supralevator inter muscular or pararectal abscess. It presents as a painful, red, hot, and tender perianal swelling. Treatment is incision and drainage with removal of the skin square.

FISTULA-IN-ANO

It is a chronic abnormal communication between anal lumen and skin **(Figs. 5A to C)**. Most fistulae are idiopathic or nonspecific, but some are due to other conditions such as tuberculosis (TB), malignancy, Crohn's disease, etc. Clinically, there is intermittent pus discharge.

Classification

Park's classification:
- *Type 1*—intersphincteric fistula—most common
- *Type 2*—transsphincteric fistula
- *Type 3*—suprasphincteric fistula
- *Type 4*—extralevator fistula
- *Low fistula*—type 1 and type 2
- *High fistula*—type 3 and type 4

Fistula can occur in the perineum in front or behind the Anu's and are according to Goodsall's rule.

The anterior fistula tract is straight. The posterior fistula tract is curved and horseshoe-shaped. The anterior fistula tract if >3.5 cm, then it goes posteriorly, so not straight; it is an exception.

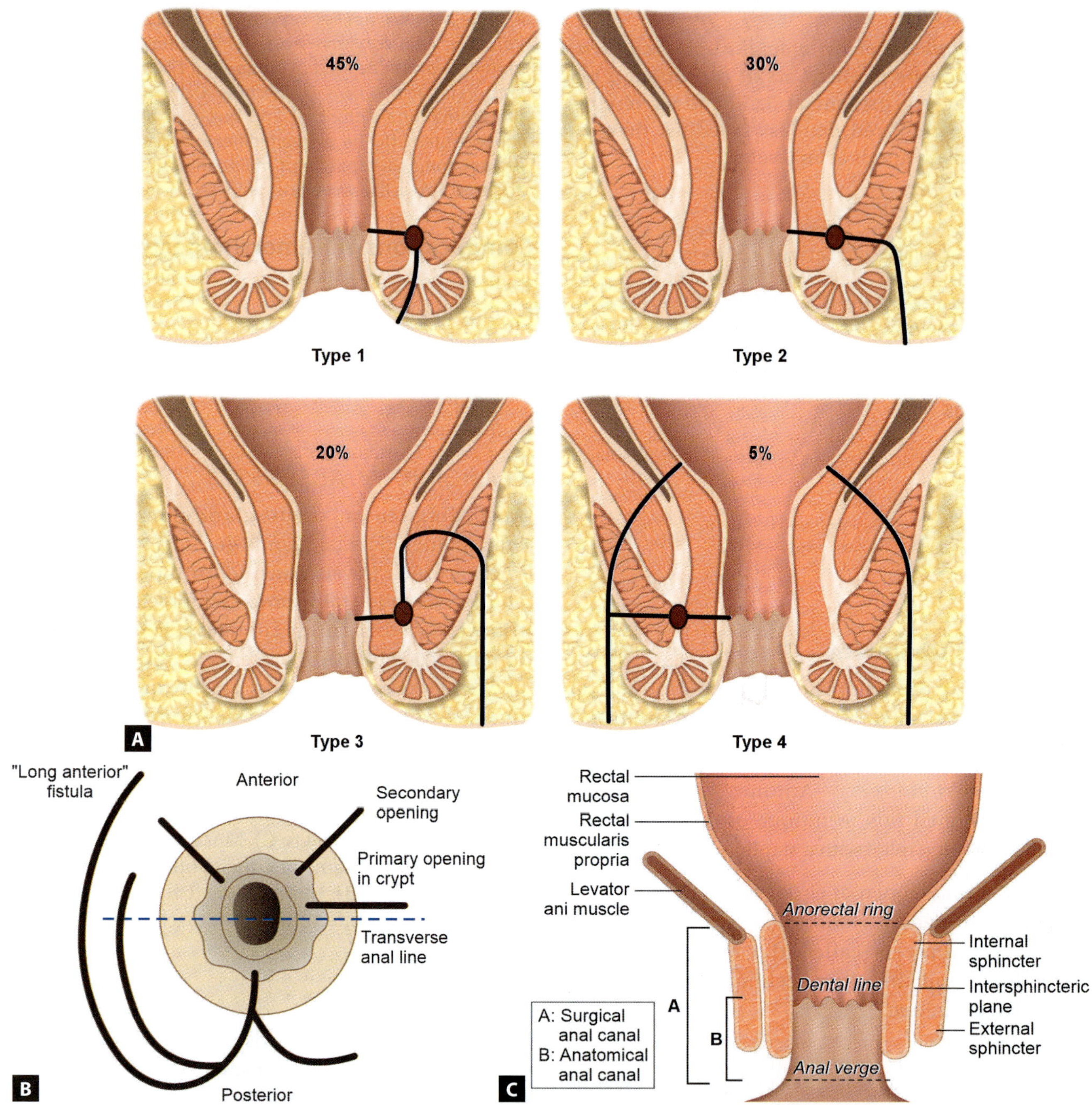

Figs. 5A to C: Fistula-in-ano. Figure B shows Goodsall's Rule or Law is a guideline to predict internal path of an anal fistula based on the location of its external opening. The law or rule explains that if the external opening is anterior to a transverse line across the anus or within 3 cm of the anal verge, the track is usually straight and radial, if opening is behind this line or further anterior, the tract follows a curved path to the posterior midline of the anal canal.

Treatment of Fistula-In-Ano

- *Low (type 1 and 2)*—fistulectomy
- *High (types 3 and 4)*—Seton application
- *Other treatment options are recently developed*: Small intestine submucosa plug (SIS), of porcine intestine, video-assisted fistula tract excision (VAFT), ligation of intersphincteric fistula tract (LIFT).
- Setons (Latin, seta = bristle) can be loose or tight (cutting). Cutting seton cuts the sphincter muscle gradually with simultaneous healing to avoid incontinence, but gives good healing.

Malignant tumors
- Cancers of anal canal and anus are squamous cell carcinoma (SCC), adenocarcinoma, and melanoma.
- Early morning diarrhea and bleeding per rectum are the main symptoms.
- Sigmoidoscopy and biopsy are the main investigation.
- MRI and CT scan show primary and metastasis well.
- Carcinoembryonic antigen (CEA) is also helpful.
- Anterior resection and abdominoperineal resection (APR) are the main operations.

TUMOR, NODE, AND METASTASIS [EIGHTH AMERICAN JOINT COMMITTEE ON CANCER (2017)] CLASSIFICATION OF ANUS AND ANAL CANAL CARCINOMA

- *T15:* Carcinoma in situ T4—invading vagina, urethra or bladder
- *T1:* ≤2 cm tumor
- *T2:* ≥2 cm but <5 cm
- *T3:* >5 cm
- *N1a:* Inguinal, mesorectal, internal iliac LNs involvement
- *N1b:* External iliac LNs involvement
- *N1c:* All above
- *M1:* Distant metastasis

Stages

- *0:* TiSN0M0
- *1:* T1 N0M0
- *IIA:* T2 N0M0
- *IIB:* T3 N0M0
- *IIIA:* T-T2 N1M0
- *IIIB:* T-4 N0M0
- *IIIC:* T3-4 N1M0
- *IV:* Any T, Any NM

Resection can be based on the site of the tumor:
- Tumor >6 cm from anal verge—AR
- Tumor >4 cm from dentate line—AR
- Tumor <6 cm from anal verge—abdominoperineal resection (APR)
- Tumor <4 cm from dentate line—APR

Some important points:
- Investigation of choice for fistula-in-ano—MRI.
- Most common site of fissure-in-ano—midline posterior.
- The most common site of extramammary Paget's disease—anogenital region.

SOME IMPORTANT QUESTIONS

Q1. A patient with carcinoma of rectum which is 5 cm from anal verge, which procedure you will prefer to perform?
a. Anterior resection
b. Abdominoperineal resection
c. Hartman's procedure
d. Defunctioning colostomy

Ans. b

Q2. All of the following are true in the management of hemorrhoids, *except*:
a. Excisional surgery is the cornerstone.
b. Fiber supplementation is effective.
c. Improvement in bowel function is helpful.
d. Ligation with a rubber band is effective.

Ans. a

Q3. The most important disadvantage of cryosurgery for hemorrhoid is:
a. Pain
b. Infection
c. Profuse watery discharge
d. Hemorrhage

Ans. a

Q4. Rectal prolapse is common in:
a. 1–3 months b. 3–5 months
c. 5–8 months d. 8–12 months

Ans. d

Q5. Delorme's procedure is used for:
a. Rectal prolapse
b. Solitary rectal ulcer
c. Rectal bilharziasis
d. Proctalgia fugax

Ans. a

Q6. The most common cause of anorectal abscess is:
a. Inflammation of anal gland
b. Folliculitis
c. Inflammation of the rectal mucosa
d. Rectum

Ans. a

Q7. An AIDS patient presents with a fistula-in-ano. His CD4 count is below 50. The treatment of choice is:
a. Seton b. Fistulectomy
c. Both d. Medical

Ans. a

Q8. Dentate line measurement from anal margin:

a. 1 cm b. 1.5 cm
c. 2 cm d. 2.5 cm

Ans. c

MULTIPLE CHOICE QUESTIONS

Grade I	*Simple*

Q1. Which of the following is the investigation of choice for assessment of depth of penetration and perirectal nodes in rectal cancer? (AIIMS November 2004)

a. Transrectal ultrasound
b. CT scan pelvis
c. MRI Scan
d. Double contrast barium enema

Q2. Not true about hemorrhoids: (AIIMS GIS May 2008)

a. First degree—no prolapse
b. Excision for externo-internal piles
c. Third degree—no surgery
d. Conservative treatment in the first degree

Q3. Hemorrhoids managed by manual reduction: (AIIMS GIS May 2011)

a. First degree b. Second degree
c. Third degree d. Fourth degree

Q4. Which of the following is not true about hemorrhoids? (PGI SS June 2007)

a. Pruritus is not common.
b. Can be palpated on digital rectal examination (DRE) in the absence of complications
c. Band ligation is most commonly done office procedure
d. Stapled hemorrhoidectomy causes less post-operative pain

Q5. True about treatment of hemorrhoids: (PGI November 2010)

a. Band ligation
b. 5% phenol in almond oil is used as a sclerosant.
c. May be resolved by diet modification
d. Hemorrhoidectomy is TOC

Q6. External hemorrhoids below the dentate line are: (AIIMS May 2012)

a. Painful
b. Ligation is done as management
c. Skin tag is not seen in these cases
d. May turn malignant

Q7. Injection sclerotherapy is ideal for the following: (All India 2004)

a. External hemorrhoids
b. Internal hemorrhoids
c. Posterior resection
d. Local resection

Q8. The most common complication following hemorrhoidectomy is: (AIIMS 1992)

a. Hemorrhage b. Infection
c. Fecal impaction d. Urinary retention

Q9. Treatment of choice in second-degree piles is: (AIIMS 1992)

a. Cryosurgery b. Sclerotherapy
c. Banding d. Surgery

Q10. The following are true of hemorrhoids, *except*: (JIPMER 2001)

a. They are arteriolar dilatation
b. They are common causes of painless bleeding
c. They cannot be per rectally palpated
d. They can be banded

Q11. Indications of hemorrhoidectomy include: (PGI May 2018)

a. Large first- and second-degree hemorrhoids
b. Third- and fourth-degree hemorrhoids
c. If not able to differentiate prolapsed hemorrhoids and lower rectal prolapse
d. Complicated by strangulations
e. Failure of conservative therapy

Q12. Treatment of rectal prolapse in childhood is: (AIIMS June 1994)

a. Lahaut's operation
b. Incision of prolapsed mucosa
c. Thiersch wiring
d. Ripstein operation

Q13. A 30-year-old male presents with complete rectal prolapse. Which of the following procedures is associated with the lowest risk of recurrence? (All India 2012)

a. Delorme's procedure
b. Thiersch procedure
c. Abdominal rectopexy
d. Altemeier's procedure

Grade II	Difficult

Q1. Most common anorectal fistula: (AIIMS GIS Dec 2009)

a. Intersphincteric
b. Transsphincteric
c. Suprasphincteric
d. Extrasphincteric

Q2. Which type of malignancy is found in anorectal fistula? (PGI June 2005)

a. Squamous cell carcinoma
b. Transitional cell carcinoma
c. Adenocarcinoma
d. Columnar carcinoma

Q3. True statement regarding "Fistula in ano" is: (All India 2001)

a. Posterior fistulae have straight tracks.
b. High fistulae can be operated on with no fear of incontinence.
c. High and low divisions are made in relation to the pelvic floor.
d. Intersphincteric is the most common type.

Q4. The treatment of choice is fistula in ano: (JIPMER 1993)

a. Anal dilatation
b. Fissurotomy
c. Fistulectomy
d. Fistulotomy

Q5. Most common site of chronic fissure in ano: (GB Pant 2011)

a. Anterior
b. Posterior
c. Lateral
d. Anterolateral

Q6. Percentage of glyceryl trinitrate (GTN) used in fissure: (GB Pant 2011)

a. 2%
b. 0.2%
c. 0.02%
d. 20%

Q7. The following statement about pilonidal sinus is true: (All India 2007)

a. More common in females
b. Mostly congenital
c. The prognosis after surgery is poor.
d. Treatment of choice is surgical excision of the sinus tract.

Q8. All of the following are true regarding pilonidal sinus, *except*: (MCI September 2009)

a. Seen predominantly in women
b. Occurs only in the sacrococcygeal region
c. Tendency for recurrence
d. Obesity is a risk factor

Q9. All are true about pilonidal sinus, *except*: (PGI November 2017)

a. More common in young females
b. It may occur due to a combination of buttock friction and shearing forces in the affected area.
c. Direction of the sinuses are cephaloid.
d. May lead to recurrent abscess formation.
e. Recurrence is common even after surgery.

Q10. Paget's disease of anal canal is: (JIPMER GIS 2011)

a. Squamous cell carcinoma in situ
b. Squamous cell adenoma
c. Intraepithelial adenocarcinoma
d. Marginal anal cell carcinoma

Q11. Which of the following is true about extramammary Paget's disease? (JIPMER 2011)

a. The most common site is the vulva.
b. The most common site is penis.
c. The most common site is vagina.
d. The most common site is the perianal region.

Grade III	Most difficult

Q1. True about melanoma of the anal canal is: (PGI June 1999)

a. Present usually as anal bleeding
b. AP resection gives better results than local excision
c. Local recurrence at the same site after resection
d. Radiosensitive

Q2. Anorectal anomalies are commonly associated with: (JIPMER 2011)

a. Cardiac anomalies
b. Duodenal atresia
c. Central nervous system (CNS) malformations
d. Abdominal

Q3. Resting tone of rectum is decreased in all, *except*: (All India 1991)

a. Micturition
b. Retained feces in the rectum
c. Prolapse rectum
d. Trauma involving the perineum

Q4. What is false regarding the dentate line? (AIIMS 1996)

a. Glands of Morgagni open below the line
b. Anal glands open at the line
c. Dentate line lies 2 cm above the anal verge
d. The transitional epithelium lies above the dentate line

Q5. Which of the following statements about the valves of Houston is true: (All India 2012)

a. The middle valve corresponds to the middle convex fold to the right.
b. The upper valve corresponds to the peritoneal reflection.
c. The valve contains all three layers of the muscle wall.
d. Valves disappear after mobilization of the rectum.

Q6. In an adult male, on per rectal examination, the following structures can be felt anteriorly, *except*: (All India 2005)

a. Internal iliac lymph nodes
b. Bulb of the penis
c. Prostate
d. The seminal vesicle, when enlarged

Q7. The following are important in the maintenance of normal fecal continence, *except*: (All India 1995)

a. Anorectal angulation
b. Rectal innervations
c. Internal sphincter
d. Haustral valve

Q8. Which of the following is not a component of the anorectal ring? (AIIMS May 2013)

a. External and sphincter
b. Puborectalis
c. Anococcygeal raphe
d. Internal anal sphincter

Q9. External anal sphincter is innervated by: (AIIMS November 2013)

a. S2, S3, S4
b. S2, S3
c. L5, S1
d. L2, L3

Q10. Hemangioma of the rectum: (PGI June 2007)

a. Common tumor
b. Fatal hemorrhage seen
c. Ulcerative colitis-like symptoms seen
d. None

Q11. Bleeding per rectum is present in all, *except*: (AIIMS June 1994)

a. Meckel's diverticulum
b. Sigmoid volvulus
c. Carcinoma rectum
d. Ulcerative colitis

ANSWERS

Grade I: 1. c (Bailey 27/e p1331); 2. c; 3. c (Bailey 27/e p1355); 4. b; 5. a, b, c, d (Bailey 27/e p1356-57); 6. a (Schwartz 10/e p1233); 7. b (Schwartz 10/e p1223); 8. d (Bailey 27/e p1360); 9. c; 10. a; 11. b, d, e; 12. c; 13. c

Grade II: 1. a (Bailey 27/e p1364); 2. a, c (Bailey 26/e p1267); 3. d (Bailey 27/e p1364); 4. d (Bailey 27/e p1365); 5. b; 6. b; 7. d; 8. a (Bailey 27/e p1347); 9. a; 10. c (Sabiston 19/e p1405); 11. a

Grade III: 1. a (Bailey 26/e p1267); 2. a; 3. b; 4. d (Bailey 27/e p1340); 5. d (Schwartz 10/e p1180); 6. a; 7. d; 8. c; 9. a (Schwartz 10/e p1179); 10. b and c (Bailey 27/e p1327); 11. b

MODEL QUESTIONS

Q1. High or low fistula in ano is termed according to its internal opening present with reference to:

a. Anal canal
b. Dentate line
c. Anorectal ring
d. Sacral promontory

Ans. c

Q2. Ideal investigation for fistula-in-ano is:

a. Endoanal ultrasound
b. Magnetic resonance imaging (MRI)
c. Fistulography
d. Computed tomography (CT) scan

Ans. b

Q3. A sentinel pile indicates:

a. Internal hemorrhoids
b. Pilonidal sinus
c. Fissure-in-ano
d. Fistula-in-ano

Ans. c

Q4. Jeep's disease is also known as:

a. Anal incontinence
b. Hemorrhoids
c. Pilonidal sinus
d. Anal fissure

Ans. c

Q5. A newborn baby presents with absent anal orifice and meconuria. What is the most appropriate management?

a. Transverse colostomy
b. Conservative
c. Posterior sagittal anorectoplasty
d. Perineal V-Y plasty

Ans. a

Q6. The length of a standard proctoscope is:

a. 4″ b. 6″
c. 8″ d. 3″

Ans. a

Q7. The internal sphincter of the rectum is formed by:

a. Levator ani
b. Puborectalis
c. Longitudinal muscle fibers condensation
d. Circular muscle fiber condensation

Ans. d

Q8. True statement about upper half of anal canal is:

a. Insensitive to pain
b. Drained by superficial inguinal lymph node
c. Lined by squamous epithelium
d. Supplied by the superior mesenteric artery

Ans. a

Q9. A patient with external hemorrhoids develops pain while passing stools. The nerve mediating this pain is:

a. Hypogastric nerve
b. Pudendal nerve
c. Splanchnic visceral nerve
d. Sympathetic plexus

Ans. b

SUGGESTED READING

1. Bailey & Love's - Short Practice of Surgery, 27th edition.
2. Schwartz's Principles of Surgery, 18th edition.
3. Textbook of Surgery by David Sabiston, 21st edition.
4. World Journal of Colorectal Surgery, Vol 9, No. 4, Oct-Dec 2020, p 64.

CHAPTER 44

Peritoneum

"Peritoneum is a membrane, a sheet of smooth tissue that lines your abdominopelvic cavity and surrounds your abdominal organs."

– Cleveland Clinic

INTRODUCTION

The abdominal cavity is actually the peritoneal cavity and is lined by peritoneum, and the peritoneum is a two-layered structure. The peritoneal cavity is the largest cavity in our body. Its area is almost equal to the area of skin **(Figs. 1A to C)**. The peritoneum has one outer layer called the parietal peritoneum, lining the abdominal wall, and an inner visceral layer lining various organs. Peritoneum has two layers in itself as a mesothelium layer lying over a layer of fibroelastic tissue, and these two layers of peritoneum are lying on stellar tissues having plexuses of capillaries and lymphatics, making it to absorb and secrete. *Normally, the peritoneal cavity has a pale yellow viscous fluid in small amounts, containing leukocytes and lymphocytes. The peritoneal fluid lubricates the viscera and helps with peristalsis.*

The parietal peritoneum is richly supplied with nerves, so its irritation causes severe pain at the site, but the visceral peritoneum is poorly supplied with nerves, so its irritation causes less severe pain, but near the midline of the abdomen. The peritoneum has a tremendous capacity to absorb a big amount of fluid, as happens in peritoneal dialysis, and to produce also big amount of fluid, as happens in ascites and in peritonitis.

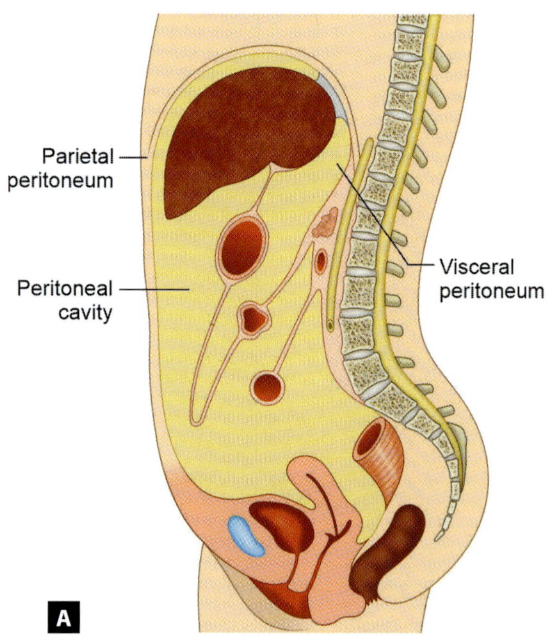

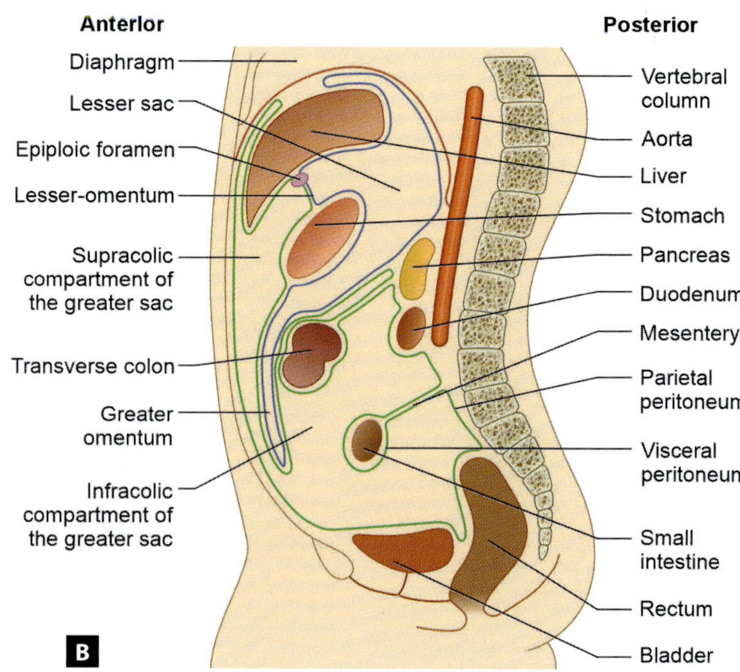

Figs. 1A and B

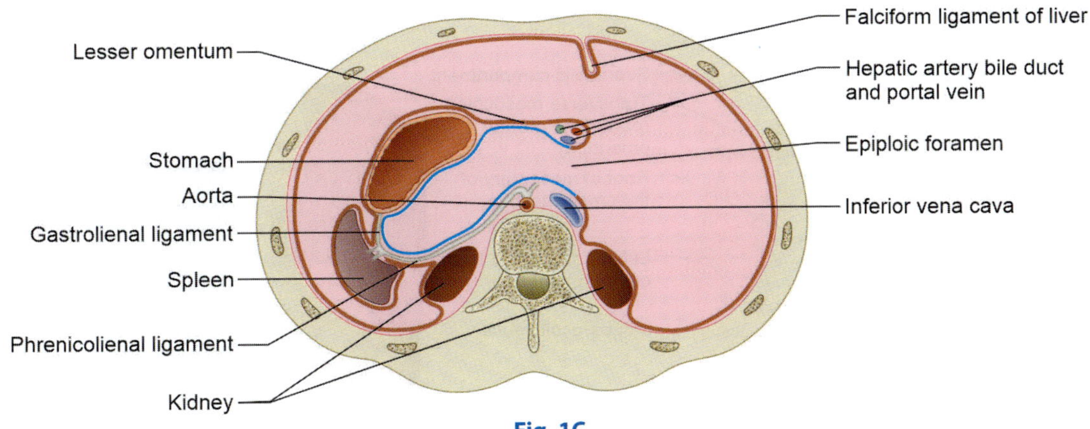

Fig. 1C

Figs. 1A to C: Peritoneum and its divisions.

> *Functions of peritoneum*:
> - Lubrication
> - Absorption
> - Perception of pain in inflammation of abdominal organs
> - Immune responses
> - Inflammatory responses
> - Fibrinolytic activity

Peritoneal cavity is divided into two cavities, the greater sac—the bigger, and the lesser sac—the smaller, communicating through the epiploic foramen **(Figs. 2 and 3)**.

PERITONEAL FLUID FLOW

Peritoneal fluid gets collected in the pelvis due to gravity and then due creation of pressure gradients by movements of the diaphragm and peristalsis, and the peritoneal fluid goes up via the right paracolic gutter mainly to Morrison's pouch and subdiaphragmatic space, and much less via the left paracolic gutter.

> *Points to remember*:
> *Liver dullness*: The percussion is done on right midaxillary line and going down you will find resonance, but it becomes dull as soon as the liver is reached and if the dullness of liver is replaced by resonance, meaning that there is gas under diaphragm from perforation of intestine. The most important cause of perforation of intestine is duodenal peptic ulcer perforation.

PERITONITIS

It is the inflammation of the peritoneum, localized or generalized.

Causes

Mn-BACTIM. B: Bacterial; A: Allergic; C: Chemical bile; T: Traumatic; I: Ischemia; M: Miscellaneous—familial Mediterranean fever.

> *Routes of peritoneal infection:*
> - Gastrointestinal (GI) or transmural perforations.
> - Translocation without perforation (primary bacterial peritonitis).
> - Exogenous contamination by trauma, drains, and dialysis.

Microorganisms

Peritonitis is caused commonly due to gastrointestinal tract (GIT) bacteria such as *Escherichia coli*, *Streptococcus*, *L Klebsiella*, etc., and other bacteria.

Localized Peritonitis

It may occur in the subphrenic space, pelvis, and main peritoneal cavity, which is divided into supra and infracolic compartments, divided by the transverse colon.

> ### Diffuse General Peritonitis
>
> *Speed of peritoneal contamination is the main factor. The inflamed hollow organ perforation sends contents to a distance with speed, and a general peritonitis develops instead local.* Virulence of the organism is also very important as it may not allow localized peritonitis to be established but develop generalized. Omentum in adult works as abdominal policeman reaching at a place of inflammation and getting attached to limit the infection avoiding the spread. *Immune deficiency as in steroid use and acquired immunodeficiency syndrome (AIDS) reduces the natural resistance and encourages generalization.*

Clinical Features

Abdominal pain, anorexia, fever, nausea, tachycardia, tenderness, rebound tenderness, rigidity, reduced bowel sounds, and may be shock. *Systemic inflammatory response*

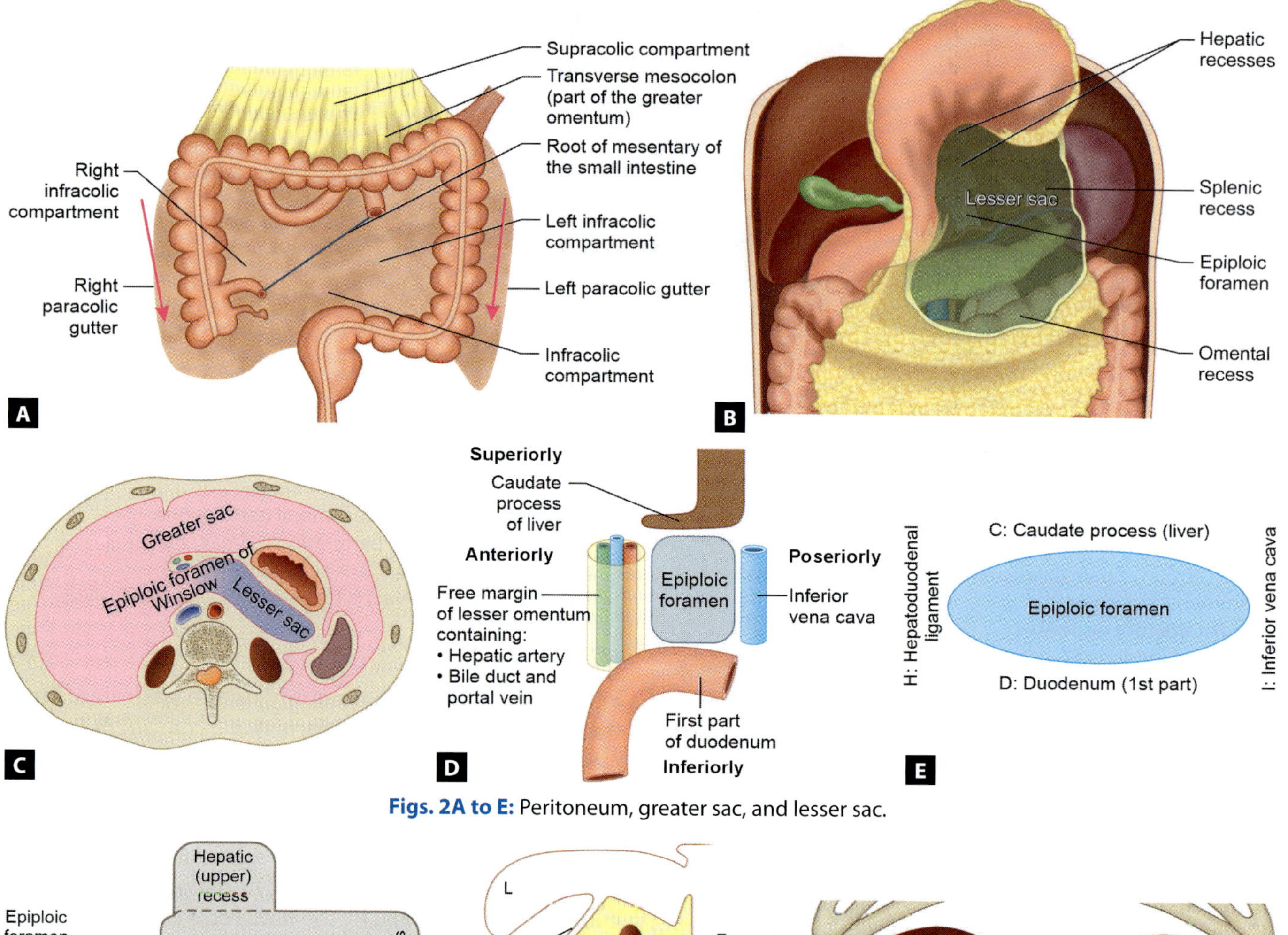

Figs. 2A to E: Peritoneum, greater sac, and lesser sac.

Figs. 3A to C: Peritoneum, lesser sac, greater sac, foramen of Winslow, and abscesses. (L: liver; S: stomach; TC: transverse colon; 1 and 3: subphrenic; 4: subhepatic; 2: lesser sac abscess)

syndrome (SIRS) and multiple organ dysfunction syndrome (MODS) can develop in an advanced stage.

Not to forget:
The perforation of GIT is diagnosed by presence of pneumoperitoneum diagnosed by plai X-ray abdomen in erect position but if patient is very weak and sick then in supine X-ray can be taken, which may show: Football sign (air in center of abdomen), cupola (large quantity of air under the diaphragm) sign, and triangle sign (air between loops of small intestine). Mesentery is a fan-shaped peritoneal fold which is attached to posterior abdominal wall and to jejunum and ileum. Root of mesentery is 15-cm long and runs to right and down. It crosses RAID, right ureter, psoas muscle, right testicular/ovarian vessels/abdominal aorta/inferior vena cava (IVC)/duodenum. Visceral pain is poorly localized, and pain of a hollow viscus is colicky.

Diagnosis

Diagnosis includes complete blood count (CBC), urine examination, electrocardiogram (ECG), urea and electrolytes, serum amylase, and imaging. Imaging includes X-ray in erect posture, ultrasound (USG), and computed tomography (CT) scan.

Management

- General care
- Fluid and electrolyte balance is to be done.
- Urinary catheterization
- Antibiotics—broad spectrum
- Ryle's tube insertion

TUBERCULAR PERITONITIS

Tuberculosis (TB) can involve peritoneum via GIT socially or mesenteric lymph nodes (LNs) or from blood. It can develop nodules with central caseation and ascites. Laparoscopic biopsy diagnoses it. It is treated by antituberculosis treatment (ATT).

INTRAPERITONEAL ABSCESSES

Clinically, these abscesses cause malaise, lethargy, anorexia, pain in the abdomen, fever, swinging pyrexia, and local tenderness.

PELVIC ABSCESS

The pelvis is the most common site of abscess development as the gravity helps the collection of pus after general peritonitis, perforation of the appendix, and after a leak postcolorectal anemic operations.

There are four common intraperitoneal abscesses:
1. *Left subphrenic space abscess*: It usually happens after an operation on the stomach, pancreas, splenic flexure, and spleen.
2. *Left subhepatic space or lesser sac abscess*: It usually happens after acute pancreatitis.
3. *Right subphrenic space abscess*: It is below the liver after cholecystitis perforation, perforated duodenal ulcer, and may be after gastrectomy.
4. *Right subhepatic space abscess*: It is below the right lobe of the liver in the Morison's pouch, it is the deepest space of all these four spaces, and it occurs after cholecystitis, appendicitis, duodenal ulcer perforation, and operations of upper abdominal structures.

Clinically, sometimes it is difficult to pinpoint, but remembering the old saying, "pus somewhere, pus nowhere, pus under the diaphragm indicates you to see under the diaphragm also, subphrenic space abscesses." The clinical symptoms are general, but specific features are also present, such as per rectal (P/R) examination shows a tender swelling in case of a pelvic abscess, which requires a transrectal approach for its drainage.

You may be asked:
Gastric and pancreatic juices are irritating to the peritoneum and cause chemical or aseptic peritonitis. The lesser sac is also called an *omental bursa*. Chylous ascites has milky ascetic fluid in the peritoneal cavity due to an excess of chylomicrons (triglycerides), and it occurs in lymphomas, nephrotic syndrome, filariasis, TB, cirrhosis, and constrictive pericarditis. Pseudochylous ascites may occur in abdominal infection or tumors.

Retroperitoneal Fibrosis

It is limited to central and paravertebral spaces between renal arteries and the sacrum, enfolding the aorta, IVC, and ureters.

Types

- Primary or idiopathic (70%) [Ormond's disease (John Kelso Ormond, 1886–1978, American Urologist, discovered in 1948) may cause renal failure].
- Secondary (30%)

  Mn-DIMAR
  D = Drugs, i.e., methysergide, methyldopa, beta-blockers, etc.
  I = Inflammatory diseases, i.e., Mn-TAP TB, actinomycosis, chronic pancreatitis.
  M = Malignancy, i.e., cancer (CA) prostate, CA stomach, etc.
  A = Autoimmune diseases, i.e., SLE, ankylosing spondylitis.
  R = Radiation

Investigation

Magnetic resonance imaging (MRI).

Treatment

- Mn-TAS
- Tamoxifen, azathioprine, and steroids.

TUMORS OF THE PERITONEUM

Primary Tumors

Mesothelioma of the peritoneum is a benign tumor, common in the pelvic peritoneum. Chemocytotoxic agents are in use for their treatment.

Secondary Tumors

Carcinomatosis Peritonei

It is the terminal happening in carcinoma stomach, colon, ovary, breast, and lungs, and causes multiple secondaries in the peritoneum with straw colored or blood-stained fluid in the peritoneal cavity. It most commonly causes discrete nodules, but multiple plaques and diffuse adhesions are also other varieties. The implantation of cells occurs due to gravity and the flow of peritoneal fluid in the peritoneal cavity. Implantation commonly occurs in the pelvis, under the surface of the diaphragm, and omentum. Debulking or cytoreductive surgery is required in most of the patients. Intraperitoneal chemotherapy is also used.

Hyperthermic intraperitoneal chemotherapy (HIPEC) is used in the main centers now.

PSEUDOMYXOMA PERITONEI

It is a rare condition in women. The peritoneal cavity is filled with large amounts of yellow jelly. It is associated with mucinous tumors of the ovary or appendix. The clinical features of this are due to its bulky amount. USG and CT scans are helpful in diagnosing the disease. Treatment by Sugarbaker (Paul Sugarbaker, American oncologist and surgeon) technique of complete cytoreduction in which the right hemicolon, spleen, gallbladder, and greater omentum are excised.

MESENTERIC CYSTS

They occur more in the small intestine mesentery than in the mesentery of the colon.

These are of four varieties:

1. Chylolymphatic
2. Enterogenous
3. Urogenital remnants
4. Dermoid cyst

Chylolymphatic Cysts

Chylolymphatic cysts are most common and arise from congenitally misplaced lymphatic tissue without any communication with the lymphatic system. Usually, solitary unipolar cysts with clear fluid or chyle are present with an independent blood supply, making enucleation possible.

Enterogenous Cysts

Enterogenous cysts develop from diverticula of the intestine, which were sequestered in embryonic life, so no communication with the lumen of the intestine is present. They contain yellow or colorless liquid. Removal with resection of the affected bowel piece is required. Clinically, these are common in adult women but are also found in children. *There appears a cystic fluctuating swelling near the umbilicus which moves freely in a plane at right angle to the attachment of the mesentery, Tillaux's (Paul Jules Tillaux, 1834-1904, French surgeon) sign.* Complications can happen as torsion, rupture, infection, and hemorrhage, in a cyst. It should be differentiated from other cysts, tubercular abscess, and Hydatid cyst. Resection or marsupialization is required.

RETROPERITONEAL FIBROSIS

Proliferation of fibrosis happens in the retroperitoneal space, encapsulating the aorta, IVC, and ureters. Most of these cases are primary or idiopathic, called Ormond's (JK Ormond, American urologist) disease. Secondary retroperitoneal fibrosis occurs due to: Mn-INDIA: I—inflammation [pancreatitis and tuberculosis (TB)], N—neoplasms (CA prostate, stomach, and carcinoids), D—drugs (methyldopa and beta blockers), I—irradiation, A—autoimmune diseases (SLE and PAN). Clinically nonspecific symptoms such as flank pain, malaise, obstructive uropathy, and effects of other structures are involved.

Investigations are: Infravesical obstruction (IVO), CT scan, and MRI.

Treatment consists of ureteral stenting, and immunosuppressant drugs (TAPS—tamoxifen, azathioprine, penicillamine, and steroids) are used.

Good to remember:

Ascites: It is called ascites when the peritoneal cavity has >150 mL of fluid. The abdomen is distended with fullness of flanks. Shifting dullness is present. Meigs' syndrome is present when a fibroma ovary is associated with pleural effusion and ascites.

Some important points:

- The most common organ involved in retroperitoneal fibrosis is the ureter.
- The most common part of the ureter involved in retroperitoneal fibrosis is the lower third.

- The most common organism in adults with spontaneous bacterial peritonitis (SBP) in adult is Klebsiella.
- The most common organism involved in children with SBP is *Streptococcus* Group A.
- The most common organism associated with peritonitis of continuous ambulatory peritoneal dialysis (CAPD)—*Staphylococcus epidermidis.*

SOME IMPORTANT QUESTIONS

Q1. Ormond's disease is:

a. Retractile testis
b. Idiopathic retroperitoneal lymphadenopathy
c. Idiopathic retroperitoneal fibrosis
d. Idiopathic mediastinitis

Ans. c

Q2. Localized idiopathic fibrosis is seen in all of the following, *except*:

a. Riedel's struma
b. Hypertrophic scar
c. Sclerosing cholangitis
d. Panniculitis

Ans. b

Q3. Primary peritonitis with *Pneumococcus* is associated with:

a. Lymphomas
b. Nephrotic syndrome
c. Carcinoids
d. None of the above

Ans. b

Q4. Generalized diffuse peritonitis has been compared to second and third-degree burns of:

a. 13%
b. 30%
c. 45%
d. 60%

Ans. c

Q5. The most common organism seen in peritonitis is:

a. *Escherichia coli*
b. *Clostridium welchii*
c. Staphylococci
d. *Klebsiella*

Ans. a

Q6. Spontaneous peritonitis occurs in cirrhosis patients; the polymorphonuclear cells are:

a. >200 cells/mm^3
b. >300 cells/mm^3
c. >400 cells/mm^3
d. >500 cells/mm^3

Ans. a

Q7. All of the following regarding the diagnosis of acute peritonitis are correct, *except*:

a. Raised white blood cell (WBC) count in peritoneal aspirate
b. Moderately raised amylase levels are diagnostic of peritonitis.
c. Computed tomography (CT) scan may aid in diagnosis.
d. Upright films show free air under the diaphragm.

Ans. b

Q8. The most common type of mesenteric cyst is:

a. Enterogenous
b. Chylolymphatic
c. Urogenital
d. Teratomatous

Ans. b

Q9. Mesenteric cyst, whose removal entrails the removal of part of the gut:

a. Chylolymphatic cyst
b. Enterogenous cyst
c. Dermoid
d. All

Ans. b

Q10. All are mesenteric cysts, *except*:

a. Dermoid cyst
b. Chylolymphatic cyst
c. Gather's cyst
d. Enterogenous cyst

Ans. c

Q11. Pseudochylous ascites occurs in:

a. Cirrhosis
b. Hyperlipidemia
c. Filariasis
d. Malignant ascites

Ans. d

Q12. In pseudomyxoma peritonei, mucinous cyst—adenocarcinoma, which of the following organs is involved?

a. Pancreas
b. Ovary
c. Kidney
d. Abdominal testis

Ans. b

MULTIPLE CHOICE QUESTIONS

Grade I	*Simple*

Q1. Retroperitoneal fibrosis most commonly presents with: (JIPMER 2011)

a. Pedal edema
b. Ascites
c. Ureteric obstruction
d. Back pain

Q2. Investigation for acute abdomen includes: (PGI May 2010)

a. Ultrasound (USG)
b. Multidetector computed tomography (CT)
c. Contrast-enhanced CT
d. X-ray abdomen
e. Echocardiography

Q3. A postoperative patient presents with peritonitis and massive contamination because of a duodenal leak. Management of choice is: (AIIMS June 2001)

a. Four-quadrant peritoneal lavage
b. Duodenostomy + feeding jejunostomy + peritoneal lavage
c. Total parenteral nutrition
d. Duodenojejunostomy

Q4. In which of the following conditions, air under both sides of the diaphragm is visualized? (PGI December 2001)

a. Perforated Meckel's diverticulum
b. Uterine rupture following illegal abortion
c. Perforation of duodenal ulcer
d. Liver abscess
e. Appendicular perforation

Q5. The most common organ involved in retroperitoneal fibrosis is: (AIIMS Nov 1993)

a. Aorta
b. Ureter
c. Inferior vena cava
d. Sympathetic nerve plexus

Q6. Emergency operation done in cases of: (PGI Nov 2010)

a. Volvulus
b. Obstructed hernia
c. Appendicular perforation with paralytic ileus
d. Toxic megacolon
e. Colonic perforation

Q7. Which of the following causes the least irritation of the peritoneal cavity? (All India 1999)

a. Bile
b. Blood
c. Gastric enzyme
d. Pancreatic enzyme

Q8. The most common cause of peritonitis in adult males is: (All India 1993)

a. Duodenal ulcer perforation
b. Abdominal tuberculosis
c. Enteric perforation
d. Perforated appendix

Q9. Apart from *Escherichia coli*, the other most common organism implicated in acute suppurative bacterial peritonitis is: (All India 2006)

a. *Bacteroides*
b. *Klebsiella*
c. *Peptostreptococcus*
d. *Pseudomonas*

Q10. The most common cause of generalized peritonitis in a 40-year-old adult male is: (AIIMS 1992)

a. Enteric perforation
b. Ruptured liver abscess
c. Duodenal ulcer perforation
d. Perforated CA stomach

Grade II	***Difficult***

Q1. True statement regarding tubercular peritonitis and ascites: (PGI Nov 2017)

a. SAAG <1.1 g/dL in ascitic fluid
b. Elevated adenosine deaminase level
c. Protein <25–30 g/L
d. The diagnosis can be made up by laparoscopy with directed biopsy of the peritoneum.

Q2. Pseudomyxoma peritonei arises from: (PGI Dec 2008)

a. Carcinoma ovary
b. Ovarian cyst
c. Ovarian dermoid
d. Adenocarcinoma colon
e. Mucocele of the appendix

Q3. All are true about pseudomyxoma peritonei, *except*: (UPPG 2007)

a. Common in males
b. Associated with ovarian tumors
c. Yellow jelly collection of fluid
d. Appendiceal appendicarcinoma

Q4. The most common site for intra-abdominal abscess following laparotomy is: (AIIMS 1992)

a. Subhepatic
b. Subphrenic
c. Pelvic
d. Paracolic

Q5. A 10-year-old female who used to use the swimming pool regularly comes with a 3-day history of vomiting, fever, and abdominal pain. On examination, abdominal tenderness and guarding are present. The liver dullness is not obliterated. Likely diagnosis is: (AIIMS 1999)

a. Gangrenous intussusceptions
b. Perforation
c. Spontaneous biliary peritonitis
d. Primary peritonitis

Q6. Sonu, a 15-year-old girl, a regular swimmer, presents with a sudden onset of pain in the abdomen, abdominal distension, and ever of 39°C and

obliteration of liver dullness. Most probable diagnosis is: (AIIMS June 2001)
a. Ruptured typhoid ulcer
b. Primary bacterial peritonitis
c. Ruptured ectopic pregnancy
d. Urinary tract infection (UTI) with pelvic inflammatory disease (PID)

Q7. True about mesenteric cyst: (PGI Dec 2005)
a. Moves perpendicular to the line of attachment.
b. Teratomatous is the most common.
c. Chylolymphatic cyst has a separate blood supply.
d. Surgical removal of the bowel along cyst is the treatment of choice for all cysts.

Q8. A part of the adjacent intestine will be removed in: (JIPMER 2012)
a. Enterogenous cyst
b. Chylolymphatic cyst
c. Dermoid cyst
d. Mesothelial cyst

Q9. Transudative ascites is/are associated with: (PGI May 2011)
a. Myxedema
b. Budd–Chiari syndrome
c. Acute pancreatitis
d. Portal vein thrombosis
e. Congestive heart failure

Q10. Mucinous ascites is seen in: (PGI June 2000)
a. Stomach CA
b. Tuberculosis (TB)
c. Nephrotic syndrome
d. Cirrhosis

Grade III | *Most difficult*

Q1. In which one of the following conditions is gas under the diaphragm not seen? (UPSC 2005)
a. Perforated duodenal ulcer
b. Typhoid perforation
c. After laparotomy
d. Spontaneous rupture of the esophagus

Q2. Lesser omentum has the following contents, *except*: (PGI 1997)
a. Hepatic vein
b. Hepatic artery
c. Portal vein
d. Bile duct

Q3. The truth about the relation of the epiploic foramen is: (AIIMS 1997)
a. Portal vein posteriorly
b. IVC inferiorly
c. Hepatic art superiorly
d. Bile duct anteriorly

Q4. Root of mesentery is crossed by: (AIIMS 2011)
a. Horizontal part of duodenum
b. Left gonadal vessels
c. Left ureter
d. Superior mesenteric artery

Q5. A patient came with ascites. Ascitic fluid analysis was done and found to have SAAG more >1.1. All of the following can be the cause, *except*: (AIIMS Nov 2017)
a. Cirrhosis
b. Liver failure
c. Metastasis to liver
d. Tubercular peritonitis

Q6. True about pseudomyxoma peritonei: (PGI June 2004)
a. Seen in males only
b. Cytoreductive surgery is needed
c. Always appendectomy is needed
d. Radiation therapy is given
e. Locally malignant tumor

Q7. False about pseudomyxoma peritonei is: (JIPMER May 2018)
a. Recurrence after surgery
b. Refractory to drugs
c. Hyperthermic intraperitoneal chemotherapy is a treatment option
d. Most commonly associated with an appendiceal tumor

Q8. Posterior perforated ulcer on pyloric antrum causes abscess formation in: (PGI June 2009)
a. Greater sac
b. Lesser sac
c. Pouch of Morrison
d. Omental bursa
e. Right subphrenic

Q9. A posteriorly perforating ulcer in the pyloric antrum of the stomach is likely to produce initial localized peritonitis or abscess formation in the: (AIIMS Nov 2004)
a. Greater sac
b. Left subhepatic and hepatorenal spaces (Pouch of Morrison)
c. Right subphrenic space
d. Lesser sac

Q10. Treatment of pneumoperitoneum, as a result of colonoscopic perforation in a young patient, is: (PGI June 1998)
a. Temporary colostomy
b. Closure + lavage
c. Permanent colostomy
d. Symptomatic

ANSWERS

Grade I: 1. d; 2. a, b, c, d (Sabiston 20/e p1126-1129); 3. c; 4. a, b, c, e (Chapman 4/e p212); 5. b; 6. a, b, c, d, e (Sabiston 20/e p1252); 7. b (Harrison 20/e p954); 8. a (Sabiston 20/e p1211); 9. a (Sabiston 20/e p1078); 10. c

Grade II: 1. a, b, d (Sabiston 20/e p1077); 2. a, d, e; 3. a; 4. c; 5. d (Sabiston 20/e p1125); 6. a; 7. a, c; 8. a; 9. a, b, d, e (Sabiston 20/e p1077); 10. a (Harrison 16/e p245)

Grade III: 1. d; 2. a; 3. d; 4. a; (Bailey 27/e p1065); 5. d (Harrison 20/e p1245); 6. b, c, e; 7. b (Schwartz 10/e p1258-1259); 8. b, d (Bailey 27/e p1056); 9. d; 10. b (Schwartz 10/e p1180)

MODEL QUESTIONS

Q1. The most common site of intraperitoneal abscess is:

a. Lesser sac b. Greater sac
c. Pelvis d. Paracolic gutter

Ans. c

Q2. The part of the peritoneal cavity that is most dependent in the supine position:

a. Right subphrenic space
b. Lesser sac
c. Supra mesocolic space
d. Right subhepatic space

Ans. d

Q3. Treatment of the pouch of Douglas abscess is:

a. Laparotomy
b. Posterior colpotomy
c. Antibiotics
d. Extraperitoneal drainage

Ans. b

Q4. Colpotomy is done to treat:

a. Ischiorectal abscess
b. Pelvic abscess
c. Appendicular abscess
d. Perianal abscess

Ans. b

Q5. The best investigation for air in the peritoneal cavity is:

a. USG
b. Laparotomy
c. Laparoscopy
d. X-ray abdomen-erect view

Ans. d

Q6. Rigler's sign is seen in:

a. Ulcerative colitis b. Crohn's disease
c. Megacolon d. Pneumoperitoneum

Ans. d

Q7. Advantages of carbon dioxide in laparoscopy are all, *except*:

a. Nonirritant b. Noninflammable
c. Minimally absorbed d. No tissue reaction
e. None

Ans. c

Q8. The most common cause of acute mesenteric adenitis is:

a. Tuberculosis
b. Brucellosis
c. Pneumococcal infection
d. Idiopathic

Ans. d

Q9. "Peritoneal mice" is:

a. Pseudomyxoma peritonei
b. Appendices epiploicae
c. Peritoneal seedings of the tumor
d. Endometriosis

Ans. b

Q10. Malignant change in lipoma is most common in:

a. Thigh b. Nape of neck
c. Retroperitoneum d. Back

Ans. c

Q11. Retractile mesenteritis may be seen in:

a. Ormond's disease b. Gardner's syndrome
c. Turner's syndrome d. Down's syndrome

Ans. a

Q12. Which is the baseline investigation in the case of an acute abdomen in this high-tech era?

a. Abdomen CT b. Abdomen X-ray
c. USG d. Colonoscopy

Ans. b

SUGGESTED READING

1. Bailey & Love's - Short Practice of Surgery, 27th edition.
2. Schwartz's Principles of Surgery, 18th edition.
3. Textbook of Surgery by David Sabiston, 21st edition.

SECTION 8

Genitourinary

CHAPTER 45

Kidneys and Ureters

"Kidney disease is not a death sentence.
You can live a very full life even if you don't have family support."

- Erica Cohen

EMBRYOLOGY

The kidney develops from the metanephros and is surrounded by a pad of fat, and the development is controlled by transcription factors, PAX2, and WT1. Ureters develop from the mesonephric duct **(Figs. 1A to D)**.

CONGENITAL ABNORMALITIES OF KIDNEY

- *Agenesis:* Unilateral or bilateral
- *Horseshoe kidney:* It can develop pelviureteric junction (PUJ) obstruction, calculi, and infection.
- *Ureterocele:* It is a cystic dilatation of the intramuscular ureter and is more common in females.
- *Ectopic kidney:* Crossed renal ectopia is happens when both kidneys are on the same side and fused **(Figs. 2A to C)**.
- *Ectopic ureter:* It is more common in women and can cause incontinence, but not in men, associated with duplex ureters.
- *Congenital megaureters:* Stones and infection are common. Whitaker (Robert H Whitaker, British urologist) test is an antegrade pressure study which excludes obstruction.
- Autosomal dominant polycystic kidney disease (ADPKD) presents at 30 years of age. Hypertension is most commonly associated with liver and pancreatic

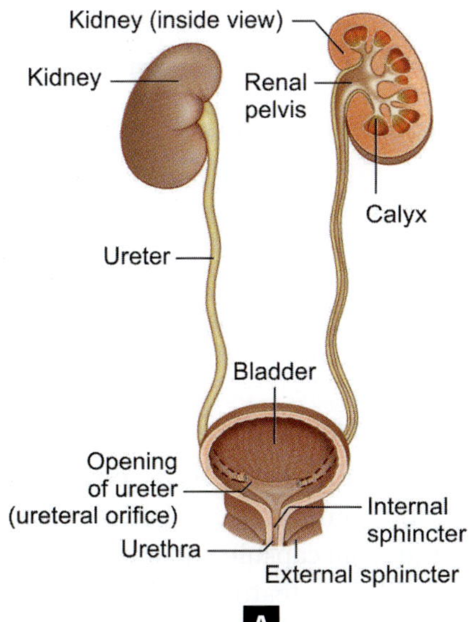

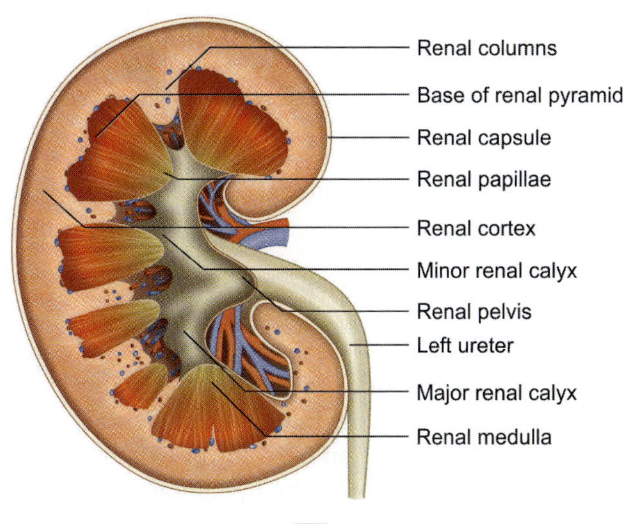

Figs. 1A and B

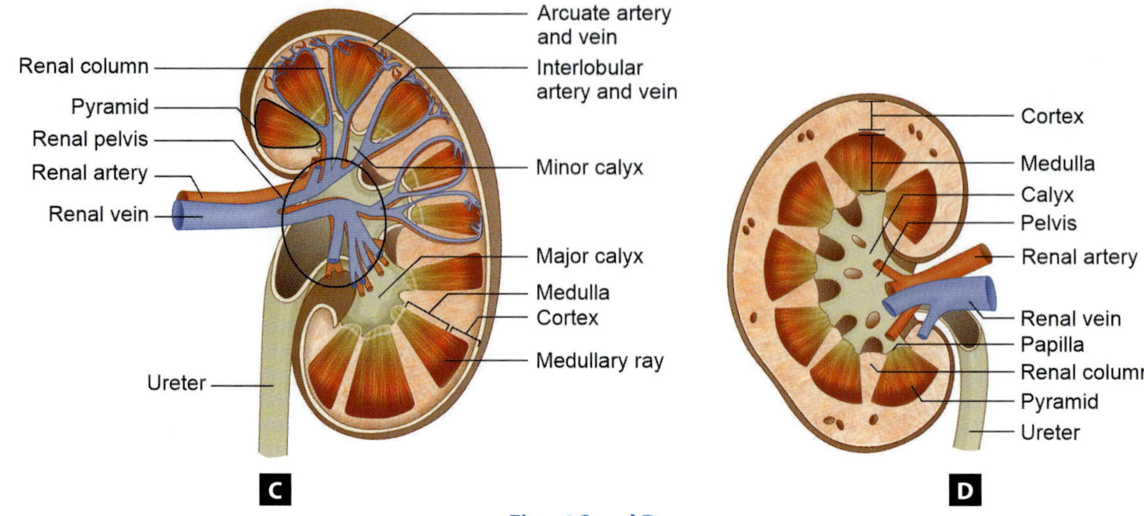

Figs. 1C and D

Figs. 1A to D: Anatomy of the kidney and ureter.

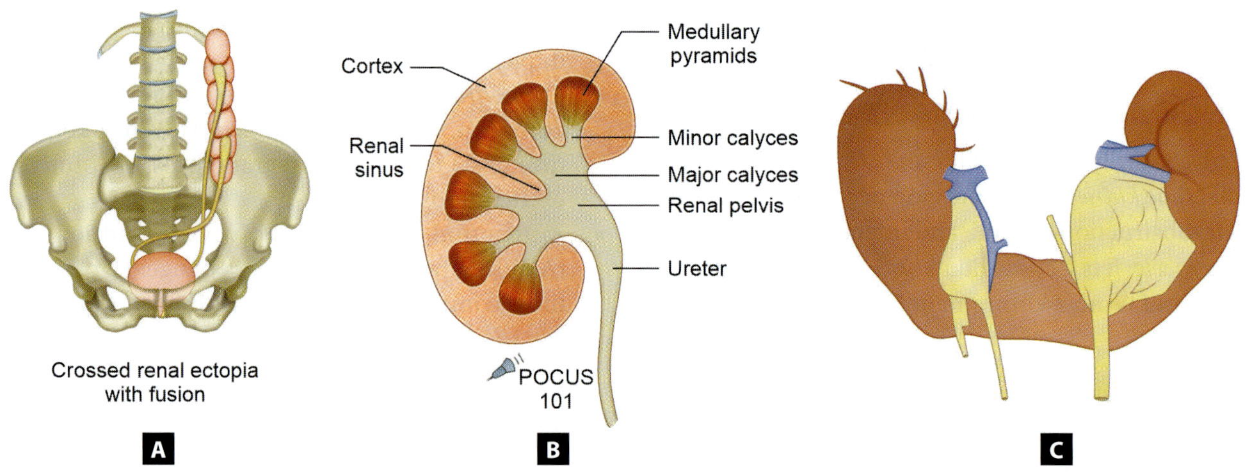

Figs. 2A to C: Anatomy of the kidney, hydronephrosis, and crossed renal ectopia.

cysts. Renal functions deteriorate and lead to renal failure more rapidly in men.

INFECTIONS OF THE URINARY TRACT

Acute Pyelonephritis

It can happen by a hematogenous route from a distant primary source as tonsillitis, skin infection, or dental infection or by ascending infection from lower urinary tract tuberculosis (TB) can happen by hematogenous route from neck, chest, and abdomen.

Clinically, high swinging fever with chills, rigors, lumbar pain, nausea, and vomiting with tenderness in the flank, especially in the costovertebral angle. The most common organism is *Escherichia coli*, but others are involved. *E. coli* with *Streptococcus* causes acidic urine, and *E. coli* with *Staphylococcus* causes alkaline urine. Pyuria is always present.

Perinephric Abscess

It develops as renal infection by ascending from lower urinary tract and commonly caused by *E. coli* infection. It perforates the renal capsule and forms abscess around and in kidney. Clinical features include fever, pain, and tenderness in costovertebral angle. It is drained through thick needle under proper ultrasound guidance. Incision and drainage of the abscess may be required.

Emphysematous Pyelonephritis

It is a necrotizing, life-threatening variant of acute pyelonephritis. Symptoms of acute pyelonephritis are present. Culture and sensitivity are done on urine. It is found more commonly having a mass that can be seen on X-ray. Drainage of the abscess is sometimes required if catheter drainage fails.

Pyonephrosis

A hydronephrotic obstructive kidney gets infected and becomes a bag of pus. Commonly caused by renal stones.

- *Investigation:* Ultrasound (USG)
- Treatment
  - Drainage (percutaneous nephrostomy)
  - Antibiotics
  - If kidney is nonfunctioning or destroyed, then nephrectomy.

> *Points to remember:*
> Anatomical anal canal extends from anal verge to dentate line. Surgical anal canal extends from anal verge to anorectal ring. It is more of a functional type. Ectopic ureters generally associated with duplex ureters, common in women (7:1), drain the upper pole of kidney. In females, it opens in urethra or vagina. Urinary tract infection (UTI) in children—in first year of life, common in girls, due to stasis of urine, VUR is common (30–40%), renal scarring may occur. All children must be investigated after the first episode of UTI.

Tuberculosis of the Urinary Tract

It is due to the blood dissemination of tubercular lesions elsewhere. Diagnosis is done by three consecutive days of morning urine. Sample identification of acid-fast bacilli with Ziehl-Neelsen stain. CT and the CT program are helpful. Treatment consists of short-term antituberculosis treatment (ATT). Kass criteria advise demonstration of 10 × 5 colony-forming units in the midstream urine sample is diagnostic of UTI in males.

Stones in the Urinary Tract

Ureter after coming out from renal hilum as renal pelvis, it course down to urinary bladder **(Fig. 3)**. During the course, ureter comes over pelvis edge and has narrowing at five sites:

1. Ureteropelvic junction
2. While crossing the iliac vessels
3. Juxtaposition of vas deferens
4. At ureterovesical junction
5. At ureters orifice

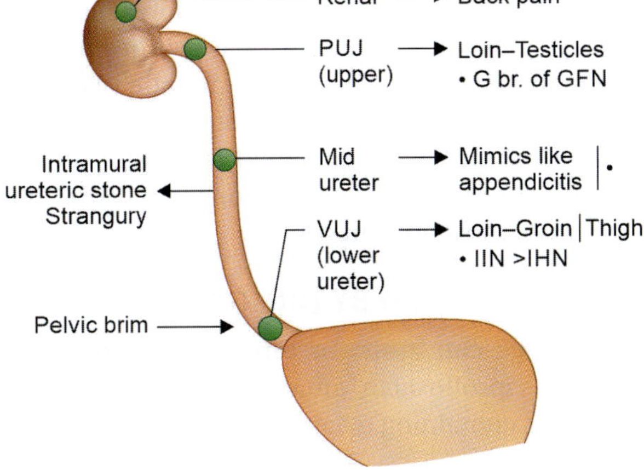

Fig. 3: Ureteric narrowing and risk for stone development.

TYPES OF URINARY STONES

- Calcium oxalate stones
- Triple phosphate stones
- Cystine stones
- Uric acid stones
- Rare stones, indinavir (HIV), are radiolucent and xanthine stones—radiolucent.

Clinical Features

Symptomatic or asymptomatic: Most of the urinary stones are asymptomatic, as they present without symptoms. The symptoms are according to the site of the stone. Pain, renal pain, is at the back of the lumbar region.

- *Pelviureteric junction stone:* Pain radiates from the flank to the testicle.
- *Midureter:* Pain is like of appendicitis.
- *Vesicoureteric junction (VUJ):* Pain radiates from the loin to the groin
- *Intramural ureter:* Pain is strangury
- Hematuria
- Frequency of micturition
- Strangury

> *Not to forget:*
> Carbuncle of kidney is renal cortical abscess. Tuberculosis of urinary tract is either reinfection or activation of old lesion. Stones in kidney pass out if size is <5 mm. Medical therapy for expulsion of stone is controversial. Surgical treatment is required in obstruction, infection, or persistent pain. Extracorporeal shockwave lithotripsy (ESWL) is a common practice now. Many sittings may be required depending upon the hardness of stone. Steinstrasse is the term given for collection of stone fragments after ESWL.

Calcium oxalate stones are also called mulberry stones, the most common stone to cause hematuria, and the hardest stone to break by extracorporeal shockwave lithotripsy (ESWL). Triple phosphate stones are called staghorn stone due to their shape, or called Jack stone, soft, and smooth stone. Cystine stones are hard and radiopaque, inspire of no calcium but a sulfur bond that makes it radiopaque; uric acid stones are radiolucent, yellow, and associated with gout.

STONES CAUSED BY DRUGS

Certain drugs can assist in renal and ureteric stone production, ciprofloxacin, antacid magnesium trisilicate, and laxatives containing magnesium.

> *Management of stones:*
> - Increase fluid intake with restriction of protein
> - ESWL
> - Dormia
> - Basket removal
> - Endoscopic removal
> - Percutaneous nephrolithotomy (PCNL)
> - Open surgeries, pyelolithotomy, ureterolithotomy, and nephrolithotomy
> - Open surgery is not much in use nowadays.

Uric Acid Stones

- 5–10% among all renal stones
- Radiolucent stone formed in acidic urine, Mn-HAL
- Treated by alkalinization of urine, hydration, and a low purine diet
- *Drug:* Allopurinol, which reduces the synthesis of uric acid by not allowing xanthine and hypoxanthine to form uric acid

Struvite Stones

- Infection stones
- Triple phosphate stones (Ca, NH4, and Mg phosphates)
- Form in alkaline urine with high ammonia content
- More common in females due to the high incidence of UTI.

Treatment

Low-calorie and low-phosphorus diet

- PCNL + ESWL
- Antibiotics to avoid recurrence

Cystine Stones

- In acidic urine, very hard and radiopaque
- Hexagonal cystine crystals in urine

Treatment

- Low methionine diet
- Alkalinization of urine
- Stone removal
- MPG (alpha-mereaptopropionylglycine)

Xanthine Stones

Brick red, round, radiolucent.

Treatment

- High fluid intake
- Allopurinol

Investigation of urinary calculi

- Urine pH
- X-ray kidney, ureter, and bladder (KUB)
- USG
- Intravenous urography (IVU)
- RGP (Retrograde pyelogram)
- Radionuclide evaluation
  - *DMSA:* Dimercaptosuccinic acid scan
  - *DTPA:* Diethylenetriaminepentaacetic acid to assess perfusion and function
  - *MAG3:* Mercaptoacetyltriglycine is best for renal perfusion assessment

Conservative treatment for (single stone ≤5 mm ureter, 4–6 weeks nondilated lower ureter stone/stone moving down)

Surgical Intervention

When conservative treatment fails

- *Stone <2 cm:* ESWL
- *Stone >2 cm:* PCNL
- Staghorn stone (PCNL + ESWL)

EXTRACORPOREAL SHOCK WAVE LITHOTRIPSY

- There are high-energy shock waves concentrated on a stone, which release energy at the stone and cause compression-induced tensile cracking of the stone.
- The best lithotripsy is "Dornier unmodified HM-e"

PERCUTANEOUS NEPHROLITHOTOMY

Stone is removed through a track or tunnel developed below the skin and the kidney that has a stone. The posterior approach is best as it avoids injury to the renal artery. Indicators of PCNL Mn-LOLO.

L = Large stone or staghorn stone
O = Obstructive uropathy
L = Lower pole calyceal stone
O = Other modalities when PCNL failure happens

Complications

Mn = BUSRI

- B = Bleeding
- U = Urinary extravasation
- S = Sepsis
- R = Retained frequency of stone
- I = Injury to other viscera, i.e., pleura

HYDRONEPHROSIS

- It may be congenital or acquired and unilateral or bilateral.
- USG, IVU, and isotope renography are helpful.
- Pyeloplasty is required.

> *You may be asked:*
> *Dietl's (Joseph Dietl, 1804–1878, Polish pathologist) crisis:* Alcoholic binge after renal colic stone leads to a swelling in loin and passage of large amount of urine with stone after few hours. Swelling also disappears. Bleeding during micturition can indicate the site of the lesion. Bleeding at beginning of urethra, bleeding at the vesical end, and bleeding mixed with urine throughout—prerenal, renal, and vertical.

POLYCYSTIC DISEASE OF ADULTS

- Autosomal dominant, 50% of offspring are affected
- Chromosomes affected 16 and 4
- Protein abnormality—polycystin
- A cause of renal failure

Presentation

- Hypertension/pain/hematuria/nocturia/CRF
- Death is due to cardiovascular disorders

Diagnosis

Ultrasound

Extrarenal Manifestation

MN = CMAC

- C = Cysts liver/spleen/pancreas/seminal vesicles
- A = Berry's aneurysm
- M = Mitral valve prolapse
- C = Colonic diverticulum

INTRAVENOUS PYELOGRAPHY

- Spider leg—due to cysts in between calyces
- Bubble appearance—calyceal distortion
- Swiss cheese appearance

Treatment

- Desoofing of cysts [Rovsing's (Niels Thorkild Rovsing, 1862-1927, Danish Surgeon)]
- Dialysis
- Renal treatment

TRAUMA

Trauma to the kidney is mostly caused by blunt trauma, but penetrating trauma can also cause renal injury.

Injuries to the kidney can be classified into five grades:

- *Grade I:* Contusion or nonenlarging subcapsular hematoma
- *Grade II:* Superficial laceration <1 cm, does not involve collecting system, nonexpanding perirenal hematoma confined to retroperitoneum.
- *Grade III:* Laceration >1 cm without extension into renal pelvis or collecting system
- *Grade IV:*
    - Laceration extends to the renal pelvis or urinary extravasation
    - Injury to a main renal artery or vein with contained hemorrhage
    - Segmental infarctions without associated lacerations
    - Expanding subcapsular hematomas comprising the kidney
- *Grade V:*
    - Shattered kidney
    - Avulsion of renal hilum
    - Ureteropelvic avulsions
    - Complete laceration or thrombus of the main renal artery or vein.

In children, the kidneys are less well protected and are at a lower level. *Contrast-enhanced computed tomography (CECT)* is helpful. Renal exploration is required. Ureteric injuries during operation, if noticed, must be repaired urgently. The *Boari (Achille Boari, an Italian urologist, performed it on a dog in 1894)* operation with forming is a tube from a strip of bladder wall to bridge the gap between the cut ureter and bladder, was required.

HYDRONEPHROSIS

It is an aseptic dilatation of the kidney.

Type

Unilateral

- *Extramural obstruction:*
  - Tumor from adjacent structures
  - Retroperitoneal fibrosis
- *Intramural obstruction:*
  - Stenosis
  - Stricture
  - Tumor
- *Intraluminal obstruction:* Calculus

Bilateral

- Congenital
  - Posterior urethral valves
  - Urethral atresia
- Acquired
  - BPH
  - Urethral stricture
  - Phimosis

PELVIURETRIC JUNCTION OBSTRUCTION

Blockage at PUJ leads to hydronephrosis.

Causes

- *Congenital:*
  - Aperistaltic segment
  - Aberrant renal vessel crosses PUJ
- *Acquired:*
  - Calculus
  - Infection
  - Iatrogenic by instrumentation

Clinical Features

- Asymptomatic
- Abdominal lump
- Abnormalities associated with it
  - PUJ obstruction on the other side
  - Vertebral abnormalities
  - Anorectal malformation

Diagnosis

- USG
- IVU
- DTPA scan
- Retrograde polygram
- *Whitaker (Roger H. Whitaker, 1939, British physician) test*—Percutaneously by a needle, contrast is injected in the kidney, and intrapelvic pressure is measured.

HORSESHOE KIDNEY

- 1:400 common in males, fusion at the lower pole
- The pelvis and ureters are anterior to the kidney
- Calyces are directed posteriorly
- The isthmus usually lies on the L3–L4 vertebrae

Associated Abnormalities

Mn = CUCAR

- C = CVS abnormalities
- U = Uterus—uni or bicarnuate
- C = CNS abnormalities
- A = Anorectal malformations
- R = Renal - PUJ obstruction

Investigations

Intravenous urography.

Treatment

It is symptomatic than pyeloplasty, if required.

RENAL CYSTS

- Solitary/multiple
- Common in men
- Bosnaik's classification
  - *Category I*: Simple benign cyst
  - *Category II*: Simple benign cyst with septation and calcification
  - *Category II F*: Calcification is more
  - *Category III*: Complicated—requires surgery
  - *Category IV*: Malignant

Treatment

Percutaneous drainage.

VESICOURETERIC REFLUX

- Autosomal dominance transmission
- 10–30%
- 75% asymptomatic

Types

- *Primary:* Alteration of the trigone of the urinary bladder with deficiency of the longitudinal muscle of the intravesical ureter leading to inadequate valvular mechanism.
- *Secondary:* Posterior urethral valve

Grading

- *Grade I:* Nondilated ureter—reflux in the ureter
- *Grade II:* Nondilated ureter—reflux in pelvis and calyces
- *Grade III:* Mild to moderate ureteric, pelvic dilatation
- *Grade IV:* Mild to moderate ureteric + blunting of fornices
- *Grade V:* Gross dilatation of ureter, pelvis, calyces

Treatment

- *Conservative:* Prophylactic antibiotics to avoid infection
- *Surgery:* Ureteric transplantation (ureterovasicoplasty).

Indications

- Failure of conservative treatment
- *Severe reflux:* Grade V
- Deterioration of renal function

Hepatorenal Syndrome

It is a functional renal failure without renal pathology, with severe liver disease.

- No blunting of fornices
- Severe renal vasoconstriction

Types

- *Type I:* Progressive renal impairment
- *Type II:* Deterioration in glomerular filtration rate (GFR) (better outcome)

Treatment

- Terlipressin is the drug of choice
- Liver transplantation

RENAL CELL CARCINOMA

It is also called the Grawitz tumor or hypernephroma. It is one of the 10 most common cancers in the world. The most common site is an upper pole. In 50–60 years of age, it originates from *proximal convoluted tubules (PCTs).*

Renal cell carcinoma is of four types:

1. *Clear cell type:* Most common
2. Papillary type
3. *Chromophobe type:* Best prognosis
4. Medullary type

Clinical Features

The most common and earliest symptom is hematuria, left-sided varicocele, and hematogenous metastasis—pulsatile skull secondaries and cannonball secondaries. CECT of the abdomen is the most important investigation. Grading is done by nuclear (Fuhrman) (Susan A Fuhrman, American pathologist, described in 1982) grading and histological scoring (Leibovich) (Bradley C Leibovich, American urologist).

Staging of Renal Cell Carcinoma

It is divided into four stages **(Fig. 4)**:

1. *Stage I:* Mass <7 cm within the kidney
2. *Stage II:* >7 cm within the kidney
3. *Stage III:* Involving renal vein, inferior vena cava (IVC), tumor not gone beyond Gerota's fascia
4. *Stage IV:* Out of Gerota's fascia

Pathology

Cut surface of tumor shows golden-yellow color, areas of hemorrhage, necrosis, and cysts. The cytoplasm is clear due to the collection of glycogen and lipids. Treatment is according to the stage. Partial and radical nephrectomies are to be considered in individual cases. Targeted treatment as tyrosine kinase inhibitors (TKIs), anti-vascular endothelial growth factor (anti-VEGF) monoclonal

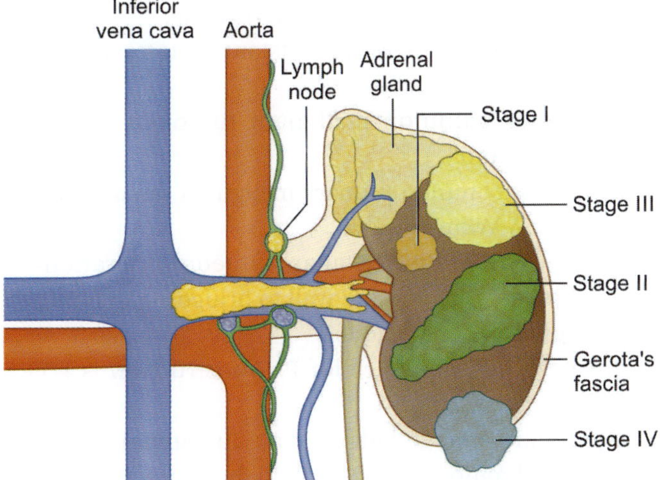

Fig. 4: Stages of renal cell carcinoma (RCC).

antibodies, and mammalian target of rapamycin (mTOR) inhibitors.

> *Good to remember:*
> An obstructed kidney must be preserved if it is contributing >20% of total renal function. Anderson-Hynes pyloroplasty is the best treatment for hydronephrosis. Bosniak's classification of renal cysts divides the cysts into four categories:
> 1. *Category I:* Simple cyst
> 2. *Category II:* Benign cysts
> 3. *Category IIF:* Complex cysts
> 4. *Category III:* Indeterminate masses
> 5. *Category IV:* Malignant cystic masses

WILMS TUMOR (NEPHROBLASTOMA)

It is usually diagnosed in the first 5 years of life, generally in one pole of the kidney, and rapidly grows. It is a big tumor. Hematuria indicates extension into the renal pelvis. Early metastasis occurs in the lungs.

Treatment is chemotherapy followed by nephrectomy.

SOME IMPORTANT POINTS

- Infectious stones are more common in females.
- Calcium oxalate stones are the most common type of renal stones.
- Acidic urine stones are Mn = UCC (urine acid, cystine, and calcium malate).
- *Alkaline urine stones are Mn = SP:* Strovite and calcium phosphate stones.
- 90% of stones are radiopaque.
- Radiolucent stones are (X-URI) uric acid/xanthine/triamterene/indinavir)
- *Hard stone to crack in ESWL:* BHOC—brushite, hydroxyapatite/calcium oxalate/cystine.
- Most common site of RCC distant metastasis—lungs (cannonball).
- The most common malignant tumor in infants—neuroblastoma.
- The most common primary malignant renal tumor in children—Wilm's tumor.
- Boari (Achille Boari, Italian surgeon) operation—a tube made from bladder wall to bridge a gap between the cut ureter and bladder.
- Investigation of choice for PUJ obstruction is DTPA scan.
- Medullary sponge kidney is an autosomal recessive defect, diagnosed by IVU, which shows Bristles on brush due to dilated ducts or Bouquet of flowers due to calcification of ectatic ducts.
- The most common anomaly of the upper urinary tract is a duplicate ureter.
- The most common congenital anomaly of the genitourinary tract is VUR.
- Urinary ascites occurs in neonates when any obstructions, such as a posterior urethral valve and urethral stricture, cause a rise in pressure in the kidney and urine extravasates into the retroperitoneal space and enters the peritoneal cavity as transudate.
- Patent urachus occurs in neonates with fluid leakage from the umbilicus. Diagnosis is done by USG/voiding cystourethrogram (VCUG).

SOME IMPORTANT QUESTIONS

Q1. The treatment of choice for a 0.5 mm renal calyx stone is:

a. Extracorporeal shock wave lithotripsy (ESWL)
b. Percutaneous nephrolithotomy (PCNL)
c. Ureteroscopy
d. Cystoscopy

Ans. a

Q2. LASER used in the treatment of ureteric calculi is:

a. Holmium b. Nd-Yag
c. Argon d. CO_2

Ans. a

Q3. The most common route of infection in kidney tuberculosis is:

a. Ascending spread b. Hematogenous
c. Lymphatic spread d. Direct invasion

Ans. b

Q4. The most common histological variant of renal cell carcinoma is:

a. Clear cell type b. Chromophobe type
c. Papillary type d. Tubular type

Ans. a

Q5. Bilateral renal cell carcinoma is seen in:

a. Eagle-Barrett syndrome
b. Beckwith-Wiedemann syndrome
c. Von Hippel-Lindau (VHL) syndrome
d. Bilateral angiomyolipoma

Ans. c

Q6. The most common site of origin of renal cell carcinoma (RCC) is:

a. Proximal convoluted tubule (PCT)
b. Distal convoluted tubule (DCT)
c. Collecting ducts
d. Loop of Henle

Ans. a

Q7. Paraneoplastic syndrome associated with RCC is all of the following, *except*:

a. Polycythemia
b. Hypercalcemia
c. Malignant hypertension
d. Cushing syndrome

Ans. None

Q8. The most common presentation of renal adenocarcinoma is:

a. Hematuria
b. Local pain
c. Mass
d. Fever

Ans. a

Q9. The most common systemic abnormality associated with renal cell carcinoma is:

a. Hypertension
b. Polycythemia
c. Elevated erythrocyte sedimentation rate (ESR)
d. Pyrexia

Ans. c

Q10. Radical nephrectomy includes all of the following, *except*:

a. Early ligation of vessels
b. Lymphadenectomy
c. Keeping fascia back in place
d. Removal of the kidney, including Gerota's fascia

Ans. c

Q11. Low and fixed specific gravity of urine is seen in:

a. Diabetes mellitus
b. Diabetes insipidus
c. Chronic renal failure
d. Acute glomerulonephritis

Ans. c

Q12. Urine incontinence is seen in all, *except*:

a. Ureterovaginal fistula
b. Vesicovaginal fistula
c. Ectopic ureter
d. Urethrovaginal fistula

Ans. d

MULTIPLE CHOICE QUESTIONS

Grade I | Simple

Q1. Renal calculi associated with *Proteus* infection: (All India 2011)

a. Uric acid
b. Triple phosphate
c. Calcium oxalate
d. Xanthine

Q2. Ureteric colic due to stone is caused by: (All India 2008)

a. Stretching of renal capsule due to back pressure
b. Increased peristalsis of a ureter to overcome the obstruction
c. Irritation of the intramural ureter
d. Extravasation of urine

Q3. The treatment of choice of ureteric colic is: (GB Pant 2010)

a. Nitrites
b. Pethidine
c. Adrenaline
d. Diclofenac

Q4. Which of the following stones is hard to break by ESWL? (All India 2010)

a. Calcium oxalate monohydrate
b. Calcium oxalate dehydrate
c. Uric acid
d. Struvite

Q5. What complication should one expect when PCNL is done through the 11th intercostal space? (All India 2010)

a. Hydrothorax
b. Hematuria
c. Damage
d. Remnant fragments

Q6. Which of the following is not a contraindication for ESWL for renal calculi? (AIIMS June 2003)

a. Uncorrected bleeding diathesis
b. Pregnancy
c. Ureteric stricture
d. Stone in a calyceal diverticulum

Q7. Which one of the following is the radiolucent stone? (MCI 2007)

a. Calcium oxalate
b. Cystine
c. Uric acid
d. Phosphate

Q8. Which of the following advises is not given to a 35-year-old female patient with recurrent renal stones? (AIIMS November 2012)

a. Increase water
b. Restrict protein
c. Restrict salt
d. Restricted calcium intake

Q9. Which of the following are radiolucent renal stones? (JIPMER 2012)

a. Uric acid stones
b. Cystine stones
c. Mixed stones
d. Calcium oxalate stones

Q10. A patient has been passing stones recurrently in urine for the past few years. All are to be restricted in diet, *except*: (AIIMS November 2010)

a. Protein restriction
b. Calcium restriction
c. Salt restricted
d. Phosphate restriction

Q11. The most common cause of emphysematous pyelonephritis is: (GB Pant 2011)

a. *Escherichia coli*
b. *Proteus*
c. *Klebsiella*
d. *Pseudomonas*

Q12. The following is true of pyonephrosis, *except*: (AIIMS 1992)

a. Commonly associated with renal calculi
b. Always unilateral
c. It is a complication of hydronephrosis.
d. Follows acute pyelonephritis

Q13. A boy is suffering from acute pyelonephritis. The most specific urinary finding will be: (AIIMS May 2012)

a. White blood cell (WBC) cast
b. Leukocyte esterase test
c. Nitrite test
d. Bacteria in the Gram stain

Q14. Chromophobe variant renal cell carcinoma is associated with: (All India 2010)

a. *VHL* gene mutations
b. Trisomy of 7 and 17 (+7, +17)
c. 3p deletions (3p-)
d. Monosomy of 1 and Y (-1, -Y)

Q15. Most important prognostic indicator for renal cell carcinoma is: (AIIMS May 2009)

a. Nuclear grade
b. Histological type
c. Size
d. Pathological staging

Q16. Not true about "struvite stones" is: (AIIMS Nov 2001)

a. Better known as staghorn calculus
b. These are triple phosphate stones
c. Common in infected urine
d. Usually seen in acidic urine

Q17. The most common stone in case of urinary tract infection (UTI): (AIIMS Nov 1997)

a. Phosphate
b. Urate
c. Cysteine
d. Calcium oxalate

Q18. Oxalate stones are found in: (PGI June 2006)

a. Ethylene glycol
b. Ethanol
c. Diethyl glycol
d. Methyl alcohol

Q19. Locate the renal stone with pain radiating to the medial side of the thigh and perineum due to slipping of the stone in males: (AIIMS June 2010)

a. At pelvic brim
b. Intramural opening of the ureter
c. Junction of the ureter and renal pelvic
d. At the crossing of the gonadal vessels and the ureter

Q20. Triad of renal colic, swelling in the loin which disappears after passing urine, is called: (All India 1996)

a. Kocher's triad
b. Saint's triad
c. Dietl's crisis
d. Charcot's triad

Grade II	***Difficult***

Q1. A 65-year-old male banker came for an ultrasound to renew his medical insurance. In the right kidney, a complex cyst was found, and the picture of the CT scan is given below. Most likely diagnosis is: (AIIMS May 2017)

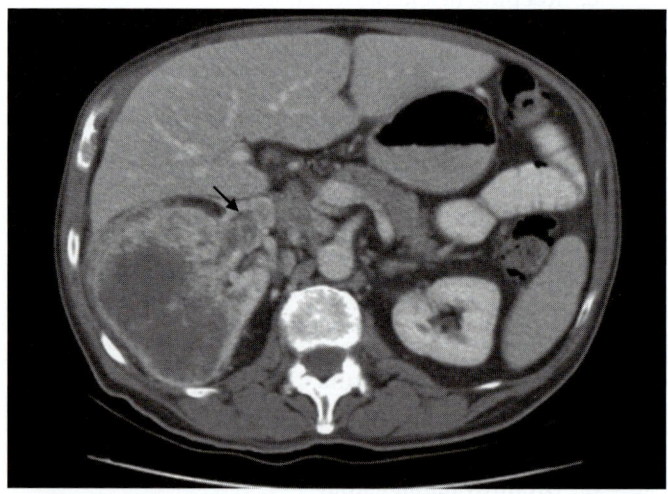

a. Oncocytoma
b. Angiomyolipoma
c. Perinephric cyst
d. Renal cell carcinoma

Q2. A patient with a suspected renal tumor/mass is diagnosed by exfoliative urinary cytology. Which of the following histological types is most likely to be diagnosed on urinary exfoliative cytology? (All India 2012)

a. Transitional cell carcinoma
b. Adenocarcinoma
c. Well-differentiated carcinoma (low grade)
d. All three types can be easily detected on exfoliative cytology.

Q3. All are true about Wilms' tumor, *except*: (All India 1997)

a. Fever and weakness are clinical features
b. Arises from primitive cells
c. Hematuria is almost always present
d. It presents as an abdominal mass

Q4. Which of the following is the treatment of choice for stage I Wilms' tumor? (All India 2012)

a. Laparoscopic nephrectomy
b. Open nephroureterectomy
c. Chemotherapy
d. Observation

Q5. Wilms' tumor chromosome is: (JIPMER 2012)

a. 13q
b. 13p14
c. 11p13
d. 17

Q6. During renal rupture, the nephrectomy is not attempted until: (UPPG 2010)

a. Fluid replacement
b. Antibiotics covers
c. Contralateral renal function is ascertained
d. Renal angiogram

Q7. Polycystic disease of the kidney may have cysts in all the following organs, *except*: (All India 2004)

a. Lungs
b. Liver
c. Pancreas
d. Spleen

Q8. All are true about polycystic kidney, *except*: (UPPG 2009)

a. Inherited as autosomal recessive
b. Hypertension and hematuria are common symptoms.
c. Spider leg deformity
d. Associated with cysts in the liver and spleen

Q9. Which one of the following statements is wrong regarding adult polycystic kidney disease? (AIIMS November 2004)

a. Mitral valve prolapse
b. Hepatic cysts
c. Splenic cysts
d. Colonic diverticulosis

Q10. Which one of the following statements is wrong regarding adult polycystic kidney disease? (AIIMS May 2004)

a. Kidneys are enlarged in size.
b. The presentation is unilateral.
c. Intracranial aneurysms may be associated.
d. Typically manifests in the third decade

Q11. Not true about congenital pelvi-ureteric junction (PUJ) obstruction is: (AIIMS November 2001)

a. Can be associated with renal agenesis
b. Can be diagnosed antenatally
c. Bilateral in 10–15% of cases
d. Aberrant vessel is the most common cause.

Q12. Most infants and children with pelvi-ureteric junction obstruction (PUJO) present with: (GB Pant 2008)

a. Pain
b. Hematuria
c. Painless abdominal mass
d. Renal failure

Q13. Best management for a symptomatic 6-year-old male with PUJ obstruction: (GB Pant 2010)

a. Endopyelotomy
b. Foley V-Y pyeloplasty
c. Dismembered pyeloplasty
d. Wait and watch

Q14. Referred pain from ureteric colic is felt in the groin due to involvement of the following nerve: (All India 2003)

a. Subcostal
b. Iliohypogastric
c. Ilioinguinal
d. Genitofemoral

Q15. The most common presentation of bilateral ureteric stones: (AIIMS 1991)

a. Chronic renal failure (CRF)
b. UTI
c. Pain
d. Hematuria

Q16. A patient present with pain and tenderness in the left iliac fossa. USG shows a 3 cm stone in the renal pelvis without any hydro-nephrosis. Most appropriate management: (AIIMS May 2012)

a. PCNL
b. ESWL
c. Diuretics
d. Medical dissolution therapy with KCI

Q17. All are radiopaque, *except* one: (AIIMS June 2000)

a. Oxalate
b. Uric acid
c. Cystine
d. Mixed

Q18. A child presents with complaints of abdominal colic and hematuria USG showed a renal stone 2.5 cm in diameter in renal pelvis the next step in management of this case: (AIIMS Nov 2000)

a. ESWL
b. Pyelolithotomy
c. Nephroureterostomy
d. Conservative

Q19. A 10 mm calculus in the right lower ureter associated with proximal hydroureteronephrosis is best treated with: (All India 2003)

a. ESWL
b. Antegrade percutaneous access
c. Open ureterolithotomy
d. Ureteroscopic retrieval

Q20. Treatment used for lower ureteric stone is: (AIIMS June 1998)

a. Endoscopic removal
b. Diuretics
c. Drug dissolution
d. Laser

Grade III | Most difficult

Q1. Which of the following is the most common renal vascular anomaly? (All India 2010)

a. Supernumerary renal arteries
b. Supernumerary renal veins
c. Double renal arteries
d. Double renal veins

Q2. Persistent fetal lobulation of adult kidney is due to: (AIIMS November 2007)

a. Congenital renal defect
b. Obstructive uropathy
c. Intrauterine infection and scar
d. Is a normal variant

Q3. All are true of an aberrant renal artery, *except*: (PGI 1993)

a. Bilateral
b. Leads to hydronephrosis
c. Common in females
d. More common on the left side

Q4. Cobra head appearance on excretory urography is suggestive of: (MCI March 2010)

a. Horseshoe kidney
b. Duplication of renal pelvis
c. Simple cyst of the kidney
d. Ureterocele

Q5. Adder head appearance on intravenous pyelography (IVP) is/are seen in: (PGI November 2011)

a. Polycystic kidney
b. Ureterocele
c. Horseshoe kidney
d. Hydronephrosis
e. Ectopic ureter

Q6. According to Weigert-Meyer's rule of duplication of ureter, the lower pole ureter in the urinary bladder is: (JIPMER November 2017)

a. Lateral and cephalad to the upper pole ureter
b. Lateral and caudal to the upper pole ureter
c. Medial and cephalad to the upper pole ureter
d. Medial and caudal to the upper pole ureter

Q7. In case of vesicoureteric reflux, which will be the investigation of choice? (AIIMS November 1998)

a. Micturating cystourethrogram
b. IVP
c. Cystography
d. Radionuclide study

Q8. In a patient suspected to be suffering from vesicoureteric reflex, which one of the following radiological investigations may confirm the diagnosis? (UPSC 2007)

a. Intravenous urography
b. Micturating cystourethrography
c. Pelvic ultrasound
d. Antegrade pyelography

Q9. Treatment of choice for grade IV vesicoureteric reflux with recurrent UTI is: (AIIMS June 2000)

a. Cotrimoxazole
b. Bilateral reimplantation of ureter
c. Injection of collagen in the ureter
d. Endoscopic resection of ureter

Q10. Features of hepatorenal syndrome are: (PGI June 2006)

a. Urine sodium <10 mEq/L
b. Normal renal histology
c. Renal functional abnormal even after liver become normal.
d. Proteinuria

Q11. First autologous renal transplantation was done: (All India 2010)

a. Hardy
b. Kavosis
c. Higgins
d. Studor

Q12. All of the following statements are correct about renal transplantation, *except*: (AIIMS November 2004)

a. Renal transplantation is heterotrophic.
b. Cyclosporine is the mainstay of immunosuppression
c. In India, organ harvesting from brain-dead patients is not permitted by law.
d. Kidney after removal is flushed with a cold perfusion solution.

Q13. After renal transplant, the most common malignancy is: (AIIMS June 1997)

a. Lymphoma
b. Renal cell carcinoma
c. Skin cancer
d. Adrenal cancer

Q14. After renal transplantation, which drug is given? (PGI June 1996)

a. Cyclophosphamide
b. Corticosteroids
c. Interferon
d. Cyclosporine

Q15. All of the following structures cross the right ureter anatomically, *except*: (All India 2012)

a. Terminal ileum
b. Vas deferens
c. Genitofemoral nerve
d. Right colic and ileocolic vessels

Q16. Ureteric construction is seen at all the following positions, *except*: (All India 2002)

a. Ureteropelvic junction
b. Ureterovesical junction
c. Crossing of the iliac artery
d. Ischial spine

Q17. Sickle cell trait is associated with which type of RCC? (JIPMER November 2017)

a. Medullary
b. Papillary
c. Chromophobe
d. Clear cell

Q18. Which of the following statements about the Holmium: YAG laser is incorrect? (AIIMS June 2004)

a. It has a wavelength of 2,100 nm
b. Its use for uric acid stones has caused deaths due to the generation of cyanide
c. It is effective against the hardest urinary stones
d. It can even cut the wire of stone baskets

Q19. All are indicated in a patient with cystinuria with multiple renal stones, *except*: (AIIMS Nov 2012)

a. Cysteamine
b. Increase fluid intake
c. Alkalinization of urine
d. Penicillamine

Q20. Which is false regarding ureteric stones? (AIIMS 1992)

a. Urine is always infected
b. Should be removed immediately
c. The source is always the kidneys
d. Pain in referred to tip of penis is intramural stones

ANSWERS

Grade I: 1. b (Bailey 27/e p1406); 2. b; 3. d; 4. a (Bailey 27/e p1408); 5. a (Bailey 27/e p1409); 6. d (Campbell 11/e p1278); 7. c; 8. d (Harrison 19/e p1870); 9. a; 10. b (Smith 18/e p253); 11. a; 12. b (Bailey 27/e p1412); 13. c (Smith 18/e p200); 14. d; 15. d; 16. d; 17. a; 18. a (Smith 18/e p254); 19. a (Bailey 27/e p1407); 20. c (Bailey 27/e p1411)

Grade II: 1. d (Bailey 27/e p1409); 2. a; 3. c; 4. b; 5. c; 6. c; 7. a; 8. a; 9. b; 10. b; 11. d; 12. c; 13. c; 14. b; 15. c; 16. a (Campbell 11/e p1236); 17. b; 18. a (Bailey 27/e p1408); 19. d (Bailey 27/e p1408); 20. a (Bailey 27/e p1408)

Grade III: 1. a (Smith 18/e p522); 2. d; 3. a; 4. d (Bailey 27/e p1401); 5. b; 6. a; 7. a (Campbell 11/e p3141); 8. b; 9. a; 10. a, b (Sabiston 20/e p1043); 11. a (Campbell 11/e p1087); 12. c (Bailey 27/e p1542); 13. c; 14. b, d; 15. c; 16. d; 17. a; 18. b (Smith 18/e p167); 19. a (Harrison 19/e p1871); 20. a, b

MODEL QUESTIONS

Q1. "Stipple sign" in transitional cell carcinoma of the renal collecting system is best demonstrated by:

a. Intravenous urography
b. Retrograde pyeloureterography
c. Radionuclide scan
d. Ultrasound scan

Ans. b

Q2. Nephroureterectomy is indicated in:

a. Renal cell carcinoma
b. Chronic pyelonephritis

c. Polycystic kidney disease
d. Transitional carcinoma of the pelvis extending till the ureter

Ans. d

Q3. What percent of cases with injury to kidney require surgical exploration?

a. 20% b. 90%
c. 50% d. 70%

Ans. a

Q4. In renal trauma, which statement is not correct?

a. Exploration is indicated in 90% of cases.
b. Hematuria is a cardinal sign.
c. Transperitoneal approach is preferred.
d. Intravenous pyelography (IVP) is urgently indicated.

Ans. a

Q5. Polycystic kidney disease is associated with all of the following, *except*:

a. Cerebral aneurysms
b. Mitral valve prolapse
c. Renal cell carcinoma
d. Hepatic cysts

Ans. c

Q6. All of the following are true about childhood polycystic kidney disease, *except*:

a. Autosomal dominant
b. Pulmonary hypoplasia may be seen.
c. Renal cysts are present at birth.
d. Congenital hepatic fibrosis may be seen.

Ans. a

Q7. All are true in PUJO, *except*:

a. Common in boys
b. Bilateral lesions occur in 10–40%
c. Right-sided lesions predominate
d. Intrinsic lesions predominate

Ans. c

Q8. Distention of the abdomen with the passage of a large amount of urine is known as:

a. Dietl's crisis
b. Anderson–Hynes crises
c. Meteorism
d. Strangury

Ans. a

Q9. The treatment of choice for ureterocele is:

a. Double-J (DJ) stent
b. Laparoscopic repair
c. LASER ablation
d. Endoscopic diathermy

Ans. d

Q10. Ectopic ureter opening is not located in:

a. Bulbar urethra b. Prostatic urethra
c. Seminal vesicle d. Bladder neck

Ans. a

Q11. Reflux into pelvis and calyces without dilatation:

a. I b. II
c. III d. IV

Ans. a

Q12. What is Bertini's column in the kidney?

a. Renal tumor
b. Tongue-like papillary projection
c. Calculus
d. None

Ans. b

Q13. Unilateral small smooth kidney is seen in:

a. Reflux nephropathy
b. Lobar infarction
c. Renal artery stenosis
d. Chronic glomerulonephritis

Ans. c

SUGGESTED READING

1. Campbell's Urology, 10th edition.
2. Smith's Urology, 18th edition.
3. Textbook of Surgery by David Sabiston, 21st edition.

CHAPTER 46

Urinary Bladder

"The length of a film should be directly proportional to the endurance of the human bladder."

- Alfred Hitchcock

ANATOMY OF THE URINARY BLADDER

The urinary bladder has transitional epithelium as the innermost layer, which rests on laminate propria having plexuses of blood vessels and lymphatics. It rests on the submucosa, which covers the detrusor muscle layer, and the outermost layer is a connective tissue layer called adventitia. The detrusor muscle hypertrophy forms trabeculations. The trigone is a triangular thin muscle to which is adherent the epithelium and is continuous with the urethra and two ureters. The urethra has two sphincters: (1) Proximal made of smooth muscle called internal sphincter, supplied by adrenergic fibers preventing retrograde ejaculation and (2) the distal is made of striated or skeletal muscle and is horseshoe-shaped which is supplied by S2–S4 through pudendal nerve and called external sphincter **(Figs. 1A to D)**.

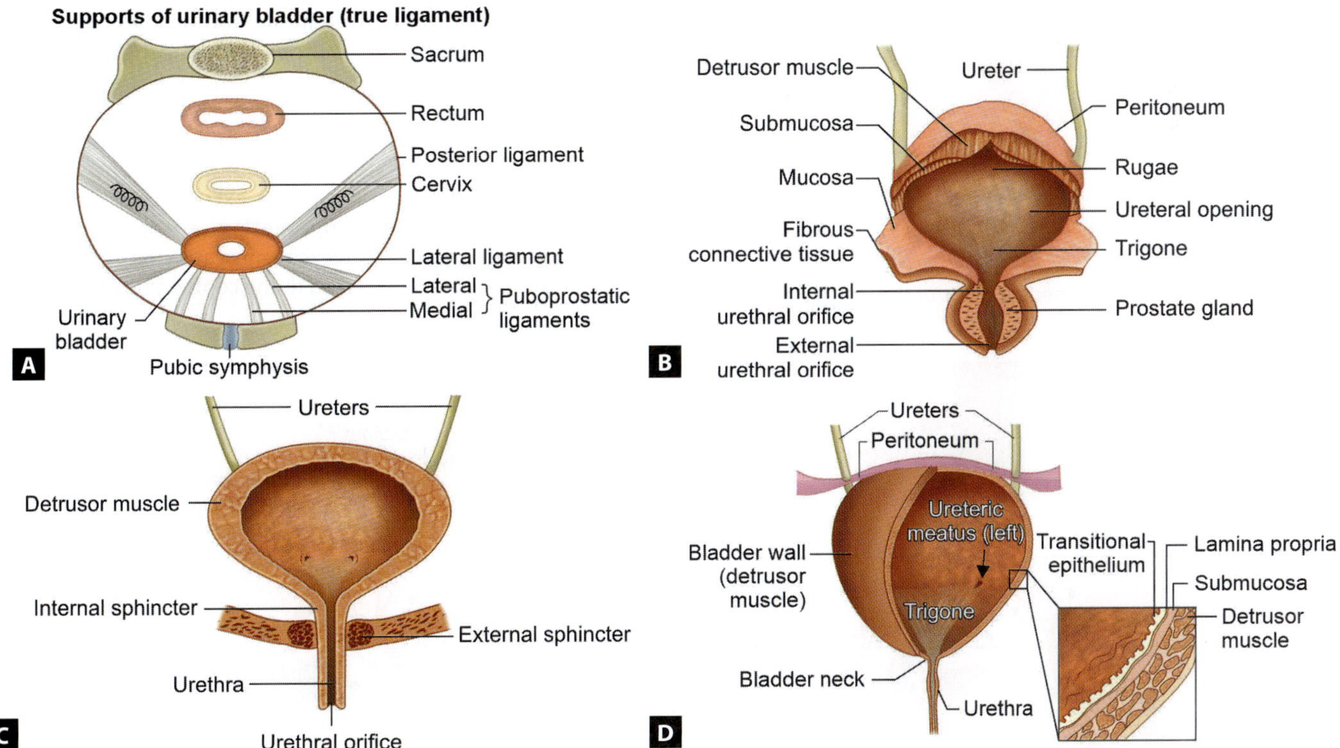

Figs. 1A to D: Anatomy of the urinary bladder.

LIGAMENTS AND OTHER SUPPORTS OF URINARY BLADDER

Ligaments and fascial support to the urinary bladder are ***(Fig. 2)***:
- The body of bladder receives support from the pelvic diaphragm from below in females and the prostate gland in males, lateral support from the obturator internus and levator ani muscles.
- Puboprostatic ligaments from the prostate to the pubis.
- The urachus and obliterated hypogastric arteries are with the peritoneal fold called the medial and lateral umbilical ligaments.

ARTERIAL SUPPLY OF THE BLADDER

The superior and inferior vesicle arteries supply the bladder after branching out from the internal iliac arteries.

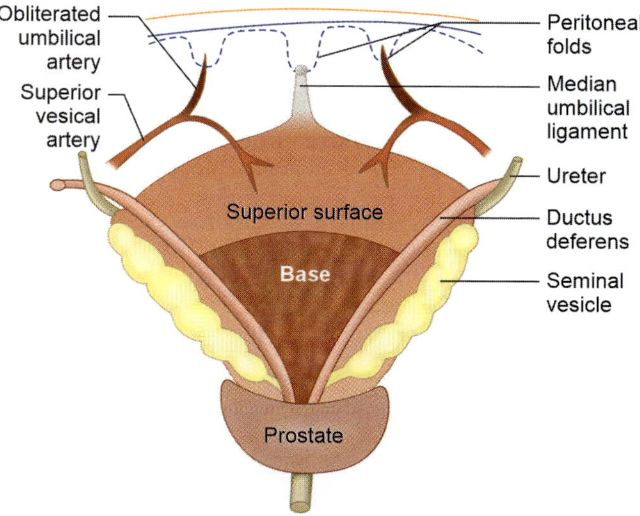

Fig. 2: Ligaments and other supports of the urinary bladder.

The urinary bladder also receives some blood supply from the obturator artery and the inferior gluteal artery.

VENOUS DRAINAGE OF BLADDER

The venous drainage from the urinary bladder starts as two large venous plexuses: (1) the vesicle and (2) the pudendal plexus. The blood is drained from the urinary bladder wall to the vesicle plexus and mainly to the pudendal plexus. Venous plexuses are a network of small veins covering the bladder, the neck of the bladder, and the proximal urethra.

LYMPHATIC DRAINAGE OF THE BLADDER

The superolateral area of the urinary bladder lymphatics drains to the external iliac lymph nodes. The fundus and neck of the urinary bladder lymphatics drain to the internal iliac, sacral, and common iliac lymph nodes. The lymphatic drainage from the proximal urethra and labia drains to the inguinal lymph nodes **(Figs. 3A and B)**.

NERVE SUPPLY OF THE BLADDER

The urinary bladder receives its nerve supply through a network of parasympathetic **(Fig. 4)**, sympathetic, and somatic nerve fibers. Parasympathetic fibers arrive from sacral spinal nerves (S2-S4) which amalgamates and forms pelvic splanchnic nerves. These nerves excite the bladder and relax the urethra so as to pass urine. Lumbar sympathetic nerves inhibit the urinary bladder and excite the base of bladder and urethra. The pudendal nerve supplies to the extraurethral sphincter. Pudendal nerve is a parasympathetic nerve which releases acetylcholine (ACh) which can excite muscarinic receptors in the bladder smooth muscles leading to the contraction of bladder.

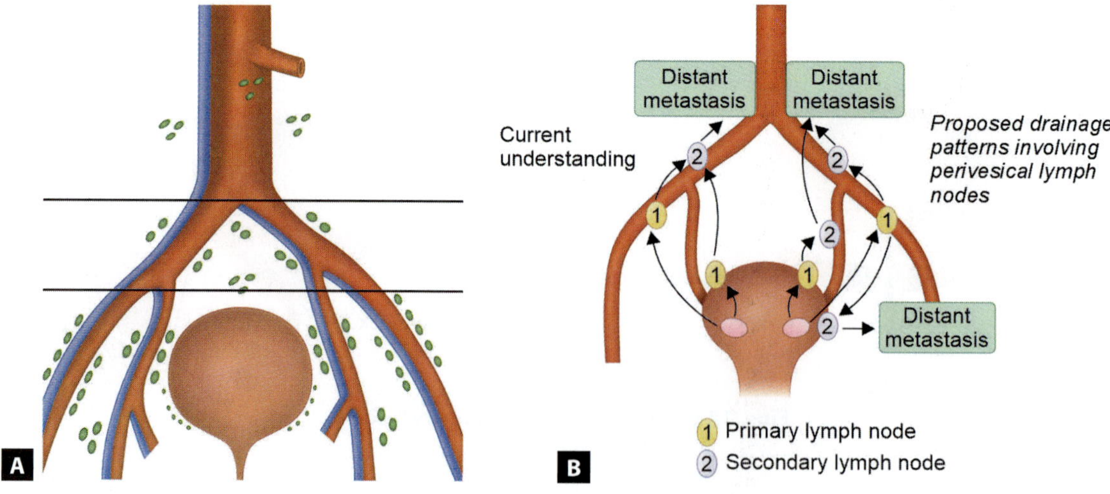

Figs. 3A and B: Lymphatic drainage of the bladder.

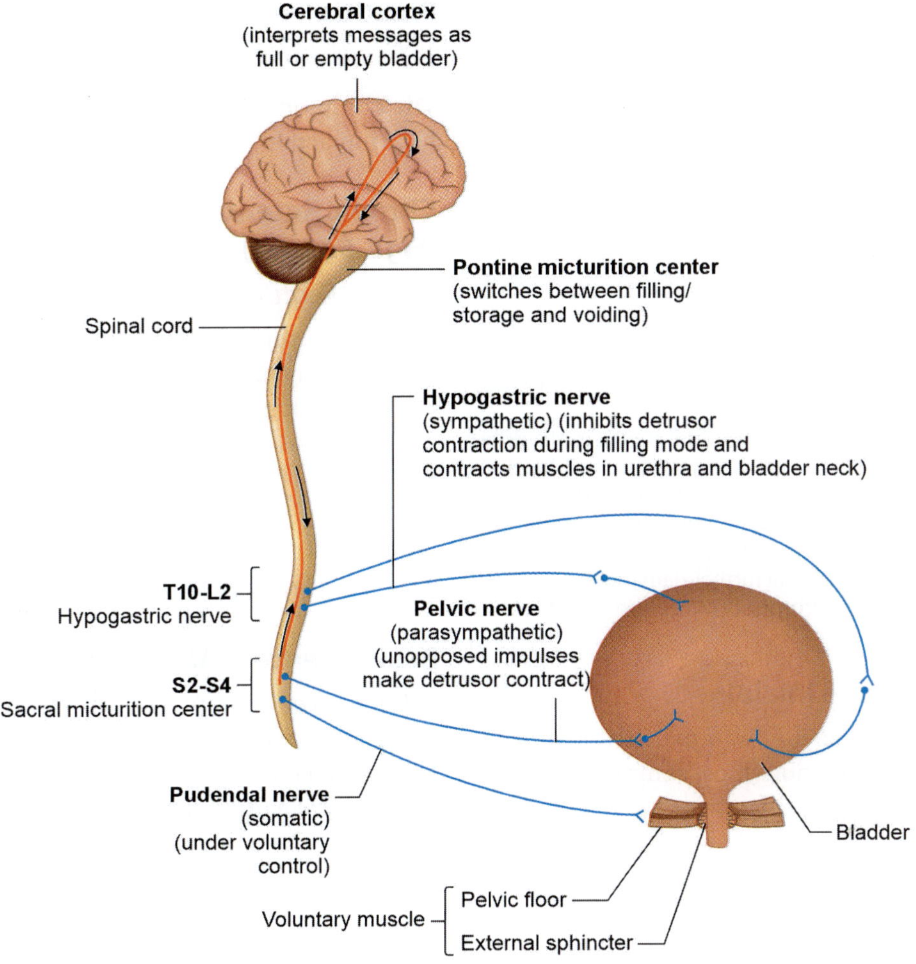

Fig. 4: Nerve supply of the bladder.

> *Points to remember:*
> *Catheterization for acute retention of urine:* Catheterization should be done with all the aseptic precautions as this procedure is known to introduce infection most commonly into the urinary tract. Before catheterization, the urethra must be anesthetized with a lignocaine jelly, after introducing the jelly in urethra the penis is either clamped or held tightly closing the urethra at the bottom of gland and massage is done from distal to proximal urethra. After catheterization, the volume of urine removed must be measured and recorded. Whenever the indwelling catheter is laced for long time, especially in old age, at the time of removal, intermittent closure should be done for 1–2 days to get away from so-called bladder disuse hypotonia.

CONGENITAL DISORDERS OF URINARY BLADDER

Bladder Exstrophy (Ectopia Vesical)

It is having total urinary incontinence with dribbling of urine. In males, it is associated with umbilical and inguinal hernia, epispadias, and undescended testis.

In females, it is associated with umbilical hernia, epispadias, split clitoris, wide labia, urinary incontinence, and wide-open pelvis with duck-like waddling gait.

Treatment

- Enterocystoplasty
- Urinary diversion with cystectomy if the bladder is small and fibrotic

Trauma to the Bladder

- It may be intraperitoneal or extraperitoneal.
- CT scan and intravenous urography (IVU) are required.
- Midline incision and repair of the bladder wound is done with 2/0 absorbable suture after catheterization.

Rupture of the Bladder

- Due to injury to a full bladder
- *Classical triad:* Suprapubic pain and tenderness + Inability to pass urine + Hematuria.

Types

Extraperitoneal:

- Due to pelvic fracture
- CT-tear drop bladder/pear sign/flame sign

Treatment: Catheterization

Intraperitoneal:

- The dome of the bladder is most commonly affected.
  - Peritonitis
  - X-Ray—ground glass appearance
  - Cystography is the investigation of choice

> *Not to forget:*
> *Urethral injury:* The most common urethral injury is straddle injury which leads to bulbar urethra injury causing blood at urethral meats and retention of urine. Membranous urethra injury occurs due to fracture of pelvis and P/R examination shows high and floating prostate gland (Vermooten sign). Never try to pass Foley's catheter as it will further damage the urethra. Suprapubically, a catheter is introduced into the bladder and cystogram done through it.

Incontinence of Urine (Male)

The common causes of retention: In males, it can occur due to bladder neck obstruction (most common), urethral stricture, phimosis, and urethritis.

Prostitis

In females, it occurs due to a retroverted gravid uterus.

The common causes in males and females are: Calculi, fecal impaction, and rupture of the urethra.

Chronic Retention of Urine (Figs. 5A to D)

Clinical Features

- Urine is not passed for a few hours.
- Pain in hypogastrium
- The bladder is palpable and visible above the pubic symphysis and dull on percussion.
- Patient is restless.

Treatment

Treatment is catheterization.

Incontinence of Urine (Female)

It is more common in women, diagnosed by history and physical examination as the initial diagnostic procedure. Urinary infection can be identified by doing a culture and sensitivity of a urine sample.

A

Bladder function

Storage and intermittent evacuation of urine are served by three structural components—bladder itself, detrusor, functional internal sphincter composed of smooth muscle, striated external sphincter or urogenital diaphragm

Urinary bladder

- Urinary bladder is a musculomembranous sac which acts as a reservoir for the urine
- The bladder is the most anterior element of the pelvic viscera
- It is entirely situated in the pelvic cavity when empty, it expands superiorly into the abdomen when full

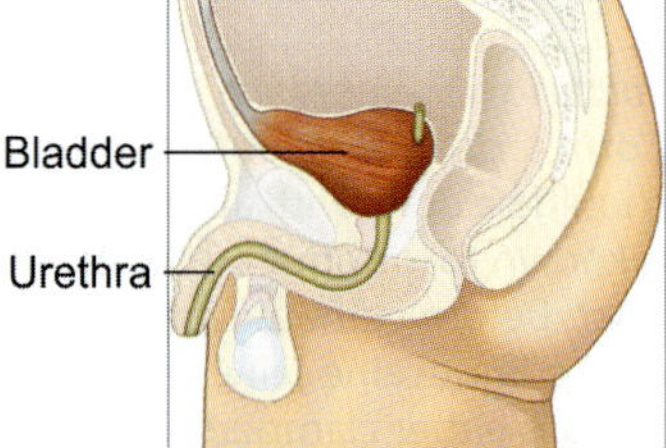

C

Structure and function

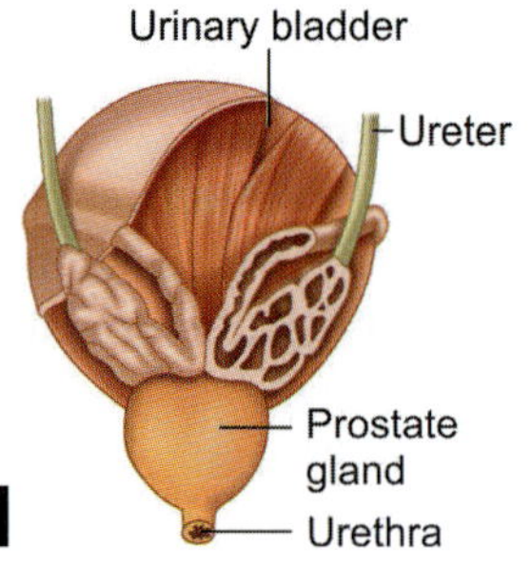

- Hollow, muscular organ that stores urine
- Sphincter muscles hold the urine in place
- Holds 300 to 400 milliliters of urine before emptying
- Walls contain epithelial tissue that stretch to allow the bladder to hold twice its capacity
- The trigone is a triangular area at the base of the bladder where the ureters enter and the urethra exits

D

Urinary bladder

- The urinary bladder is posterior to the pubic symphysis
- The shape of urinary bladder depends on how much urine is contain, when empty, it look like a deflated balloon
- Capacity-700–800 mL
- Smaller in female because, uterus occupies the space superior to the urinary bladder
- Toward the base of urinary bladder, the ureter drains into the urinary bladder via the ureteral opening

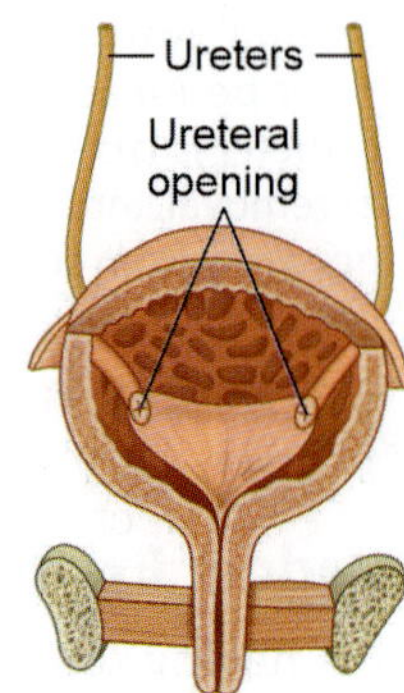

Figs. 5A to D: Structure and function related to the retention of urine.

> *You may be asked:*
> *Urinary fistula*: The most common fistula here is vesicovaginal fistula due to obstetric trauma. Three swab tests, (1) vaginoscopy, (2) cystoscopy, and (3) intravenous urography (IVU) should be done. Surgical procedure of repair is required as a conservative treatment and is rarely successful. The secret of a successful surgical repair is the removal of all diseased tissues and tension-free repair.

Urodynamic testing is the main test for the urinary tract, especially of the bladder. This can find out stress incontinence as in coughing, leakage of urine occurs and detrusor instability. The normal adult bladder can accommodate 400–550 mL of urine. Normal voiding pressure is around and <60 cmH_2O in males and 40 cmH_2O in females. The overactive bladder is due to an overactive detrusor, and a physical increase in pressure gives urgency and urge incontinence. Genuine stress incontinence (GSI) is actually urinary leakage during increased bladder pressure when this is solely due to increased abdominal pressure. It is caused by a weak sphincter.

Causes of Incontinence

- Impaired social perception
- Small bladder/small functional capacity of the bladder.
- Bladder emptying is defective.
- Weak sphincter

Uses of Urodynamic Testing

- Investigation of incontinence
- To differentiate GSI from detrusor instability in women
- To differentiate bladder outflow obstruction (BOO) from idiopathic detrusor instability (IDI) in men. Male incontinence is due to chronic urinary retention with overflow and prostatectomy. Female incontinence is stress incontinence. Incontinence is common in males and females and is due to congenital, aging, infection, trauma, and neoplasm.

Treatment of Incontinence

- Pelvic floor exercises
- Bladder training
- Catheterization—indwelling
- Enterocystoplasty in a small bladder
- Prostatectomy
- Colposuspension
- Urinary diversions
- Bladder substitution
- *Clam enterocystoplasty:* It was developed by Bramble (Frank James Bramble, British urologist) for nocturnal enuresis, but now for idiopathic detrusor instability (IDI).

> *Good to remember:*
> Urinary tract infection (UTI) is more common in females than males. A shorter urethra is probably a factor. Common investigations are urine examinations and culture, and sensitivity tests. Imaging of the upper urinary tract and cystoscopy are required in almost every case if it is recurrent. Sterile pyuria presence indicates infection by tuberculosis (TB), *Neisseria gonorrhoeae*, and *Mycoplasma genitalium*. Frequency-dysuria syndrome, or urethral syndrome, is having lower UTIs with negative urine culture.

URINARY BLADDER STONE (VESICAL CALCULUS)

Primary bladder stone develops in sterile urine and it usually comes down from kidney but secondary stone occurs due to BOO and infection. Bladder stones are more common in Asian countries than in Western countries. Oxalate stone is most common. Bladder stones move freely in the bladder. Clinically, stones of the bladder are either symptomatic or asymptomatic and are more common in men (8:1).

- Pain in lower abdomen, suprapubic region, and pelvis, and at tip of penis.
- Strangury
- Sense of incomplete emptying
- Hematuria
- UTI symptoms
- Interruption in urinary stream

Ultrasonography (USG) and computed tomography (CT) are the main investigations.

Treatment is by lithotripsy and percutaneous suprapubic litholapaxy.

Malakoplakia

It is an inflammatory disease of the urinary bladder due to defective phagolysosomal activity of macrophages or monocytes. It can also involve the ureters and kidneys.

Risk Factors

- Immunosuppressors
- Diabetes

Investigation

USG/CT

Treatment

- Trimethoprim-sulfamethoxazole (TMP-SMX)
- Fluoroquinolones

BLADDER DIVERTICULA

- These are either congenital due to urachus or acquired propulsion due to BOO.
- Usually, it is 2–5 cm in size, lined by bladder mucosa, situated above and lateral to the ureteric orifice.

Normal intravesical pressure during voiding is 35–50 cmH_2O, but pressure up to 150 cmH_2O can be tolerated by a hypertrophied bladder; however, more than that pushes the mucosa through the muscles, forming diverticulae.

Complications

- Recurrent UTI
- Stone formation
- Hydronephrosis and hydroureter due to fibrosis around a ureteral orifice.

Clinical Features

Usually, a male adult with symptoms of UTI and hematuria. Cancer can occur in a diverticulum in <5% of cases. Most frequently diagnosed incidentally while doing a cystoscopy. Treatment is by diverticulectomy, intravesical, and extravesical.

URINARY FISTULAE

- Ectopia vesicle, patent urachus, with imperforate anus.
- Traumatic fistulae.
- Generally, after surgery or radiation.

VESICOVAGINAL FISTULAE

It can develop from:

- Obstetric causes, such as neglected labor.
- Gynecological causes, such as complications of total hysterectomy.
- Radiotherapy
- Neoplastic invasions

Clinically, there is urine leak which can be seen with vaginal speculum. Three swab tests: one swab is kept in vagina, methylene blue dye is injected in urethra, and the vaginal swab becomes colored. Surgical repair is required. Lower UTI and cystitis. Infection of the urinary bladder is called "cystitis."

Risk factors for lower UTI:
- BOO
- Stone
- Foreign body
- Pregnancy
- Vesicoureteric reflux in children
- Diabetes mellitus
- *Other causes:* Tumor and perianal infection

Routes of Infection

- Ascending from the urethra and descending from the kidney.
- Organisms commonly involved are *Escherichia coli, Proteus mirabilis, Staphylococcus epidermidis, Streptococcus faecalis, Pseudomonas, Klebsiella, Mycobacterium tuberculosis*, and *Neisseria gonorrhoea.*
- Clinically, a patient has frequency, pain, hematuria, and pyuria. Treatment is by antibiotics after a culture and sensitivity test.

URETHRAL SYNDROME

- It has symptoms of lower UTI with a negative urine culture.
- Hunner's (Guy Leroy Hunner, American gynecologist, 1868–1957, described in 1914).
- Ulcer (interstitial cystitis).

Symptoms of pain and frequency are absent after micturition. Hematuria is present. Symptoms increase by overdistention and jolts of travel; chronic pancystitis leads to ulceration, fibrosis, and reduced size of the bladder. Linear bleeding ulcers are characteristic of it, developing after distention of the bladder after an anesthesia. Cystoscopy reveals it, and decompression of the bladder after cystoscopy causes bleeding. No specific treatment is available, but one can get some relief by hydrostatic dilatation.

SCHISTOSOMIASIS BILHARZIASIS OF URINARY BLADDER

It is common in Egypt and other Arab countries. Lifecycle: Bathing in infected water cercariae (embryos) penetrate skin and enter circulation and go to liver and develop into adult male and female worms, leave liver and enter portal vein then reach vertical plexus of veins and female gives 20 ova in a chain form which penetrate vessel wall and appear in urine and reach fresh water and enter into the snail as the intermediate host. Clinically, swimmers' itch, fever, sweating, pain, and intermittent painless terminal hematuria are present.

Types

- *Schistosoma hematobium*: Urinary affects blades
- *Schistosoma japonicum*: Liver and small bowel
- *Schistosoma mansoni*: Large intestine

X-ray

- Fetal head appearance—calcification in the wall of the urinary bladder.
- Linear or parallel calcification due to the calcification of the distal ureters.

EGGS IN URINE

Eggs, miracidium and cercaria move to venous plexus of urinary bladder.

- Katayama fever is due to acute schistosomiasis [(Mn = HALF) fever, allergy, hepatosplenomegaly, lymphadenopathy].

> Diagnosis is done by examining the early morning last few mm of urine for a few consecutive days. Cystoscopy reveals Bilharzial (Theodor Maximilian Bilharz, 1825–1862, Egyptian zoologist) tubercles, nodules, sandy patches, ulcers, and papilloma.
>
> Complications can occur, which may require treatment of fibrosis of the bladder, calculi, stricture of the urethra and ureters, and seminal vesiculitis. *Squamous cell carcinoma (SCC)* can develop. *Treatment* is by praziquantel, 20 mg/kg, 4 hourly for three doses.

SOME IMPORTANT POINTS

- The most common stone in sterile urine is uric acid stone.
- The most common stone in infected urine is struvite stones.
- The most common renal stone is calcium oxalate stone.
- The most common bladder stone is a uric acid stone.
- The most common primary bladder stone is ammonium urate.
- The most bladder stones are secondary stones.
- Complications of bladder diverticula Mn-NISH.
  H = Hydronephrosis and hydroureter
  I = Infection
  S = Stone
  N = Neoplasm
- The most common benign mesenchymal tumor of the urinary bladder is leiomyoma.
- The most common malignant mesenchymal tumor of the urinary bladder is leiomyosarcoma.
- The most common malignant mesenchymal tumor in children is embryonal rhabdomyosarcoma.
- A kiss ulcer is a noninvasive papillary tumor of the bladder.

CARCINOMA OF THE URINARY BLADDER

Types

- Transitional cell carcinoma (90%) (TCC).
- Squamous cell carcinoma (Bilharzial carcinoma) (5–10%) (SCC).
- Adenocarcinoma (20%) (AC).

RISK FACTORS FOR URINARY BLADDER CARCINOMA

A. TCC-Mn = SIC SID
   S = Smoking
   I = Industry, i.e., dye, petroleum, and leather
   C = Chemical, i.e., Naphthalamine and aniline dye
   S = *Schistosoma haematobium*
   I = Irradiation
   D = Drug, i.e., phenacetin
B. SCC: Bilharziasis
C. AC: Urachal remnant

CARCINOMA IN SITU IS MALIGNANT

Cystitis

Painless hematuria is the most common symptom

- Metastasis—lymphatic—pelvic lymph node.
- Metastasis—hematogenesis—liver.

Diagnosis

- Cystoscopy + Biopsy
- *Exfoliated markers:* BTA/NMP22/hyaluronidase

Treatment

- TUR
- *Chemotherapy:* MVAC (Methotrexate/Vinblastine/Adriamycin/Cisplatin)

TNM (8TH AMERICAN JOINT COMMITTEE ON CANCER, 2017) CLASSIFICATION

Primary Tumor

- Ta = Noninvasive papillary carcinoma
- T1S = Flat tumor

- T1 = Invades subepithelial connective tissue
- T2a = Invades superficial muscularis propria (inner half)
- T2b = Invades deep muscularis propria (outer half)
- T3a = Microscopic extension in perivesical fat
- T3b = Macroscopic extension in perivesical fat
- T4a = Pelvic viscera
- T4b = Side soft and bony walls
- N = Regional LNs
- N1 = Single LN involvement
- N2 = Multiple LN involvement
- N3 = Common iliac LN involvement
- M = Distant metastasis
- M0 = No
- M1 = Yes

Treatment

- Tis = Intravesical Bacillus Calmette-Guérin (BCG)
- Ta = TUR
- T9 = TUR + Chemo or immunotherapy
- T2–T4
    - Radical cystectomy
    - Neoadjuvant chemotherapy
    - Radiotherapy

Any TNM: Systemic chemotherapy followed by surgery or radiotherapy.

BACILLUS CALMETTE–GUÉRIN

It is an attenuated strain of *Mycobacterium bovis* that immunologically acts by eliciting a T response. It is best used intravesically.

Contraindications of Bacillus Calmette–Guérin

Mn = HILT

- H = Gross hematuria
- I = Immunosuppression
- L = Liver function deranged
- T = Tuberculosis (TB)

Types

- Primary—without known cause
- Secondary:
    - F = Foreign body
    - I = Infection
    - O = Obstruction
    - Endemic bladder calculi are found in certain areas among children due to high intake of oxalate-rich vegetables with low phosphate and dehydration as in Rajasthan.

SOME IMPORTANT QUESTIONS

Q1. In ectopia vesicae, the bone divided is:

a. Pubic bone b. Sacrum
c. Coccyx d. Iliac bone

Ans. d

Q2. Ectopia vesicae includes all, *except*:

a. Hypospadias
b. Exstrophy of the bladder
c. Defective abdominal wall
d. Bifid clitoris

Ans. a

Q3. Secondary vesical calculus refers to stones formed due to:

a. Hypercalciuria
b. Injury
c. Infection
d. Migrating from above

Ans. c

Q4. Jackstone calculi is seen in which anatomic part:

a. Prostate b. Kidney
c. Ureter d. Bladder

Ans. d

Q5. Malakoplakia of the urinary bladder is considered to be associated with:

a. Tuberculosis (TB)
b. Urothelial carcinoma
c. Schistosomiasis
d. Defect in phagocytosis

Ans. d

Q6. True about malakoplakia is:

a. Benign lesion of the urinary bladder
b. May turn into malignancy
c. Michaelis-Gutmann bodies are a characteristic feature.
d. May cause severe hematuria and lead to death

Ans. c

Q7. Metrifonate is effective against:

a. Amebiasis b. Leishmaniasis
c. Schistosomiasis d. Giardiasis

Ans. c

Q8. Carcinoma is common in dye industry workers:

a. Skin
b. Scrotum
c. Urinary bladder
d. Maxilla

Ans. c

Q9. Transitional cell carcinoma can be seen in:

a. Analgesic nephropathy
b. Urate nephropathy
c. Pulmonary infections
d. Myocardial infarction

Ans. a

Q10. The following is true about bladder stones:

a. Girls more than boys
b. Treatment is litholapexy
c. Always forms in the kidneys and passes down to the bladder
d. Usually asymptomatic

Ans. b

MULTIPLE CHOICE QUESTIONS

Grade I	*Simple*

Q1. What is the diagnosis based on the given image? (JIPMER November 2017)

a. Gastroschisis
b. Omphalocele
c. Umbilical hernia
d. Ectopia vesicae

Q2. For the treatment of the ectopia vesicae, which of the following bones is divided to reach the site? (UPPG 2004)

a. Pubic rami
b. Iliac bone
c. Ischium bone
d. Symphysis

Q3. Regarding urinary bladder stone, one is not true: (AIIMS June 1998)

a. Common in pediatric patients in the tropics than that of nontropical areas
b. Uric acid stones are dropped from above.
c. Jackstone is due to urea-splitting bacteria.
d. Commonly distal passage obstruction causes stone

Q4. Not true about bladder stones is: (AIIMS November 2001)

a. Rare in Indian children
b. Primary stones are rare.
c. Small stones can be removed per urethra.
d. Maximum stones are radiopaque.

Q5. A patient, Ramu, presents with hematuria for many days. On investigations, he is found to have renal calculi, calcifications in the wall of the urinary bladder, and a small contracted bladder; the most probable cause is: (AIIMS November 2001)

a. Schistosomiasis
b. Amyloidosis
c. Tuberculosis
d. Carcinoma (CA) of the urinary bladder

Q6. Squamous cell tumor of the urinary bladder is due to: (PGI June 1997)

a. Stone
b. Schistosomiasis
c. Chronic cystitis
d. Diabetes mellitus

Q7. All of the following are features of exstrophy of the bladder, *except*: (All India 1997)

a. Epispadias
b. Cloacal membrane is present
c. Posterior bladder wall protrudes through the defects
d. Umbilical and inguinal hernia

Q8. About ectopia vesicae, the following is true, *except*: (PGI June 1998)

a. Cancer (CA) bladder may occur
b. Ventral curvature of penis
c. Incontinence of urine
d. Visible ureterovesical efflux

Q9. Which of the following is false regarding endemic bladder stones? (AIIMS Nov 2013)

a. Always associated with recurrence
b. High incidence in cereal-based diet
c. Peak incidence in 3-year-old children in India
d. The most common type is ammonium urate or calcium oxalate

Q10. Cystoscopic findings in TB bladder are all *except*: (PGI Dec 1997)

a. Cobblestone mucosa
b. Thimble bladder
c. Golf hole ureter
d. Whitish efflux from the ureteric holes

Grade II	*Difficult*

Q1. Squamous cell carcinoma of the urinary bladder is predisposed to by: (PGI June 2002)

a. Urolithiasis
b. Persistent urachus
c. Schistosomiasis
d. Polyp
e. Smoking

Q2. True about transitional cell carcinoma of the urinary bladder: (PGI December 2003)
a. Smoking predisposes
b. Schistosoma infection predisposes
c. Aniline dye workers
d. Radiation

Q3. Associated with urinary bladder carcinoma are all of the following, *except*: (MCI September 2009)
a. Smoking
b. Human papillomavirus (HPV) infection
c. Schistosomiasis
d. Cyclophosphamide

Q4. Squamous cell carcinoma (SCC) of the bladder is best treated by: (GB Pant 2011)
a. Chemotherapy
b. Radical cystectomy
c. Radiotherapy
d. Transurethral resection (TUR)

Q5. The most common bladder tumor is: (GB Pant 2011)
a. Transitional cell carcinoma (TCC)
b. SCC
c. Rhabdomyosarcoma
d. Sarcoma

Q6. A 55-year-old smoker presents with a history of five episodes of macroscopic hematuria, each lasting for about 4–5 days in the past 5 years. Which of the following investigations should be performed to evaluate the suspected diagnosis? (All India 2011)
a. Urine microscopy and cytology
b. X-ray kidney, ureter, and bladder (KUB)
c. Ultrasound KUB
d. Diethylenetriaminepentaacetic acid (DTPA) scan

Q7. A 67-year-old chronic heavy smoker presents with a 2-week history of frank hematuria. Ultrasound pelvis shows a filling defect. Most probable diagnosis: (JIPMER May 2018)
a. Bladder diverticulae
b. Adenocarcinoma of the bladder
c. Squamous cell carcinoma of the bladder
d. Transitional cell carcinoma of the bladder

Q8. A 60-year-old smoker came with a history of painless gross hematuria for 1 day. Most logical investigation would be: (All India 2007)
a. Urine routine
b. Plain X-ray KUB
c. USG KUB
d. Urine microscopy for malignant cytology

Q9. A 60-year-old smoker came with the history of painless gross hematuria for 1 day. The investigation of choice would be: (AIIMS November 2006)
a. Urine routine and microscopy
b. Plain X-ray KUB
c. USB KUB
d. Urine for malignant cytology

Q10. False statement regarding urothelial bladder tumor is: (PGI May 2018)
a. Most common variety
b. Schistosomiasis is not a risk factor.
c. Strongly related to smoking
d. Pain is the most common presenting feature
e. The most common site is the trigone.

Grade III	*Most difficult*

Q1. Treatment of choice for low-grade superficial bladder carcinoma: (JIPMER 2011)
a. Local excision
b. Radical cystectomy
c. Intravesical Bacillus Calmette-Guérin (BCG)
d. Chemotherapy

Q2. Which of the following is the most effective intravesical therapy for superficial bladder cancer? (AIIMS November 2005)
a. Mitomycin
b. Adriamycin
c. Thiotepa
d. BCG

Q3. BCG is used in tumor therapy: (JIPMER 1998)
a. Bladder
b. Stomach
c. Esophagus
d. Colon

Q4. A 60-year-old female presented with hematuria and was diagnosed with transitional cell carcinoma of the bladder stage T1N1M0. Best treatment modality is: (UPPG 2008)

a. Transurethral resection
b. Transurethral resection and intravesical chemoimmunotherapy
c. Total cystectomy and pelvic lymphadenectomy
d. Systemic chemotherapy

Q5. Catheterization of the bladder done in: (PGI December 2006)
a. CA of prostate
b. Postoperative retention
c. Preoperative evaluation before taking the patient for appendicitis
d. Stricture
e. Rupture

Q6. A young lady presents with symptoms of a urinary tract infection. All of the following findings on a midstream urine sample support the diagnosis of uncomplicated acute cystitis, *except*: (All India 2011)
a. Positive nitrite test
b. Colony-forming unit (CFU) count < 1,000/mL
c. Detection of one bacteria/field on Gram stain
d. >10 white blood cells (WBCs)/high-power field (HPF)

Q7. In the Boari operation: (GB Pant 2011)
a. Ureteric retransplant
b. Lower ureteric reconstruction
c. Diversion
d. Bowel interposition

Q8. After a surgery, the surgeon asked the intern to remove the Foley's catheter, but he could not do it. The surgeon himself tried to remove the Foley's catheter, but he was unsuccessful. What should be done next? (AIIMS May 2016)
a. Computer tomography (CT)-guided rupture of the bulb of Foley's
b. Inject ether to dissolve the balloon and pull it out
c. Inject water to overdistend the balloon until it bursts, and the Foley's catheter can be removed.
d. Use ultrasound guidance to locate the prick the balloon and then remove the catheter.

Q9. An elderly male presents with one episode of gross hematuria. All of the following investigations are recommended for this patient, *except*: (All India 2007)
a. Cystoscopy
b. Urine microscopy for malignant cells
c. Urine tumor markers
d. Intravenous pyelogram

Q10. A 60-year-old male smoker patient presents with painless gross hematuria for 1 day. Intravenous urography (IVU) shows a 1.2 cm filling defect at the lower pole of the infundibulum. Which is the next best investigation to be done? (MCI November 2017)
a. Cystoscopy
b. Urine cytology
c. USG abdomen
d. Dimercaptosuccinic acid (DMSA) scan

ANSWERS

Grade I: 1. d; 2. b; 3. b (Bailey 27/e p1434); 4. d (Bailey 27/e p1435); 5. a (Bailey 27/e p1442); 6. a, b, c; 7. b; 8. b; 9. a (Bailey 27/e p1434); 10. d (Bailey 27/e p1442)

Grade II: 1. a, c; 2. a, b, c, d; 3. b; 4. b (Bailey 27/e p1451); 5. a; 6. a (Bailey 27/e p1447); 7. d; 8. d; 9. d; 10. b, d

Grade III: 1. a (Bailey 27/e p1451); 2. d (Campbell 11/e p2212-2216); 3. a; 4. c; 5. a (Bailey 27/e p1437); 6. a (Smith 18/e p200); 7. b; 8. d; 9. c; 10. a

MODEL QUESTIONS

Q1. The most common tumor of the urinary bladder is:
a. Squamous cell carcinoma
b. Adenocarcinoma
c. Transitional carcinoma
d. Stratified squamous carcinoma

Ans. c

Q2. Urinary cytology is a useful screening test for the diagnosis of:
a. Renal cell carcinoma
b. Wilms' tumor
c. Urothelial carcinoma
d. Carcinoma prostate

Ans. c

Q3. Which of the following is a tumor marker for bladder cancer?
a. α-fetoprotein (AFP)

b. Carcinoembryonic antigen (CEA)
c. Bladder surface protein
d. NMP22

Ans. d

Q4. BCG is used in the treatment of:
a. Carcinoma cervix
b. Carcinoma colon
c. Carcinoma of the urinary bladder
d. All

Ans. c

Q5. pT2, pT3, or CIS carcinoma of the bladder not responding to BCG is best treated by:
a. Intravesical mitomycin-C and interferon
b. Systemic chemotherapy
c. Cystoscopic
d. Radical cystectomy

Ans. d

Q6. Treatment of choice for bladder pTa:
a. Endoscopic tumor resection
b. Endoscopic tumor resection and intravesical chemotherapy
c. Partial cystectomy with intravesical
d. Radical cystectomy with or without radical radiotherapy, BCG

Ans. a

Q7. Identify the false statement regarding urothelial cell carcinoma of the bladder.
a. Ileal conduit diversion is required after cystectomy.
b. Intravesical chemotherapy and immunotherapy are not found to be beneficial in nonmuscular invasive bladder cancer (NMIBC).
c. Radical cystectomy following chemotherapy has been shown to be beneficial in muscle-invasive bladder cancer.
d. Strongly associated with smoking and *Schistosoma haematobium*

Ans. b

Q8. Urinary diversion is indicated in the following, *except*?
a. Ectopia vesicae
b. Carcinoma of the bladder
c. Neurogenic bladder
d. Bladder hematoma

Ans. d

Q9. Postmicturition dribbling is due to:
a. Detrusor
b. Dribbling decreased in the case of urethral stricture
c. Collection of urine in "U"-shaped curve of bulb of penis
d. Neurogenic bladder

Ans. c

Q10. What is Boari flap surgery?
a. Ureterostomy
b. Double-J (DJ) stent in situ
c. Bowel interposition
d. Flap of the bladder wall fashioned into a tube to replace lower ureter

Ans. d

SUGGESTED READING

1. Bailey & Love's - Short Practice of Surgery, 27th edition.
2. Campbell's Urology, 10th edition.
3. Textbook of Surgery by David Sabiston, 21st edition.

CHAPTER 47

Prostate and Seminal Vesicles

"I recently formed a foundation to raise awareness for prostate cancer. I feel it's very necessary that men be more aware about prostate cancer and their health in general."

– Herbie Mann

INTRODUCTION

The prostate gland develops from the primitive urethra as several epithelial buds, which become canalized, and the surrounding mesenchymal tissue gives muscle and connective tissues of the gland.

SURGICAL ANATOMY

The prostate gland is divided into three zones: (1) Transitional zone (TZ)—from this zone most of benign prostatic hyperplasia (BPH) arise, (2) central zone (CZ) is situated behind the urethra and above the ejaculatory ducts as they pass through prostate, (3) the peripheral zone (PZ) is placed posteriorly and carcinoma arises from this zone **(Figs. 1A to C)**.

The glands of PZ are long and branched and open on either side of the verumontanum.

The glands of CZ and TZ are short and unbranched and open in the prostatic urethra. PZ is also known as the cancerous zone, and TZ and CZ are known as the adenomatous zone.

> *Points to remember:*
> *The vesicoureteric reflux in children is:*
> - *Grade I*: Reflux in the ureter.
> - *Grade II*: Reflux into the ureter and renal pelvis.
> - *Grade III*: Reflux associated with mild or moderate dilatation on an intravenous urography (IVU).
> - *Grade IV*: Additional blunting for ices.
> - *Grade V*: Absent papillary impressions.

There are two capsules in the prostate gland:

1. True capsule made up of endopelvic fascia
2. False capsule made by compression of PZ by enlarging the adenoma.

Enucleation is done for hyperplastic nodules and venous plexus, and both capsules are left behind **(Fig. 2)**.

The arterial supply to the prostate is mainly from the internal iliac artery. The inferior vertical artery is the main artery. The middle rectal artery and the internal pudendal artery also supply blood to the prostate gland.

Venous drainage of the prostate is through the venous plexus, which goes to the internal iliac vein. The lymphatic

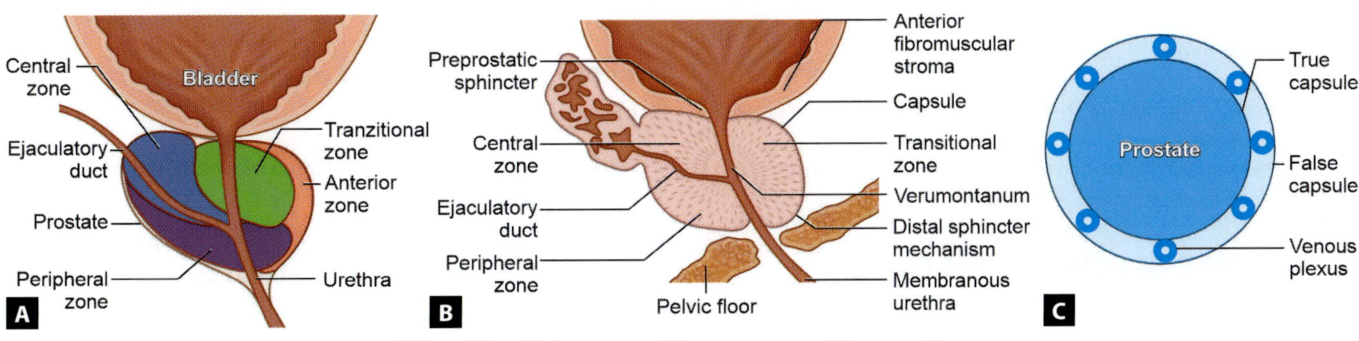

Figs. 1A to C: Anatomy of the prostate and its capsules.

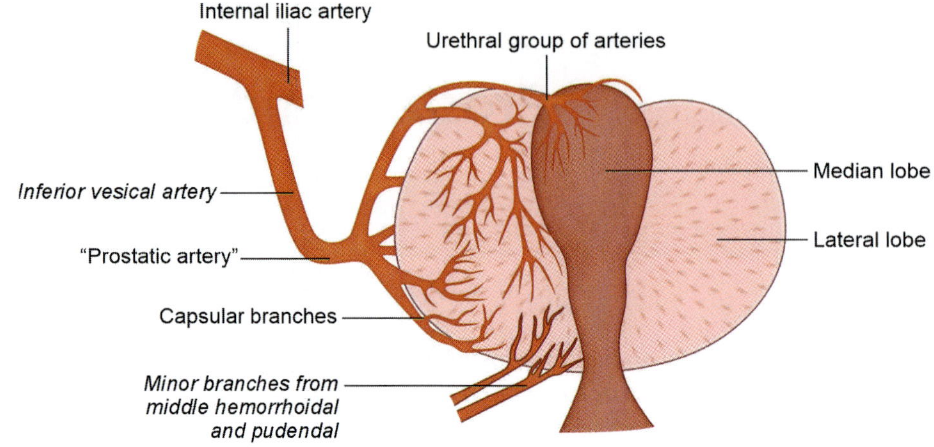

Fig. 2: Arterial supply of the prostate.

drainage of the prostate is mainly to the internal iliac lymph nodes (LNs). External iliac LNs receive a smaller portion of the lymphatic drainage.

PHYSIOLOGY OF THE PROSTATE GLAND

The prostate is a gland of the male reproductive system that has many functions, such as semen production, nourishment of spermatozoa, and ejaculation of semen. The most important function of the prostate gland production of a fluid that, together with the sperm from the testicles and fluid from the other glands, forms semen. The muscles of the gland help to push the semen into the urethra and then to expel out during ejaculation.

The prostate gland has five lobes: anterior, posterior, two lateral, and one median lobe.

The female prostate gland is Skene's (Alexander Johnston Chalmers Skene, 1837–1900, American gynecologist) glands as it develops from the same cells that become the prostate gland.

Not to forget:
Treatment strategies:
- *Low-risk disease*: Conservative treatment
- *Intermediate-risk disease*: Radical prostatectomy, as the patient is young and fit.
- *High-risk patient*: Androgen ablation with radiotherapy
- *Metastatic disease*: Androgen ablation

PROSTATE-SPECIFIC ANTIGEN

- It helps in the liquefaction of semen but also acts as a marker for prostate diseases.
- Normally, the prostate-specific antigen (PSA) remains <0.4 ng/mL

The seminal vesicles are a pair of glands in the pelvis of a male **(Figs. 3A and B)**. *The fluid produced by the seminal vesicles contributes to the constituents of the semen.* They are also called seminal glands or vesicular glands. Their contribution to the total volume of semen is approximately 70%. The fluid secreted by the seminal vesicle is viscous and contains:
- *Fructose*—provides energy to sperm.
- *Prostaglandins*—help in the mobility and viability of sperm.
- *Proteins*—cause a coagulation reaction in semen after ejaculation.

Benign prostatic hyperplasia: BPH is the most common disease of prostate gland. It occurs in men above 50 years of age, and 50% of men above the age of 60 years are positive histologically for BPH.

Theory of BPH development: As we age, the testosterone secretion in our body gradually decreases but the secretion and body levels of estrogenic steroids are not much affected. So, the estrogenic effects take upper hand and prostate gland enlarges. It usually affects the glands of TZ area of submucosal glands. If the CZ area is affected then median lobe develops which projects inside the bladder.

EFFECTS OF BENIGN PROSTATIC HYPERPLASIA

- *Urethra:* It is lengthened, the curvature increases, and it is distorted.
- *Bladder:* Hypertrophic trabeculae and engorgement of veins at the base leading to hematuria.
- Lower urinary tract symptoms (LUTS) can be described as:
  - Idiopathic overactivity of the bladder.
  - Bladder outlet obstruction (BOO)

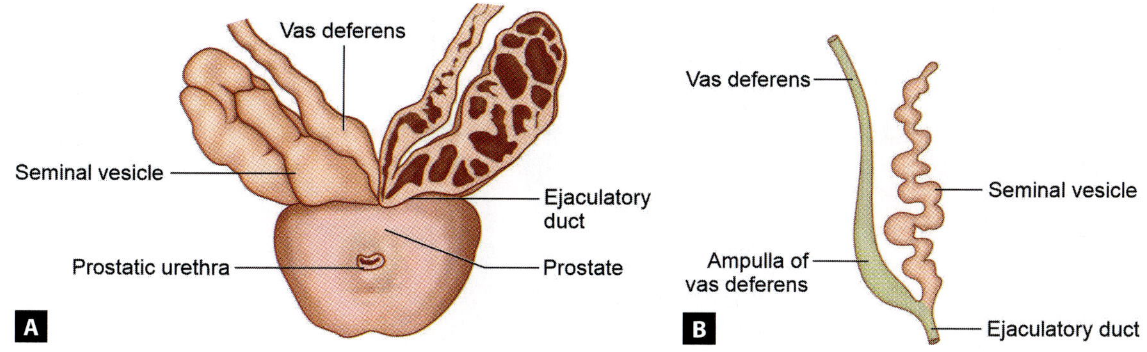

Figs. 3A and B: Anatomy of seminal vesicles.

- *Symptoms with voiding:* Hesitancy, poor flow, intermittent interruption in urine flow, dribbling, and near retention.
- *Symptoms with storage:* Frequency, urgency, nocturnal, enuresis, and urge incontinence.

Bladder Outlet Obstruction

It is positively diagnosed by pressure flow studies.

Causes of BOO: Causes include BPH, bladder neck obstruction, urethral stricture, cancer of prostate, and neurological causes.

Pathological effects on urinary bladder: Reduced urinary flow rate, increased voiding pressure, and irritable bladder.

> *Bladder outlet obstruction can produce complications:*
> - Acute retention of urine—commonly due to postponement of micturition
> - Chronic retention of urine—when the residual volume of urine is >250 mL.
> - Impaired bladder emptying—a large volume of residual urine keeps continuous pressure on the walls of the bladder, which leads to disturbed bladder functioning, leading to impaired bladder emptying too.
> - Hematuria
> - Pain may develop as a complication of BOO due to infection.

Investigations in Lower Urinary Tract Symptoms

- Urine examination to detect glucose, blood, and protein.
- Urine for culture and sensitivity
- Urine flow rate
- Serum creatinine
- PSA
- Pressure flow

> ### *Flow Rate Measurement*
> It is done by a flow meter. Voiding volume of urine should be >150 mL, and three recordings should be done. The flow rate of <10 mL/s is sufficient to start treatment. Decreased flow rate is seen in BOO, detrusor instability, weak bladder contraction (low pressure flow voiding)

Cystourethroscopy

Management of Bladder Outlet Obstruction

Prostatectomy is the treatment.

Indications of prostatectomy:

- Acute retention of urine
- Chronic retention of urine
- *Complications of BOO*: Calculus, infection, and diverticulum.
- Elective prostatectomy for BPH with disturbing symptoms.
- Heavy hematuria

Out of all indications of prostatectomy, 60% are done for BPH with disturbing symptoms, 25% are done for BPH with acute retention of urine, and 25% are done for BPH with chronic retention of urine **(Fig. 4)**.

> ### *Drug Treatment for Bladder Outlet Obstruction*
> Drug treatment for BPH patients who do not want surgery is a quite good option. α-adrenergic blocking agents lead to the relaxation of smooth muscle in the prostate, which helps in the micturition flow of urine and also reduces the nocturnal frequency of micturition.

The other group of drugs, 5α predicate inhibitors, which reduce the conversation of testosterone to more active form dihydrotestosterone (DHT) cause shrinkage of

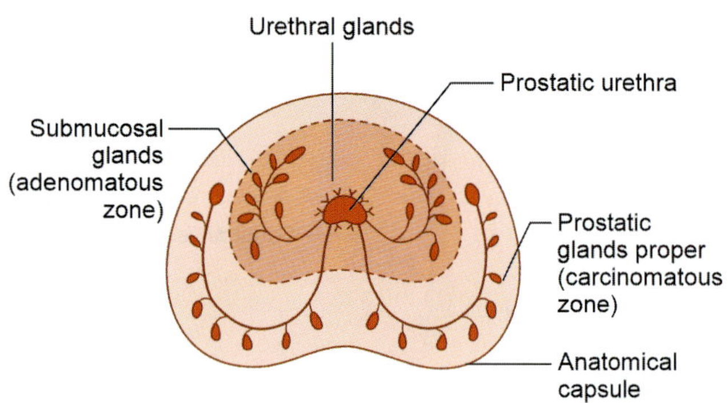

Fig. 4: Zones and glands of the prostate.

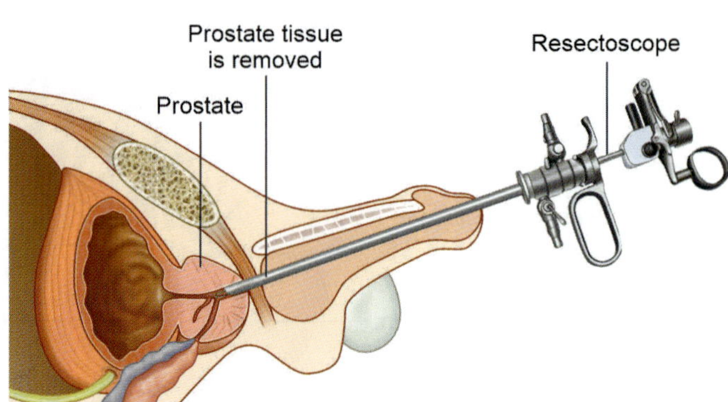

Fig. 5: Transurethral resection of the prostate (TURP).

prostate gland but it takes time which should be properly explained to the patient, action of these drugs takes 6–8 weeks to start and 1 year use causes approximately 25% reduction in size of prostate gland.

Medical explanations and counseling with patients going to undergo prostatectomy. These patients must be explained and convinced of some problems occurring after prostatectomy:

- Success rate of the operation—most patients with severe symptoms and BOO undergoing elective prostatectomy do very well (90%).
- Recurrence after transurethral resection of the prostate (TURP)—approximately occurs in 15% of cases after about 10 years
- *Morbidity and mortality:* Death after TURP is very low (0.5%). Morbidity after TURP varies from 3 to 20%.
- Retrograde ejaculation
- Erectile impotence

> *Types of prostatectomy:*
> - Transurethral (TURP)
> - Retropubic (RPP)
> - Transvesical (TVP)
> - Through the perineum

Transurethral resection of the prostate:

- The resection is done from the bladder neck to the verumontanum.
- High-frequency current is used for cutting the tissue and coagulation is bone at the same time. It is the most commonly used prostatectomy procedure.
- Retropubic prostatectomy or Millin's (Terence John Millin, 1903–1980, British surgeon) prostatectomy. It is rarely performed today.

> *You may be asked:*
> - The growth of the prostate gland is under control by androgenic hormones.
> - Most of our testosterone hormone is secreted by Leydig cells of the testes and is under the control of *luteinizing hormone (LH)* secreted from the anterior pituitary.
> - Testosterone is converted to a more active form, DHT (it is five times more active) by the enzyme 5α-reductase type II. It is found in high concentration in the prostate gland.

TRANSVESICAL PROSTATECTOMY

This operation is rarely performed nowadays **(Fig. 5)**.

Complications of Prostatectomy (Figs. 6A and B)

- Hemorrhage
- Perforation of the bladder
- Sepsis
- Incontinence
- Retrograde ejaculation
- Bladder neck contracture
- Reoperation

> *Bladder outflow obstruction:*
> - It is common in males and usually develops after TURP at the bladder neck.
> - Clinical symptoms are either due to muscle hypertrophy or due to fibrosis.
> - Treatment by α-blockers alfuzosin and doxazosin.
> - Transurethral incision of the bladder neck is the operation of choice.

CARCINOMA OF THE PROSTATE

It is the most common malignancy in persons above 65 years of age.

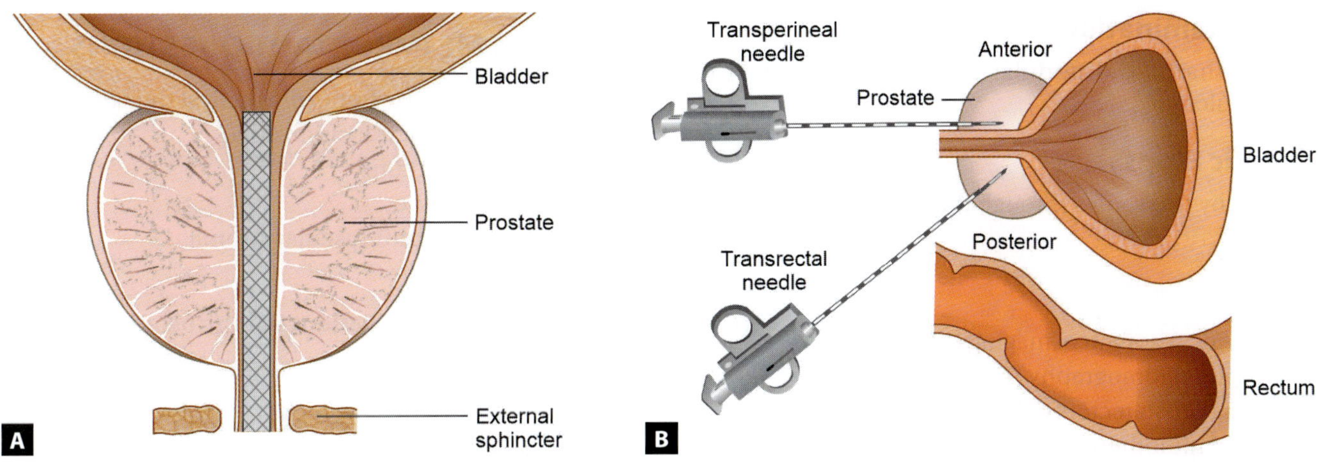

Figs. 6A and B: Prostatic urethra and sphincters.

Pathology

The following are the types of prostate cancer:

- Microscopic latent cancer
- Tumor found incidentally
- Early localized prostate cancer
- Advanced localized cancer
- Metastatic disease

Gleason (Donald F Gleason, 1920-2008, American pathologist, published in 1966) score:

- *Grade 1:* Small uniform glands
- *Grade 2:* More space between glands and an increase in stroma
- *Grade 3:* Distinct infiltration of the cell margin
- *Grade 4:* Irregular masses of neoplastic cells
- *Grade 5:* Lack of glandular pattern
- Old score is grade 1–5.
- The new score is from 1 to 10.
  Local spread—involves surrounding structures.
  Spread by blood circulation involves the skeleton.
  Lymphatic spread goes to the LN—internal iliac LNs and external iliac LNs.

TUMOR, NODE, AND METASTASIS CLASSIFICATION (FIG. 7)

- *Tla, Tlb, and Tlc:* These are incidental tumors found in specimens after TURP.
- *T2a and T2b:* Presence of a nodule in one lobe and in two lobes.
- *T3:* Extension of tumor to capsule in one or two lobes.
- *T4:* Tumor fixed to adjacent structures.

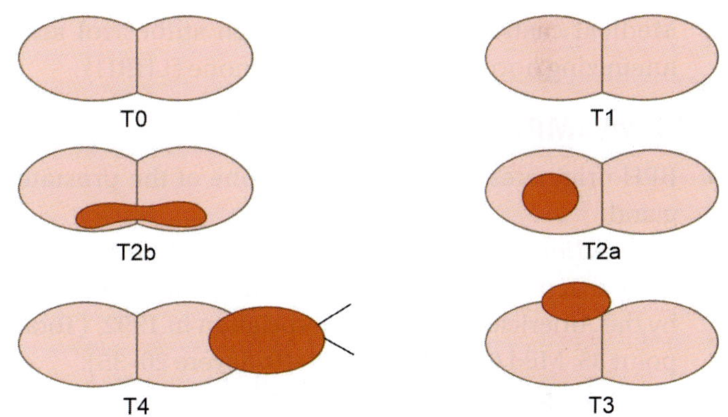

Fig. 7: Stages of carcinoma of prostate.

Clinical Features

- BOO
- Pain
- Hematuria
- Bone pain
- Arthritis
- Anemia

> *Good to remember:*
> *Prostate-specific antigen:*
> - PSA is a protein, synthesized by normal and cancerous cells of prostate gland.
> - Though the normal levels of PSA should be below 4 ng/L in elderly patient but it is decided that a normal PSA should be below 1.5 units per liter.
> - Dangerous level is >10 ng/L which indicates localized cancer.
> - Metastatic level is >35 ng/L, it indicates that metastatic cancer is present.
> - PSA level also increases after a prostatic massage and prostate biopsy. However, the PSA levels can be around 4 even in cancer of prostate patients and may be high in a normal individual.
> - Green tea, cranberry juice, and other berries.

Rectal Examination

Irregular, hard, and nodular gland obliteration of the median sulcus.

Prostatic Biopsy

It is done by two routes through the rectum or perineum.

Imaging

- TRUS
- Magnetic resonance imaging (MRI)
- Computed tomography (CT)
- Radical prostatectomy
- Radical radiotherapy
- Brachytherapy
- Orchidectomy
- Medical castration is done through stilbestrol and luteinizing hormone-releasing hormone (LHRH)

SOME IMPORTANT POINTS

- BPH originates in the transition zone of the prostate gland.
- *International prostate symptom score (IPSS):* It is a score that measures the severity of LUTS. It was created by the American Urological Association in 1992. (Total point 35, Mild 0–7, Moderate 8–19, Severe 20–35).
- The most common cancer in men.
- It is the most common cause of bone metastasis.
- African-Americans have the highest incidence of prostate cancer.
- *What can decrease risk of CA prostate:* Mn = LEAST (Lycopene/Vit E/Vit A/Selenium/Tomatoes.
- The most common type of prostate CA is adenocarcinoma (TCC).
- Tumor markers of CA prostate are Mn = PAPAHD.
- (PSA/Alkaline phosphatase/prostate acid phosphatase/alpha-methyl co-A racemase/Hepsin/DD3
- New drugs to treat CA prostate, even with metastasis-cabazitaxel/sipuleucel-T.
- *Minimum requirement in semen analysis*:
    - Volume 1.5–5.5 mL
    - Count 20 million/mL
    - Mortality >50%
- *Abnormalities in semen*:
    - Volume—ejaculatory duct obstruction or androgen deficiency.
    - Count—azoospermia—testicular failure/obstruction.
    - Fructose absence—obstruction or seminal vesicle (SV) agenesis.

SOME IMPORTANT QUESTIONS

Q1. Benign prostatic hyperplasia first develops in the:
a. Periurethral transition zone
b. Peripheral zone
c. Central zone
d. Anterior fibromuscular stroma

Ans. a

Q2. Assessment of a patient with prostatism includes all, *except*:
a. Rectal examination
b. Serum prostate-specific antigen
c. Pressure flow urodynamic studies
d. Transrectal ultrasound scanning

Ans. d

Q3. What of the following is an absolute indication for surgery in cases of benign prostatic hyperplasia?
a. Bilateral hydroureteronephrosis
b. Nocturnal frequency
c. Recurrent urinary tract infection
d. Voiding bladder pressure >50 cmH_2O

Ans. a and c

Q4. The drug that has the fastest onset of action in benign prostatic hyperplasia is:
a. Finasteride b. Tamsulosin
c. Dutasteride d. Flutamide

Ans. b

Q5. In the management of symptomatic benign prostatic hyperplasia with finasteride, the period of trial required for determining a satisfactory response is:
a. 1 month b. 2 months
c. 4 months d. 6 months

Ans. d

Q6. The most common complication of transurethral resection of the prostate (TURP) is:
a. Erectile dysfunction
b. Retrograde ejaculation
c. Urinary incontinence
d. Impotence

Ans. b

Q7. Which of the following is true about prostate cancer screening?
a. Digital screening along with prostate-specific antigen (PSA) is additive

b. Prostate cancer is common among young males
c. Tumor markers are diagnostic
d. Bleeding per rectum is the earliest manifestation of the disease

Ans. a

Q8. Gleason scoring is done for:
a. Prostatic cancer
b. Lung cancer
c. Bladder cancer
d. Hodgkin's lymphoma

Ans. a

Q9. True about prostate cancer (CA) is:
a. Arises in the periurethral zone
b. Extremely radiosensitive
c. Obturator nodes are most commonly involved
d. PSA is not used in the workup

Ans. c

Q10. Treatment for metastatic CA prostate:
a. Gonadotropin-releasing hormone (GnRH) analog
b. Estrogen therapy
c. Radiotherapy with chemotherapy
d. Radiotherapy

Ans. a

MULTIPLE CHOICE QUESTIONS

Grade I	*Simple*

Q1. Which of the following is an absolute indication for surgery in cases of benign prostatic hyperplasia (BPH)? (All India 2003)
a. Bilateral hydroureteronephrosis
b. Nocturnal frequency
c. Recurrent urinary tract infection (UTI)
d. Voiding bladder pressure >50 cm of water

Q2. Which of the following lasers is used for the treatment of BPH as well as urinary calculi? (All India 2003)
a. CO_2 laser
b. Excimer laser
c. Ho:YAG laser
d. Nd:YAG laser

Q3. The following statements regarding finasteride are true, *except*: (All India 2005)
a. It is used in the medical treatment of benign prostatic hypertrophy
b. Impotence is well documented after its use
c. It blocks the conversion of dihydrotestosterone to testosterone
d. It is a 5α-reductase inhibitor

Q4. In follow-up of BPH, the most important indication of surgery is: (AIIMS November 2010)
a. Prostate size >75 g
b. Single episode of UTI requiring 3 days of antibiotics
c. Cannot use medication due to hypertension
d. Bilateral hydronephrosis

Q5. Which of the following drugs can decrease the size of the prostate? (AIIMS November 2017)
a. Tamsulosin
b. Sildenafil
c. Finasteride
d. Prazosin

Q6. Delirium, mental confusion, and nausea in patients who had undergone TURP suggest: (MCI November 2017)
a. Hypernatremia
b. Sepsis
c. Hepatic coma
d. Water retention

Q7. In BPH most common lobe involved is: (AIIMS June 2000)
a. Lateral
b. Posterior
c. Median
d. Anterior

Q8. A 60-year-old diabetic and hypertensive with a second-grade prostate, admitted for prostatectomy, developed a myocardial infarction. Treatment now would be: (All India 1999)
a. Finasteride
b. Terazosin
c. Finasteride and terazosin
d. Diethyl stilbestrol

Q9. What is the reason for the following set of symptoms after prostatic surgery—restlessness, vomiting, and change in sensorium? (AIIMS June 1999)
a. Electrolyte imbalance
b. Bladder neck obstruction
c. Acute pyelonephritis
d. Ureter stenosis

Q10. The most common cause of periumbilical pain after 30 minutes of TURP done under spinal anesthesia with bupivacaine: (AIIMS June 2000)
a. Meteorism
b. Perforation of the bladder
c. Recovery from bupivacaine anesthesia
d. Mesentery artery ischemia

Grade II	Difficult

Q1. Which of the following is the most common cause of delayed urinary tract obstructive symptoms after TURP? (All India 2011)

a. Stricture of the navicular fossa
b. Stricture of the membranous urethra
c. Stricture of the bulb of the urethra
d. Bladder neck stenosis

Q2. During TURP, the surgeon takes care of dissecting above the verumontanum to prevent injury of: (All India 2011)

a. External urethral sphincter
b. Urethral crest
c. Prostatic utricle
d. Trigone of the bladder

Q3. TURP was done in an old patient of BHP, after which he developed altered sensorium cause is: (MCI June 2018)

a. Hypernatremia
b. Hypokalemia
c. Hyponatremia
d. Hypomagnesemia

Q4. Which of the following substances is not used as an irrigant during TURP? (AIIMS November 2003)

a. Normal saline
b. 1.5% glycine
c. 5% dextrose
d. Distilled water

Q5. True about TURP is: (PGI November 2017)

a. More morbidity than retropubic prostatectomy
b. Can cause retrograde ejaculation
c. Open prostatectomy is preferred in larger obstructive masses.
d. Less risk of bleeding in transurethral laser vaporization than in TURP
e. The resectoscope is passed through the urethra, and the prostate is resected into multiple pieces and removed.

Q6. Screening of prostate cancer (CA) is commonly done by: (PGI November 2010)

a. Digital rectal examination (DRE)
b. Ultrasound (USG)
c. Magnetic resonance imaging (MRI)
d. Prostate-specific antigen (PSA)
e. Computed tomography (CT) scan

Q7. Transrectal ultrasonogram in evaluation of prostate carcinoma is most useful for: (All India 2008)

a. Taking guided biopsy
b. Identifying seminal vesicle invasion
c. Nodal sampling
d. Measuring the extent of invasion

Q8. Gleason score: all are true, *except:* (AIIMS May 2011)

a. Used for grading prostate cancer
b. Scores range from 1 to 10
c. The higher the score, the poorer the prognosis
d. Helps in planning and management

Q9. Osteoblastic metastasis commonly arises from: (JIPMER 2014)

a. Breasts
b. Prostate
c. Lung
d. Renal cell carcinoma (RCC)

Q10. All of the following can be seen after transurethral resection of the prostate, *except:* (AIIMS November 2000)

a. Congestive cardiac failure
b. Transient blindness
c. Convulsions
d. Hypernatremia

Grade III	Most difficult

Q1. Treatment for metastatic prostate carcinoma: (JIPMER 2011)

a. Gonadotropin-releasing hormone (GnRH) analog
b. Estrogen therapy
c. Radiotherapy with chemotherapy
d. Radiotherapy

Q2. Which of the following is the most troublesome source of bleeding during a radical retropubic prostatectomy? (All India 2005)

a. Dorsal venous complex
b. Inferior vesical pedicle
c. Superior vesical pedicle
d. Seminal vesicular artery

Q3. A 70-year-old man with prostate cancer was given radiotherapy. The recurrence of the cancer is monitored biochemically by: (AIIMS November 2012)

a. Androgens only
b. Prostate-specific antigen and carcinoembryonic antigen
c. Prostate-specific antigen only
d. Alkaline phosphatase (ALP) and carcinoembryonic antigen (CEA)

Q4. Treatment of metastatic prostate carcinoma is: (JIPMER 2011)

a. Radiotherapy
b. Estrogen only
c. GnRH analogs
d. Radiotherapy with chemotherapy

Q5. Which of the following drugs is useful for the treatment of advanced prostate cancer? (AIIMS November 2014)

a. Goserelin b. Ganirelix
c. Cetrorelix d. Abarelix

Q6. A 60-year-old male presented with fever, chills, and dysuria. The patient was hospitalized in the emergency department for 5 days. PSA level was 7.4. The next best step in this patient is: (AIIMS November 2013)

a. Repeat PSA
b. TURP
c. TRUS-guided biopsy
d. Antibiotics and admit

Q7. Absence of fructose in semen indicates: (PGI December 2008)

a. Obstruction to the seminal vesicles
b. Obstruction at the prostatic urethra
c. Vas deferens obstruction
d. Testicular failure

Q8. Which of the following is true about obstructive azoospermia? (All India 2011)

a. Increased follicle-stimulating hormone (FSH) and luteinizing hormone (LH)
b. Normal FSH and LH
c. Increased LH and normal FSH
d. Increased FSH and normal LH

Q9. Hot flush is not associated with: (PGI December 2008)

a. Medical castration
b. Surgical castration
c. Ketoconazole therapy
d. Androgen receptor blockade
e. Radical prostatectomy

Q10. Transurethral resection (TUR) syndrome is due to: (UPSC 1995)

a. Hyponatremia b. Hypokalemia
c. Hypovolemia d. Hypoxia

ANSWERS

Grade I: 1. a, c (Bailey 27/e p1463); 2. c (Smith 18/e p356); 3. c; 4. d; 5. c (Goodman Gilman 12/e p308); 6. d; 7. c; 8. b (Bailey 27/e p1464); 9. a; 10. b (Bailey 27/e p1466)

Grade II: 1. d; 2. a; 3. c; 4. a (Campbell 11/e p2510); 5. b, c, d, e; 6. a, d; 7. a; 8. b (Bailey 27/e p1472); 9. b; 10. d

Grade III: 1. a; 2. a; 3. c (Harrison 19/e p581); 4. c; 5. a; 6. d; 7. a; 8. b; 9. e; 10. a

MODEL QUESTIONS

Q1. A 70-year-old patient with benign prostatic hyperplasia (BPH) underwent transurethral resection of the prostate (TURP) under spinal anesthesia. 1 hour later, he developed vomiting and altered sensorium. The most probable cause is:

a. Overdosage of spinal anesthetic agent
b. Rupture of the bladder
c. Hyperkalemia
d. Water intoxication

Ans. d

Q2. Which one of the following is used as an irrigation solution during TURP?

a. 1.5% glycine b. Physiological saline
c. Ringer's lactate d. 5% dextrose

Ans. a

Q3. The normal level of prostate-specific antigen (PSA) in males is:

a. <4 ng/mL
b. 4–10 ng/mL
c. >10 ng/mL
d. PSA is not produced by normal males.

Ans. a

Q4. Management of prostate carcinoma in a 50-year-old man revealed after TRUP os:

a. No treatment required
b. Hormonal therapy
c. Bilateral subcapsular orchidectomy
d. Radical prostatectomy

Ans. d

Q5. Regarding prostatectomy, which one of the statements is false?

a. Water intoxication and hyponatremia can give rise to congestive heart failure (CHF).
b. Perineal prostatectomy (Young) is a commonly done surgical procedure.
c. Retrograde ejaculation occurs in about 65% of men
d. Intraurethral stents are helpful in the management of men who are grossly unfit [the American Society of Anaesthesiologists (ASA) grade 4].

Ans. b

Q6. Corpora amylacea is seen in:

a. Thymus
b. Lymph node
c. Spleen
d. Prostate

Ans. d

Q7. Which is the earliest symptom of benign hypertrophy of the prostate?

a. Frequency
b. Hematuria
c. Incontinence
d. Strangury

Ans. a

Q8. Indications for surgery in benign prostatic hypertrophy are all, *except*:

a. Prostatism
b. Chronic retention
c. Hemorrhage
d. Enlarged prostate

Ans. d

Q9. The most important use of transrectal ultrasonography (TRUS) is for:

a. Screening for cancer (CA) prostate
b. Distinguishing prostate cancer from BPH
c. Systematic prostate biopsy in suspected prostate cancer
d. Guiding transurethral resection of prostate cancer

Ans. c

Q10. The most common site of development of carcinoma of the prostate is:

a. Peripheral zone
b. Central zone
c. Transitional zone
d. Fibromuscular stroma

Ans. a

SUGGESTED READING

1. Bailey & Love's - Short Practice of Surgery, 27th edition.
2. Schwartz's Principles of Surgery, 18th edition.
3. Smith's Urology, 18th edition.

CHAPTER 48

Urethra and Penis

"The aim of the art of medicine is health, but its end is the possession of health. Doctors have to know by which means to bring about health, when it is absent, and by which means to preserve it, when it is present."

- Galen

ANATOMY OF MALE URETHRA

It is about 7–8 cm long, which extends from the bladder neck to the external urethral meatus. It has four parts: (1) Prostatic, (2) membranous, (3) bulbar, and (4) penile urethra. The prostatic urethra extends from the bladder neck to verumontanum, the membranous urethra extends from verumontanum to where the urethra penetrates the pelvic floor, the bulbar urethra extends from here to the penoscrotal junction, and the penile urethra is beyond this point.

The external urethral sphincter is made up of circular striated muscles, and the internal urethral sphincter is made up of smooth muscles **(Figs. 1A to D)**.

ANATOMY OF PENIS

It is made up of three tubular structures. Upper two are called corpora cavernosa and are highly vascular and cause erection. The two corpora cavernosa are attached to the pubic rami. The lower one is single, corpus spongiosum, which contains urethra, and it expands at distal end forming the glans penis.

Corpora cavernosa are covered by tunica albuginea. The main arterial supply of penis is through internal pudendal artery which is a branch of internal iliac artery. *Common penile artery gives three branches: (1) dorsal, (2) cavernous, and (3) bulb urethral artery* **(Fig. 2)**.

VEINS OF PENIS

Superficial vein of penis lies in superficial fascia and drains into superficial external pudendal vein. Deep dorsal vein of penis passes between perineal membrane and pubic symphysis and drains into prostatic plexus of veins. Fascia of penis is superficial and deep. The deepest layer of superficial fascia is called "Buck's fascia." It surrounds all three tubular structures.

SUPPORTS OF BODY OF PENIS

- *Fundiform ligament:* It runs down from linea alba and splits and encloses the penis.
- *Suspensory ligament:* It runs down from pubic symphysis and blends with fascia of penis on each side.

Not to forget:

- *Malacoplakia:* It is characterized by the presence of foamy histiocytes (von Hansemann cells).
- *Peyronie's (François Gigot de la Peyronie, 1678–1747, French Surgeon, described in 1743) disease:* It is an entity with pain on eruption, ED, penile plaques, and penile deformity. The deformity is dorsal curvature on erection. It is also called penile fibromatosis, a part of the process called superficial fibromatosis. (Dupuytren's contracture and plantar fibromatosis are part of the same process). Nesbitt's operation is required to straighten the penis.
- *Priapism:* It is a painful erection of penis. It is of two types:
  1. *High-flow type:* It is due to increased arterial blood flow than normal, as happens in spinal cord injury or after papaverine injection. It is less dangerous than the other.
  2. *Low-flow type (Ischemic):* It is due to venous return obstruction. It can lead to compartment syndrome.

Treatment

- Injection of phenylephrine
- *Operation:* Winter's (George D Winter) operation—cavernoglandular shunt

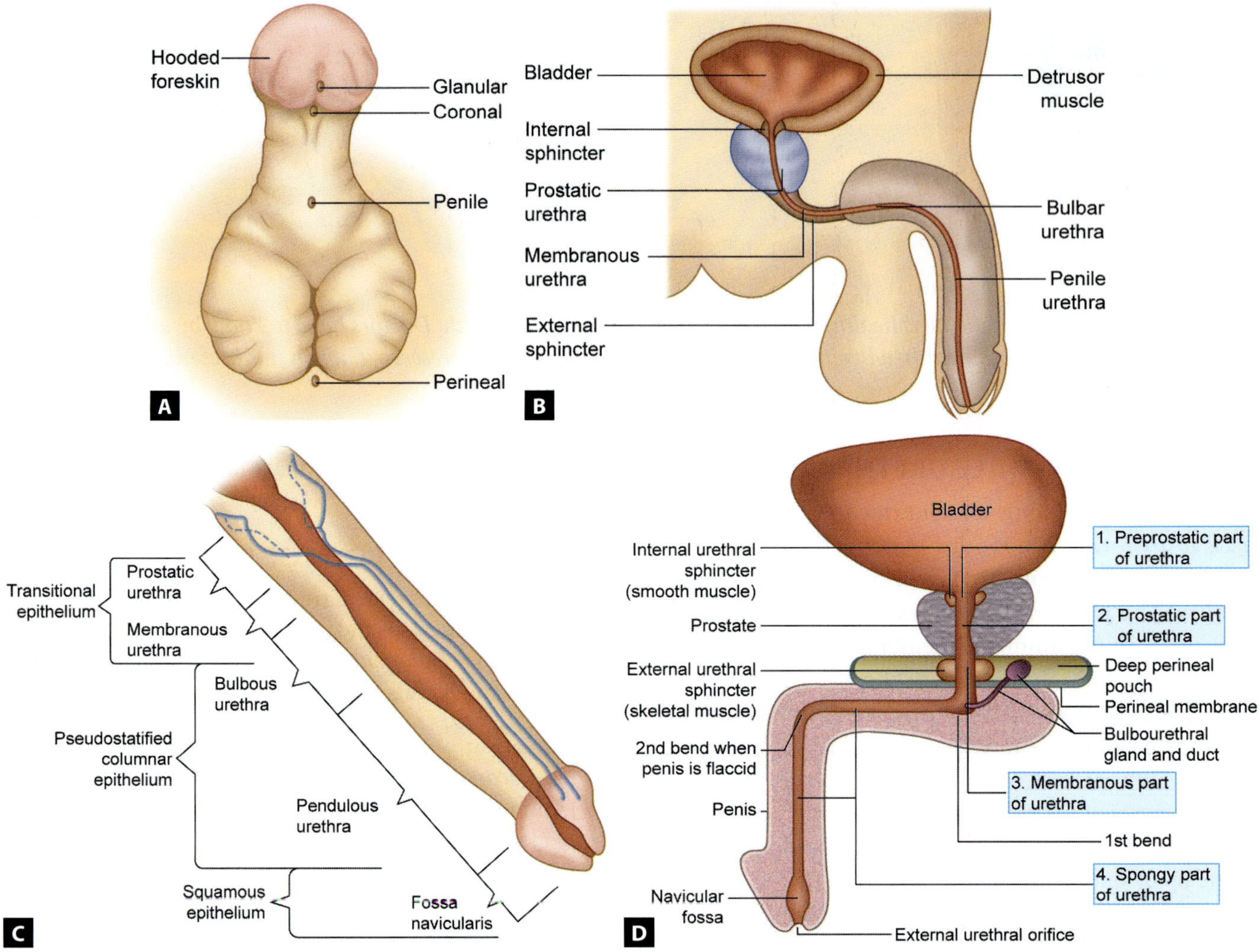

Figs. 1A to D: Anatomy of the urethra and its parts.

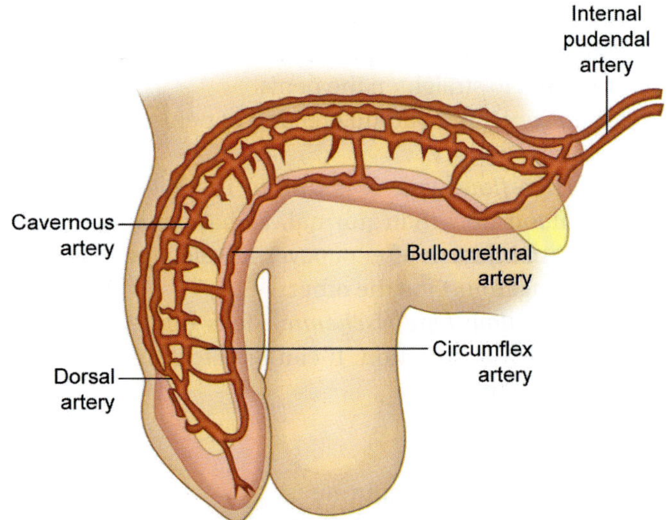

Fig. 2: Arterial supply of penis.

Lymphatic Drainage of Penis

- Lymphatics from glans penis drain to deep inguinal lymph nodes (LNs)
- Lymphatics from rest of the parts of penis drain to superficial inguinal LNs

You may be asked:

- Amputation of penis is called penectomy.
- Cancer in situ of glans penis is called erythroplasia of Queyrat.
- Cancer in situ of shaft of penis is called Bowen's disease.
- *Clinical or Jackson's staging of carcinoma of penis:*
  - I: Glans and prepuce are only involved.
  - II: Shaft involved
  - III: Nodes involved
  - IV: Metastasis present
- *Fowler's syndrome:* Clinically, this condition, which is common in women, is simulated with urethral stricture. There is an abnormal myotonic discharge in the striated muscle containing the urethral sphincter, which can be detected by electromyography of the sphincter.

- Urethral dilatation is of no help, and intermittent self-catheterization is required.
- *Caruncle:* It is a common problem in elderly women. There is a pedunculated mass from the posterior wall of urethra near external meatus. Treatment is diathermy excision.

Nerve Supply of Penis

- The sensory nerve supply of penis is from dorsal nerve of penis and ilioinguinal nerve.
- Autonomic nerves are from the prostatic plexus. The sympathetic nerves are vasoconstrictors, and the parasympathetic nerves are vasodilators.

Erection of Penis

Dilatation of helicine arteries pours in plenty of blood in penis and filling of vascular spaces in erectile tissue causes enlargement of penis. Erection is controlled by parasympathetic nerves.

CONGENITAL ABNORMALITIES OF URETHRA

- Posterior urethral (PU) valve
- It is common in males, a membrane distal to the verumontanum, and to be detected early to avoid renal failure. Antenatal diagnosis is made by ultrasound (USG), as bilateral hydronephrosis and a distended bladder.

Treatment

Treatment is removal of valve by endoscopy.

These valves cause urinary obstruction and itemize. If not detected antenatally, the baby has recurrent *urinary tract infection (UTI)* and retention of urine.

HYPOSPADIAS

It is 1 in 300 births, and urethral opening is not at the top of penis but over undersurface of penis.

Three abnormal characteristics are:

1. Abnormal site of the external urinary meatus
2. The ventral aspect of the prepuce is poorly developed.
3. Ventral deformity of penis in erect penis is called "chordee."

Meatus classification is based on different positions of the meatus:

- Glandular
- Coronal
- Penile and penoscrotal
- Perineal hypospadias

Points to remember:

Semen analysis: Semen is produced in testis and mixes with secretion of seminal vesicles and travels via vascular deferens and reaches to prostatic urethra and ejaculated. Sperms are counted and observed for motility. Azoospermia is either due to obstruction or failure of production. If obstruction is found, vasography is done and treatment is decided, and for other, testicular biopsy is required.

Treatment

Treatment is by plastic surgery.

EPISPADIAS

It is a very rare congenital abnormality. The meatus is situated on dorsal surface of penis and there is upward chordee.

Operations

- Denis Brown (Sir Denis John Wolko Browne, 1892–1967, British pediatric surgeon) operation—it is performed in two states (chordee correction and urethroplasty)
- MAGPI for coronal or subcoronal hypospadias (meatal advancement and glanduloplasty, integrated).

Rupture of Urethra

Injuries to the urethra are either caused by instrumentation or trauma.

Rupture of the Bulbar Urethra

The most common injury is falling astride, and the bulbar urethra is crushed between the pubic bone and the blow.

There appears to be a bruise in the perineum and acute retention of urine.

Treatment consists of suprapubic catheterization with all aseptic precautions.

Rupture of the membranous urethra.

It is usually accompanies fracture of the pelvis.

The complications of these injuries are:

- Urinary incontinence
- Erectile dysfunction (ED)
- Urethral disruption injuries

Management

- Antibiotics and appropriate anal
- Analgesics are given.
- Extravasation of urine
- It usually occurs in extraperitoneal rupture of the bladder and pelvic fracture, urethral disruption.
- Treatment is by suprapubic cystoscopy and definitive repair later.

Urethral Strictures

Commonly caused by:
- Inflammatory
- Idiopathic
- Iatrogenic
- Traumatic

Iatrogenic conditions are caused by urethral instrumentation, transurethral resection of the prostate (TURP), secondary to radical prostatectomy, and radiation for prostatic cancer.

Clinical Features

Clinically, there is straining, hesitancy, and poor stream. The voiding period is prolonged and dribbling also occurs. Investigations are uroflowmetry, urethroscopy, and USG.

Complications

Infection of the urinary tract is the main complication. Diverticulum is also developed due to effects of bladder outlet obstruction (BOO).

Treatment

Treatment consists of:
- Urethral dilatation with bogies
- Urethroplasty
- Internal urethrotomy

FEMALE URETHRA

The female urethra is 2–3 cm long, from the bladder neck to the external urethral meatus. Abnormalities of the female urethra include: Prolapse, diverticulum, stricture, and carbuncle, and Fowler's syndrome.

Good to remember:
- *Fracture of penis:*
  - It is an accidental injury caused by forceful bending of erected penis during sexual intercourse.
  - Emergency repair is required.
- *Erectile dysfunction:* It is not a disease but a psychological symptom associated with diabetes mellitus, hypertension, dyslipidemia, smoking, spinal cord injury, multiple sclerosis, pituitary tumor, and after radical prostatectomy.
- *Reuter's (Hans Conrad Julius Reiter, 1881–1969, German hygiene specialist) disease:* It is a triad of urethritis, conjunctivitis, and polyarthritis. It is treated with symptomatic therapy and antibiotics.
- *Buschke–Löwenstein tumor:* It is like vertigo in carcinoma without metastasis, and so local excision is sufficient.

PHIMOSIS

It is a condition in which the foreskin becomes tight and it cannot be pulled back over glans penis. It is a result of balanitis (inflammation of glans penis) and posthitis (inflammation of foreskin). *Balanitis xerotica obliterans (BXO)* can also cause phimosis.

Treatment

Treatment is circumcision.

Paraphimosis: A tight foreskin if retracted beyond glans penis cannot be returned. Injection of hyaluronidase may reduce edema, and the prepuce is returned back. If it fails then dorsal slit or circumcision is considered.

POSTERIOR URETHRAL VALVE

- It is an anomaly of the male urethra specifically
- It is of three types, Type I, II, III (5%) (Hugh Hampton Young, American Surgeon and Urologist, 1870–1945, described in 1919) according to Young's criteria.
- Type I is most common.
- It is an abnormal membranous fold in the posterior urethra.
- Causes urinary obstruction but allows a catheter
- Palpable kidneys and bladder as abdominal lumps.
- Vesicoureteral reflux (VUR) is common, in 50%
- Pulmonary hypoplasia also develops with PUV and becomes a cause for mortality
- Prenatal USG—keyhole sign—investigation—USG—cystoscopy.

Management

Catheterize for a few days, and when serum creatinine becomes normal, fulguration of value is done endoscopically.

CARCINOMA OF PENIS

It is less common in Western countries and more common in Asian, Africa, and South America.

Etiology

The causes include human papillomavirus (HPV) infection, BXO, smoking, balanoposthitis, phimosis, paraphimosis, and leucoplakia. Circumcision soon after birth gives immunity from carcinoma for 2 years, but delayed operation does not provide any immunity.

TNM classification:
The most common classification:
- T1 is confined to the skin
- T2 invades corpus spongiosum
- T3 invades the corpus cavernosum
- T4 invades adjacent structures
- N1 and N2 are for the involvement of inguinal LNs
- N3 is for iliac LNs.

Clinical Features

It usually occurs after 40 years of age. Growth becomes infected secondarily, and a foul-smelling discharge with blood is common. Approximately 50% of patients have nodal enlargement, and infection also contributes.

Treatment

- Excision of the primary tumor is the main treatment. Penile conservative surgery is now done against the 2 cm margin principle.
- Treatment of secondary LNs is managed by block dissection, but it should be done 3 weeks after primary resection, as infection will subside with antibiotics. LN involvement is a poor prognostic sign. Disease confined to only penis is having 5-year survival rate as 80% and disease with LNs involvement as 40%.

SOME IMPORTANT POINTS

- Hypospadias is the most common congenital abnormality of the urethra
- The optimal time for surgical repair of hypospadias is 6–12 months of age
- Galezia's triad is a combination of Dupuytren's contracture, Peyronie's disease, and retroperitoneal fibrosis.

SOME IMPORTANT QUESTIONS

Q1. Circumcision is contraindicated in:

a. Paraphimosis b. Meatal stenosis
c. Hypospadias d. Phimosis

Ans. c

Q2. The most common congenital anomaly of the urethra is:

a. Hypospadias
b. Epispadias
c. Meatal stenosis
d. Posterior urethral (PU) valve

Ans. a

Q3. The most common hypospadias is:

a. Penile b. Glandular
c. Scrotal d. A or C

Ans. b

Q4. Which of the following is true regarding hypospadias?

a. It is attributed to the failure of complete urethral tubularization in the fetus.
b. The urethral opening is most common in the perineum.
c. Urethra opens proximally and dorsally
d. It is seen in 1 in 1,500 boys.

Ans. a

Q5. Which of the following developmental defects of the urogenital sinuses never occurs in the female?

a. All these defects can occur
b. Hypospadias
c. Ectopia vesicae
d. Epispadias

Ans. b

Q6. For the PU valve, the investigation of choice is:

a. Cystoscopy
b. Micturating cystourethrogram (MCU)
c. Cystourethroscopy
d. Retrograde urethroscopy

Ans. b

Q7. Most common location of PU valve:

a. Proximal to verumontanum
b. Distal to verumontanum
c. At the level of verumontanum
d. At the bladder neck

Ans. b

Q8. Posterior urethral valve is usually seen:

a. Above verumontanum
b. Below the verumontanum
c. At the level of the bladder neck
d. At the level of the verumontanum

Ans. b

Q9. Which of the following are *true* regarding the picture depicted here of a patient who underwent a Foley's catheterization?

- P: Obstruction of venous and lymphatic return from the glans
- Q: Commonly due to sickle cell anemia

- R: The condition occurred due to the doctor forgetting to replace the retracted prepuce
- S: Previous circumcision is the cause of this condition here.

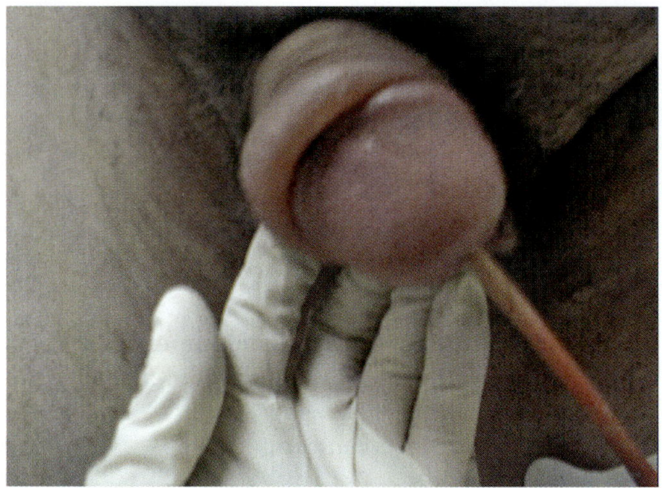

a. PQRS are all true b. Only R and S are true
c. Only P and R are true d. Only P and S are true

Ans. c

Q10. Indications of circumcision are all, *except*:
a. Chronic balanoposthitis
b. Jewish religion
c. Carcinoma penis
d. Paraphimosis

Ans. c

Q11. Persistent priapism is rarely seen as a consequence of:
a. Sickle cell disease
b. Leukemia
c. Spinal cord disease
d. Prolonged sexual activity

Ans. c

MULTIPLE CHOICE QUESTIONS

Grade I	*Simple*

Q1. True about hypospadias: (JIPMER 2011)
a. Associated with chordee
b. 50% associated with undescended testis
c. Due to the failure of fusion of the posterior wall of the urethra
d. Circumcision done immediately

Q2. True about hypospadias is: (PGI May 2010)
a. Defect seen in ventral penis
b. Always associated with chordee
c. Associated with hooded prepuce
d. Circumcision should be avoided.

Q3. All are true about hypospadias, *except:* (AIIMS June 1993)
a. Circumcision in infancy is contraindicated
b. Avoid surgery till puberty
c. No treatment required in glandular variety
d. If associated chordee is present, a two-stage operation is done

Q4. Order of correction of hypospadias: (JIPMER November 2017)
a. Straightening of penis—balanoplasty—urethroplasty
b. Urethroplasty—balanoplasty—straightening
c. Straightening—urethroplasty—balanoplasty
d. Balanoplasty—urethroplasty—straightening

Q5. Epispadias is associated with: (All India 2008)
a. Bifid pubic symphysis
b. Chordee
c. Anal atresia
d. Intestinal obstruction

Q6. All are true about posterior urethral valve, *except*: (GB Pant 2011)
a. Most common in boys
b. Can be detected by prenatal USG
c. Early catheterization should be done.
d. Diagnosed by early urethroscopy

Q7. The most common uropathic obstruction in children is: (UPPG 2009)
a. Stricture
b. Stones
c. Posterior urethral valve
d. Anterior urethral valve

Q8. The recommended treatment for preputial adhesions producing ballooning of the prepuce during micturition in a 2-year-old boy is: (AIIMS June 2003)
a. Wait and watch policy
b. Circumcision
c. Dorsal slit
d. Preputial adhesions release and dilatation

Q9. The best time for surgery of hypospadias is: **(All India 2003)**

a. 1–4 months of age
b. 6–10 months of age
c. 12–18 months of age
d. 2–4 years of age

Q10. Features of hypospadias are all, *except*: **(All India 1998)**

a. Chordee
b. Hooded prepuce
c. No treatment required with glandular variety
d. Cryptorchidism

Grade II	***Difficult***

Q1. All are true regarding circumcision, *except*: **(JIPMER November 2017)**

a. Hemorrhage due to bleeding from the frenular artery
b. Increases sexual drive
c. Avoid correction of congenital anomaly
d. Reduces sexually transmitted infections

Q2. The Grayhack shunt is established between: **(All India 2010)**

a. Corpora cavernosa and corpora spongiosa
b. Corpora cavernosa and saphenous vein
c. Corpora cavernosa and dorsal vein
d. Corpora cavernosa and glans

Q3. The following statements are true about Peyronie's disease, *except*: **(AIIMS November 2002)**

a. Patient presents with complaints of painful erection
b. Condition affects adolescent males
c. The condition can be associated with Dupuytren's contracture of the tendon of the hand
d. Spontaneous regression occurs in 50% of the cases.

Q4. All are true about Peyronie's disease, *except*: **(UPPG 2007)**

a. Self-limiting
b. Medical treatment is effective.
c. Association with Dupuytren's contracture
d. Calcified plaques

Q5. A child suffering from recurrent urinary tract infection is most likely to show: **(All India 2005)**

a. Posterior urethral valves
b. Vesicoureteric reflux
c. Neurogenic bladder
d. Renal and ureteric calculi

Q6. Urinary retention in a child is most commonly caused by: **(PGI December 2003)**

a. Metal scab with ulceration
b. Posterior urethral valve
c. Urethral stricture
d. Epispadias
e. Congenital short penis

Q7. Not true about urethral injuries is: **(AIIMS November 2001)**

a. Catheterize the patient immediately
b. Can be associated with a fracture pelvis
c. Bladder injury is associated with posturethral injuries
d. Blood at the external urethral meatus is an important feature.

Q8. Urine extravasation occurs in the following in case of penile urethral rupture, *except*: **(JIPMER 2003)**

a. Ischiorectal fossa
b. Scrotum
c. Abdominis
d. Below superficial fascia of penis

Q9. A young man gets into a fight after taking a beer and is kicked by the lower abdomen. There was a pelvic fracture. Blood at the meatus. Most likely cause is: **(MCI November 2017)**

a. Rupture of the membranous urethra
b. Bulbar urethral injury
c. Kidney laceration
d. Ureteric injury

Q10. In hypospadias, all are seen, *except*: **(PGI Dec 1999)**

a. Hooded penis
b. Dorsal chordee
c. Spatulated glans
d. Meatal stenosis

Grade III	***Most difficult***

Q1. With the knowledge of anatomy of the pelvis and perineum, which of the following is true regarding the collection of urine in a urethral rupture above the deep perineal pouch? **(AIIMS November 2012)**

a. Medial aspect of thigh
b. Scrotum
c. True pelvis only
d. Anterior abdominal wall

Testes and Scrotum

"Edward Gibbon, the author of 'The Decline and Fall of the Roman Empire,' was greatly embarrassed by a large hydrocele. The second time that it was tapped it became infected, and Gibbon died a few days later. The hydrocele was associated with a large scrotal hernia, which had probably been punctured."

– Bailey and Love

EMBRYOLOGY

The testis develops in the retroperitoneal space below the kidney. Gubernaculum developed in the fold of the peritoneum with the upper part attached to the developing testis and the lower part with the peritoneum. Simultaneously, another process develops beside the gubernaculum called processus vaginalis, which brings the gubernaculum and testis down. The left testis is at a lower level. The testis is oval-shaped and is 3.5 × 2.5 cm and about 15 g in weight. The epididymis lies along its posterior border along its lateral part. The testis is covered by three coverings, from out to in as tunica vaginalis, tunica albuginea, and tunica vasculosa **(Figs. 1A to C)**.

STRUCTURE OF TESTIS

Testis contains 200–300 lobules, and each lobule contains 2–3 seminiferous coiled tubules, 60 cm in length and 0.2 mm in diameter, lined with spermatozoa in stages of development. Seminiferous tubules end in 20–30 straight tubes and enter the mediastinum, forming a network of tubules called the rete testis. 20–30 efferent ductules come out of the rete testis and enter the epididymis and end as a single tubule, continuous with the vas deferens.

Arterial supply (venous drainage and lymphatic drainage) of testis:
- Testicular artery is a branch of abdominal aorta and it originates from just below the renal arteries in retroperitoneum. Testicular vein drains in renal vein on left side and inferior vena cava (IVC) on right side. The artery and vein run parallel to the ureter on the same side. Lymphatics drain into para-aortic lymph nodes (LNs).
- Epididymis has head, body, and tail.

UNDESCENDED TESTIS

The incomplete descent of the testis is the arrest of the testis at any site during its normal path to the scrotum. Ectopic testis is an abnormally placed testis outside this path. 4% of males are born with undescended testes. It occurs on one side, the right side is more common, or bilaterally (20%). It can occur at any of these sites:
- Intra-abdominal, extraperitoneally
- In the inguinal canal
- Extracanalicular—at the neck of scrotum
- Ectopic—anywhere outside this path.

In the early period, the testis is on the same side as the opposite side by puberty, it becomes smaller.

Pathology

Microscopic changes develop in the undescended testis after about 2 years with a reduction of Leydig cells, degeneration of Sertoli cells, and reduced spermatogenesis. The pathological changes are according to the level or arrest of descent; the higher the testis, the higher the pathological changes.

Consequences and Complications

- Infertility
- Hernia
- *Malignancy:* 5–10 times more chances than normal. Seminole is the most common cancer. Orchidopexy reduces the number of malignancies which is not clear.
- Testicular torsion

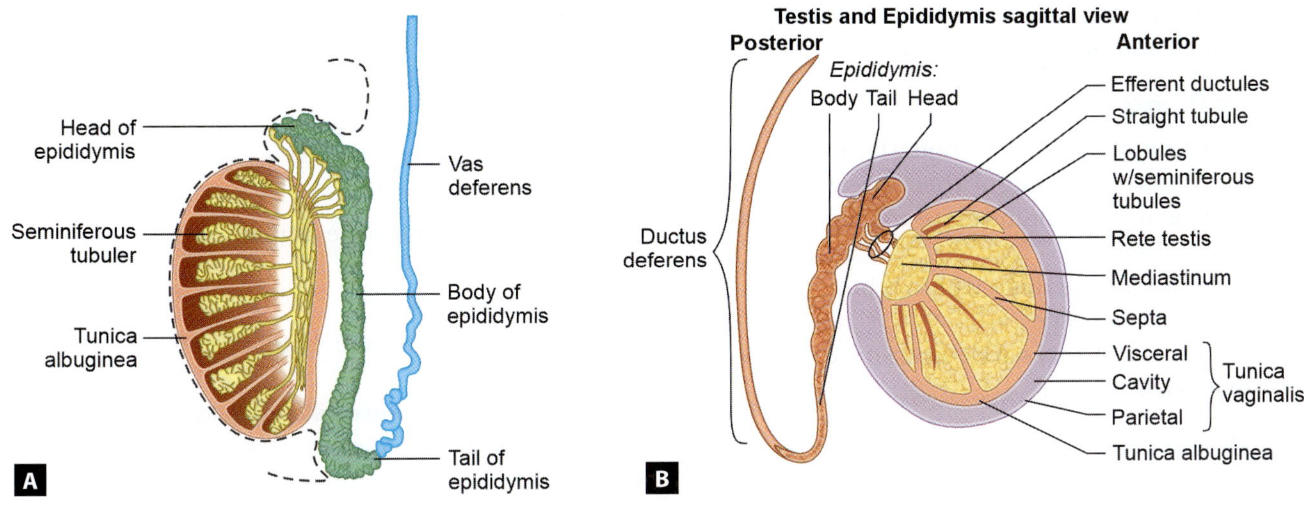

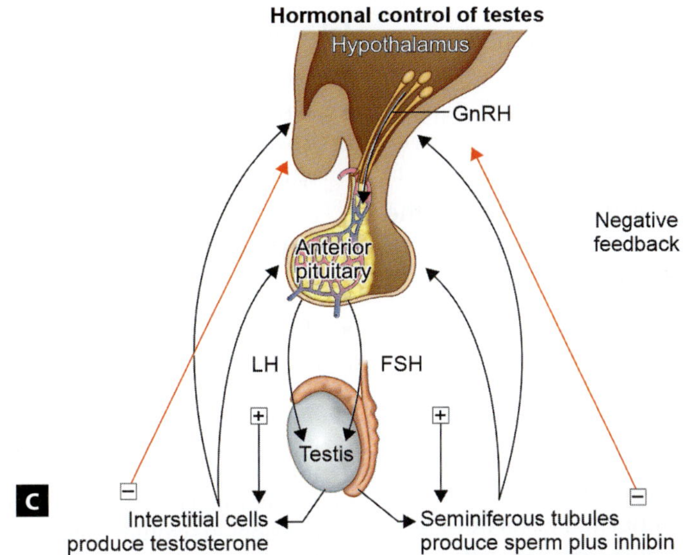

Figs. 1A to C: Anatomy of scrotum and testis. (FSH: follicle-stimulating hormone; GnRH: gonadotropin-releasing hormone; LH: luteinizing hormone)

Clinical Features

- Testing is impalpable.
- Ultrasonography (USG) is diagnostic.

Treatment

- Orchidopexy is required.
- When bringing the testis down to the scrotum, it is difficult or not possible. Orchidectomy is considered.

Points to remember:
Why is varicocele common on the left side?
- Left testicular vein drains at a right angle into the left renal vein
- The left testicular vein is longer.
- The loaded sigmoid colon compresses the left testicular vein
- Renal cell carcinoma (RCC) can invade the left renal vein and block the left testicular vein.

To differentiate torsion from orchitis:
Mn: DAP
- D: Deming sign—involved testis lies higher than the others
- A: Angel sign—normal testis lying horizontally
- P: Prehn's sign—lifting of the testis causes pain—torsion
- Pain decreases—orchitis

Epididymal cyst: It is a congenital, multilocular, clear fluid-filled, located behind the testis.

Spermatocele: It is an acquired condition, filled with barley water color fluid containing sperms, commonly unilateral, when gets enlarged, looking like three testicles.

RETRACTILE TESTIS

In retractile testis, the scrotum is normal, whereas in the case of an undescended testis, the scrotum is underdeveloped.

In retractile testis, the testis can be brought to the scrotum, but if undescended, it cannot.

Alerting Points

- Sudden contraction of the cremaster muscle causes torsion as in a blow, lifting of a heavy weight with a jerk, straining at defecation in severe constipation, sexual activity, and sports.
- Untwisting must be done within 6 hours, and 100% chance of full recovery.
- There are more chances of ischemia if the rotation is of 72° than 360°.

Clinical Features

- Sudden severe pain in the groin and lower abdomen
- Nausea and vomiting
- The scrotum is swollen and tender, and the testis is placed high.
- Apyrexia

Differential Diagnosis

- Epididymo-orchitis—elevation of the testis reduces the pain in epididymo-orchitis, but increases in torsion.
- Torsion of the appendix of the testis
- Small strangulated inguinal hernia
- Treatment is exploration and untwisting.

TORSION OF TESTIS

It is a surgical emergency. The testis twists and the blood supply gets compromised, and if left untreated, then the testis gets necrosed and dies out. A normal testis does not get torsioned, but some abnormalities can cause it.

- High investment of tunica vaginalis causes the testis to hang like a clapper in bell, and the torsion becomes easy. It is the most common cause.
- *Inversion of testis:* Testis rotates and occupies a transverse or upside-down position.
- There is separation of testis from epididymis and it rotates on this site.

VARICOCELE

It is a varicose dilatation of veins draining the testis.

Veins draining the testis and epididymis go up and form a plexus of veins called the pampiniform plexus, which goes up through the inguinal canal and comes out into the abdomen as one or two veins that pass up in the retroperitoneal space. The left testicular vein enters the left renal vein, and the right testicular vein enters the IVC.

Etiology

It affects 15–20% of adult males and is most common on the left side (90%).

- Absence or incompetence of valves in the proximal testicular veins
- Idiopathic
- Obstruction of the left testicular vein by a renal tumor

Clinical Features

It is usually asymptomatic, but if symptoms are present, then:

- A dragging sensation on standing at the end of the day.
- On standing, the left scrotum hangs lower than the right.
- On standing, the scrotum is palpable as a bag of worms.

Grades of Varicocele

- *Grade I:* Impalpable
- *Grade II:* Palpable
- *Grade III:* Visible

  Varicocele can cause subfertility.

Treatment

- Percutaneous embolization of gonadal veins
- Ligation of the testicular veins is the right treatment.

Not to forget:

Gubernaculum testis:

- It is a fibromuscular cord which guides and pull-up testis to the scrotum.
- It is attached from lower pole of testis to skin of groin which develops in scrotum later on.
- It is also called scrotal ligament.

Gubernaculum has five tails: Pubic tail, perineal tail, femoral tail, inguinal tail, and gubernaculum tail reaching the scrotum.

Locations of ectopic testis:

Mn: S3PF

- S: Superficial inguinal pouch
- S: Suprapubic
- S: Scrotum, contralateral
- P: Perineum
- F: Femoral canal

HYDROCELE

It is an abnormal collection of fluid in the tunica vaginalis.

Etiology of Hydrocele (Figs. 2A to D)

- Congenital hydrocele is due to the connection of the peritoneal cavity via the patent processus vaginalis.

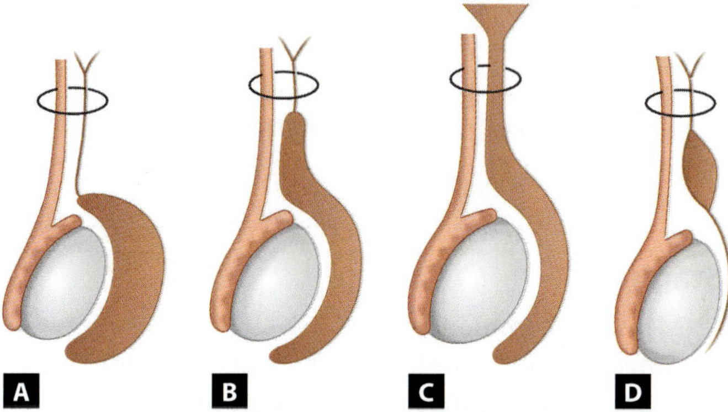

Figs. 2A to D: Various types of hydroceles.

- Secondary hydrocele is caused by excessive production of fluid within the sac.
- Vaginal hydrocele is by defective absorption of fluid.
- Interference with the lymphatic drainage of the scrotum.

Clinical Features

- It is a transilluminant swelling of the scrotum.
- You can get above the swelling. It differentiates from inguinoscrotal hernia.
- Painless
- It cannot palpate the testis due to the surrounding fluid.
- In congenital hydrocele, you can see hydrocele disappears when the baby lies down, as fluid from the scrotum goes to the peritoneal cavity through the patent processus vaginalis.
- Encysted hydrocele of cord is felt above testis and can be mistaken for inguinal hernia.
- Hydrocele of canal of Nuck (Anton Nuck, 1650–1692, Dutch physician and anatomist) is found in females in relation to the round ligament and is in inguinal canal always even partially.

Treatment

- *Eversion of sac or Jaboulay's (Mathieu Jaboulay, 1860–1913, French surgeon) operation:* The sac is everted and sutured.
- *Lord's operation of plications:* A series of interrupted sutures are used to plicate the redundant tunica vaginalis.
- *Window operation*

EPIDIDYMO-ORCHITIS

It is the inflammation of the testis and epididymis. Rule—epididymitis arises in sexually active young men from a sexually transmitted general infection, while in older men it is more usually arises from a urinary infection or may be secondary to an indwelling urethral catheter. Infection starts in the tail of the epididymis, then spreads to the whole epididymis, and then to the testis.

Clinical Features

- Fever with pain in the groin
- Scrotum becomes red, swollen, shiny, tender, and edematous.

Investigations

- Urine analysis
- Urethral swab
- Nucleic acid amplification testing (NAAT)
- USG

Treatment

- *Doxycycline:* 100–300 mg daily for 2 weeks.
- Quinolones are better for elderly patients.
- IV antibiotics are better than oral as recovery is required fast to avoid irreversible tissue loss.
- Plenty of oral fluids to keep hydrated.
- Scrotal support reduces pain.
- Analgesics

TUMORS OF TESTIS

They coin for approximately 1% of all male malignancy and are increasing for past few decades. Most common is germ cell tumor occurring between 40 and 50 years whereas nonseminomatous germ cell tumor (NSGCT) occurs between 39 and 40 years.

Classification

- *Germ cell tumors (90–95%):* Seminole, teratoma, embryonic cell carcinoma, yolk cell tumor, and choriocarcinoma.
- *Interstitial tumor:* Leydig cell tumor.
- Lymphoma
- Other tumors

SEMINOMA

Cut surface is homogeneous pink. Oval cells with clear cytoplasm and large rounded nuclei with spermatozoa resembling cells. Histologically, it is of two types: One with more anaplastic features and other with spermatozoa development stages. Active lymphocytic infiltration shows good prognosis.

TERATOMA

The components are derived from all three: (1) Ectoderm, (2) endoderm, and (3) mesoderm. It may arise from mature (well-differentiated) or immature (undifferentiated).

INTERSTITIAL CELL TUMOR

Tumors of Leydig (Franz von Leydig, 1821–1908, German anatomist) cells are masculinizes, and tumors of Sertoli (Enrico Sertoli, 1842–1910, Italian physiologist) cells are feminizing. About 10% are malignant.

You may be asked:
Tumor markers for testicular tumors:
- α-fetoprotein (AFP)
- β-human chorionic gonadotropin (β-hCG)
- Lactate dehydrogenase (LDH)
- Placental alkaline phosphatase (PLAP)
- γ-glutamyl transferase (GGT)

Most common testicular tumor in infants and children is yolk sac tumor.
Yolk sac tumor has three microscopic patterns:
1. Microcystic
2. Endodermal sinus
3. Solid

Chimney sweeper's cancer:
- It is a SCC of scrotum caused by environmental carcinogens in chimney soot.
- Diagnosis is done by biopsy of scrotal skin.
- Treatment is excision by 2 cm margin.

Clinical Features

- Painless testicular mass
- Sensation of heaviness
- Rarely pain
- Lung metastasis is usually asymptomatic but may cause chest pains, dyspnea, and hemoptysis.
- A solid mass is felt in the scrotum, with difficult to feel epididymis separate.

Investigations

- USG
- Tumor markers are raised in 50% of cases—AFP and human chorionic gonadotropin (hCG)
- X-ray chest
- CT abdomen

Staging

TNM is most commonly used.
- *Stage I:* Tumor is confined to the testis and epididymis.
- *Stage II:* Nodal disease is present but confined to nodes below the diaphragm.
- *Stage III:* Nodes are present above the diaphragm.
- *Stage IV:* Nonlymphatic metastatic disease (most typically within the lungs).

Treatment

- *Suspected case:* Scrotal exploration and Orchidectomy
- Seminoma is radiosensitive and NSGCT is not.
- Tumors are treated according to their category.
- Platinum-based chemotherapy has excellent potential.

Good to remember:
Male infertility: 30% cases of infertility show defect in women and 30% show defect in men, and 30% cannot show any abnormality.
Vasectomy:
- It is an operation of family planning.
- Precautions must be taken for some time till two negative semen analysis reports are negative.

SOME IMPORTANT QUESTIONS

Q1. Surgery for undescended testis is recommended at what age?

a. 6 months b. 12 months
c. 24 months d. 36 months

Ans. a

Q2. All are true regarding torsion of the testis, *except*:

a. Common in adolescents and young adults
b. Inversion of the testis is the most common predisposing cause.
c. Elevation of the testis reduces the pain
d. If diagnosis is doubtful, prompt exploration is the rule.

Ans. c

Q3. All the following statements are true regarding torsion of the testis, *except*:
a. Most common between 10 and 25 years of age
b. Prompt exploration and twisting, and fixation is the only way to save the torted testis
c. Anatomical abnormality is unilateral, and the contralateral testis should not be fixed
d. Inversion of the testis is the most common predisposing cause

Ans. c

Q4. In the treatment of varicocele, testicular vein ligation is done at the level of:
a. Above inguinal ligament
b. Below inguinal ligament
c. Neck of the sac
d. Scrotum

Ans. a

Q5. Which of the following is true about varicocele, *except*:
a. Incompetent valves of the testicular vein are responsible for varicocele
b. 90% are on the left side
c. Asymptomatic cases require surgery
d. Femoral catheterization with spermatic vein ablation is done in recurrence.

Ans. c

Q6. After varicocele surgery, venous drainage occurs by:
a. Cremasteric veins
b. Penile veins
c. Ectopic in the iliac fossa
d. Present at the usual location

Ans. a

Q7. The true about varicocele is:
a. More common on the right side
b. Can cause oligospermia
c. No effect on Valsalva
d. Lies anterior on testis

Ans. b

Q8. Congenital hydrocele is best treated by:
a. Eversion of sac
b. Excision of sac
c. Lord's procedure
d. Herniotomy

Ans. d

Q9. Subcapsular orchidectomy is done for cancer of:
a. Testes
b. Prostate
c. Penis
d. Urethra

Ans. b

Q10. Ligation of the cord in orchidectomy for the treatment of testicular tumors is done at:
a. External ring
b. Internal ring
c. Base of scrotum
d. Just above the epididymis

Ans. b

MULTIPLE CHOICE QUESTIONS

Grade I	*Simple*

Q1. Stephen Fowler's surgery is done for: **(GB Pant 2010)**
a. Ectopic testis
b. Undescended testis
c. Hypospadias
d. Epispadias

Q2. Which of the following investigations is used to confirm anorchia? **(AIIMS November 2013)**
a. Positron emission tomography (PET)
b. Magnetic resonance imaging (MRI)
c. Laparoscopy
d. Ultrasonography (USG)

Q3. Orchidopexy is done in cases of undescended testes at the age of: **(AIIMS June 2006)**
a. Infancy
b. 1–2 years
c. 5 years
d. Puberty

Q4. True about incompletely descended testis are all of the following, *except*: **(MCI March 2008)**
a. Early repositioning can preserve function
b. It may lead to sterility if bilateral.
c. Poorly developed secondary sexual characters
d. May be associated with indirect inguinal hernia

Q5. Testis does not descend beyond: **(JIPMER 2012)**
a. 2 months
b. 4 months
c. 6 months
d. 8 months

Q6. The most common site of ectopic testis is: **(GB Pant 2010)**
a. Superficial inguinal pouch
b. Root of penis
c. Femoral triangle
d. Perineum

MODEL QUESTIONS

Q1. What do these images depict?

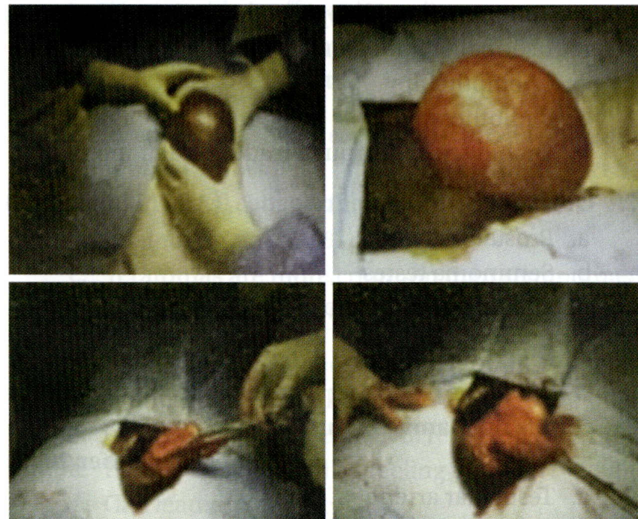

a. Jaboulay's operation
b. Hernia repair
c. Surgery for Fournier's gangrene
d. Lord's plication for hydrocele

Ans. a

Q2. Which of the following statements is true regarding acute epididymitis?

a. All the statements are true.
b. Mostly bilateral
c. Absence of blood flow on Doppler examination
d. Occurs in young sexually active men and is commonly due to *Chlamydia trachomatis*

Ans. d

Q3. All are features of Fournier's gangrene, *except*:

a. Testicles are involved.
b. Obliterative arteritis seen
c. Hemolytic streptococci, isolated
d. Necrotizing fasciitis

Ans. a

Q4. Carcinoma testis, the lymphatic metastasis goes to the first site seen in:

a. Para-aortic lymph nodes
b. Superficial inguinal nodes
c. Deep inguinal nodes
d. Internal iliac nodes

Ans. a

Q5. All are true regarding seminoma, *except*:

a. Common in age between 35 and 45 years
b. Metastasis to lymphatics
c. Radioresistant
d. Not seen before puberty

Ans. c

Q6. High inguinal orchidectomy specimen showed teratoma testis with involvement of epididymis; the stage is:

a. T1
b. T2
c. T3
d. T4b

Ans. a

Q7. Which of the following is a known complication of modified RPLND (retroperitoneal lymph node dissection) done for nonseminomatous germ cell tumor of the testis?

a. Impotence
b. Bladder atony
c. Dry ejaculation
d. Retrograde ejaculation

Ans. d

Q8. Not true of Sertoli cell tumor is:

a. Poor response to radiotherapy
b. Prominent lymphocytes in section
c. Common in adults
d. Can be malignant in 10–20% of cases

Ans. b

Q9. The lymph nodes first involved in cancer of the skin of the scrotum are:

a. Superficial inguinal
b. External iliac
c. Para-aortic
d. Gland of Cloquet

Ans. a

Q10. Orchiectomy is not indicated in:

a. Seminoma testis
b. Prostatic carcinoma
c. Tubercular epididymitis
d. Male breast cancer

Ans. c

SUGGESTED READING

1. Bailey & Love's - Short Practice of Surgery, 27th edition.
2. Schwartz's Principles of Surgery, 18th edition.
3. Campbell's Urology, 10th edition.
4. Urology, November 1984, Vol. XXIV, No. 5. pp. 481-482.

SECTION 9

Vascular System

CHAPTER 50

Arterial Disorders

"Joy and pain, they are but two arteries of the one heart that pumps through all those who don't numb themselves to really living."

– Ann Voskamp

ARTERIAL DISORDERS

Arterial stenosis and occlusion

This is usually caused by:

- Atherosclerosis
- Thromboembolic disease
- Trauma

DISEASES CAUSING PERIPHERAL ARTERIAL OCCLUSION

Common Causes

Mn = ABAI

- A = Atherosclerosis
- B = Buerger's disease (thromboangiitis obliterans)
- A = Arteritis
  - Takayasu disease
  - Systemic lupus erythematosus (SLE)
  - Trauma
- I = Injury/irradiation

Uncommon Causes

Mn = CAD

- C = Compression
  - Popliteal artery entrapment
  - TOS
- A = Anomalies—coarctation of the aorta
- D = Disorders of the arterial wall
  - Retroperitoneal fibrosis
  - Cystic medial necrosis

ATHEROSCLEROSIS

- The most common cause of arterial occlusion.
- It is a disease of medium and large arteries.
- It is due to deposition of atheroma (lipid complex) on the intima arteria.
- It is common at the bifurcation of an artery.
- It causes narrowing of the lumen, leading to ischemic changes.
- Embolism results due to plaque dislodgment in the brain and other organs.
- Transient ischemic attack (TIA) results due to small emboli.
- Aneurysm can occur due to weakness of the wall of the artery caused by atheromatous plaques, common in the lower abdominal aorta.
- The most common age is below 60–70 years.

Pulseless Disease or Aortoarteritis or Takayasu Arteritis

It is an inflammatory disease of medium and large-sized arteries causing stenosis. It is common among young women in Asia. Investigation of choice is computed tomography (CT) angiography. Treatment by steroids and, if required, bypass surgery.

Clinical Features of Chronic Arterial Stenosis

- *Intermittent claudication:*
  - Debilitating cramp-like pain on walking, making forcing one to stop. Pain is relieved by rest in the standing and sitting position, generally within 5 minutes.
  - Claudication distance is the distance walked without pain. The claudication distance is reduced when walking uphill or at higher speeds, and if the disease is worsening.
  - *Leriche's (René Leriche, 1879–1955, French surgeon) syndrome* is buttock claudication associated with

sexual impotence due to arterial insufficiency and absent femoral pulse.

- *Rest pain:* As the disease progresses, the claudication distance reduces, and pain happens on rest on with little exertion.
- Ulceration
- Gangrene
- *Color:* On elevation, the limb becomes paler, and on hanging from the bed, it is reddish, called the sunset foot sign.
- *Temperature of the limb:* Initially, the limb feels warm on touching.
- Sensations are intact.
- Movements are not affected, and there is no paralysis.
- *Arterial pulses:* Pulse diminishing is appreciated by compairing with the other side.
- Arterial bruit is heard on auscultation.
- Capillary filling is slow.

Investigations

- CBC
- ECG
- Doppler (Christian Johann Doppler, 1803–1853, Austrian physicist, gave the Doppler principle in 1842), ultrasound. It is one of the best tests to detect obstructive lesions of arteries.
- Duplex scanning
- Digital subtraction percutaneous angiography.

Treatment

General

Stopping smoking and reducing alcohol will help a lot. Diabetes, hypertension, and hyperlipidemia are to be treated well. Lifestyle modifications are required.

Medication

Aspirin (75 mg/day) and clopidogrel (75 mg/day) are to be started. Percutaneous transluminal angioplasty (PTA).

Operations

Bypass surgery is done if symptoms are severe and PTA fails.

Gangrene

Gangrene develops at the most distal part of a limb. Dry gangrene occurs when the obstruction occurs slowly, and wet gangrene occurs when occlusion occurs suddenly in diabetes and infection develops. Amputation is required when it becomes life-threatening.

VASCULAR GRAFTS

Autologous

- Autograft (e.g., saphenous vein)
- Allograft (Homograft)
- Xenograft (Hetrograft)
- Tissue-engineered

Synthetic

- *Textile:* Dacron
- *Nontextile:* Polytetrafluoroethylene (PTFE)

Best graft for AFB: Dacron
Best graft for FPB: Saphenous vein

ANEURYSM

Dilatation of a segment of an artery >50% of its diameter is called "aneurysm," and <50% is known as "ectasia." Aneurysm is of two types: (1) True (all three layers of the wall are present, intimate, media, and adventitia) and (2) false (pseudoaneurysm, single layer of fibrous tissue). They are either fusiform or saccular. The most common site of a pseudoaneurysm is the femoral artery. True aneurysm most commonly occurs in the abdominal aorta and the popliteal artery.

Etiology

- Atheromatous (90%)
- Mycotic
- Collagen disease (Marfan's syndrome)
- Traumatic

Investigations

- General
- Complete blood count (CBC), electrolytes, and ultrasound CT scan
- Magnetic resonance imaging (MRI)

Clinical Features

- Most of the aneurysms are asymptomatic.
- Abdominal aortic aneurysm

Operations

- Open repair of an aneurysm.
- Endovascular aneurysm repair (EVAR).

ABDOMINAL AORTIC ANEURYSM

- Enlargement or focal dilatation of the aorta, 1.5 times of its diameter (or more than 3 cm)
- The most common site is infrarenal
- 90% due to atherosclerosis
- More common in males
- Pain in the abdomen with abdominal aortic aneurysm (AAA) is an indication that AAA is going to rupture, which is life-threatening
- *Investigation:* Contrast-enhanced computed tomography (CECT)
- *Treatment:*
  - Indication of surgery based on size: AAA ≥ 5.5 cm.
  - Repair of the aneurysm with a graft.
    - *Ruptured AAA:* Triad—shock, pain in abdomen, and pulsating abdominal mass.
    - Planned surgery of AAA mortality rate is 1–2%, and in acute rupture, 45–50%
    - *Treatment of pseudoaneurysm:* It is common in the femoral artery. Injection of thrombin to cause thrombosis of the aneurysm under U/S guidance.
    - Mycotic aneurysms are caused by bacterial infection and not by fungi, so it is a misnomer. It does not commonly occur in the femoral artery and is caused by *Staphylococcus.*
- Transperitoneal approach
- Retroperitoneal approach—especially when a history of multiple abdominal operations.

- *Advantages:* Less risk of postoperative gastrointestinal (GI) and lung complications.
- *Disadvantages:* Difficult to approach the right renal artery.

- *Complications:*
  - Myocardial dysfunction
  - Renal failure

Dissecting aneurysm of the aorta: It is aortic dissection by a circumferential or, less commonly, transverse tear of the intima. Most commonly occurs at the right lateral wall of the ascending aorta and then less commonly at the descending thoracic aorta. It is common in the sixth and seventh decades. Other common causes are Marian's syndrome, Takayasu arteritis, and coarctation of the aorta. Clinically, it presents as severe pain and hypertension. X-ray chest shows widening of the mediastinum. Investigation of choice is CECT.

DeBakey classification divides it into three types:

- *Type I:* Ascending, arch, and descending aorta involved.
- *Type II:* Ascending aorta alone involved.
- *Type III:* Descending aorta alone involved.

Boyd's clinical classification of claudication:

- *Grade I:* Pain relieved on continued walking.
- *Grade II:* Walks in pain with a limp.
- *Grade III:* Pain compels to sit.
- *Grade IV:* Rest pain

Ankle-brachial pressure index (ABPI) = AP/BP = 0.9–1.1 (normal). If AP is less than BP, stenosis of the vessel:

- <0.9—claudication
- <0.5—rest pain
- <0.3—imminent necrosis

THROMBOANGIITIS OBLITERANS/ BUERGER'S DISEASE

In this disease, the occlusion occurs due to sympathetic overactivity, leading to vasospasm in the infrapopliteal arteries bilaterally. It is a segmental inflammatory disease of small and medium-sized arteries of the limbs. In advanced cases, arteries, veins, and nerves also get involved by fibrosis. There is a history of smoking, <50 years of age, infrapopliteal lesion only, unilateral involvement, and superficial phlebitis is present.

Investigations

- Color Doppler
- *Arteriography:* Angiography reveals well-developed collaterals as corkscrew, tree root, and spider leg collaterals.
- Biopsy

Clinical Features

Mn = RIT

- *R* = Raynaud's phenomenon
- *I* = Intermittent claudication
- *T* = Thrombophlebitis, which is superficial and migratory

Treatment

- Calcium channel blockers.
- Stop smoking and change your lifestyle. Lumber sympathectomy is indicated, especially if rest pain. Ulcer or gangrene is present.

IMPORTANT POINTS IN BUERGER'S DISEASE

- Revascularization surgery is not required.
- The bypass surgery role is minimal.
- The pulsation in brachial and popliteal arteries are reduced or absent, but in radial, ulnar, and tibial arteries are present.
- Ileoprost (It is a prostacyclin mimetic) acts as a potent vasodilator, reducing the pain of Buerger's disease.
- Intermittent pneumatic compression is used especially in critical limb ischemia.

LUMBAR SYMPATHECTOMY

The lumbar sympathetic chain is a ganglionated chain on the side of the bodies of the lumbar vertebrae. There are five ganglions, but the first and second are fused, so there are only four ganglions. Usually, L1 to L3 ganglia are removed if done on one side, but if bilateral is required, then the first ganglion is spared to avoid retrograde ejaculation.

Indications of Lumbar Sympathectomy

Mn = BARC BPH

- *B* = Buerger's disease
- *A* = Artherosclerosis
- *R* = Raynaud's disease
- *C* = Cyanosis (acrocyanosis/erythrocyanosis)
- *B* = Frostbite
- *P* = Peripheral vascular insufficiency
- *H* = Hyperhidrosis

> *You may be asked:*
> *Arteriovenous fistula and due to trauma*: The most common cause of acquired arteriovenous fistula (AVF) is iatrogenic. Cimino fistula—cephalic vein and radial artery fistula rested for dialysis. The most common type is congenital.
>
> *Pathology:* There is arterialization of the vein, higher temperature on that limb than the other, pulse rate is high on the concerned limb, and machinery murmur (continuous thrill). Pressure on the proximal limb of a fistula diminishes swelling and pulse rate and disappears murmur and thrill, it is called Branham's sign.
>
> *Fontaine classification of limb ischemia:*
> - *Stage I:* Asymptomatic
> - *Stage IIa:* Mild claudication
> - *Stage IIb:* Moderate-to-severe claudication
> - *Stage IV:* Ischemic rest pain
> - *Stage V:* Ulceration or gangrene

Types

- Bressica: Cimino
    - *F:* Radial artery and cephalic vein.
- Feinberg F—radial artery and basilic vein.
- Snuff box F—posterior branch of radial artery and cephalic vein.

Diabetic Foot

It is due to, Mn = TIL

- T = Trophic changes due to neuropathy
- I = Ischemia (due to atherosclerosis)
- L = Low resistance to infection due to tissue hyperglycemia.

Neuropathy causes 'stocking and glove' diminished sensations. Infection leads to the destruction of tissues, leading to ulcers.

Treatment

- Control diabetes with diet and drugs
- Debridement

TEMPORAL ARTERITIS (GIANT CELL ARTERITIS)

- It is an inflammatory disease of the superficial temporal artery in more female patients of >50 years.
- Clinically has a headache, facial claudication, and can sometimes cause blindness as a complication.
- *Treatment:* Steroids.

CELIAC PLEXUS OR SOLAR PLEXUS BLOCK

- It is done to reduce severe pain in pancreatitis or CA pancreas.
- It is done by injecting alcohol bilaterally.

ACUTE LIMB ISCHEMIA

It is an emergency, and after 6 hours, it becomes irreversible.

Clinically, it is 6P, pain, pallor, paralysis, pulsation loss, poikilothermia (unable to maintain a constant temperature), and paresthesia.

CRITICAL LIMB ISCHEMIA

It is associated with rest pain in the distal part of the foot, ischemic nonhealing ulcers, or gangrene. It is a severe arterial occlusive disease.

Treatment

- IV heparin
- Embolectomy
- Thrombolysis

Pseudoclaudication

It is neurogenic claudication occurring in lumbar canal stenosis, mimicking intermittent claudication of PVD. Symptoms can occur even while standing alone without walking.

> *Points to remember:*
> - Most common cause of aneurysm is atherosclerosis.
> - Most common site of aneurysm is in circle of Willis.
> - Most common aneurysm of peripheral artery is popliteal artery.
> - Most common site of visceral artery aneurysm is splenic artery.
> - Most common site of mycotic aneurysm is femoral artery.
> - Mycotic aneurysm is a misnomer. It is bacterial.
> - Saccular aneurysm has high chances of rupture than fusiform aneurysm.
> - Most common site of abdominal aortic aneurysm (AAA) is infrarenal.
> - Most common presentation of AAA is back pain.
> - Most are asymptomatic till burst.
> - Aortoiliac occlusive disease (AIOD) differs femoropopliteal (FPOD) as it is rarely limb sacrificing as good collaterals develop quickly.
> - Limb revascularization techniques are used in AIOD and FPOD, such as aortofemoral and iliofemoral bypass.

RUPTURED ABDOMINAL AORTIC ANEURYSM

Abdominal aortic aneurysm rupture happens in the peritoneal cavity in 20% of cases, whereas in 80% of cases in the retroperitoneal space. It is a surgical emergency.

Thoracic Outlet Syndrome

It is a compression of the subclavian vessels and brachial plexus nerves at the thoracic inlet. It is common in middle-aged women with neurological symptoms most commonly. Though the neurovascular bundle is compressed but symptoms present depend upon the individual structure involved. It is caused by cervical rib, long transverse process of C7, abnormal first rib, fibrous band, trauma, osteoarthritis, scalene muscle shortness, or spasm. Ulnar nerve involvement is most common. Treatment is by division of the cervical rib, first rib, or division of the scalene muscle.

Proactive Tests for Diagnosis

Mn = *WHAR*

- *W* = Weight test (hyperabduction test 180° arm is hyperabducted = Neurocompression occurs.
- *H* = Halsted test (costoclavicular test) draw shoulder backs and down—nerves compressed between the clavicle and the first rib (costoclavicular space).
- *A* = Adson test (Scalene test)—patient should inspire maximum, hold breath, extend neck and head to be turned toward affected side—ipsilateral radial pulse decreases, due to reduction of space between scalenus anticus and medius, causing pressure on subclavian artery and brachial plexus.
- *R* = ROOS test (Arm claudication test) Patient extends his arm at 90° with external rotation of the shoulder—compression on nerves happens.

Treatment

- Early diagnosis
- Immediate resuscitation
- Maintain systolic blood pressure (BP)
- Urinary catheter
- Crossmatch 6 units of blood

> *Good to remember:*
> *Raynaud's phenomenon:* It is episodic digital (fingers and toes) ischemia when exposure to cold is done, or a stressful emotional episode happens. Mn-BC Roy: B—blanching, C—cyanosis, R—redness (rubor). There are three stages: (1) Stage of local syncope (White), (2) stage of local asphyxia (Blue), and (3) stage of recovery (Red), so called as triphasic color response.

Types

- Primary: Raynaud's disease
- Secondary: *Mn* = *NPC TOMB*
- *N* = Neurological causes—spinal cord disorders
- *P* = Pulmonary—hypertension
- *C* = Collagen vascular disease—scleroderma
- *T* = Trauma—vibration injuries
- *O* = Occlusive arterial disease—atherosclerosis
- *M* = Medicines—Ergot derivatives
- *B* = Blood dyscrasias—cold agglutinins

Raynaud's Disease

When secondary causes of Raynaud's phenomenon are ruled out. Most of the patients are women below 40 years of age. Fingers are more involved than toes. Treatment is palliative. Vasodilation drugs are used. Diltiazem are the drug of choice.

Allen (A) Test

It is done to detect patency of both radial and ulnar arteries, which form a palmar arch. Both arteries are pressed and then, while one artery pressure is released, if this artery is blocked, then pallor remains, then do the same with the other artery.

TINEL'S SIGN

The trapping of a nerve causes tingling or pins and needles due to nerve compression. It is done in TOS also.

PHALEN'S SIGN

Flexion of the elbow or wrist on an abducted arm at 90° causes compression on nerves, leading to tingling in the hand.

SUBCLAVIAN STEAL SYNDROME

It is due to atherosclerotic obstruction of the first part of the subclavian artery, and this leads to reversal of blood flow in the vertebral artery, which provides blood to the aorta through the postocclusive subclavian artery segment. When the arm exercise is done, blood is stolen from the blood flow of the brain stem, which reduces pressure in the posterior cerebral circulation and may lead to transient vertebrobasilar ischemia.

SOME IMPORTANT QUESTIONS

Q1. Which among the following is not a feature of peripheral arterial occlusion?

a. Shock
b. Pallor
c. Pain
d. Pulselessness

Ans. a

Q2. Buerger's disease usually affects all of the following, *except*:

a. Small-sized arteries
b. Medium-sized arteries
c. Large arteries
d. Deep veins

Ans. c

Q3. True about ischemic rest pain:

a. More at night
b. Most common (MC) in calf muscle
c. Increase upon elevation of limbs
d. Relieved by dependent position
e. Often associated with trophic changes

Ans: a, b, c, d, and e

Q4. An adult patient with leg pain and gangrene of the toe. His ankle to brachial arterial pressure ratio would be less than:

a. 1
b. 0.3
c. 0.5
d. 0.8

Ans. b

Q5. The definition of critical limb ischemia includes:

a. Rest/night pain
b. Ankle blood pressure >50 mm Hg
c. Intermittent claudication
d. Well-preserved tissues

Ans. a

Q6. Dissecting aneurysm is best diagnosed by:

a. Computed tomography (CT)
b. Magnetic resonance imaging (MRI)
c. Angiography
d. USG

Ans. b

Q7. Allen's test is useful in evaluating:

a. Thoracic outlet compression
b. Presence of cervical rib
c. Integrity of palmar arch
d. Digital blood flow

Ans. c

Q8. Butcher's thigh is:

a. Vastus lateralis rupture
b. Subcutaneous lipodermatosclerosis
c. Bursa in the adductor canal
d. Accidental injury to major vessels in the thigh or groin

Ans. d

Q9. What is the best way to control external hemorrhage?

a. Direct pressure
b. Elevation
c. Proximal tourniquet
d. Artery forceps

Ans. a

Q10. Intermittent claudication is defined as:

a. Pain in the muscle at rest only
b. Pain in a muscle on the first step
c. Pain in the muscle on exercise only
d. Pain in a muscle on the last step

Ans. c

MULTIPLE CHOICE QUESTIONS

Grade I	Simple

Q1. Acute vascular ischemia manifests as: (PGI December 2008)

a. Pulselessness
b. Paralysis
c. Flushing
d. Anesthesia
e. Coolness

Q2. Clinical feature of acute arterial embolism is: (PGI November 2017)

a. Pulselessness
b. Pain
c. Erythema of distal part
d. Numbness
e. Sensory loss

Q3. In a subclavian artery block at the outer border of the first rib, all of the following arteries help in maintaining the circulation to the upper limb, *except*: (AIIMS May 2011)

a. Subscapular artery
b. Superior thoracic artery
c. Thyrocervical trunk
d. Suprascapular artery

Q4. Both arterial and venous thrombosis occur in: (PGI November 2011)

a. Antiphospholipid antibodies
b. Antithrombin III deficiency
c. Hyperhomocysteinemia
d. Protein C deficiency
e. A mutation in the factor V gene

Q5. Which of the following is the most common symptom of aortoiliac occlusive disease? (AIIMS November 2016)

a. Calf claudication
b. Gluteal claudication
c. Impotence
d. Symptomless

Q6. Not included in the treatment of Buerger's disease: (PGI May 2011)

a. Lumbar sympathectomy
b. Endovascular stent
c. Rheostatic agent
d. Extra-anatomical bypass

Q7. All are true about intermittent claudication, *except*: (PGI May 2010)

a. Most common in the calf muscle
b. Pain in the positional
c. Atherosclerosis is an important predisposing factor
d. Relieved by rest

Q8. Which of the following is true about Buerger's disease? (AIIMS November 2012)

a. Atherosclerotic
b. Neural involvement present
c. Ulnar artery and peroneal arteries are involved
d. Only the arteriole is involved

Q9. Which of the following is spared in lumbar sympathectomy? (JIPMER November 2017)

a. L1
b. L2
c. L3
d. L4

Q10. The most common cause of peripheral limb ischemia in India is: (AIIMS Nov 2005)

a. Trauma
b. Atherosclerosis
c. Buerger's disease
d. Takayasu disease

Grade II	Difficult

Q1. Which of the following statements is not true? (AIIMS November 2011)

a. Ankle-brachial index <0.5 indicates critical limb ischemia
b. Ankle-brachial index changes during exercise and rest
c. Ankle-brachial index >1 is normal
d. Smoking is more specific for peripheral vascular disease than coronary artery disease.

Q2. True regarding leg ulcers and their location is/are: (PGI May 2018)

a. Arterial insufficiency—tip of the toes
b. Arterial insufficiency—medial side of leg
c. Venous insufficiency—above medial malleolus
d. Diabetic neuropathic ulcer—plantar aspect of metatarsal head
e. Pressure ulcer—heel

Q3. All are true about arteriovenous fistula, *except*: (PGI November 2017)

a. Trauma is the most common cause of acquired fistula.
b. Congenital fistula is easier to repair by surgery than acquired fistula.
c. Artificial fistula is a surgically created fistula for hemodialysis access.
d. High blood pressure from artery results in arterializations of the vein.
e. A large A-V fistula may cause thrombocytopenia.

Q4. The most common age group affected in thoracic outlet obstruction syndrome is: (DNB 2014)

a. 10–25 years
b. 25–45 years
c. 45–65 years
d. >65 years

Q5. All of the following are true regarding Raynaud's phenomenon, *except*: (AIIMS November 2012)

a. It involves the acral parts of fingers.
b. Migratory thrombophlebitis is seen only in Raynaud's phenomenon.
c. Drugs acting by inhibiting the β receptors in blood vessels also play a role.
d. Emotional stress may also precipitate Raynaud's phenomenon.

Q6. Which of the following is true about celiac plexus block? (AIIMS May 2013)

a. Located retroperitoneally at the level of L3
b. Usually done unilaterally
c. Useful for the painful conditions of the lower abdomen
d. A most common side effect is diarrhea and hypotension

Q7. True about visceral aneurysms: (JIPMER May 2018)

a. Splenic artery is most commonly involved.
b. Hepatic aneurysm is operated on irrespective of symptoms.
c. Splenic artery aneurysm is most commonly followed by trauma.
d. True aneurysms are more common nowadays with increasing abdominal trauma.

Q8. After doing a graft repair of a thoracoabdominal aneurysm, the patients developed weakness. Most probable cause for this: (AIIMS May 2012)

a. Decreased blood supply to the lower limb
b. Thoracosplanchnic injury
c. Discontinuation of arteria radicularis magna
d. Lumbosacral nerve injury

Q9. All of the following are true about aortic aneurysm, *except*: (JIPMER 2013)

a. Saccular aneurysm involves the whole circumference
b. True aneurysm involves all three layers
c. Atherosclerosis is the most common cause
d. False aneurysm is not covered by all three layers.

Q10. Treatment of femoral artery aneurysm: (PGI June 2007)

a. Ultrasound-guided compression of the neck of an aneurysm
b. Thrombin injection
c. Bypass graft repair
d. Ligation of the involved vessel

Grade III	Most difficult

Q1. Oliver's sign is seen in: (JIPMER November 2017)

a. Ascending aortic aneurysm
b. Aortic arch aneurysm
c. Descending aortic aneurysm
d. Aortic dissection

Q2. Most common site of peripheral aneurysm: (MCI June 2018)

a. Femoral artery
b. Radial artery
c. Popliteal artery
d. Brachial artery

Q3. Best graft for aortic dissection: (JIPMER May 2018)

a. Dacron
b. Autologous vein
c. Autologous artery
d. Polytetrafluoroethylene (PTFE)

Q4. Radiological findings of a torn thoracic aorta is/are: (PGI November 2011)

a. Mediastinal widening
b. Abnormal aortic contour
c. Right apical pleural cap
d. Right paratracheal stripe thickening
e. Left apical pleural cap

Q5. Seldinger needle is used for: (MCI March 2010)

a. Suturing muscles
b. Arteriography
c. Pulmonary biopsy
d. Lymphangiography

Q6. Which is not true about femoral artery cannulation? (AIIMS May 2011)

a. The common femoral artery is cannulated.
b. Single-wall puncture is indicated in those with a normal coagulation profile.
c. The femoral artery is catheterized at the medial third of the femoral head.
d. The Seldinger technique is used both for the femoral artery and vein.

Q7. Which of the following is a feature of temporal arteritis? (AIIMS November 2012)

a. Giant cell arteritis
b. Granulomatous vasculitis
c. Necrotizing vasculitis
d. Leukocytoclastic vasculitis

Q8. Which of the following is true about celiac plexus block? (AIIMS May 2013)

a. Located retroperitoneally at the level of L3
b. Usually done unilaterally
c. Useful for the painful conditions of the lower abdomen
d. A most common side effect is diarrhea and hypertension.

Q9. Not a temporary embolization agent is: (JIPMER May 2018)

a. Collagen
b. Gel foam
c. Thrombin
d. Onyx

Q10. Bilateral pulseless disease in upper limbs is caused by: (PGI June 1997)

a. Aortoarteritis
b. Coarctation of the aorta
c. Fibromuscular dysplasia
d. Buerger's disease

ANSWERS

Grade I: 1. a, b, d, e (Sabiston 20/e p1756); 2. a, b, d, e; 3. b; 4. a, c (Harrison 20/e p841); 5. b; 6. b, d (Bailey 27/e p967); 7. b; 8. b (Sabiston 20/e p1780); 9. a (Sabiston 20/e p1780); 10. b

Grade II: 1. d (Schwartz 10/e p881-900); 2. a, c, d, e; 3. b; 4. b; 5. b (Bailey 27/e p967); 6. d; 7. a; 8. c (Sabiston 20/e p1781); 9. a; 10. a, b, and c (Bailey 27/e p966)

Grade III: 1. b; 2. c (Sabiston 20/e p1782); 3. a; 4. a, b, d, e (Chapman 4/e p163-164); 5. b (Bailey 26/e p190); 6. b; 7. a (Harrison 20/e p2583); 8. d; 9. d; 10. a (Schwartz 10/e p788)

MODEL QUESTIONS

Q1. Drug used for Buerger's disease:

a. Xanthinol nicotinate
b. Propranolol
c. GTN
d. All of the above

Ans. a

Q2. True statements of Buerger's disease is/are:

a. Small and medium-sized vessels involved
b. Commonly involves the upper limb than the lower limbs
c. Common in male
d. Common in females

Ans. a and c

Q3. Superficial thrombophlebitis is seen in:

a. Arteriovenous (AV) fistula
b. Raynaud's disease
c. Buerger's disease
d. Aneurysm

Ans. c

Q4. The most common site of thromboangiitis obliterans is:

a. Femoral artery
b. Popliteal artery
c. Iliac artery
d. Pelvic vessels

Ans. None

Q5. The following are used in the treatment of Buerger's disease, *except*:

a. Trental
b. Anticoagulation
c. Sympathectomy
d. Antiplatelets

Ans. b

Q6. Indications for sympathectomy are all, *except*:

a. Intermittent claudication
b. Ischemic pains

c. Rest pain
d. Buerger's disease

Ans. a

Q7. Lumbar sympathectomy is of value in the management of:

a. Intermittent claudication
b. Distal ischemia affecting the skin of the toes
c. Arteriovenous fistula
d. Back pain

Ans. b

Q8. In all of the following, sympathectomy is effective, *except one*:

a. Intermittent claudication
b. Hyperhidrosis
c. Raynaud's disease
d. Causalgia

Ans. a

Q9. Lumbar sympathectomy is not indicated in:

a. Healing of the ulcer over the great toe
b. Claudication
c. Rest pain
d. Buerger's disease

Ans. b

Q10. Which of the following best responds to sympathectomy?

a. Buerger's disease
b. Hyperhidrosis
c. Raynaud's disease
d. Acrocyanosis

Ans. b

SUGGESTED READING

1. Bailey & Love's - Short Practice of Surgery, 27th edition.
2. Schwartz's Principles of Surgery, 18th edition.
3. Textbook of Surgery by David Sabiston, 21st edition.

CHAPTER 51

Venous Disorders

"Love is the blood that flows through my veins."

– Lailah Gifty Akita

INTRODUCTION

The venous system of the lower limb is divided into superficial and deep veins **(Figs. 1A to D)**. Blood is drained from superficial veins and then flows to deep veins through junctions or perforators, and deep veins then take this blood to the right atrium of the heart. Anterior tibial, posterior tibial, and perineal veins formed in leg join popliteal vein in the leg. The popliteal vein goes up through the adductor hiatus in the subsartorial canal as the femoral vein (FV). FV goes further up through the femoral triangle, and while passing behind the inguinal ligament, changes to the external iliac vein. The internal iliac vein combines with the external iliac vein and forms the common iliac vein in the pelvis. Two common iliac veins join to form the inferior vena cava (IVC) and run up on the right to the aorta, ending in the right atrium **(Fig. 2)**.

The venous drainage in the lower limb starts from the dorsal venous arch, which runs in subcutaneous tissue at the level of metatarsals **(Figs. 3A to C)**. The medial end of the arch goes up as the great saphenous vein (GSV), which is the longest vein in the body. GSV passes in front of the medial malleolus and ascends in the leg along with

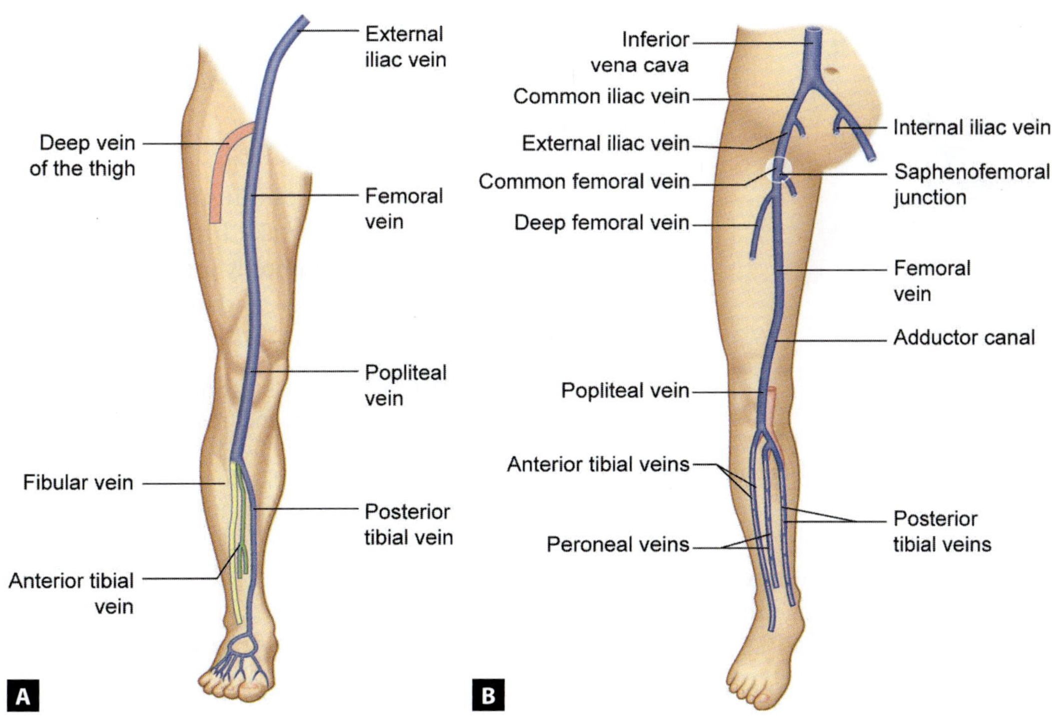

Figs. 1A and B

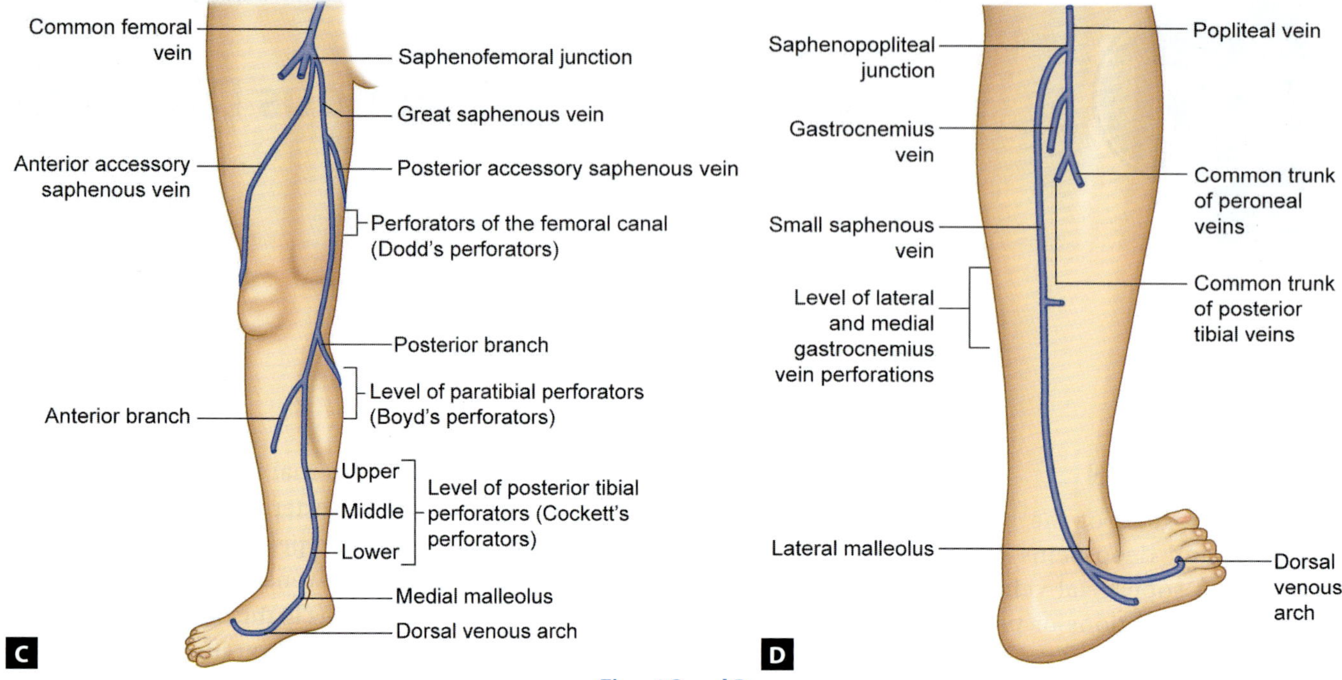

Figs. 1C and D

Figs. 1A to D: Veins of the lower limb.

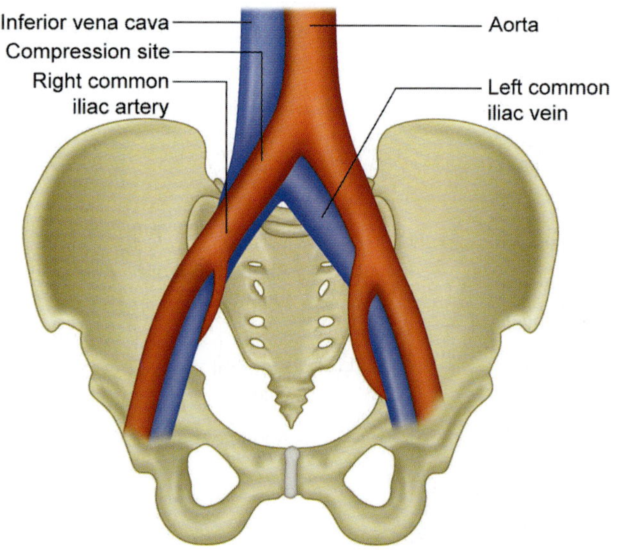

Fig. 2: Internal iliac veins and internal iliac arteries crossing.

the saphenous nerve goes up behind the medial condyle of the femur and runs up on medial side of the thigh and takes a few tributaries before piercing the cribriform fascia to join the common femoral vein (CFV).

The great saphenous vein joins the CFV at the saphenofemoral junction.

The small saphenous vein (SSV) originates from the lateral side of the arch and goes up in leg. It passes behind the lateral malleolus, then runs up in the middle of the leg between the two heads of the gastrocnemius muscle, pierces the fascia at the popliteal fossa, and joins the popliteal vein at the saphenopopliteal junction.

Perforators

There are a few communicating valved vessels called perforators which take blood from superficial to deep veins, they are commonly present at the medial and lateral calf, around the knee, and mid thigh.

> *Points to remember:*
> *Foam sclerotherapy:* USG shows dilated veins, and sclerosing agents are injected by the Tessari method.
> Sodium tetradecyl sulfate is most commonly used for sclerosis.
> In Tessari's method, a foam is created by taking 4 mL of sclerosant in a 10 mL syringe and 16 mL of air in two 10 mL syringes. All are mixed 20 times by opening and closing three-way taps, and the foam is ready.

PATHOPHYSIOLOGY

Blood is pumped out by the heart, and it returns to it after getting oxygenated. 60% of the body's blood lies in veins.

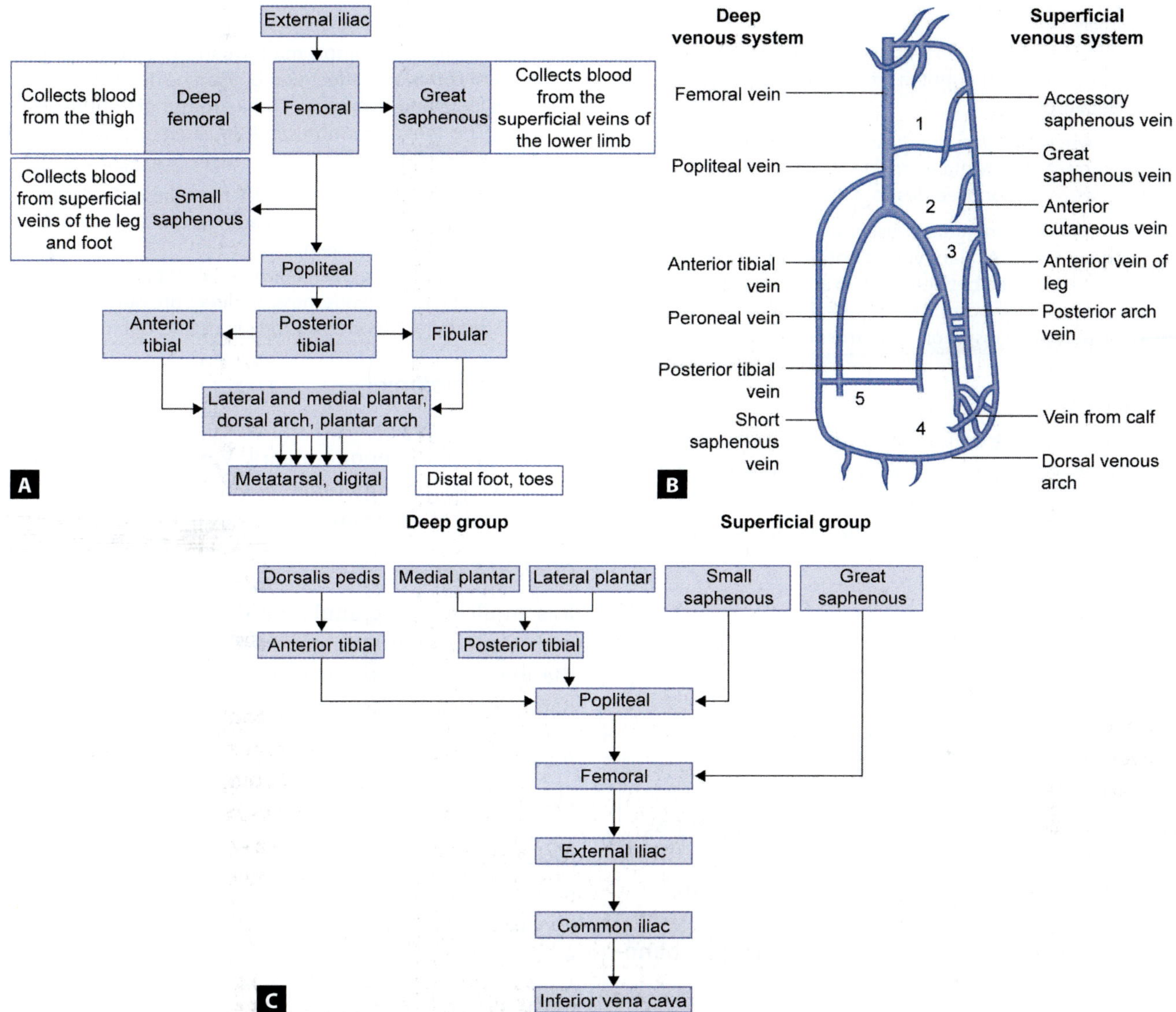

Figs. 3A to C: Veins of the lower limb—venous circulation.

The return of blood to the heart is to run against gravity. So, it has two mechanisms:

1. During inspiration, thorax expands and creates negative pressure which sucks the blood up (pulling effect)
2. The calf muscles contract and pump the blood up (pushing effect). It is called the calf muscle pump and the second heart.

CLINICAL FEATURES OF VENOUS HYPERTENSION

- Varicose veins
- Telangiectasia
- Saphena varicose
- Edema
- Pigmentation
- Venous ulcer
- Eczema
- Lipodermatosclerosis—woody leg

Classification of chronic venous disorders: CEAP classification is based on clinical, etiological, anatomy, and pathophysiological factors.

Varicose Veins

It is commonly found more in women, in middle age, with high body mass index (BMI), increases chances during pregnancy, and in smokers.

Not to forget:

Endovenous laser ablation (EVLA): A laser catheter is placed inside the dilated vein, and the intima with some superficial tissue is destroyed completely.

Radiofrequency ablation (RFA): An electromagnetic coil for passing current is introduced inside the dilated vein and the thermal energy so produced destroys the vein.

Venous entrapment syndrome: It usually occurs with the axillary and popliteal veins. Axillary vein is entrapped at the thoracic outlet and compressed between first rib and the clavicle. Axillary vein thrombosis may occur. The popliteal vein gets entrapped due to the abnormal insertion of gastrocnemius muscle.

Clinical Features

Heaviness, burning sensation, and pain are commonly found, but discoloration and ulcerations develop gradually if treatment is not properly done. Dilated GSV and SSV are seen clearly. They are dilated, elongated, and tortuous veins.

Investigations

Duplex scanning.

Management

- Compression stockings
- Endothermal ablation
- Laser ablation/endovenous laser ablation (EVLA)
- Radiofrequency ablation
- Nonendothermal and nontumescent ablation
- Ultrasound-guided foam sclerotherapy
- Catheter-directed sclerotherapy and mechano-chemical ablation
- Endovenous glue
- *Open surgery*:
  - Saphenofemoral ligation
  - Saphenopopliteal ligation
  - Multiple vein ligation

Complications of Varicose Vein Surgery

- Wound infection
- Hemorrhage
- Nerve injury
- Lymph leak
- Venous thromboembolic problems
- Recurrence

Venous Leg Ulcers

The venous ulcers are common ulcers of the leg, 85% of all leg ulcers.

You may be asked:
- *Venous tumors:* Common malformations and hemangioma are most commonly affect skin but can be deep also.
- Leiomyoma and leiomyosarcoma are tumors of the walls of veins. The most common genetic cause of thrombophilia is factor V Leiden.

The most common site of deep venous thrombosis (DVT) calf:
- The most common site of DVT leading to pulmonary embolism is the femoropopliteal vein.
- The most common presentation of DVT is pain and swelling.
- Moses's sign is calf tenderness on direct pressure on calf.
- Pratt's sign is calf tenderness on squeezing calf from side.

Pathophysiology

The ambulatory venous hypertension is now believed as the cause of venous ulcers. Venous hypertension is due to valve incompetence of GSV or SSV or due to the obstruction of deep veins.

Clinical Features

It is an ulcer with granulation tissue at the base covered with some slough and exudate. These usually occur at the lower area of the leg, posteriorly or laterally, with hemosiderosis or pigmentation surrounding it.

Investigations

Duplex scan.

Management

- Compression
- Superficial venous ablation
- Surgical procedures

VENOUS THROMBOEMBOLISM

It is one of the most common causes of death in surgical cases. It is called superficial venous thromboembolism (SVTE) when superficial veins are affected, and called deep venous thrombosis (DVT) when deep veins are involved.

Etiology

Virchow's triad (Rudolph Virchow, 1821–1902, German pathologist), mentioned over a century is still valuable. It consists of three features:

1. Contact of blood with an abnormal surface (endothelial damage)
2. Abnormal flow (stasis)
3. Abnormal blood (thrombophilia)

There are various causing factors and risk factors, such as obesity, immobility, pregnancy, history of (H/O) DVT, and surgical procedures, but immobility remains the most important factor.

A thrombus is formed due to platelet aggregation, and then red cells and fibrin form a bigger thrombus blocking the lumen of the vein and extending further to a bigger vein, and a part of it gets detached and, with circulation, reaches the lungs, causing pulmonary embolism.

Clinical Features

Pain and swelling of the leg, discoloration (phlegmasia alba dolens and cerulea dolens), stiff calf, pitting edema at ankle, tenderness at the calf, *Homan's (John Homans, 1877–1954, American surgeon) sign*, pyrexia, cyano, dyspnea, etc.

Investigations

The modified Wells criteria is used to predict the chances of DVT. It is based on physical signs. Venous duplex ultrasound is used nowadays, especially by compression, as a vein with DVT will not be well compressed. Ascending venography is not performed today.

PROPHYLAXIS

- Aspirin
- Low-molecular-weight heparin (LMWH) is a very effective good way of prophylaxis, given once a day subcutaneously.
- Graduated elastic compression stockings

TREATMENT

- Low molecular weight heparin (LMWH)
- Thrombolysis
- Thromboembolectomy
- Newer devices disrupting the thrombus and simultaneously doing lysis are told to cause a significant reduction in *post-thrombotic syndrome (PTS).*

Post-thrombotic Syndrome

Perforators:
Most of the perforators are situated on the medial side of the lower limb **(Figs. 4A and B)**:
- *Hunterian or adductor canal perforator:* It connects GSV to FV at midthigh.
- *Dodd or above knee perforator:* It connects GSV to FV
- *Boyd or below knee perforator:* It connects GSV to the proximal thigh (PT)
- *Cockett or lower leg perforator:* It connects the posterior arch vein (a branch of GSV) to the PT.
- Kuster or ankle perforator.

BRITISH CLASSIFICATION OF STOCKINGS

These are divided according to their pressure they apply. Class I is used for prophylaxis, and Class III for treatment. Class I gives 14–17 mm Hg pressure, Class II 18–24, and Class III 25–35 mm Hg.

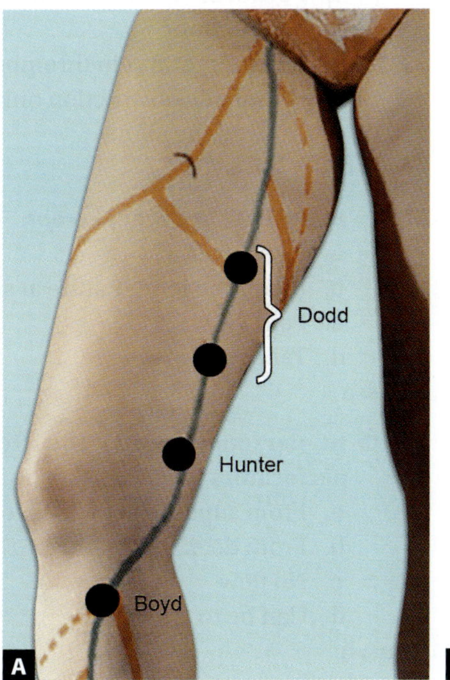

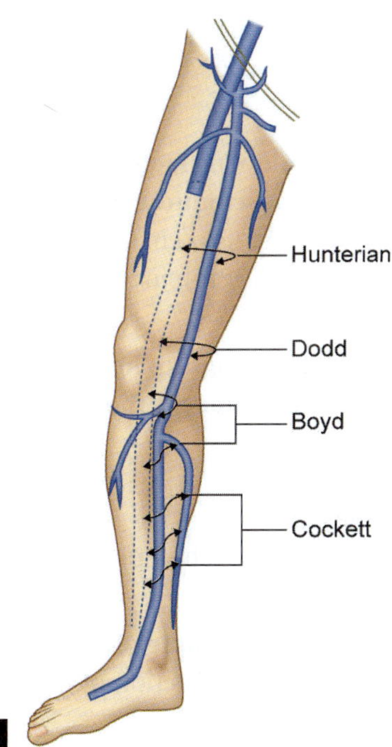

Figs. 4A and B: Various perforators.

BISGAARD METHOD OF VENOUS ULCER TREATMENT

- Keep the leg lifted
- Pus for culture and sensitivity (C&S) test
- Antibiotics according to the culture report
- Four-layer bandage dressing: cotton wool, cotton Elastocrepe bandage, elastic bandage, and cohesive bandage

> *Good to remember:*
> In saphenofemoral junction flush ligation, the all four tributaries are divided and they are:
> 1. Superficial inferior epigastric
> 2. Superficial circumflex iliac
> 3. Deep external pudendal
> 4. Superficial external pudendal
>
> Marjolin's ulcer develops on a venous ulcer.
> *Migratory superficial (Trousseau Sign) thrombophlebitis:* It commonly occurs in a few malignancies:
> - Pancreatic cancer
> - Gastrointestinal malignancies
> - Carcinoma of the lungs.
> - Cancer of the prostate gland
> - Cancer of the ovary
> - Lymphoma

SOME IMPORTANT QUESTIONS

Q1. All of the following disorders are inherited, *except*:
a. Protein S deficiency
b. Antiphospholipid antibody syndrome
c. Protein C deficiency
d. Factor V Leiden mutation

Ans. b

Q2. The deficiency of all the following factors increases the incidence of thrombus formation, *except*:
a. Lipoprotein A
b. Protein C
c. Antithrombin III
d. Protein S

Ans. a

Q3. The patient falls in a high-risk group for deep vein thrombosis (DVT) and pulmonary embolism after:
a. Major burns
b. Major surgery age <40 years
c. Major medical illness/cancer
d. Major orthopedic surgery/fracture pelvis

Ans. c

Q4. TRIVEX is a percutaneous technique of:
a. Intravenous intraluminal destruction of the vein by ablation catheter
b. Intravenous intraluminal injection of a sclerosant like sodium tetradecyl sulfate
c. Removal of vein by suction following injection of fluid
d. Striping of veins

Ans. c

Q5. Cockett and Dodd's operation is for:
a. Saphenofemoral flush ligation
b. Subfascial ligation
c. Deep vein thrombosis
d. Diabetic foot

Ans. b

Q6. Lipodermatosclerosis is most commonly seen at:
a. Anterior aspect of leg
b. Medial aspect of leg
c. Anterior aspect of the thigh
d. Posterior aspect of the thigh

Ans. b

Q7. In CEAP classification for chronic venous disorders, CO stands, CO (zero) for:
a. No signs of venous disease
b. Reticular veins
c. Varicose veins
d. Edema

Ans. a

Q8. White leg is due to:
a. Femoral vein thrombosis and lymphatic obstruction
b. Deep femoral vein thrombosis
c. Lymphatic obstruction only
d. None of the above

Ans. b

Q9. In DVT, all are seen, *except*: (CMC 2001)
a. High fever
b. Increased temperature at site
c. Pain
d. Tenderness

Ans. a

Q10. In varicose veins, the flow in incompetent perforators is:
a. From superficial to deep to
b. From deep to superficial
c. No flow
d. Can be to and for

Ans. b

MULTIPLE CHOICE QUESTIONS

Grade I	*Simple*

Q1. Congenital causes of hypercoagulable states are all, *except*: (AIIMS November 2010)

a. Protein C deficiency
b. Protein S deficiency
c. MTHFR mutation
d. Lupus anticoagulant

Q2. All of the following are acquired causes of hypercoagulability, *except*: (All India 2009)

a. Infection
b. Inflammatory bowel disease
c. Myeloproliferative disorders
d. Prolonged surgery

Q3. Deep vein thrombosis (DVT) prophylaxis is indicated in all, *except*: (PGI May 2011)

a. Abdominal surgery for malignant disease and high-risk patients
b. All patients with age >40 years
c. Patient undergoing major orthopedic surgery
d. Systemic heparin is the only method for DVT prophylaxis
e. 10% of patients with calf vein thrombosis progress to pulmonary embolism

Q4. A patient is admitted with the third episode of Deep venous thrombosis. There is no history of any associated medial illness.
All of the following investigations are required for establishing the diagnosis, *except*: (AIIMS Nov 2004)

a. Protein C deficiency
b. Antithrombin II deficiency
c. Antibodies to factor VIII
d. Antibodies to cardiolipin

Q5. Which of the following is associated with Virchow's triad? (MCI Sept 2005)

a. Hypercoagulability
b. Disseminated malignancy
c. DVT
d. All of the above

Q6. Deep vein thrombosis occurs most commonly after: (AIIMS Feb 1997)

a. Total hip replacement
b. Gastrectomy
c. Prostatic operation
d. Brain surgery

Q7. The most common cause of pulmonary embolism is: (All India 1999)

a. Thrombosis of leg veins
b. Thrombosis of prostatic veins
c. Inferior vena cava (IVC) thrombosis
d. Thrombosis of the internal pudendal artery

Q8. DVT, investigation of choice is: (PGI Dec 1997)

a. Doppler
b. Plethysmography
c. Venography
d. X-ray

Q9. For prophylaxis of deep vein thrombosis used is: (PGI June 1997)

a. Warfarin
b. Heparin
c. Pneumatic shock garment
d. Graded stocking

Q10. The earliest sign of deep vein thrombosis is: (AIIMS 1987)

a. Calf tenderness
b. Rise in temperature
c. Swelling of the calf muscle
d. Homan's sign

Grade II	*Difficult*

Q1. A patient undergoes surgery in the pelvic region. Which vein is most likely to result in thrombosis? (JIPMER November 2017)

a. Iliac vein
b. Femoral vein
c. Calf vein
d. IVC

Q2. The device, whose image is given below, is used for: (AIIMS November 2018)

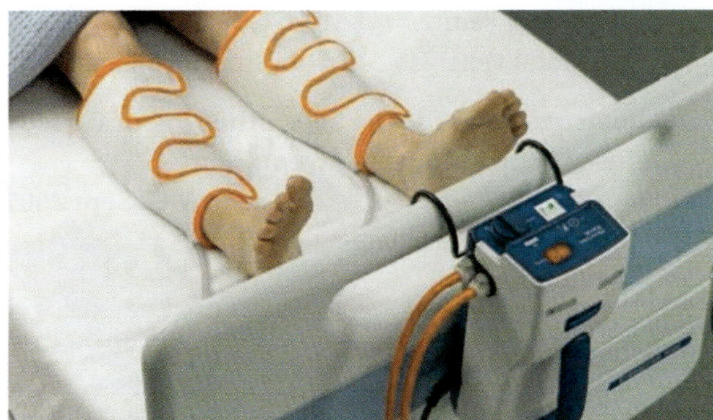

a. Pneumatic compression shocking to prevention of DVT
b. Varicose vein
c. Hypothermia
d. Cellulitis

Q3. True about compression stockings are: (PGI May 2018)
- a. Worn even after the ulcer heals to prevent recurrence
- b. Worn in the morning and taken off at night before bedtime
- c. Compression occurs maximum at the calf
- d. Worn only at edema sites
- e. Provide a calf pump

Q4. "SEPS" is a procedure used for: (All India 2009)
- a. Veins
- b. Arteries
- c. Lymphatics
- d. Arteriovenous (AV) fistula

Q5. The most common complication of varicose vein stripping is: (DPG 2011)
- a. Infection
- b. Hemorrhage
- c. Ecchymosis
- d. Thromboembolism

Q6. True about venous ulcer: (PGI November 2010)
- a. Always stripping is done
- b. Always examine the deep venous system
- c. A biopsy should be taken from a chronic ulcer.
- d. Associated with Klippel–Trenaunay syndrome

Q7. All of the following are seen in deep vein thrombosis, *except*: (All India 1990)
- a. Pain
- b. Discoloration
- c. Swelling
- d. Claudication

Q8. Most common site for venous thrombosis: (JIPMER 1998)
- a. Popliteal vein
- b. Soleal vein
- c. Femoral vein
- d. Internal iliac vein

Q9. The drugs used for the sclerotherapy of varicose veins are the following, *except*: (MCI Sept 2007)
- a. Ethanolamine oleate
- b. Polidocanol
- c. Ethanol
- d. Sodium tetradecyl sulfate

Q10. Most commonly, varicose veins are seen with: (AIIMS June 1999)
- a. Long saphenous vein
- b. Short saphenous vein
- c. Both
- d. Popliteal and femoral vein

Grade III	*Most difficult*

Q1. The patient presents with varicose veins with saphenofemoral incompetence and normal perforators. Management options include all of the following, *except*: (AIIMS November 2012)
- a. Endovascular stripping
- b. Sclerotherapy
- c. Saphenofemoral flush ligament
- d. Saphenofemoral flush ligation with stripping

Q2. Klippel–Trenaunay syndrome associated with all, *except*: (JIPMER November 2017)
- a. Port-wine stain
- b. Varicose veins
- c. Limb lengthening
- d. Fused vertebra

Q3. True about Kasabach syndrome: (PGI November 2009)
- a. May be due to complications of port-wine stain
- b. Coagulopathy occurs
- c. Due to complication of hemangioma
- d. Thrombocytopenia present

Q4. The most common cause of superficial thrombophlebitis is: (All India 2009)
- a. Intravenous catheters/infusion
- b. DVT
- c. Varicose veins
- d. Trauma

Q5. Regarding varicose veins, which one of the following statements is true: (AIIMS Nov 2000)
- a. Over 20% are recurrent varicosities
- b. The sural nerve is in danger during stripping of the long saphenous vein
- c. The saphenous nerve is closely associated with the short saphenous vein
- d. 5% oily phenol is an appropriate sclerosant for venous sclerotherapy

Q6. Surgery in varicose veins is not attempted in the presence of: (AIIMS Nov 1993)
- a. Deep vein thrombosis
- b. Multiple incompetent perforators
- c. Varicose veins with leg ulcer
- d. All of the above

Q7. Which is true regarding the Trendelenburg operation? (PGI Dec 2001)
- a. Stripping of the superficial varicose vein
- b. Flush ligation of the superficial varicose vein
- c. Ligation of the perforators

d. Ligation of small tributaries at the distal end of the superficial varicose vein
e. Ligation of the short saphenous vein

Q8. The first treatment of rupture of varicose veins at the ankle should be: (All India 2004)
a. Rest in the prone position of the patient
b. Application of a tourniquet proximally
c. Application of a tourniquet distally
d. Direct pressure and elevation

Q9. Perforators are not present at: (AIIMS Nov 2007)
a. Ankle
b. Medial calf
c. Distal to calf
d. Below inguinal ligament

Q10. A patient presented with pulsating varicose veins of the lower limb. Most probable diagnosis is: (AIIMS Nov 2001)
a. Klippel-Trenaunay syndrome
b. Tricuspid regurgitation
c. DVT
d. Right ventricular failure

ANSWERS

Grade I: 1. d; 2. None; 3. d (Bailey 27/e p989-990); 4. c. 5. a (Harrison 20/e p1910); 6. a; 7. a; 8. a; 9. b, c, d; 10. a

Grade II: 1. c; 2. a (Bailey 27/e p989); 3. a, b, e (Sabiston 20/e p1843); 4. a; 5. c; 6. b, c, d; 7. d; 8. b; 9. c (Schwartz 10/e p929); 10. a (Bailey 27/e p975)

Grade III: 1. b (Sabiston 20/e p1835); 2. d; 3. b, c, d; 4. a; 5. d; 6. a (Bailey 27/e p976); 7. b (Schwartz 10/e p917-918); 8. d; 9. d (Bailey 26/e p902); 10. a (Schwartz 10/e p1850)

MODEL QUESTIONS

Q1. Venous air embolism is most common in which position in surgery?
a. Sitting
b. Prone
c. Lateral
d. Lithotomy

Ans. a

Q2. May Thurner or Cockett syndrome involve:
a. Common iliac artery obstruction
b. Internal iliac artery obstruction
c. Internal iliac vein obstruction
d. Left iliac vein compression

Ans. d

Q3. Harvey's sign is:
a. Transmitted pressure wave on coughing in a varicose vein
b. Related to the use of venous filling after emptying a length of vein
c. Loss of hair from eyebrows
d. None of the above

Ans. b

Q4. An elderly male has a 0.5 mm dilated tortuous vein in the posterior part of the right calf. What is a stage as per the CEAP classification?
a. C0
b. C1
c. C2
d. C3

Ans. b

Q5. Contraindications for surgery in varicose veins:
a. DVT
b. Multiple incompetent perforators
c. Ulcer at ankle
d. None

Ans. a

Q6. Bisgaard treatment is for:
a. Arterial ulcer
b. Venous ulcer
c. Thromboangiitis obliterans (TAO)
d. Raynaud's phenomenon

Ans. b

Q7. The gold standard diagnostic test in varicose veins is:
a. Photoplethysmography
b. Duplex imaging
c. Ultrasonography
d. Radio-labeled fibrinogen study

Ans. b

Q8. An operated case of varicose veins has a recurrence rate of:

a. About 10%
b. About 25%
c. About 50%
d. Over 60%

Ans. a

Q9. The following is the most common site for a venous ulcer:

a. Instep of foot
b. Lower one-third leg and ankle
c. Lower two-thirds of leg
d. The middle one-third of the leg

Ans. b

Q10. Injection sclerotherapy for varicose veins is performed by using:

a. Phenol
b. Absolute alcohol
c. 70% alcohol
d. Ethanolamine oleate

Ans. a, d

SUGGESTED READING

1. Bailey & Love's - Short Practice of Surgery, 27th edition.
2. Schwartz's Principles of Surgery, 18th edition.
3. Textbook of Surgery by David Sabiston, 21st edition.

CHAPTER 52

Lymphatic Disorders

"Lymph is like a sewage system that carries all of the toxins out of your body."

- Valentina Zelyaeva

INTRODUCTION

The main function of lymphatics is to return back the protein-rich fluid to the circulation via the lymphaticovenous route.

The lymphatic system contains **(Figs. 1 and 2)***:*

- Lymphatic channels
- *Lymphoid organs:* Tonsils, thymus, spleen, Peyer's patches, and lymph nodes (LNs).
- *Circulating elements:* Lymphocytes and other mononuclear immune cells.

Microanatomy and physiology:
- Microanatomy includes various small but significant structures.
- Lymphatic capillaries.
- They originate as endothelialized (initial lymphatics) or nonendothelialized spaces of Disse (Joseph Disse, 1852–1912, German anatomist).
- The initial capillaries are blind-ended, much larger, allow molecules up to 1,000 kDa in size, and they are anchored to an interstitial matrix by filaments.

TERMINAL LYMPHATICS

The initial lymphatics enter terminal (collecting) lymphatics, which have valves, contractile protein action, and are surrounded by muscles. The valves in a lymphatic divide it into segments called "lymphangions."

LYMPH TRUNKS

Terminal lymphatics enter lymph trunks, and about 10% of lymph from a limb is carried by these trunks.

STARLING FORCES

The distribution of fluid and proteins, and other important structures in interstitial fluid (ISF) and vascular compartment depends upon hydrostatic and oncotic pressures [Starling's (Earnest Henry Starling, 1866–1927, British physiologist) forces].

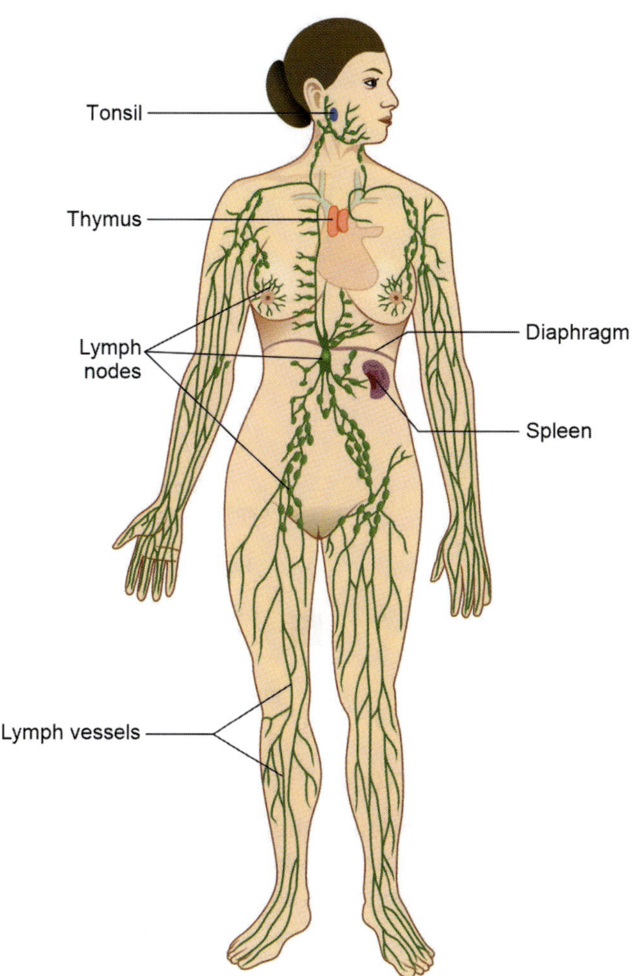

Fig. 1A

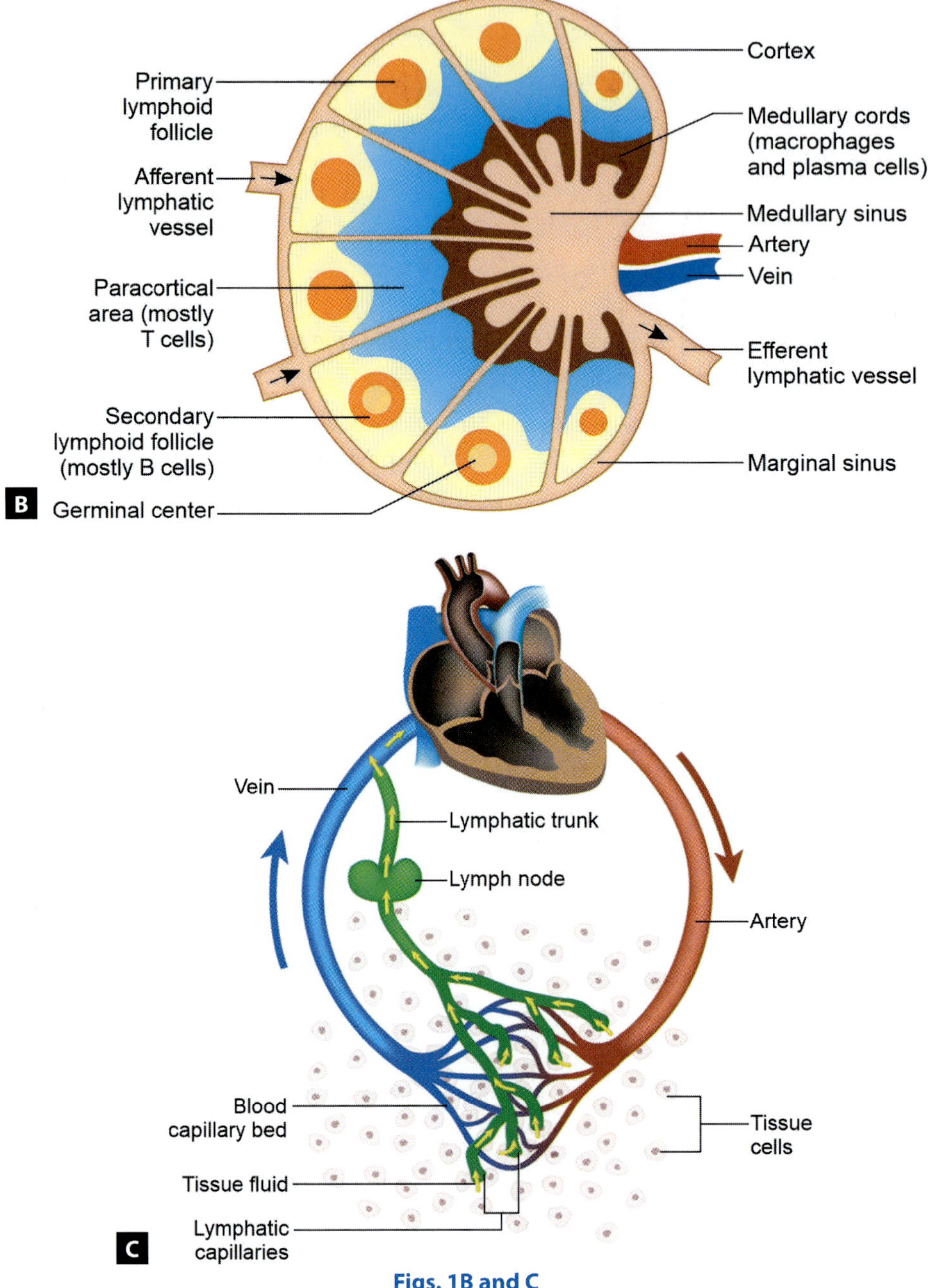

Figs. 1B and C

Figs. 1A to C: Structure of lymph nodes and lymph circulation.

TRANSPORTATION

Particles are transported as they enter through interendothelial spaces or intraendothelial pores, or if large, by phagocytosis by macrophages and travel.

Lymphangions act as a heart, so they respond to increased lymph flow, which depends upon:

- Increase in interstitial pressure by muscular and external compression.

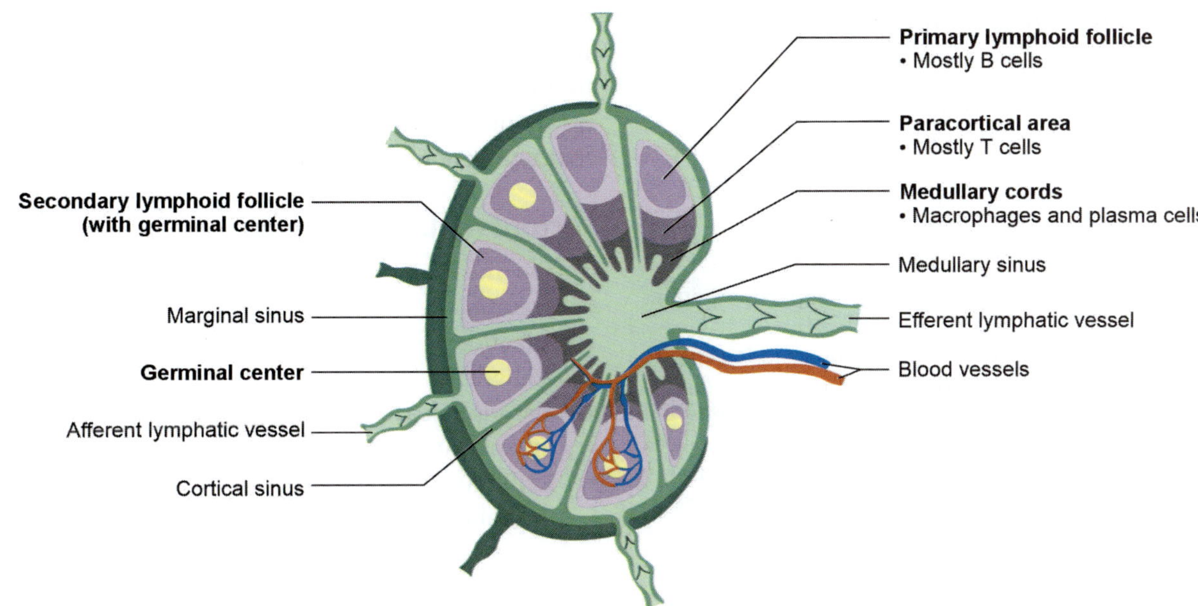

Fig. 2: Structure of a lymph node.

- Contraction and relaxation of lymphangions.
- Prevention of reflux by valves.

LYMPHEDEMA

It is an abnormal limb swelling caused by the accumulation of increased amounts of high-protein ISF secondary to defective lymphatic drainage in the presence of near-normal net capillary filtration.

Symptoms

Swelling, dull ache, cramps, burning and bursting sensations, pins and needles, and skin problems.

Pathophysiology

In a body of 70 kg ISF compartment contains 10–22 L of fluid, which is 50% of the weight of wet skin and subcutaneous tissue. To produce visible lymphedema, it has to be doubled. Our body produces 8 L of lymph each day. Lymphedema is usually caused by lymphatic plasma or hypoplasia and obliteration of lymphatics by inflammation, neoplastic infiltration, or surgical procedures.

Classification of Lymphedema

- *Primary*—unknown—probably congenital lymphatic dysplasia.
- *Secondary or acquired*—underlying causes.

Primary are familial [Nonne–Milroy's (William Forsyth Milroy, 1855–1942, American physician, described in 1892) disease and Letessier–Meige's disease]

Causes of secondary are parasitic and fungal infections, surgery, radiotherapy, malignancy, trauma, and DVT.

Points to remember:
- *Lymphangioma:*
  - Having blisters filled with clear fluid.
  - Long-lasting lymphangioma gets thrombosed and forms nodules, which are called according to local or generalized variety. Lymphangioma circumscribes when localized and big, >2 cm in size, and lymphangioma diffuse if generalized. A lymph discharging lymphangioma is called weeping lymphangioma. Lymphangiomas are capillary or simple lymphangioma and cavernous or cystic lymphangioma. Treatment of lymphangioma is surgical excision.
- *Chyluria:* It is the passage of milky white urine without pain and is commonly seen in filariasis. Ascariasis and malaria may also cause chyluria. A lymphourinary fistula can be identified by intravenous urography (IVU) or lymphangiography. Sclerotherapy or surgical ligation of dilated lymph vessels is required.

Brunner's Grading

- *Subclinical or latent:* Histological disorders present but no clinical signs.
- *Grade I*: Pitting edema
- *Grade II*: No pitting edema
- *Grade III*: Edema with irreversible skin changes

Risk Factors for Lymphedema

Upper Limb and Trunk

- Surgical procedures as axillary LN dissection
- Radiotherapy
- Obesity
- *Others:* Trauma, chronic skin disease, etc.

> *Not to forget:*
> - *P 5 signs of acute limb ischemia:* Pain, pallor, paralysis, pulselessness, and paresthesia
> - *Trophic ulcer:* It is an ulcer commonly found in leg due to poor blood flow, poor nutrition, and poor nerve supply (neurological deficit). It is caused commonly by diabetes but neuritis, syphilis, and leprosy can also cause. It is usually caused by immobility and develops on pressure points as bedsores. Stemmer's pinch sign—subcutaneous tissue in lymphedema cannot be pinched.

Lower Limb

- All as in upper limb plus
- Malignancy and poor nutrition

Malignancies Associated with Lymphedema

Malignancies associated with lymphedema are lymphangiosarcoma, Kaposi's sarcoma, squamous cell carcinoma (SCC), liposarcoma, malignant melanoma, malignant fibrous histiosarcoma, basal cell carcinoma (BCC), and lymphoma.

> **Primary Lymphedema**
> - It is mostly congenital, as congenital lymphatic dysplasia, but can occur due to other causes, with almost normally developed lymphatics.
> - In primary lymphedema, genetic mutation can be inherited as an autosomal dominant, recessive, or c-linked pattern. *Milroy's disease as a congenital unilateral lymphedema has mutations in FMS-like tyrosine kinase 4 (FLT4) or vascular endothelial growth factor C (VEGF-C).*
>
> *Age at which it occurs:*
> - Lymphedema congenita—within 2 years of birth.
> - Lymphedema praecox—2–35 years of age.
> - Lymphedema tarda—after 35 years of age.

Browse (Sir Norman Leslie Browse, 1931, British surgeon) has given a lymphangiographic classification of primary lymphedema into congenital hyperplasia (10%), distal obliteration (80%), and proximal obliteration (10%).

In congenital hyperplasia, lymphatics are increased in numbers, and also LNs, chloasma, and chylous ascites are present. In distal obliteration, superficial lymphatics are reduced or absent. In proximal obliteration, there is obstruction at the level of the aortoiliac or inguinal LNs.

Secondary Lymphedema

It is the most common type of lymphedema. Its causes are:

- Trauma
- Infection
- Malignancy
- Venous disease
- Inflammation
- Endocrine/myxedema
- Immobility

> **FILARIASIS**
>
> *It is the most common cause of lymphedema all over the world. Wuchereria bancrofti nematode has man as the only host. It is responsible for 90% of cases.* It spreads by mosquito. Parasite enters blood and settles in lymph nodes. Immature parasites called microfilariae enter blood at night and so can be detected in peripheral blood smears. Diethylcarbamazine destroys the parasites.

Clinical Features

- Acute fever, headache, inguinal and axillary lymphadenitis, lymphatics, and epididymoorchitis.
- Chronic lymphedema legs, hydrocele, chyluria, etc.

Investigations of Lymphedema

- *General*: Complete blood count (CBC), liver function test (LFT), renal function test (RFT), and blood smears at night
- Lymphangiography
- Lymphoscintigraphy
- CT
- Magnetic resonance imaging (MRI)
- USG
- Lymphofluoroscopy

> *You may be asked:*
> - *Multilayer lymphedema bandaging (MLLB):* It is advised for lymphedema but it is contraindicated in severe arterial insufficiency, uncontrolled heart failure, and severe peripheral neuropathy.

MLLB works as:
- Reduces edema
- Restores the shape of the area affected
- Reduces skin changes
- Eliminates lymphorrhea
- Supports skin
- Softens subcutaneous tissue

Management

- General care
- Pain relief
- Care of skin
- Lymph drainage
- Compression garments
- Exercise
- Drugs
- *Surgery:*
  - Bypass procedures
  - Liposuction
  - Limb reduction procedures
  - *Sistrunk (Walter Ellis Sistrunk, 1880–1933, American surgeon):* A wedge of skin and subcutaneous tissue is excised, and the wound is sutured.
  - *Homans Thompson (John Homans, 1877–1957, American surgeon/Frederick Thompson, 1910–1975, British plastic surgeon):* It is a modification of Homan's procedure to increase the connection between superficial and deep systems.
  - *Charles (Sir Richard Havelock Charles, 1858–1934, British surgeon):* Removal of skin and subcutaneous tissue, and then split skin grafts applied.

Good to remember:
Endemic elephantiasis: It is also called podoconiosis, commonly seen in tropical regions specifically in Africa, barefoot cultivation leads this as silica in soil damages foot lymphatics. Silica particles can be seen in macrophages of inguinal LNs. It can be prevented by wearing shoes.

SOME IMPORTANT QUESTIONS

Q1. Which of the following is not an operation for congenital lymphedema?
a. Homan's operation
b. Charles' operation
c. De Quervain's cross red operation
d. Sistrunk's operation

Ans. c

Q2. In Neibulowitz surgery, what is done?
a. Skin bridge
b. Lymph node with vein anastomosis
c. Ileal mucosal patch
d. All of the above

Ans. b

Q3. The most common type of primary lymphedema is:
a. Lymphedema congenital
b. Lymphedema precox
c. Lymphedema tarda
d. None

Ans. b

Q4. In India, what is the most common cause of unilateral lymphedema of the lower limb?
a. Lymphedema tarda
b. Carcinoma of penis with metastatic nodes
c. Filariasis
d. Tubercular lymphadenopathy

Ans. c

Q5. The most common bacterial infection in lymphedema is:
a. *Staphylococcus*
b. *Streptococcus*
c. *Escherichia coli*
d. *Pseudomonas*

Ans. a

Q6. Popcorn type of Reed–Sternberg cell is seen in the following type of Hodgkin's lymphoma:
a. Lymphocyte rich
b. Mixed cellularity
c. Lymphocyte predominance
d. Lymphocyte depletion

Ans. c

MULTIPLE CHOICE QUESTIONS

Grade I	*Simple*

Q1. True about primary lymphedema:
(PGI November 2010)
a. Lymphangiosarcoma may occur.
b. Associated with Milroy's disease
c. Onset between 2 and 35 years indicates lymphedema tarda
d. Onset >35 years indicates the praecox variety
e. Prevalence is 2%

Q2. All are true about congenital lymphedema, *except*: (All India 1991)

a. It is bilateral
b. Involve lower limb
c. Almost always manifests before puberty
d. Acute lymphangitis may occur

Q3. True about primary lymphedema: (PGI November 2010)

a. Prevalence is 2%
b. Onset between 2 and 35 years indicates lymphedema tarda
c. Onset >35 years indicates praecox type
d. Associated with Milroy's disease
e. Lymphangiosarcoma may occur

Q4. Milroy's disease is: (JIPMER 1992)

a. Edema due to filariasis
b. Postcellulitic lymphedema
c. Congenital lymphedema
d. Lymphedema following surgery

Q5. The most common cause of unilateral pedal edema in India is: (All India 1990)

a. Filariasis
b. Post-traumatic
c. Postirradiation
d. Milroy's disease

Q6. The commonest cause for lymphedema of the upper limb is: (All India 1992)

a. Filariasis
b. Congenital
c. Neck surgery
d. Postmastectomy irradiation

Grade II — Difficult

Q1. Hydrocele and edema in food occur in: (PGI November 2011)

a. *Wuchereria bancrofti*
b. *Brugia malayi*
c. *Brugia timori*
d. *Onchocerca volvulus*
e. Guinea worm

Q2. Chronic lymphedema of the limb predisposes to all of the following, *except*: (All India 2004)

a. Thickening of the skin
b. Recurrent soft-tissue infections
c. Marjolin's ulcer
d. Sarcoma

Q3. A 45-year-old man presents with progressive cervical lymph nodes enlargement, since 3 months; the most diagnostic investigation is: (All India 2001)

a. X-ray soft tissue
b. Fine-needle aspiration cytology (FNAC)
c. Lymph node biopsy
d. None of the above

Q4. Grade I lymphedema means: (JIPMER 2000)

a. Pitting edema up to the ankle
b. Pitting edema up to the knee
c. Nonpitting edema
d. Edema disappears after overnight rest

Q5. The most common presentation of Hodgkin's lymphoma is: (All India 1999)

a. Painless enlargement of lymph node
b. Pruritus
c. Fever
d. Leukocytosis

Q6. The most common site of enlargement of the lymph nodes in Hodgkin's lymphoma is: (All India 1995)

a. Mediastinal
b. Axillary
c. Cervical
d. Abdominal

Grade III — Most difficult

Q1. True statement regarding lymphedema is: (PGI May 2018)

a. Can be complicated by cellulitis
b. A familial version of congenital lymphedema is known as Milroy's disease.
c. Commonly caused by *W. bancrofti*
d. Lymphedema congenital is more likely to be unilateral
e. Lymphedema precox is more common in males.

Q2. Carcinoma in which surgery is rarely indicated: (PGI November 2009)

a. Osteosarcoma
b. Wilms' tumor
c. Neuroblastoma
d. Rhabdomyosarcoma
e. Hodgkin's lymphoma

Q3. Lymphovenous anastomosis is done for: (PGI December 1997)

a. Filarial lymphedema
b. Lymphoid cyst
c. Cystic hygroma
d. Malignant lymphedema

Q4. True about lymphangioma: (PGI June 2003)
a. It is a malignant tumor.
b. It is a congenital sequestration of lymphatic.
c. Laser excision is done
d. Sclerotherapy is commonly done

Q5. Investigation of choice in detecting small para-aortic lymph node is: (JIPMER 1992)
a. Ultrasound scan
b. CT scan
c. Lymphangiography
d. Arteriography

Q6. Treatment of acute lymphangitis requires: (JIPMER 1981)
a. Antibiotic and rest
b. Immediate lymphangiography
c. Immediate multiple incisions
d. No special treatment

ANSWERS

Grade I: 1. a, b, e; 2. None (Schwartz 10/e p934); 3. d (Sabiston 20/e p1845-50); 4. c (Bailey 27/e p998); 5. a (Bailey 27/e p1003); 6. a (Bailey 27/e p909)

Grade II: 1. a, b, c; 2. c; 3. c (Harrison 19/e p409); 4. d (Bailey 27/e p998); 5. a (Bailey 27/e p741); 6. a (Harrison 19/e p708)

Grade III: 1. a, b, c; 2. e; 3. a (Bailey 27/e p1011); 4. b (Bailey 27/e p999); 5. b (Sutton's Radiology 7/e p515); 6. a (Bailey 27/e p998)

MODEL QUESTIONS

Q1. The most common type of primary lymphoma is:
a. Lymphedema of lymphoma
b. Lymphedema praecox
c. Lymphedema tarda
d. Lymphangioma

Ans. b

Q2. Lymphedema precox all are true, *except:*
a. One sided
b. More common in men
c. Affects the legs
d. 2–35 years of age

Ans. b

Q3. Lymphangiosarcoma occurs in:
a. Filarial edema
b. Lymphedema
c. Lymphoma
d. Millroy's disease

Ans. b

Q4. The common site of lymphangiosarcoma is:
a. Liver
b. Spleen
c. Postmastectomy edema of the arm
d. Retroperitoneum

Ans. c

Q5. Lymph drainage is increased from the lower limbs by:
a. Massaging b. Standing
c. Aerobics d. Sleeping

Ans. a

Q6. Stemmer's sign is seen in:
a. Lymphedema b. Venous disease
c. Factitious lymphedema d. Arterial disease

Ans. a

SUGGESTED READING

1. Bailey & Love's - Short Practice of Surgery, 27th edition.
2. Harrison's Principles of Internal Medicine, 15th edition.
3. Schwartz's Principles of Surgery, 18th edition.
4. Textbook of Surgery by David Sabiston, 21st edition.

Thorax and Lungs

"As long as there's breath in our lungs, our story is still being written."

– Bart Millard

CHEST WALL DEFORMITIES

Pectus Excavatum

- It is also called funnel chest.
- It is the most common chest deformity.
- Males are more affected than females.
- 1 in 400 births.
- It is due to the excessive growth of the lower costal cartilages.
- There is a displacement of mediastinal strictures due to a depressed sternum.
- Clinically, there are no symptoms in most of cases, but others show respiratory symptoms.

Investigations

Pulmonary function test (PFT)/echocardiogram (ECHO)/ computed tomography (CT) chest/Haller index ratio of the width of the chest wall and the distance between the sternum and the vertebral column.

Treatment

2–8 years of age, Revitech operation, open procedure, NUSS procedure (Minimal invasive problem).

PECTUS CARINATUM

- It is also called pigeon chest as the prominence of the chest looks like the back of a parrot.
- The upper chest is projected out.
- Common in males
- Usually asymptomatic
- May be associated with mitral valve disorders and coarctation of the aorta.

Treatment

Surgery is usually done due to cosmetic reasons.

MEDIASTINUM

The mediastinum is the space between the two lungs, and it has three parts:

1. Anterior mediastinum—anterior to the pericardium and trachea
2. Middle mediastinum—pericardium and trachea
3. Posterior mediastinum—posterior to the pericardium and trachea

Lumps of Mediastinum

- Anterior mediastinum—thymoma + GALT (Germ cell tumor, aneurysm, lymphoma, thyroid lesion).
- Middle mediastinum—cysts (pericardial and bronchogenic) + *MAL* (Mesenchymal tumor, aneurysm, lymphoma)
- *Posterior mediastinum—Mn-BELM*

Neurogenic tumors + BELM (Bochdalek hernia, enterogenic cyst, lymphoma, and mesenchymal cyst).

Common Mediastinal Tumors in Children

- Germ cell tumors
- Neurogenic tumors
- Lymphomas
- Cysts

THYMOMA

- It is a neoplasm of the thymus gland.
- It is of three types: (1) *Mn-LEL* (Lymphocyte 25%, (2) epithelial 25%, and (3) lymphoepithelial 50%)

- It is usually asymptomatic.
- If symptomatic, then *Mn-DDS* [Dyspnea/Dysphagia/Syndromes (Superior vena cava syndrome/Para neoplastic syndrome)]; *Mn-HAN* (Hematological—cytopenia, Autoimmune—SLE, Neuromuscular—myasthenia gravis)

Investigation

Computed tomography scan.

Staging—Masaoka (A Masaoka, Japanese Doctor, Given in 1981) Staging

- *Ia*—completely capsulated.
- *IIa*—microscopic invasion of capsule.
- *IIb*—macroscopic invasion of capsule.
- *III*—macroscopic invasion of adjacent structure.
- *IVa*—pleural and pericardial implants.
- *IVb*—lymphatic and hematogenous metastasis.

PLEURAL EFFUSION

- The pleural cavity contains a serous fluid, also at 10–20 mL/kg of body weight, which is produced by the parietal pleura.
- At least 500 mL of fluid in the pleural cavity is required to be diagnosed clinically, though 300 mL of pleural fluid is sufficient to demonstrate blunting of the costophrenic angle on erect X-ray.

Causes of Pleural Effusion

- Exudate—(Due to inflammation)—due to local factors causing increased formation of flow or reduced absorption (total serum protein <3 g/dL and pleural fluid protein/serum protein <0.5)
- Transudate—(Due to pressure filtration)—due to systemic factors (total serum protein >3 g/dL and pleural fluid protein/serum protein >0.5)

Treatment

Intracostal tube drainage through the fifth intercostal space (fourth to sixth) through the triangle of safety (Lateral border of pectoralis major, anterior border of latissimus dorsi, and superior border of the sixth rib).

PNEUMOTHORAX

- Pressure of air in the pleural cavity.
- *Types*:
    - Closed pneumothorax (spontaneous pneumothorax)
        - Primary pneumothorax
        - Secondary pneumothorax
    - Open pneumothorax

Primary Spontaneous Pneumothorax

- It is due to rupture of the subpleural bulla without any lung disease.
- It is common in male smokers.
- It occurs suddenly with pain in the chest and dyspnea.

Investigation

Plain X-ray chest and noncontrast computed tomography (NCCT) chest.

Treatment

Treatment is by needle aspiration, and if recurrent, then endoscopic bleb resection and pleurodesis.

Secondary Spontaneous Pneumothorax

- There is an underlying lung disease, such as chronic obstructive pulmonary disease (COPD)/asthma.
- More severe presentation than primary spontaneous pneumothorax (PSP).

Treatment

The treatment includes intercostal drainage (ICD).

Open Pneumothorax

- Sucking chest wound.
- Open wound on chest wall.
- Air is sucked in the pleural cavity causing dyspnea and hypoxia.

Treatment

- Closure of the wound.
- ICD—away from the wound.

Tension Pneumothorax

- When one way valve develops either from the lung to the pleural cavity or from outside to the pleural cavity.
- Pneumothorax causes collapse of the same side of the lung with displacement of the mediastinum, compressing the other lung.

Causes

- Trauma
- Penetrating
- Blunt
- While doing subclavian vein puncture, the lung is punctured.

Clinical Features

Sudden tachypnea, dyspnea, and hyperresonant chest.

Investigation

X-ray

Treatment

First needle puncture with a No 16 needle of the second ICS in the midclavicular line with ICD.

ACUTE RESPIRATORY DISTRESS SYNDROME

- Sudden severe dyspnea, hypoxia, and respiratory failure
- Cause—diffuse lung injury causing diffuse alveolar damage.
- It may be direct lung injury, like—PAP (pulmonary contusion, aspiration, and pneumonia), or indirect lung injury—SBS (Severe trauma, burns, sepsis).
- Clinical course occurs in three phases. *Exudating phase* (edema), *proliferative phase* (Proliferation of Type II pneumocytes), and *fibrotic phase* (long-term healing with fibrosis).

Treatment

- Mechanical ventilation with fluid and electrolyte control.
- *5Ps:* (*P*erfusion/*p*ositioning/*p*rotective lung ventilation/*p*rotocol weaning/*p*reventing complications.

CARCINOMA LUNG

- It is also called bronchogenic carcinoma.
- It originates from the epithelium of alveoli, bronchioles, and bronchi.

Causes

Mn: RAISE

- *S:* Smoking
- *A:* Air pollution
- *E:* Exposure to asbestos and uranium, etc.
- *I:* Scars of the lung due to old injury or infarcts.
- *R:* Radiation exposure

Types

Small Cell Carcinoma

Due to overexpression of:

Mn = Mycobacterium tuberculosis

- *M*—myc
- *B*—bcl-2
- *T*—Tumorigenesis

Nonsmall Cell Carcinoma

Due to overexpression of:

Mn = Kox TB

- *B*—bcl-2
- *T*—telomerase
- *K*—K-ras mutation is most common mutation (90%)

Clinical Features

- Cough, wheeze, stridor, and dyspnea.
- Hemoptysis
- Pain due to involvement of the pleura or chest wall.
- *Features due to metastasis:* Mn = HERPS [Horner's syndrome/Pancoast syndrome/SVC syndrome (most common)/RLN paralysis/Malignant pleural effusion]
- Metastasis to Mn = B2L2AKE (Brain/Bone/Lung/Liver/Adrenal/Kidney/Esophagus)

Diagnosis

- Biopsy—Bronchoscopic
- Positron emission tomography (PET)/CT

8th American Joint Committee on Cancer (2017) TNM Classification of Lung Cancer

- *Tis:* Carcinoma in situ
- *T1a:* Tumor ≤1 cm
- *T1b:* Tumor >1 cm
- *T1c:* Tuor >2 cm
- T2*:* Tumor >3 cm
- *T2a:* Tumor >3 cm but ≤4 cm in greatest dimension
- *T2b:* Tumor >4 cm but ≤5 cm in greatest dimension
- *T3:* Tumor >5 cm but ≤7 cm in greatest dimension

- *T4:* Tumor >7 cm or of any size that invades the surrounding stricture.
- *N1:* Metastasis in ipsilateral peribronchial and/or ipsilateral hilar lymph nodes.
- *N2:* Metastasis in ipsilateral mediastinal and/or subcranial lymph nodes.
- *N3:* Metastasis in contralateral mediastinal, contralateral hilar, ipsilateral or contralateral scalene, or supraclavicular lymph nodes.
- *M1a:* Separate tumor nodule(s) in a contralateral lobe.
- *M1b:* Single extrathoracic metastasis in a single or multiple organs **(Tables 1 and 2)**.

TABLE 1: 8th American Joint Committee on Cancer (AJCC) (2017) TNM stage groupings.

Stage	*T*	*N*	*M*
Occult cancer	TX	N0	M0
0	Tis	N0	M0
IA	T1	N0	M0
IA1	T1mi-T1a	N0	M0
IA2	T1b	N0	M0
IA3	T1c	N0	M0
IB	T2a	N0	M0
IIA	T2b	N0	M0
IIB	T1a-c, T2a-b	N1	M0
	T3	N0	
IIIA	T1a-c, T2a-b	N2	M0
	T3	N1	
	T4	N0-1	
IIIB	T1a-c, T2a-b	N3	M0
	T3, T4	N2	
IIIC	T3, T4	N3	M0
IVA	Any T	Any N	M1a/b
IVB	Any T	Any N	M1c

- *M1c:* Multiple extrathoracic metastasis in single or multiple organs.

Not to forget:

- *Chylothorax:*
  - Chyle is stored in the pleural cavity due to thoracic duct damage, i.e., trauma
  - Mostly on the right side with pain and dyspnea
- *Investigation*—Chest X-ray
- *Treatment:*
  - Octreotide administration
  - Ligation of the thoracic duct if injured

HEMOTHORAX

- Presence of blood in the pleural cavity.
- *Cause*: Mn-TTT (Trauma/Tumor/Tuberculosis).
- *Investigation:* X-ray chest—needle aspiration
- *Treatment*: ICD (Supine position is better than erect) position, as the domes of the diaphragm or thoracotomy can conceal 0.5 L of blood).

When to do a thoracotomy?

If ICD is >1 L in penetrating injury of the chest and >1.5 L in blind injury, and then if >200 mL/h × 3–4 hours.

You may be asked about

- Thoracic duct injury (TDI)
- *Causes*: Trauma [Accidental/iatrogenic (most common) during thoracic operation]
- *Clinical feature:* Chylothorax and chyle from the drain.
- TDI leads to Mn = DIL (Dehydration/Immunity reduction/Loss of protein and electrolytes)
- *Treatment:* Video-assisted thoracoscopic surgical ligation of the thoracic duct.
- Poirier's triangle is between the arch of the aorta, the left subclavian artery, and the vertebral column. The thoracic duct travels through this triangle.

TABLE 2: WHO classification of lung carcinoma.

Adenocarcinoma	*Squamous cell carcinoma*	*Small cell carcinoma*	*Large cell carcinoma*
• MC histological type • MC in nonsmokers, young patients, females • Located peripherally • Slow growth • Metastasize more frequently to the CNS	• MC in smokers • MC type in India • Central in distribution • Associated with the best prognosis	• Most malignant, strongly related to smoking • Associated with massive hilar, mediastinal lymphadenopathy • MC variety associated with paraneoplastic syndrome	• Highly undifferentiated with cavitating nature • Metastasize early with a poor prognosis

(CNS: central nervous system; MC: most common; WHO: World Health Organization)

Q8. The most common symptom of carcinoma bronchus is:

a. Hemoptysis b. Dyspnea
c. Cough d. Wheezing
e. Pain

Ans. c

Q9. Hoarseness secondary to bronchogenic carcinoma is usually due to extension of the tumor into:

a. Vocal cord
b. Superior laryngeal nerve
c. Left recurrent laryngeal nerve
d. Right vagus nerve

Ans. c

Q10. In small cell carcinoma of the lung, one of the following is not seen:

a. Hypercalcemia b. Hyponatremia
c. Watery diarrhea d. Hypokalemia

Ans. c

Q11. Clinical manifestations of bronchogenic carcinoma include the following, *except*:

a. Hoarseness of voice due to involvement of left recurrent laryngeal nerve
b. Horner's syndrome
c. Diaphragmatic palsy due to infiltration of the phrenic nerve
d. Gastroparesis due to vagal involvement

Ans. d

Q12. A 60-year-old male was diagnosed with carcinoma right lung. On contrast-enhanced computed tomography (CECT) chest, there was a tumor of 5 × 5 cm in the upper lobe and another 2 × 2 cm size tumor nodule in the middle lobe. The primary modality of treatment is:

a. Radiotherapy
b. Chemotherapy
c. Surgery
d. Supportive treatment

Ans. c

Q13. The lung tumor responding best to radiotherapy:

a. Small cell anaplastic
b. Squamous cell cancer (CA)
c. Adeno CA
d. All respond equally well

Ans. a

Q14. The first step when doing a pneumonectomy for cancer of the bronchus is to:

a. Ligate the pulmonary vein
b. Ligate the pulmonary artery
c. Divide the bronchus
d. Perform lymph node clearance

Ans. b

Q15. Structures pierced during pleural tapping are:

a. Endothoracic fascia
b. Pulmonary pleura
c. Skin
d. Intercoastal muscle

Ans. b

MULTIPLE CHOICE QUESTIONS

Grade I | ***Simple***

Q1. In thymoma, all are seen, *except*: **(AIIMS June 2001)**

a. Hypogammaglobulinemia
b. Hyperalbuminemia
c. Red cell aplasia
d. Myasthenia gravis

Q2. Not a posterior mediastinal tumor: **(AIIMS Nov 1998)**

a. Neurofibroma b. Lymphoma
c. Thymoma d. Gastroenteric cyst

Q3. Anterior mediastinal tumors are: **(PGI June 2004)**

a. Thymoma b. Aortic aneurysm
c. Bronchogenic cyst d. Lymphoma
e. Bochdalek hernia

Q4. Posterior mediastinal tumors: **(PGI June 2003)**

a. Neuroblastoma
b. Bronchogenic cyst
c. Neuroenteric cyst
d. Lymphoma
e. Anterior thoracic meningioma

Q5. The majority of lung cysts occur in: **(AIIMS Nov 1994)**

a. Mediastinum
b. Near Carina
c. Base of the lung
d. Peribronchial tissue

Q6. Which tumor among the following is not found in the anterior mediastinum: (AIIMS Nov 1995)
a. Retrosternal goiter b. Thymoma
c. Teratomatous mass d. Neurogenic tumor

Q7. The most common anterior mediastinum tumor is: (AIIMS Nov 1998)
a. Thymoma b. Neurogenic fibroma
c. Lymphoma d. Meningocele

Q8. The most common tumor in the posterior mediastinum is: (All India 2008)
a. Neurofibroma b. Teratoma
c. Lymphoma d. Bronchogenic cyst

Q9. Most common site for putting chest drain in case of pleural effusion: (AIIMS June 2000)
a. Second intercostal space midclavicular line
b. Seventh intercostal space midaxillary line
c. Fifth intercostal space midclavicular line
d. Fifth IC space just lateral to the vertebral column

Q10. A 44-year-old male underwent video-assisted thoracic surgery (VATS) thymectomy for Myasthenia gravis. During surgery, the pleura was accidentally injured. The surgeon decided to put a drain in the pleural cavity. Which of these statements is correct about the timing of the removal of an intercostal chest tube? (AIIMS Nov 2016)
a. After partial expansion of lungs and <50 mL output from the drain for 2 consecutive days.
b. After complete expansion of lungs and <30 mL output from the drain for 2 consecutive days.
c. On the fourth day, irrespective of the output from the drain and lung expansion
d. After complete expansion of lungs and <200 mL from the drain for 2 consecutive days.

Q11. Complications of empyema are: (PGI Dec 1999)
a. Empyema necessitans
b. Bronchopleural fistula
c. Osteomyelitis
d. Pneumonia

Q12. The ideal treatment for hemothorax of blood loss >500 mL/h: (PGI June 1999)
a. Wait and watch
b. Needle aspiration
c. Intercostal tube
d. Open thoracotomy with ligation of a vessel

Q13. About hemothorax. (PGI Dec 2002)
a. Seen in choriocarcinoma
b. Supine posture is better than erect posture
c. Needle aspiration may be needed for diagnosis
d. Thoracotomy is always done

Q14. Excessive bleeding during hemothorax is usually caused by: (AIIMS June 1994)
a. Vena cava
b. Internal mammary artery
c. Heart
d. Major artery

Q15. For open pneumothorax, which of the following is M/n of choice? (AIIMS June 1997)
a. Intermittent positive pressure ventilation (IPPV)
b. Intercostal drain (ICD) with underwater seal
c. Thoracostomy and close the rent
d. Wait and watch

Grade II	*Difficult*

Q1. A case of spontaneous pneumothorax comes to you. What will be the earliest treatment of choice? (AIIMS June 1997)
a. IPPV b. Needle aspiration
c. ICD d. Wait and watch

Q2. Spontaneous pneumothorax exceeding ..... % of chest cavity should have a chest tube inserted: (AIIMS 1984)
a. 10 b. 25
c. 45 d. 60

Q3. A patient after a road traffic accident presents with respiratory distress, hypotension, and dilated, bulging neck veins. On examination, absent breath sounds and contralateral tracheal shift is found. What would be the first line of management? (AIIMS Nov 2018)
a. Emergency thoracotomy
b. Immediate chest X-ray
c. CT scan
d. Insert a wide-bore needle in the second intercostal space

Q4. Intralobar sequestration of lung takes its blood supply from: (AIIMS Nov 1994)
a. Internal mammary artery
b. Descending abdominal aorta
c. Pulmonary artery
d. None of the above

Q5. Lung sequestration occurs most commonly in which lobe: (AIIMS June 1993)
a. Apical
b. Left posterior basal
c. Left posterosuperior
d. Right lateral basal

Q6. Diagnosis of lung sequestration by: (JIPMER 2000)
a. CT
b. Angiography
c. MRI
d. X-ray

Q7. The most common cause of lung abscess is: (AIIMS Nov 1996)
a. Aspiration
b. Hematogenous spread from a distant site
c. Direct contact
d. Lymphatic spread

Q8. The least common site of lung abscess is: (PGI June 1999)
a. Left upper lobe
b. Left lower lobe
c. Right upper lobe
d. Right lower lobe

Q9. Which is true regarding hydatid cyst of the lung: (AIIMS June 2002)
a. Nerve ruptures
b. Calcification is common
c. Always associated with cyst in the liver
d. More common in the lower lobes

Q10. The most common cause of amoebic lung abscess is: (AIIMS Nov 1994)
a. Direct extension from the liver
b. Hematogenous spread
c. Lymphatic spread
d. By inhalation

Q11. Foreign body aspiration in the supine position causes which of the following parts of the lung to be commonly affected: (AIIMS June 2002)
a. Apical left lobe
b. Apical lobe of right lung
c. Apical part of the lower lobe
d. Posterobasal segment of the left lung

Q12. A foreign body completely obstructing the right main bronchus causes: (PGI June 1999)
a. Decreased ventilation perfusion ratio
b. Increased ventilation in the left lung
c. Perfusion doubles in right lung
d. Increased ventilation/perfusion (VF) ratio in the right lung

Q13. In video-assisted thoracoscopic surgery for better vision, the space in the operative field is created by: (AIIMS June 2002)
a. Self-retaining retractor
b. CO_2 insufflations
c. Collapse of ipsilateral lung
d. Rib spacing

Q14. Muscle not cut in posterolateral thoracotomy is: (PGI Dec 1998)
a. Serratus anterior
b. Latissimus dorsi
c. Rhomboid major
d. Pectoralis major

Q15. Which is not an indication of thoracotomy? (AIIMS Nov 1998)
a. Massive pneumothorax
b. Pulmonary contusion
c. Bleeding >200 mL/h in thoracotomy tube
d. Esophageal rupture

Grade III	Most difficult

Q1. In Pancoast tumor, the following is seen, *except*: (PGI June 1998)
a. Horner's syndrome
b. Rib erosion
c. Hemoptysis
d. Pain in the shoulder and arm

Q2. In pulmonary embolism, fibrinolytic therapy is responsible for: (PGI Dec 1997)
a. Risk of hemorrhage
b. Prognosis good
c. Massive emboli
d. All of the above

Q3. A patient presented to the casualty with massive life-threatening Hemoptysis. Which of the following procedures is least useful? (AIIMS May 2017)
a. Lobectomy of the affected segment
b. Bronchoscopic laser cauterization
c. Pulmonary artery embolization
d. Bronchial artery embolization

Q4. A young man with pulmonary tuberculosis presents with massive recurrent hemoptysis. For angiographic treatment, which vascular structure should be evaluated first? (All India 2004)
a. Pulmonary artery
b. Bronchial artery
c. Pulmonary vein
d. Superior vena cava

Q5. All are elaborated by small cell carcinoma lung, *except*: (PGI June 2000)
a. Antidiuretic hormone (ADH)
b. Adrenocorticotropic hormone (ACTH)
c. 5-hydroxytryptamine (5-HT)
d. Noradrenaline

Q6. In case of CA lung, which among the following will be contraindicated for surgical resection? (AIIMS Nov 2000)
a. Malignant pleural effusion
b. Hilar lymphadenopathy
c. Consolidation of one lobe
d. Involvement of the visceral pleura

Q7. A 50-year-old male smoker presents with pain along the left arm and ptosis. His chest radiograph shows a soft tissue opacity at the left lung apex with destruction of adjacent ribs. The picture is suggestive of: (AIIMS Nov 2003)
a. Adenocarcinoma lung
b. Bronchial carcinoid
c. Pancoast tumor
d. Bronchoalveolar carcinoma

Q8. Coronary artery bypass graft surgery (CABG) is done for all of the following indications, *except*: (All India 1999)
a. To reduce symptoms
b. To prevent further catastrophes
c. To prolong life
d. To prevent the progress of native blood vessel disease

Q9. Absolute contraindications of heart transplantation: (PGI Dec 2000)
a. Human immunodeficiency virus (HIV) infection
b. Age >60 years
c. Irreversible pulmonary hypertension
d. Significant pulmonary vascular disease
e. Malignancy

Q10. Regarding pectus excavatum, all are true, *except*: (PGI Dec 1997)
a. Gross central venous system (CVS) dysfunction
b. Decrease in lung capacity
c. Cosmetic deformity
d. Depression in the chest

Q11. Superior vena cava syndrome is caused most commonly by: (AIIMS Nov 1995)
a. Adenocarcinoma
b. Squamous cell carcinoma
c. Small cell carcinoma
d. Large cell carcinoma

Q12. Which of the following incisions in the diaphragm is the safest? (AIIMS May 2015)
a. Radial
b. Circumferential
c. Horizontal
d. Vertical

Q13. About Diaphragmatic injury, the true statement is: (AIIMS June 1998)
a. Treatment is conservative
b. Resolves spontaneously
c. The left side is more common
d. Associated with pneumothorax

Q14. The most common symptom of bronchial adenoma is: (All India 1996)
a. Chest pain
b. Cough
c. Recurrent hemoptysis
d. Weight loss

Q15. True about bronchial adenoma: (All India 1998)
a. 10–15% of all lung tumors
b. Mostly malignant
c. Recurrent hemoptysis
d. Peripherally located

ANSWERS

Grade I: 1. b; 2. c (Schwartz 10/e p673); 3. a, b, d (Schwartz 10/e p673); 4. a, b, c, d (Schwartz 10/e p673); 5. a (Bailey 27/e p936); 6. d (Schwartz 10/e p679); 7. a (Schwartz 10/e p673); 8. a; 9. b (Sabiston 20/e p1604); 10. d; 11. d (Bailey 27/e p922); 12. d; 13. a, b, c (Schwartz 10/e p166-8); 14. d; 15. b

Grade II: 1. b (Sabiston 20/e p1607); 2. b; 3. d; 4. b; 5. b (CSDT 13/e p337); 6. a; 7. a (Harrison 19/e p813); 8. a (Schwartz 10/e p650); 9. d (Bailey 27/e p67); 10. a (Bailey 27/e p58); 11. c; 12. a; 13. c; 14. c, d (Farquharson's Op. Surgery 9/e p132); 15. b

Grade III: 1. c (Schwartz 10/e p623); 2. a; 3. c (Sabiston 20/e p1598); 4. b; 5. d (Harrison 19/e p608); 6. a (Sabiston 20/e p1584); 7. c (Harrison 19/e p510); 8. d; 9. a, c, e; 10. a (Bailey 27/e p939); 11. c; 12. b; 13. c (Bailey 27/e p938); 14. c; 15. c

MODEL QUESTIONS

Q1. In a patient with one episode of spontaneous pneumothorax, which is advised:

a. Stop diving
b. Stop smoking
c. Stop flying
d. All

Ans. d

Q2. Intralobar sequestration of the lung is commonest in the:

a. Apical segment of upper lobe
b. Medial segment of the middle lobe
c. Lateral basal segment of the lower lobe
d. Posterior basal segment of the lower lobe

Ans. d

Q3. A young man with pulmonary tuberculosis presents with massive recurrent hemoptysis. For angiographic treatment, which vascular structure should be evaluated first?

a. Pulmonary artery
b. Bronchial artery
c. Pulmonary vein
d. Superior vena cava

Ans. b

Q4. Coronary artery bypass graft surgery (CABG) is done for all of the following indications, *except*:

a. To reduce symptoms
b. To prevent further catastrophes
c. To prolong life
d. To prevent the progress of native blood vessel disease

Ans. d

Q5. A neonate with a scaphoid abdomen and respiratory distress has:

a. Congenital pyloric stenosis
b. Diaphragmatic hernia
c. Volvulus
d. Wilm's tumor

Ans. b

Q6. Valvuloplasty is done in the following, *except*:

a. Coarctation of the aorta
b. Pulmonary stenosis (PS)
c. Mitral stenosis (MS)
d. Aortic stenosis (AS)

Ans. a

Q7. About diaphragmatic injury, the true statement is:

a. Treatment is conservative
b. Resolves spontaneously
c. The left side is more common
d. Associated with pneumothorax

Ans. c

Q8. The inferior vena cava (IVC) filter is used in the following, *except*:

a. Massive emboli
b. Negligible size of emboli
c. Repeated emboli
d. None

Ans. b

Q9. Pleural mesothelioma is associated with:

a. Asbestosis
b. Beryllіosis
c. Silicosis
d. Bagassosis

Ans. a

Q10. Chylothorax means the pleural cavity contains:

a. Lymph
b. Blood
c. Air
d. Pus

Ans. a

Q11. Coronary graft is most commonly taken from:

a. Axillary vein
b. Cubital vein
c. Saphenous vein
d. Femoral vein

Ans. c

Q12. Morgagni hernia:

a. Hernia between the costal and sternal part of the diaphragm
b. Hernia through the pleuroperitoneal canal
c. Hernia through the lumbar triangle
d. Hernia through the inguinal canal

Ans. a

Q13. Steering wheel injury on the chest of a young man reveals multiple fractures of ribs and paradoxical movement with severe respiratory distress. X-ray shows pulmonary contusion on the right side without pneumothorax. What is the initial treatment of choice?

a. Immediate internal fixation
b. Endotracheal intubation and mechanical ventilation
c. Thoracic epidural analgesia and Q2 therapy
d. Stabilization with towel clips

Ans. b

Q14. Which needle is used for a pleural biopsy?

a. Vin Silvermann's
b. Abram's
c. Abraham's
d. Osgood's

Ans. b

Q15. An 80-year-old male presented with a lung abscess in the left upper zone. The best treatment modality is:

a. Antibiotics according to the organisms
b. Surgical drainage
c. Tube thoracostomy
d. Wait and watch

Ans. a

SUGGESTED READING

1. Bailey & Love's - Short Practice of Surgery, 27th edition.
2. Schwartz's Principles of Surgery, 18th edition.
3. Textbook of Surgery by David Sabiston, 21st edition.

CHAPTER 54

Tumors

"Cancer cannot cripple love, it cannot shatter hope, it cannot conquer the spirit."

- Unknown

INTRODUCTION

The word cancer is from the Greek word meaning crab. *Rudolf Virchow (Rudolf Ludwig Carl Virchow, 1821–1902, German pathologist)* was the first to show that cancer is a disease of cells, and it proliferates abnormally by saying, omnis cellula e cellula meaning "every cell from a cell."

FEATURES OF MALIGNANT TRANSFORMATION (BAILEY AND LOVE)

- Establish an autonomous lineage.
- Obtain replicative immortality.
- Evade apoptosis and detection/elimination.
- Acquire antigenic competence, ability to invade, ability to disseminate, and implant.
- Evocation of inflammation
- Jettison excess baggage.
- Subvert communication to and from the cellular environment.
- Develop ability to change energy metabolism.

In 1953, Watson (James Dewey Watson, 1928, American biologist) and Crick (Francis Harry Compton Crick, 1916–2004, British molecular biologist) described the structure of deoxyribonucleic acid (DNA), and the way to the research for molecular biology of cancer opened.

Points to remember:
- *Tumor lysis syndrome:* It is the rapid destruction of neoplastic cells. It is commonly associated with Burkitt's lymphoma, leukemia, and some other lymphomas.
- *Abnormalities associated are* hyperuricemia, hypokalemia, hypophosphoric, hypocalcemia, lactic acidosis, and acute renal failure.
- *Treatment* is by rehydration, allopurinol, rasburicase, and if required hemodialysis.

How does a cell become malignant?

Mutation is the main process for malignant transformation. Usually, multiple mutations are required. Actually, the cancer is a clonal process; a malignant cell is capable of giving an infinite number of identical cells fully malignant.

Not to forget:
Chemoport: It is a device to deliver chemotherapy drugs. Chemotherapy drugs are highly irritant and corrosive so should not be given by any other route than chemoport. The most common site for chemoport is below the clavicle.

HYPERCALCEMIA OF MALIGNANCY

It is caused either by increased release of calcium or increased reabsorption of calcium, usually due to parathyroid hormone (PTH).

Two mechanisms are mainly responsible for malignant transformation:

1. Genomic instability
2. Tumor-related inflammation

Cancer starts from a single transformed cell, which can make a tumor mass. *Gompertzian (Benjamin Gompers, 1779–1865, insurance actuary) growth.* Growth rate reduces exponentially as the population approaches its maximum.

You may be asked:
- *Screening for cancer:*
  - It is to recognize and treat cancer at the earliest.
  - Tests for screening should be free or inexpensive.
  - Tests should be specific and related to the disease.
  - The benefits of screening programs should outweigh the difficulties faced by people.

Common screening programs are as follows:

- *CA breast:*
    - *BSE/clinical examination of breast:* Monthly
    - *BSE/clinical examination of breast:* Every 3 years after 20, every 5 years after 40
    - Mammography—yearly after 40
- *CA cervix:* Pap test—starts at 21 years or after first intercourse
- *CA prostate:*
    - DRE—annually at 50 years
    - PSA—annually at 50 years
- *Colorectal CA:*
    - Fecal occult blood test (FOBT)—yearly at 50 years
    - Sigmoidoscopy—5 yearly at 50 years
    - DCBE (Double contrast barium enema)—5 yearly at 50 years
    - Colonoscopy—10 yearly—5 yearly at 50 years

MANAGEMENT OF CANCER

- Prevention
- Screening
- Diagnosis
- Investigations
- Classification and staging
- Surgery
- Radiotherapy
- Chemotherapy
- Combined therapy
- Palliative therapy

RADIOSENSITIVE TUMORS

Highly RS - Mn = WeSMEL: Wilm's tumor, seminoma, myeloma, Ewings sarcoma, and lymphoma

Highly radioresistant: Mn = MOP: Melanoma, Osteocarcoma, Pancreatic CA

- The body's most radiosensitive tissue: Bone marrow
- The body's least radiosensitive tissue: Nervous tissue
- The body's most radiosensitive blood all lymphocytes
- The body's least radiosensitive platelets
- Ionizing radiation is of two types:
    1. Particulate (Mn EPNA: Electron, Proton, Neutron, Alpha particles with maximum effect).
    2. Electromagnetic—X-ray and gamma rays (most penetrating).

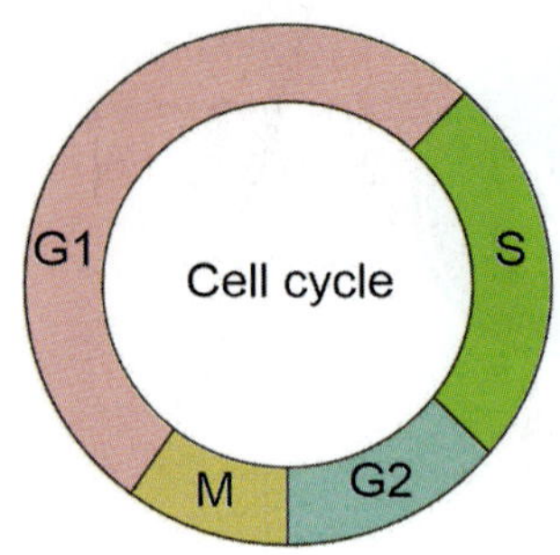
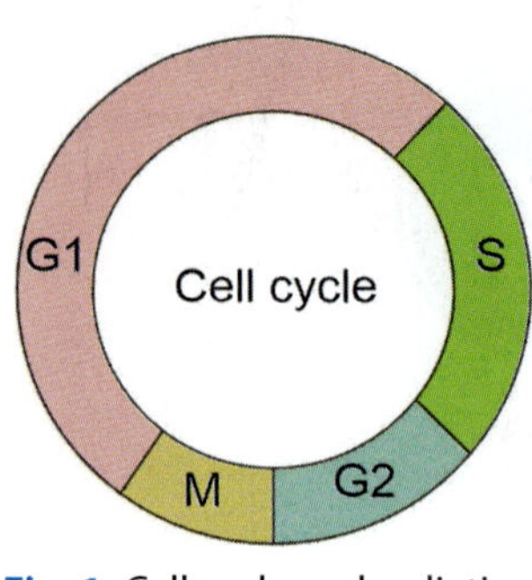

Fig. 1: Cell cycle and radiation.

RADIOTHERAPY

- X-rays—produced by a linear accelerator.
- *Gamma rays are:* Usually, produced by the decay of Cobalt (Cobalt-60) nucleoli (radioisotope).

Cell Cycle and Radiation

Cell cycle and radiation shown in **Figure 1**.

Types of Radiotherapy

- Teletherapy—radiation is generated at a distance.
- Brachytherapy—implanted inside the organ or in adjacent tissue.
- Systemic therapy.

INTENSITY MODULATED RADIATION THERAPY

- Applying high radiation while minimizing the surrounding normal tissue.
    - *Indications*: *3P—Prostate CA, Pancreatic CA, and Primary brain tumors*
- O_2 application increases the radiosensitivity of tissue
- Tissue hypoxia makes it radioresistant.

CHEMOTHERAPY

- Highly chemosensitive tumors
  Mn = WHEAT
    - *W:* Wilm's tumor
    - *H:* Hodgkin's lymphoma
    - *E:* Ewing's tumor
    - *A:* ALL
    - *T:* Testicular teratoma

CHEMORESISTANT TUMORS

Mn = Maybe the Sun Hot

- Melanoma
- Thyroid carcinoma
- SCC
- HCC

Good to remember:
- Tumor markers are substances that can indicate the presence of cancer or certain cancerous conditions. These are cellular, biochemical, molecular or genetic changes. Examples are:
  - Alpha-fetoprotein (AFP)—liver cancer
  - CA 125—ovarian cancer
  - Carcinoembryonic antigen (CEA)—colon cancer
  - CA 27–29—breast cancer
  - Estrogen and progesterone receptors—breast cancer
- *Most common sets of bone metastasis:* Mn BPO (Breast, Prostate, Others (RCC, lung, thyroid, urinary bladder)
- The most common cause of osteoblastic secondaries in males—CA prostate/in females—CA breast.
- The most common osteolytic secondaries are from the kidney and total leukocyte count (TLC) (thyroid, lung, and GI tumor).
- Metastasis in lymph nodes, e.g., Rother's LN (CA breast—interpectoral LNs), Sister Joseph (Nodes periumbilical metastatic nodes).

SOME IMPORTANT QUESTIONS

Q1. Which one of the following is the most common tumor to produce metastasis to cervical lymph nodes?

a. Glottic carcinoma
b. Nasopharyngeal carcinoma
c. Carcinoma base of tongue
d. Carcinoma lip

Ans. b

Q2. Delphian nodes are:

a. Pretracheal b. Paratracheal
c. Supraclavicular d. Posterior triangle

Ans. a

Q3. The most common cause of skeletal metastasis is:

a. Kidney b. Prostate
c. Breast d. Thyroid

Ans. c

Q4. The most common primary of metastatic bone tumor in a male is:

a. Lung b. Liver
c. Bone d. Brain

Ans. a

Q5. Tumor lysis syndrome is associated with all of the following laboratory features, *except*:

a. Hyperkalemia b. Hypercalcemia
c. Hyperuricemia d. Hyperphosphatemia

Ans. b

Q6. The most common site of lymphoma in the gastrointestinal system is:

a. Small bowel b. Stomach
c. Large intestine d. Esophagus

Ans. b

Q7. Sentinel lymph node biopsy is done in all, *except*:

a. Cancer of the breast b. Cancer of penis
c. Malignant melanoma d. Cancer of the colon

Ans. d

Q8. Which of the following malignant tumors is radioresistant?

a. Ewing's sarcoma b. Retinoblastoma
c. Osteosarcoma d. Neuroblastoma

Ans. c

Q9. Craniospinal irradiation is employed in the treatment of:

a. Oligodendroglioma
b. Mixed oligoastrocytoma
c. Pilocytic astrocytoma
d. Medulloblastoma
e. Glioblastoma

Ans. d and e

Q10. Which of the following is the most radiosensitive phase of the cell cycle?

a. G_2M b. G_2
c. S d. G_1

Ans. a

Q11. The most common intra-abdominal tumor between 2 and 5 years:

a. Neuroblastoma b. Wilm's tumor
c. Hepatoblastoma d. Lymphoma

Ans. a

Q12. Kaposi's sarcoma.

a. Does not occur in non-human immunodeficiency virus (HIV) positive persons
b. Has an increasing incidence among AIDS patients
c. No gastrointestinal (GI) bleeding
d. Uncommon among homosexual HIV positive

Ans. b

Q13. Which one of the following is a rare site for metastasis?

a. Vertebrae b. Skull
c. Pelvis d. Forearm and leg bones

Ans. d

Q14. The most common site of lymphoma in the gastrointestinal system is:

a. Small bowel
b. Stomach
c. Large intestine
d. Esophagus

Ans. b

Q15. Which one of the following is the most common tumor to produce metastasis to cervical lymph nodes?

a. Glottic carcinoma
b. Nasopharyngeal carcinoma
c. Carcinoma base of tongue
d. Carcinoma lip

Ans. b

MULTIPLE CHOICE QUESTIONS

Grade I	*Simple*

Q1. The following is a marker of Paget's disease of the mammary gland: (All India 2007)

a. S-100
b. HMB-45
c. CEA
d. Neuron-specific enolase

Q2. In which of the following tumors alpha fetoprotein is elevated? (AIIMS November 2005)

a. Choriocarcinoma
b. Neuroblastoma
c. Hepatocellular carcinoma
d. Seminoma

Q3. Which of the following tumors secretes erythropoietin? (PGI June 2010)

a. Pheochromocytoma
b. Hepatoma
c. Renal cell carcinoma (RCC)
d. Adrenal adenoma
e. Breast cancer

Q4. CA-125 is associated with: (PGI June 2007)

a. Pregnancy
b. Breast carcinoma
c. Tuberculosis (TB)
d. Endometrial carcinoma
e. Endometriosis

Q5. Which of the following is a marker of carcinoma? (All India 2012)

a. Cytokeratin
b. Vimentin
c. Calcitonin
d. CD-45

Q6. CEA is increased in all, *except*: (AIIMS May 2007)

a. Lung cancer
b. Breast cancer
c. Colon cancer
d. Osteogenic sarcoma

Q7. In which of the following diseases, the overall survival is increased by a screening procedure? (All India 2005)

a. Prostate cancer
b. Lung cancer
c. Colon cancer
d. Ovarian cancer

Q8. Screening increases life span in which of the following carcinomas? (PGI June 2007)

a. Breast
b. Colon
c. Prostate
d. Lung

Q9. Screening is useful for: (PGI November 2011)

a. Carcinoma lung
b. Carcinoma breast
c. Carcinoma skin
d. Carcinoma ovary

Q10. In which of the following head and neck cancers is lymph node metastasis least common? (AIIMS May 2008)

a. Tongue
b. Buccal mucosa
c. Hard palate
d. Lower alveolus

Q11. Which carcinoma most commonly metastasizes to cervical lymph nodes? (AIIMS June 1993)

a. Maxillary sinus
b. Posterior tongue
c. Cheek
d. Hard palate

Q12. Lymph node metastasis is a common feature with the following variant of soft tissue sarcoma: (All India 1997)

a. Fibrosarcoma
b. Angiosarcoma
c. Liposarcoma
d. Neurofibrosarcoma

Q13. A 65-year-old smoker presents with hoarseness, hemoptysis, and a hard, painless lump in the left supraclavicular fossa. Which of the following is the most appropriate diagnostic step? (AIIMS June 2004)

a. Undertake an open biopsy of the neck lump
b. Undertake a radical neck dissection
c. Do fine-needle aspiration cytology
d. Give a trial of antituberculous therapy

Q14. Upper GI endoscopy and biopsy from the lower esophagus in a 48-year-old lady with chronic heartburn shows the presence of columnar epithelium with goblet cells. The feature is most likely consistent with: (AIIMS June 2003)

a. Dysplasia
b. Hyperplasia
c. Carcinoma in situ
d. Metaplasia

Q15. A 55-year-old chronic smoker presents with complaints of hoarseness of voice and a single enlarged, painless lymph node in the left supraclavicular region. Next step to be done: (AIIMS Nov 2000)

a. CT scan of chest
b. Sputum exam for acid-fast bacilli (AFB)
c. Laryngoscopy and chest X-ray
d. Excision biopsy of the node

Grade II	*Difficult*

Q1. Treatment of bony metastasis is by: (JIPMER 2011)

a. Samarium-153
b. I-131 with tositumomab
c. P-32
d. Yttrium

Q2. Best investigation for bone metastasis is: (All India 2012)

a. Magnetic resonance imaging (MRI)
b. Computed tomography (CT)
c. Bone scan
d. X-ray

Q3. A malignant tumor of childhood that metastasizes to bones most often is: (All India 2006)

a. Wilm's tumor
b. Neuroblastoma
c. Adrenal gland tumors
d. Granulosa cell tumor of ovary

Q4. Features of tumor lysis syndrome: (PGI May 2011)

a. Hyperuricemia
b. Hypercalcemia
c. Hypophosphatemia
d. Hyperphosphatemia
e. Hyperkalemia

Q5. Tumor lysis syndrome is characterized by all, *except*: (AIIMS November 2017)

a. Hyperuricemia
b. Hypercalcemia
c. Hyperkalemia
d. Hyperphosphatemia

Q6. A 53-year-old patient was admitted with complaints of dyspnea. On examination, he has a puffy face with engorged veins over the chest. Superior vena cava (SVC) obstruction is suspected. Chest X-ray shows mediastinal enlargement. What is the next step? (AIIMS November 2017)

a. Total blood count with peripheral smear
b. CT thorax
c. Start cyclophosphamide
d. Urgent referral to radiotherapy

Q7. Sentinel lymph node biopsy is an important part of the management of which of the following conditions? (All India 2002)

a. Carcinoma prostate
b. Carcinoma breast
c. Carcinoma lung
d. Carcinoma nasopharynx

Q8. Sentinel lymph node biopsy is most useful for: (AIIMS November 2018)

a. Carcinoma cervix
b. Carcinoma endometrium
c. Carcinoma vulva
d. Carcinoma vagina

Q9. Upper GI endoscopy and biopsy from the lower esophagus in a 48-year-old lady with chronic heartburn shows the presence of columnar epithelium with goblet cells. The feature is most likely consistent with: (AIIMS June 2005)

a. Dysplasia
b. Hyperplasia
c. Carcinoma in situ
d. Metaplasia

Q10. Spontaneously regressing tumors are: (PGI 2006)

a. Malignant melanoma
b. Neuroblastoma
c. Ewing's sarcoma
d. Wilm's tumor

Q11. A patient comes with a stony hard, painless lymph node in the left supraclavicular fossa. A biopsy report shows squamous cell carcinoma. What is the diagnosis? (AIIMS Nov 1999)

a. Stomach carcinoma b. Breast carcinoma
c. Lung carcinoma d. Pancreas carcinoma

Q12. By mucosal resection which carcinoma can be diagnosed early: (AIIMS June 1998)

a. Esophageal carcinoma
b. Anal carcinoma
c. Colon carcinoma
d. Pancreatic carcinoma

Q13. The most favorable prognosis after radiotherapy is in: (PGI June 1997)

a. Melanoma b. Teratoma
c. Seminoma d. Desmoid

Q14. Spontaneously regressing tumors are: (PGI June 2006)

a. Malignant melanoma b. Neuroblastoma
c. Ewing's sarcoma d. Wilm's tumor

Q15. All of the following about gastrointestinal carcinoid tumors are true, *except*: (All India 2010)

a. Small intestine and appendix account for almost 60% of all gastrointestinal carcinoids.
b. 5-year survival for carcinoid tumors is >60%
c. Rectum is spared.
d. Appendiceal carcinoids are more common in females than males.

Grade III	***Most difficult***

Q1. All of the following are pure beta emitters, *except*: (AIIMS May 2011)

a. Yttrium-90 b. Phosphorus-32
c. Strontrium-90 d. Samarium-153

Q2. Which of the following imaging techniques gives maximum radiation exposure to the patient? (All India 2006)

a. Chest X-ray b. MRI
c. CT scan d. Bone scan

Q3. Which of the following elements is obsolete in radiotherapy? (AIIMS 2009)

a. Cesium-137 b. Cobalt-60
c. Radium-226 d. Iridium-192

Q4. Amifostine protects all of the following, *except*: (All India 2009)

a. Central nervous system (CNS)
b. Salivary glands
c. Kidneys
d. Gastrointestinal (GIT)

Q5. High energy linear accelerators use: (PGI 2006)

a. X-rays b. Gamma-rays
c. Alpha-rays d. Infrared-rays
e. Beta-rays

Q6. Amifostine is: (AIIMS May 2012)

a. Radiosensitizer b. Radioprotector
c. Radiomodifier d. Radiomimetic

Q7. Small deposits of neuroendocrine cell hyperplasia in scarred lungs are known as: (JIPMER 2014)

a. Teratoma b. Tumor let
c. Carcinoid d. Hamartoma

Q8. A 24-year-old man presented with a retroperitoneal, necrotic, heterogenous enhancing mass on CT near the hilum of the left kidney. What is the most probable diagnosis? (AIIMS November 2010)

a. Metastatic germ cell tumor
b. Metastatic melanoma
c. Lymphoma
d. Metastatic transitional cell tumor

Q9. Octreotide is used in all, *except*: (AIIMS May 2011)

a. Insulinoma b. Glucagonoma
c. Glioma d. Carcinoids

Q10. Which of the following is the most beneficial technique of using chemotherapy with a course of radiotherapy in head and neck malignancies? (AIIMS Nov 2004)

a. Neo-adjuvant chemotherapy
b. Adjuvant chemotherapy
c. Concurrent chemotherapy
d. Alternating chemotherapy and radiotherapy

Q11. True about sentinel lymph node biopsy: (PGI June 2004)

a. Special OT is required.
b. Blue dyes were injected.
c. Contraindicated if axillary LN is involved.
d. It is done to avoid inadvertent axillary LN biopsy.
e. Radioactive dye is used.

Q12. The most common malignant tumor of adult males in India is: (All India 2004)

a. Oropharyngeal carcinoma
b. Gastric carcinoma
c. Colo-rectal carcinoma
d. Lung cancer

Q13. Bony metastasis is common with all of the following, *except*: (All India 1998)

a. Cancer breast
b. Cancer lung
c. Cancer testis
d. Cancer prostate

Q14. Lymph node metastasis is a common feature with the following variant of soft tissue sarcoma: (All India 1997)

a. Fibrosarcoma
b. Angiosarcoma
c. Liposarcoma
d. Neurofibrosarcoma

Q15. Not true about bone metastasis: (AIIMS June 1998)

a. Uncommon distal to the elbow and knee
b. Breast secondary may be osteoblastic
c. Renal cell carcinoma secondary are expansile
d. Soft tissue sarcoma causes bony metastasis

ANSWERS

Grade I: 1. c (Harrison 20/e p532); 2. c; 3. b, c (Harrison 20/e p666); 4. a, b, d, e; 5. a; 6. d; 7. c (Schwartz 10/e p298); 8. b; 9. b, d; 10. c (Bailey 27/e p764-765); 11. b; 12. b; 13. a (Harrison 17/e p371); 14. d; 15. d (Harrison 17/e p371)

Grade II: 1. a; 2. c (Sutton 7/e p1251); 3. b (Harrison 20/e p454); 4. a, d, e; 5. b (Sabiston 20/e p90); 6. b; 7. b; 8. c; 9. d; 10. a, b; 11. c; 12. a (Bailey 26/e p1004); 13. c; 14. a, b; 15. c (Sabiston 19/e p1259)

Grade III: 1. d; 2. c; 3. c; 4. a; 5. a; 6. b; 7. b; 8. a; 9. c; 10. c (Harrison 17/e p550); 11. b, d, e (Schwartz 10/e p305); 12. a (Bailey 26/e p706); 13. c (Harrison 17/e p601); 14. b; 15. d (Harrison 18/e p820)

MODEL QUESTIONS

Q1. The half-life of radioactive cobalt-60 is:

a. 2.26 years
b. 3.26 years
c. 5.26 years
d. 7.26 years

Ans. c

Q2. Which does not have an underlying malignancy?

a. Paget's disease of bone
b. Paget's disease of the nipple
c. Paget's disease of the vulva
d. Paget's disease of anal region

Ans. a

Q3. The most common site of carcinoma in India:

a. Lung
b. Oral cavity
c. Breast
d. Uterus

Ans. b

Q4. In which of the following locations is the carcinoid tumor most common?

a. Esophagus
b. Stomach
c. Small bowel
d. Appendix

Ans. c

Q5. Radiation exposure during infancy has been linked to which one of the following carcinomas:

a. Breast
b. Melanoma
c. Thyroid
d. Lung

Ans. c

Q6. Elderly male with icterus having a large painless gallbladder lump, diagnosis is:

a. Acute hepatitis
b. Carcinoma head of the pancreas
c. CBD stone
d. Cholelithiasis

Ans. b

Q7. Erythroplasia of Queyrat occurs in:

a. Scrotum
b. Testes
c. Penis
d. Bladder

Ans. c

Q8. Carcinoma is common in dye industry workers:

a. Skin
b. Scrotum
c. Urinary bladder
d. Maxilla

Ans. c

Q9. Which of the following is not a neuroglial tumor?

a. Schwannoma
b. Astrocytoma
c. Medulloblastoma
d. Ependymoma

Ans. a

Q10. Buschke–Lowenstein tumor is:

a. Molluscum contagiosum
b. Condyloma lata
c. Giant condyloma accuminata
d. Metastasis

Ans. c

Q11. Which one of the following is a frequent cause of serum alpha-fetoprotein level >10 times the normal upper limit?

a. Seminoma
b. Metastatic carcinoma of the liver
c. Cirrhosis of the liver
d. Oat cell tumor of the lung

Ans. b

Q12. Duke's classification is used for:

a. Pancreas carcinoma
b. Gastric carcinoma
c. Urinary bladder carcinoma
d. Colo-rectal carcinoma

Ans. d

Q13. What is the treatment of choice for desmoid tumors?

a. Irradiation
b. Wide excision
c. Local excision
d. Local excision following radiation

Ans. b

Q14. Which cancer develops in a chronic ulcer?

a. Malignant melanoma
b. Basal cell CA
c. Squamous cell CA
d. Kaposi sarcoma

Ans. c

Q15. Ringertz tumor is commonly seen in:

a. Nose and sinuses
b. Stomach
c. Upper part of neck
d. Mediastinum

Ans. a

SUGGESTED READING

1. Bailey & Love's - Short Practice of Surgery, 27th edition.
2. Harrison's Principles of Internal Medicine, 16th edition.
3. Schwartz's Principles of Surgery, 18th edition.
4. Textbook of Surgery by David Sabiston, 21st edition.

Transplantation

CHAPTER 55

Kidney

"Live life after death—pledge to donate your body"

– Amit Abraham

TRANSPLANTATION

Mathieu Jaboulay (Mathieu Jaboulay, 1860–1913, French surgeon) and Alexis Carrel (1874–1944, French surgeon) developed the technique for anastomosis of blood vessels, which laid the foundation of organ transplant in the 1950s. Joseph Murray (1919–2012, American surgeon) performed the first kidney transplantation in 1945. Tom Starzi (Thomas Earl Starzi, American surgeon) performed the first liver transplantation in 1963. Christian Bernard performed the first human heart transplant in 1967. Fritz Derom performed the first lung transplant in 1968. Bruce Reitz and Norman Shumway performed the first heart–lung transplantation in 1981. In 1995, Lloyd Ratner performed the first laparoscopic living donor nephrectomy.

Points to remember:

- *Maastricht classification of donation after cardiac death (DCD):* Categories are five, divided on the basis of brought dead, cardiac arrest, brain dead, and effect of resuscitation in hospital.
- *Optimum cold ischemic time:* Kidney <28 hours, liver <23 hours, heart <3 hours, lungs <3 hours, pancreas <10 hours, small intestine >4 hours.

- *Allograft:* An organ or tissue transplanted from one individual to another.
- *Xenograft:* A graft performed between different species
- *Orthotopic graft:* A graft is placed into a normal anatomical site.
- *Heterotrophic graft:* A graft placed in a site different from that where the organ is normally located
- *Alloantigen:* Transplant antigen
- *All antibodies:* Transplant antibodies
- Human leukocyte antigen (HLA) is, main trigger to graft rejection

GRAFT REJECTION

Allograft stimulates an immune response, which leads to rejection unless this response is suppressed by strong immunosuppressive therapy. This strong rejection response is due to the differences between tissue antigens specifically ABO and HLAs.

HUMAN LEUKOCYTE ANTIGEN

These are the most common causes of rejection. They act as antigen recognition units. They are highly polymorphic as amino acid sequence differs widely between individuals. *HLA-A, HLA-B, HLA-C (Class I), and -DR, -DP, -DQ (Class II) have the most important role in organ transplantation.*

TYPES OF DONORS

- Live donors
- Brain-dead donors
- Donor after cardiac death (DCD)
- Xenograft donors

Who cannot donate organ?

- Human immunodeficiency virus (HIV) and hepatitis B virus (HBV) patients
- Patient with malignancy
- Creutzfeldt–Jakob (CJ) disease
- Death due to sepsis

DONOR MATCHING OF ABO BLOOD GROUPS

- Rh system is not involved, so not tested.
- The AB group is a universal recipient.

Q4. Renal transplantation is most commonly done in:
a. Chronic glomerulonephritis
b. Bilateral staghorn calculus
c. Horseshoe kidney
d. Oxalosis

Q5. The highest chance of success in renal transplant is seen when the donor is the: (JIPMER 1987)
a. Identical twin b. Father
c. Mother d. Sister
e. Husband

Q6. An isograft indicates transfer of tissues between: (All India 1993)
a. Unrelated donors
b. Related donors
c. Monozygotic twins
d. From the same individual

Q7. Human leukocyte antigen (HLA) matching is not necessary in which of the following organ transplantations? (JIPMER 2002)
a. Liver b. Bone marrow
c. Pancreas d. Kidney

Q8. Hyperacute rejection of graft is seen in: (All India 2003)
a. Lung b. Liver
c. Kidney d. Pancreas

Grade II	***Difficult***

Q1. The most common malignancy in renal transplant recipients is: (AIIMS Nov 1995)
a. Skin cancer
b. Renal cell carcinoma
c. Non-Hodgkin's lymphoma
d. Hodgkin's lymphoma

Q2. Steroids are used in transplantation: (TN 2003)
a. To prevent graft rejection
b. To prevent infection
c. To speed up recovery
d. To enhance immunity

Q3. Hyperacute rejection is due to: (AIIMS Nov 2012)
a. Performed antibodies
b. Cytotoxic T-lymphocyte-medicated injury
c. Circulating macrophage-mediated injury
d. Endothelitis caused by donor antibodies

Q4. The most common complication of immunosuppression is: (All India 1988)
a. Malignancy b. Graft rejection
c. Infection d. Thrombocytopenia

Q5. Amputated digits are preserved in: (All India 1992)
a. Cold saline b. Cold Ringer Lactate
c. Plastic bag in ice d. Deep freezer

Q6. A patient had undergone a renal transplantation 2 months back and now presented with difficulty breathing. The X-ray showed bilateral diffuse interstitial pneumonia. The probable etiologic agent would be: (AIIMS June 2002)
a. *Cytomegalovirus (CMV)*
b. *Histoplasma*
c. *Candida*
d. *Pneumocystis carinii*

Q7. Expanded criteria for liver donation include all of the following, *except*: (All India 2012)
a. Taken from a diseased individual after brain death
b. Hepatitis B serology positive
c. Age of donor may be >70 years
d. Can be taken from an individual with mild hepatic steatosis

Q8. Extended criteria for liver donation include all of the following, *except*: (AIIMS GIS Dec 2011)
a. Donor age >70 years
b. Hepatitis B surface antigen (HBsAg) positive donor
c. Mild hepatic steatosis
d. Donor after cardiac death

Grade III	***Most difficult***

Q1. Transplantation of which one of the following organs is most often associated with hyperacute rejection? (UPSC 2006)
a. Heart b. Kidney
c. Lungs d. Liver

Q2. The most common disease caused by CMV in postrenal transplant patients: (JIPMER 2011)
a. Pyelonephritis
b. Meningitis
c. Pneumonia
d. Gastrointestinal (GI) ulceration

Q3. An elderly male presents 2 months after renal transplantation with nephropathy. Which of the following can be a viral etiological agent? (AIIMS May 2014)

a. Polymoavirus BK
b. Human herpes virus type 6
c. Hepatitis C
d. Human papillomavirus, high-risk types

Q4. Allopurinol is used in organ preservation as: (AIIMS May 2009)

a. Antioxidant
b. Preservative
c. Free radical scavenger
d. Precursor for energy metabolism

Q5. Graft from sister to brother is: (JIPMER 1990)

a. Isograft
b. Allograft
c. Autograft
d. Heterograft

Q6. Indications of liver transplantation are all, *except*: (PGI June 2005)

a. Biliary
b. Sclerosing cholangitis
c. Hepatitis A
d. Cirrhosis
e. Fulminant hepatic failure

Q7. Auxiliary orthotopic liver transplant is indicated for: (AIIMS May 2008)

a. Metabolic liver disease
b. As a standby procedure until finding a suitable donor
c. Drug-induced hepatic failure
d. Acute fulminant liver failure for any cause

Q8. The advantage of bladder drainage over enteric drainage after pancreatic transplantation is better monitoring of: (All India 2009)

a. HBA_1C levels
b. Amylase levels
c. Glucose levels
d. Electrolyte levels

ANSWERS

Grade I: 1. b (Bailey 26/e p1408); 2. a; 3. c; 4. a (Smith's Urology 17/e p539); 5. a (Harrison 17/e p1777); 6. c; 7. a; 8. c

Grade II: 1. a (Schwartz 10/e p330); 2. a (Bailey 26/e p1413); 3. a; 4. c (Bailey 26/e p1415); 5. None (Schwartz 10/e p1800); 6. a (Sabiston 20/e p657); 7. a (Sabiston 20/e p644); 8. b

Grade III: 1. b (Bailey 26/e p1410); 2. c; 3. a (Harrison 20/e p508); 4. c (Schwartz 10/e p332); 5. b; 6. c (Harrison 19/e p2068); 7. a,d; 8. b (Sabiston 20/e p660);

MODEL QUESTIONS

Q1. Renal transplantation expanded criteria donor (ECD) is:

a. Donors with extremes of age
b. Donors with excess alcohol intake
c. Donors with a history of cerebrovascular accident
d. All of the above

Ans. d

Q2. Postrenal transplant immunosuppressant regimen:

a. Calcineurin inhibitors + Purine antagonists + Glucocorticoids
b. Glucocorticoids + Purine antagonists + Glucocorticoids
c. Glucocorticoids + Cyclophosphamide + Basiliximab
d. Calcineurin inhibitors + Purine antagonists + Basiliximab

Ans. a

Q3. The cold ischemia time of the kidney should be around:

a. 3 hours
b. 6 hours
c. 12 hours
d. 18 hours

Ans. c

Q4. An elderly male presents 2 months after renal transplantation with nephropathy. Which of the following can be a viral etiological agent?

a. Hepatitis C
b. Polyoma BK virus
c. Human papilloma virus
d. Human herpes virus

Ans. b

Q5. Hyperacute graft rejection is caused by:

a. Preformed antibodies
b. T—lymphocytes
c. Macrophages
d. B—lymphocytes
e. Mast cells

Ans. a

Q6. Minimum rejection in transplant is seen in:

a. Allograft
b. Isograft
c. Xenograft
d. Heterotopic graft

Ans. b

Q7. Skin grafting done on the wound following major skin loss taken from the twin brother is:

a. Orthotopic graft
b. Allograft
c. Isograft
d. Xenograft

Ans. c

Q8. Tissue transplanted between two people of identical genetic makeup is called:

a. Heterotopic graft
b. Allograft
c. Isograft
d. Xenograft

Ans. c

SUGGESTED READING

1. Bailey & Love's - Short Practice of Surgery, 27th edition.
2. Harrison's Principles of Internal Medicine, 16th edition.
3. Schwartz's Principles of Surgery, 18th edition.
4. Textbook of Surgery by David Sabiston, 21st edition.

CHAPTER 56

Liver

"Transplant is a life-changing experience. Organ donation transforms lives. It is torture for you, torment for you as an individual in need."

– Andy Cole

CRITERIA FOR LIVER TRANSPLANT

Model for end-stage liver disease (MELD) criteria is a model to give a number to a person to determine whether they can be put on the liver transplant waiting list (LTWL). Number 26 is the entry point. It is to avoid mortality and reduce morbidity in both the transplanted and donor.

LIVER TRANSPLANTATION

The first liver transplantation was done in 1963 by Starzl.

Most common indications of liver transplantation are: *Mn = ABCD*

- *A:* Alcoholic liver diseases
- *B:* Biliary atresia
- *C:* Hepatitis C virus (HCV)-induced cirrhosis
- *D:* Drug toxicity, i.e., paracetamol and acetaminophen

Common contraindication of liver transplantation: *Mn = MASC*

- *M:* Metastatic liver malignancy
- *A:* Active alcohol abuse
- *S:* Advanced sepsis
- *C:* Advanced cardiopulmonary disease

Types of liver transplantation:
Mn = OH APSARA

- *O: Orthotopic:* Transplanted liver is placed in the site of the liver
- *H: Heterotopic:* Transplanted liver is placed in some other site
- *A: Auxiliary:* Native liver remains in its normal place, and the transplanted liver is added
- *P:* Piggyback LT
- *S: Split liver transplant:* Cadaveric liver is divided and given to two persons
- *A: APOLT:* Auxiliary Partial Orthotopic Liver Transplantation: Left lobe is excised, and the transplanted liver is placed here.
- *R: Reduced liver transplantation:* The Liver is reduced to an approximate size according to the place in the recipient.
- *A: Auxiliary heterotrophic:* Transplanted liver is placed in the subhepatic space

You may be asked:

- *Split liver transplant:* Segments 2 and 3 are sufficient for children, and segments 5, 6, 7, and 8 can be given to adults.
- *Reduced liver transplant:* The liver is removed from an adult body, then it is made suitable for the body of a child by trimming and removal of some fat, etc.
- *Domino liver transplant:* The transplanted liver can be transplanted to other recipients.

PIGGYBACK TRANSPLANT

If the inferior vena cava (IVC) is preserved, then without removal of the recipient liver, the donor liver is transplanted above the recipient liver as piggyback.

What should be the outcome after a transplant?

- Quality of life must be better with proper mobility.
- Complications must be reduced.
- The graft survival period must be increased.
- Chronic rejection should be diminished in its incidence, as it is the most notorious cause of rejection.

SOME IMPORTANT POINTS

- The first liver transplant was done by Starzl (Thomas Starzl, 1926–2017, American physician) in 1963, in Colorado, USA.

- The most common cause of death in liver transplant is multiple organ failure due to sepsis.
- A combined liver and heart transplant is done in amyloidosis.
- Combined liver and lung transplantation was done in cystic fibrosis.
- The most common indication of liver transplantation is HCV-induced cirrhosis.
- The operative sequence of liver transplantation. Mn = Should I Plan Heartbreaking
  S: Suprahepatic IVC
  I: Infrahepatic IVC
  P: Portal vein
  H: Hepatic artery
  B: Bile duct

COMPLICATIONS OF LIVER TRANSPLANTATION

Mn = *P*ost *A*lcoholic *C*irrhosis *S*ilently *H*eals
P: Portal vein thrombosis
A: Anastomotic leak
C: Chronic liver graft rejection
S: Stricture in the bile duct
H: Hepatic artery thrombosis

SOME IMPORTANT QUESTIONS

Q1. Dr Christian Bernard is associated with:
a. Heart transplant b. Renal transplant
c. Liver transplant d. Hair transplant

Ans. a

Q2. The cold ischemic time of the kidney should ideally be below:
a. 2 hours b. 6 hours
c. 12 hours d. 24 hours

Ans. None

Q3. The length of time for which an organ can be cold stored before transplantation is maximum with:
a. Liver b. Pancreas
c. Kidney d. Small intestine

Ans. c

Q4. Skin grafting was done on the wound following major skin taken from a twin brother:
a. Isograft b. Allograft
c. Autograft d. Xenograft

Ans. a

Q5. Concordant xenograft if:
a. Between closely related different species
b. Between the same species of different races
c. Between the same species
d. Between nonidentical twins

Ans. a

MULTIPLE CHOICE QUESTIONS

Grade I ***Simple***

Q1. Expanded criteria for liver donation include all of the following, *except*: (All India 2012)
a. Taken from a diseased individual after brain death
b. Hepatitis B serology positive
c. Age of donor may be >70 years
d. Can be taken from an individual with mild hepatic steatosis

Q2. Extended criteria for liver donation include all of the following, *except*: (AIIMS Dec 2011)
a. Donor age >70 years
b. HBsAg-positive donor
c. Mild hepatic steatosis
d. Donor after cardiac death

Q3. Reduced liver transplants: (GB Pant 2011)
a. Give to two recipients after dividing into two parts
b. Left lateral lobe divided and given to child
c. The left lateral segment was divided from segment 2 and given to child
d. Part of the liver segment is transplanted into the recipient, depending upon

Grade II ***Difficult***

Q1. The advantage of bladder drainage over enteric drainage after pancreatic transplantation is better monitoring of: (All India 2009)
a. HBA_1C levels
b. Amylase levels
c. Glucose levels
d. Electrolyte levels

Q2. All are true about intestinal transplant, *except*: (JIPMER GIS 2011)
a. The principal barrier to widespread application is vigorous rejection reactions.

b. Severe form of GVHD occurs when T cells of the graft respond to foreign human leukocyte antigen (HLA) cells.
c. Uniquely dangerous complication is loss of protective mucosal barrier, bacterial translocation, and severe sepsis.
d. The majority of intestinal grafts are multivisceral grafts.

Q3. Auxiliary orthotopic liver transplant is indicated for: (AIIMS May 2008)
a. Metabolic liver disease
b. As a standby procedure until finding a suitable donor
c. Drug-induced hepatic failure
d. Acute fulminant liver failure for any cause

Grade III	*Most difficult*

Q1. Post-transplant lymphoma is most commonly associated with: (AIIMS May 2012)
a. Epstein–Barr virus (EBV)
b. Cytomegalovirus (CMV)
c. Herpes simplex
d. HHV-6

Q2. Which of the following organs/tissues are presently not being used for organ/tissue transplantation? (All India 2011)
a. Blood vessels
b. Lung
c. Liver
d. Urinary bladder

Q3. Indications of liver transplantation are all, *except*: (PGI June 2005)
a. Biliary
b. Hepatitis A
c. Clerosing cholangitis
d. Cirrhosis
e. Fulminant hepatic failure

ANSWERS

Grade I: 1. a (Sabiston 20/e p644); 2. b; 3. d
Grade II: 1. b (Bailey 27/e p1552); 2. d (Schwartz 10/e p352-354); 3. a, d (Blumgart 5/e p1689-1693)
Grade III: 1. a (Sabiston 20/e p672); 2. d (Lawrence 4/e p475); 3. b (Harrison 10/e p2068)

MODEL QUESTIONS

Q1. The most common indication of liver transplantation in children:
a. Biliary atresia
b. Wilson's disease
c. Hemochromatosis
d. Primary biliary cirrhosis

Ans. a

Q2. All are scoring systems used in liver transplant, *except*:
a. Child-Turcotte-Pugh (CTP)
b. Percutaneous endoscopic lumbar discectomy (PELD)
c. Model for end-stage liver disease (MELD)
d. Multidimensional prognostic index (MPI)

Ans. d

Q3. Liver transplant was first done by:
a. Starzl
b. Huggins
c. Carrel
d. Christian Bernard

Ans. a

Q4. All are marginal liver donors, *except*:
a. Older donor
b. Hepatitis B virus (HBV) core antibody-positive donors
c. Moderate steatosis
d. Severe hepatitis

Ans. d

Q5. Which of the following is not an indication for liver transplantation?
a. Fatty liver
b. HIV
c. Wilson's disease
d. Primary hyperoxaluria

Ans. b

SUGGESTED READING

1. Bailey & Love's - Short Practice of Surgery, 27th edition.
2. Schwartz's Principles of Surgery, 18th edition.
3. Textbook of Surgery by David Sabiston, 21st edition.

Pediatric Surgery

CHAPTER 57

Pediatric Surgery

Pediatric surgery is about preserving futures, where "by saving the life of one child, we are adding atleast 50-70 years of life," and surgeons aim to give children "hope and a better future" by treating congenital issues, with the ultimate reward being "the smile on the face of these children."

– C Everett Koop

TRAUMA

Advanced trauma life support (ATLS) has given some important points about trauma in children.

- Nonoperative treatment is often possible in splenic and liver injuries.
- Blood pressure is normal until 25% of blood volume is lost.
- Cardiorespiratory arrest is due to hypoxia and not due to vascular disease.

Overextension of the neck can compromise airways. Cervical spine injury can be present without radiographic signs. Lung contusion can occur without rib fractures.

Points to remember:

- Most common cancer of childhood is leukemia, and second most common is brain tumor, astrocytoma.
- Neuroblastoma is the most common abdominal tumor after Wilm's tumor.
- Rhabdomyosarcoma is the most common soft tissue sarcoma in children.
- Neuroblastoma is the most common pediatric tumor producing metastasis.

INGUINAL HERNIA

- Inguinal hernias are more common in premature babies more in boys.
- Indirect inguinal hernia with patent processus vaginalis is most common, more on the right side, but 15% are bilateral.
- Mostly, inguinal hernias in infants are transilluminant.
- In children, herniotomy is done.

UNDESCENDED TESTIS

- It may be palpable or improbable.
- Ectopic testis lies outside the route of descent.
- *Orchidopexy, if done before the age of 1 year, improves chances of fertility and reduces the risk of malignancy.* Acute scrotum must be treated as torsion of the testis, and urgent surgery is required.

Not to forget:

Neuroblastoma is characterized by features:

- *Crosses midline*
- Calcification
- *Extensive metastasis*
- Invades spinal cord
- *Elevated VMA*

Staging system divides in three stages: Low-risk patients, intermediate patients, and high-risk patients.

- Hypospadias and phimosis are common.
- Recurrent balanoposthitis, paraphimosis, and scarring causing phimosis are indications for circumcision.

You may be asked:

Causes of rectal bleeding in children:

- Necrotizing enterocolitis is a life-threatening disease of newborns.
- Intussusception in older children
- Others, polyps, gastroenteritis, anal fissures, etc.

UMBILICAL HERNIA

It is due to incomplete closure of the umbilical ring; strangulation is very rare, and it gets resolved by the age of 4 years.

HYPERTROPHIC PYLORIC STENOSIS

It commonly affects boys. Projectile vomiting after feeds, an ultrasound (US) can diagnose; pyloromyotomy is required.

INTUSSUSCEPTION

Classic presentation of bilious vomiting, colicky pain, and bloody stools, common before the age of 2 years.

Good to remember:

Preparation of children for operation and operative techniques:

- Nothing by mouth (NPO) 2 hours for clear fluids and 4 hours for breast milk, and 6 hours for solids.
- Gentle handling of tissues.
- Closure of abdominal incisions with absorbable sutures.
- Skin should be closed with absorbable subcuticular sutures.

The diagnosis is confirmed by ultrasonography (USG), conservatively air enema can be used, but surgical procedures are required if other methods fail.

ACUTE APPENDICITIS

For anorexia, vomiting, fever, right iliac fossa (RIF) tenderness, and guarding, surgery is the treatment.

CONGENITAL CAUSES OF INTESTINAL OBSTRUCTION IN CHILDREN

Intestinal atresia, cystic fibrosis, bands, volvulus, intussusception, Hirschsprung's disease, and imperforate anus are the main causes.

SOME IMPORTANT QUESTIONS

Q1. Sacrococcygeal teratoma is an embryological remnant of:

a. Neural tube b. Allantois
c. Notochord d. Primitive streak

Ans. d

Q2. Primitive streak remnants give rise to:

a. Neuroblastoma
b. Wilm's tumors
c. Sacrococcygeal teratoma
d. Hepatoblastoma

Ans. c

Q3. The most common intra-abdominal tumor in infants:

a. Neuroblastoma
b. Wilm's tumor
c. Hepatocellular carcinoma (HCC)
d. Hypernephroma

Ans. a

Q4. The most common renal tumor in children:

a. Renal cyst
b. Congenital mesoblastic nephroblastoma
c. Neuroblastoma
d. Nephroblastoma

Ans. b

Q5. Signe-de-Dance is:

a. Empty right iliac fossa in intussusception
b. Pincer-shaped appearance in barium enema in intussusception
c. Tenderness at the McBurney's Point
d. Passing of large quantities of urine in hydronephrosis

Ans. a

MULTIPLE CHOICE QUESTIONS

Grade I	Simple

Q1. A 6-year-old female presents with constipation and urinary retention. On examination, a presacral mass is noted. Most probable diagnosis is: (AIIMS May 2008)

a. Pelvic neuroblastoma
b. Rectal duplication cyst
c. Sacrococcygeal teratoma
d. Anterior sacral meningocele

Q2. The following are true about William Halsted: (PGI June 2008)

a. First person to receive the Nobel Prize in surgery
b. Pioneered the introduction of gloves
c. Promoted a radical approach for breast surgery
d. Pioneered the role of antibiotics

Q3. Quant's sign (a T-shaped depression in the occipital bone) may be present in: (Gujarat 2014)

a. Down's syndrome b. Head injury
c. Rickets d. Scurvy

Q4. Nezelof's syndrome is recurrent episodes of: (Gujarat, 2014)

a. Appendicitis b. Cholecystitis
c. Intestinal obstruction d. Pneumonia

Q5. The most common cause of fresh bleeding per rectum in a 5-year-old child is: (AIIMS May 2013)

a. Volvulus
b. Trauma
c. Worm infestation
d. Rectal polyp

Grade II	*Difficult*

Q1. A 1-month-old female child has swelling over the back in the sacral region. There is no cough impulse in the swelling. X-ray examination shows erosion of the coccyx. The most likely clinical diagnosis would be: (UPSC 1995)

a. Meningocele
b. Lipoma
c. Sacrococcygeal teratoma
d. Neurofibroma

Q2. The most common tumor among children aged 1–5 years in South Africa is: (TN 1996)

a. Neuroblastoma
b. Wilm's tumor
c. Neurofibroma
d. Burkitt's lymphoma

Q3. In sickle cell anemia sudden onset of pancytopenia with hemolysis and no rise of reticulocyte count occurs in: (JIPMER 2004)

a. Sequestration crisis
b. Aplastic crisis
c. Hemolytic crisis
d. Vaso-occlusive crisis

Q4. Cells from the neural crest are involved in all, *except*: (AIIMS June 2003)

a. Hirschsprung's disease
b. Neuroblastoma
c. Primitive neuroectodermal tumor
d. Wilms' tumor

Q5. A child presents with an expansile swelling on the medial side of the nose. Likely diagnosis is: (All India 2001)

a. Teratoma
b. Meningocele
c. Dermoid cyst
d. Lipoma

Grade III	*Most difficult*

Q1. Which of the following is the most common tumor in newborns? (All India 2012)

a. Neuroblastoma
b. Wilm's tumors
c. Leukemia
d. Sacrococcygeal teratoma

Q2. Sonu, a 15-year-old girl, a regular swimmer, presents with a sudden onset of pain in the abdomen, abdominal distension, and fever of 39°C and obliteration of the liver dullness. Most probable diagnosis is: (AIIMS June 2001)

a. Ruptured typhoid ulcer
b. Primary bacterial peritonitis
c. Ruptured ectopic pregnancy
d. Urinary tract infection (UTI) with pelvic inflammatory disease (PID)

Q3. Which of the following abdominal structures will be responsible for sharp pain while doing abdominal surgery? (AIIMS Nov 2000)

a. Parietal peritoneum
b. Liver parenchyma
c. Small intestine
d. Colon

Q4. A 10-year-old child with pain and mass in the right lumbar region with no fever, with the right hip flexed, and X-ray shows spine changes. Most probable diagnosis is: (AIIMS Nov 2017)

a. Psoas abscess
b. Pyonephrosis
c. Appendicitis in retrocecal position
d. Torsion of Right Undecided testis

Q5. A newborn child has not passed meconium for 48 hours. What is the diagnostic procedure of choice? (All India 2008)

a. Ultrasonography (USG)
b. Contrast enema
c. Computed tomography (CT)
d. Magnetic resonance imaging (MRI)

ANSWERS

Grade I: 1. d (Sabiston 20/e p1932); 2. b, c; 3. c; 4. d; 5. d (Harrison 18/e p321)

Grade II: 1. c; 2. d; 3. a (Harrison 20/e p693); 4. d; 5. b (Short cases surgery by Das 2/e p88)

Grade III: 1. d (Surgery of Childhood Tumors (Springer) 2008/49); 2. a (S. Das Manual of clinical surgery 4/e p344); 3. a; 4. a (Bailey 27/e p1065); 5. b

MODEL QUESTIONS

Q1. First, meconium is said to be formed during the month of fetal life:

a. Second
b. Fourth
c. Seventh
d. Ninth

Ans. a

Q2. The most common solid malignant tumor of infancy:

a. Neuroblastoma
b. Nephroblastoma
c. Germ cell tumor
d. Rhabdomyosarcoma

Ans. a

Q3. The most common posterior mediastinal mass in children is:

a. Hodgkin's disease
b. Neuroblastoma
c. Esophageal duplication cyst
d. Bronchogenic cyst

Ans. b

Q4. Malignant tumor of childhood that metastasizes to bone most often is:

a. Neuroblastoma
b. Nephroblastoma
c. Adrenal gland tumors
d. Ovarian granulose cell tumor

Ans. a

Q5. Snowstorm ascites is seen in:

a. Meconium ileus
b. Hirschsprung disease
c. Ileocecal tuberculosis
d. Pseudomyxoma peritonei

Ans. a

SUGGESTED READING

1. Bailey & Love's - Short Practice of Surgery, 27th edition.
2. Schwartz's Principles of Surgery, 18th edition.
3. Textbook of Surgery by David Sabiston, 21st edition.

SECTION 13

Miscellaneous

Miscellaneous Subjects Multiple Choice Questions

SOME IMPORTANT QUESTIONS

Q1. A cricoid hook is used particularly:
a. In thyroidectomy
b. In block dissection of the neck
c. For retracting the superior laryngeal nerve
d. In tracheostomy

Ans. d

Q2. Aminopeptidase is elevated in obstruction of:
a. Ureter
b. Urethra
c. CBD
d. Bladder

Ans. c

Q3. Hormonal treatment is given for which of the following malignancies?
a. Choriocarcinoma
b. Carcinoma prostate
c. Hepatoma
d. Teratoma
e. Granulosa cell tumor

Ans. b

Q4. First neurosurgeon of India:
a. Jacob Chandy
b. Jacob Abraham
c. KV Mathal
d. Mathew Candy

Ans. a

Q5. All are true about long flexor tendons, *except*:
a. Flexor digitorum profundus inserted to the distal phalanx bas.
b. Flexor digitorum superficialis attached to the sides of the middle phalanx.
c. Damage to the tendons involves the formation of tenoma during repair.
d. Good repair results if the tendon sheath is damaged.

Ans. d

Q6. Failure of migration of neural crest cells is seen in:
a. Albinism
b. Congenital megacolon
c. Odontomas
d. Adrenal tumor

Ans. b

Q7. The most sensitive qualitative method for the detection of air embolism is:
a. Doppler ultrasound
b. Electrocardiogram
c. Arterial pressure
d. End expiratory carbon dioxide content

Ans. d

Q8. Who said these words: To study the phenomenon of disease without books is to sail an uncharted sea, while to study books without patients is not to go to sea at all?
a. Hamilton Bailey
b. Sir Robert Hutchison
c. Sir William Osler
d. JB Murphy

Ans. c

Q9. Lamina dura lining the alveolus is:
a. Cancellous bone
b. Ligament
c. Dense cortical bone
d. Muscle

Ans. c

Q10. Orthobaric oxygen is used in:
a. Carbon monoxide poisoning
b. Ventilation failure
c. Anaerobic infection
d. Gangrene

Ans. a

Q11. Potato nodes are a feature of:
a. Sarcoidosis
b. Tuberculosis
c. Carcinoid
d. Lymphoma

Ans. a

MULTIPLE CHOICE QUESTIONS

Grade I	Simple

Q1. The most important technical consideration at the time of doing below-knee amputation is: **(AIIMS Nov 2000)**

a. Posterior flap should be longer than the anterior flap
b. Stump should be long
c. Stump should be short
d. The anterior flap should be longer than the posterior flap.

Q2. Referred pain from all of the following conditions may be felt along the inner side of the right thigh, *except*: **(All India 2006)**

a. Inflamed pelvic appendix
b. Inflamed ovaries
c. Stone in the pelvic ureter
d. Pelvic abscess

Q3. Fine-needle aspiration cytology (FNAC) needle size: **(AIIMS Nov 2007)**

a. 18–22
b. 22–26
c. 27–29
d. 16–18

Q4. Subcutaneous calcification are seen in: **(JIPMER 1993)**

a. Gout
b. Hyperparathyroidism
c. Ochronosis
d. Malignancies

Q5. In polycythemia vera, the most common postoperative complication following major surgery is: **(PGI 1991)**

a. Thrombosis
b. Gastric ulcer
c. Diabetes insipidus
d. Hemorrhage

Q6. 'Sterile needle test' helps in differentiating: **(Gujarat 2014)**

a. Healing process
b. Depth of burns
c. Degenerative process
d. Infection

Q7. Van Buchem syndrome is characterized by all, *except*: **(Gujarat 2014)**

a. Overgrowth
b. Distortion of mandible
c. Facial palsy
d. Increased acid phosphatase

Q8. Hickey–Hare test is used to diagnose: **(Gujarat 2014)**

a. Congenital pyloric stenosis
b. Duodenal atresia
c. Achalasia cardia
d. Diabetes insipidus

Q9. Bolognini's symptom (a feeling of crepitation occurring from gradually increasing pressure on the abdomen) is seen in: **(Gujarat 2014)**

a. Congenital pyloric stenosis
b. Gastric polyp
c. Duodenal atresia
d. Measles

Q10. Mauriac's syndrome is characterized by the following, *except*: **(Gujarat 2014)**

a. Diabetes
b. Obesity
c. Dwarfism
d. Cardiomegaly

Grade II	Difficult

Q1. During endotracheal intubation, unilateral breath sounds, no air heard entering the stomach, and no gastric distension are suggestive of entry of the endotracheal tube into: **(UPSC 1996)**

a. Right main bronchus
b. Esophagus
c. Midtrachea
d. Left main bronchus

Q2. A female patient complains of periumbilical pain and nausea, particularly after taking food. The diagnosis is: **(UPPG 1995)**

a. Meckel's diverticulum
b. Peptic ulcer syndrome
c. Lactose intolerance
d. None

Q3. Hypothermia is used in all, *except*: **(PGI 1998)**

a. Cardiac surgery
b. Neonatal ischemia
c. Heat stroke
d. Cardiac arrhythmia

Q4. About congenital torticollis, all are *except*: **(AIIMS Nov 2006)**

a. Always associated with breech extraction
b. Spontaneous resolution in most cases
c. Two-thirds of cases have palpable neck mass at birth
d. Uncorrected cases develop plagiocephaly

Q5. Dye used in chromoendoscopy for detection of cancer: (AIIMS May 2009)
a. Gentian violet
b. Toluidine blue
c. Hematoxylin and eosin
d. Methylene blue

Q6. Concomitant chemoradiotherapy is indicated in all of the following, *except*: (All India 2009)
a. Stage IIIB CA cervix
b. T2 N0 M0 anal cancer
c. T2 N0 M0 glottic cancer
d. T1 N2 M0 Nasopharyngeal cancer

Q7. Smoking may be associated with all of the following cancers, *except*: (All India 2009)
a. CA larynx
b. CA nasopharynx
c. CA bladder
d. CA esophagus

Q8. Frozen sections is/are used for: (PGI Nov 2009)
a. Enzyme
b. Intraoperative histopathological examination
c. Fat
d. Acid fast bacilli
e. To check the surgical margin in tumor surgery

Q9. Conditions associated with panniculitis is/are (PGI Nov 2009)
a. Pancreas cancer
b. Chronic pancreatitis
c. Acute pancreatitis
d. Pancreatic divisum
e. Post-traumatic pancreatitis

Q10. True about apocrine gland: (PGI June 2009)
a. Modified sweat gland
b. Modified sebaceous gland
c. Present in axilla and groin
d. Hidradenitis suppurativa is an infection of the apocrine gland

Grade III	Most difficult

Q1. Not associated with fat necrosis: (PGI June 2009)
a. Liposuction
b. Radiotherapy
c. Mammoplasty
d. Carcinoma breast
e. Following trauma

Q2. Aflatoxins are produced by: (All India 2011)
a. *Aspergillus flavus*
b. *Aspergillus niger*
c. *Aspergillus fumigates*
d. *Candida*

Q3. Axillary abscess is safely drained by which approach? (AIIMS May 2011)
a. Medial
b. Posterior
c. Lateral
d. Floor

Q4. Topical mitomycin C is used in: (AIIMS May 2011)
a. Basal skull carcinoma
b. Tracheal stenosis
c. Skull base osteomyelitis
d. Angiofibroma

Q5. Fixative used in histopathology: (AIIMS May 2012)
a. 10% buffered neutral formalin
b. Bouin's fixative
c. Glutaraldehyde
d. Ethyl alcohol

Q6. In the preoperative patient surgical checklist, which of the following is not required? (AIIMS Nov 2017)
a. Oral consent
b. Doctor's signature
c. Site marking
d. Confirming the patient's identity

Q7. How to measure nasogastric tube length? (AIIMS Nov 2017)
a. Tip of nose to ear to xiphisternum
b. Tip of nose to angle of ear to umbilicus
c. Mouth to ear to umbilicus
d. Mouth to ear to midway between the xiphisternum and the umbilicus

Q8. Kraissl's lines are: (AIIMS May 2017)
a. Collagen and elastin lines in stab wounds
b. Point of maximum tension in a fracture
c. Point of tension in hanging
d. Relaxed tension lines in skin

Q9. One French size of angiographic catheter corresponds to: (PGI Nov 2017)
a. 0.33 mm
b. 1.67 mm
c. 0.133″
d. 0.013″
e. 0.057″

Q10. Reverse Trendelenburg position is not used for: (PGI Nov 2017)
a. Prophylaxis against thromboembolism
b. High intracranial tension
c. Thyroid surgery
d. Parathyroid surgery

ANSWERS

Grade I: 1. a (Sabiston 20/e p1769); 2. d; 3. b; 4. b, d; 5. a (Harrison 20/e p735); 6. b (Schwartz 10/c p229); 7. b; 8. d; 9. d; 10. d

Grade II: 1. a; 2. a; 3. b, d (Schwartz 10/e p393); 4. a (Bailey 27/e p582); 5. d; 6. c (Harrison 20/e p535); 7. None (Harrison 20/e p3293); 8. a, b, c, e (Bailey 25/e p169-170); 9. a, c, d (Harrison 20/e p352); 10. a, c, d (Bailey 27/e p593)

Grade III: 1. d; 2. a (Ananthnarayan 7/e p625); 3. d (BDC 4/e pl/58); 4. b (Dillon 3/e p67); 5. a; 6. b (Sabiston 20/e p232); 7. a; 8. d; 9. a, d; 10. a

MODEL QUESTIONS

Q1. Not a premalignant ulcer:

a. Bazin's ulcer
b. Paget's disease of the nipple
c. Marjolin's ulcer
d. Lupus vulgaris

Ans. a

Q2. Sappey's line denotes a line:

a. Encircling the neck at the C6 vertebra level
b. Encircling the trunk just above the umbilicus
c. Encircling the salpigian tubes
d. None of the above

Ans. b

Q3. Local anesthetics cannot be used at the site of infection because they cause:

a. Spread of infection
b. Lowered efficiency
c. Both
d. None

Ans. c

Q4. No man's land in palm corresponds:

a. Zone I
b. Zone II
c. Zone III
d. Zone IV

Ans. b

Q5. The most common symptom postoperatively seen is:

a. Depression
b. Psychosis
c. Euphoria
d. None of the above

Ans. d

Q6. A depressed bridge of the nose can be due to any of the following, *except*:

a. Leprosy
b. Syphilis
c. Thalassemia
d. Acromegaly

Ans. d

Q7. In the acronym "Swelling" used for the history and examination of a lump or swelling, the letter "N" stands for:

a. Nodes
b. Noise (thrill/bruit)
c. Numbness
d. Neurological effects

Ans. b

Q8. Vidian neurectomy is indicated in:

a. Glossopharyngeal neuralgia
b. Trigeminal neuralgia
c. Vasomotor rhinitis
d. Atrophic rhinitis

Ans. c

Q9. "Tennis elbow" is characterized by:

a. Tenderness over the medial epicondyle
b. Tendinitis of the common extensor origin
c. Tendinitis of the common flexor origin
d. Painful flexion and extension

Ans. b

Q10. Hutchinson and Pepper syndrome is a feature of:

a. Von Recklinghausen's
b. Neuroblastoma
c. Renal cell carcinoma
d. Meningioma

Ans. b

Q11. Moure's sign is seen in:

a. Carcinoma
b. Appendicitis
c. Varicose vein
d. Pancreatitis

Ans. a

SUGGESTED READING

1. Bailey & Love's - Short Practice of Surgery, 27th edition.
2. Schwartz's Principles of Surgery, 18th edition.
3. Textbook of Surgery by David Sabiston, 21st edition.

Index

Page numbers followed by *b* refer to box, *f* refer to figure, *fc* refer to flowchart, and *t* refer to table.

A

B

C

D

E

F

G

H

I

J

K

M

P

T

U

V

W

X

Y

Z